EMERGING INFECTIOUS DISEASES

TRENDS AND ISSUES

Second Edition

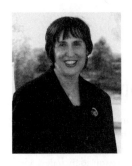

Felissa R. Lashley (formerly Cohen), RN, PhD, ACRN, FACMG, FAAN, is a professor and dean of the College of Nursing at Rutgers, The State University of New Jersey, an appointment she assumed in November 2002, as well as the interim director of the Nursing Center for Bioterrorism and Emerging Infectious Diseases Preparedness. She received the BS degree in nursing from Adelphi College, the MA degree in medical surgical nursing/higher education from New York University, and the PhD degree in human genetics from Illinois State University. She has a certificate in medical genetics from Jackson Laboratories. Dr. Lashley is certified as a PhD medical geneticist by the American Board of Medical Genetics (the first nurse to be so certified), an acquired immunodeficiency syndrome (AIDS) certified registered nurse, and a founding fellow of the American College of Medical Genetics. She is a fellow of the American Academy of Nursing.

Dr. Lashley has authored more than 300 publications and has presented nationally and internationally on a variety of topics, most recently at Yamaguchi University in Ube, Japan. The first and second editions of her book *Clinical Genetics in Nursing Practice* received Book of the Year Awards from the *American Journal of Nursing*. Three of her other books have won *AJN* Book of the Year awards: *The Person With AIDS: Nursing Perspectives* (Durham and Cohen, Eds.), *Women, Children and HIV/AIDS* (Cohen and Durham), and *Emerging Infectious Diseases: Trends and Issues* (Lashley and Durham), which was also a *Choice* awardee, while *Tuberculosis: A Sourcebook for Nursing Practice* (Cohen and Durham) won a Book of the Year Award from *The Nurse Practitioner*. She created a Web page for nurses to share biopreparedness and emerging infectious diseases information and initiated an annual interdisciplinary conference on emerging infectious diseases. Dr. Lashley has given over 350 presentations, most recently on emerging infectious diseases and avian influenza. She has been interviewed on avian influenza for television, radio, newspapers, and *O, the Oprah Magazine* (June 2006).

She also has long experience as a grant reviewer and was a member of the charter AIDS Research Review Committee at the National Institute of Allergy and Infectious Disease, National Institutes of Health (NIH). She was a member of the invited interdisciplinary working group assembled to advise the National Institute of Nursing Research, NIH, on research opportunities and challenges in emerging infections. She was a member of the NIH consensus panel *Phenylketonuria: Screening and Management*.

Dr. Lashley received the 2000 Research Recognition Award for Outstanding Research from the Association of Nurses in AIDS Care and received the Member of the Year recognition for SLANAC in 2002. In March 2003 she received the Distinguished Alumni Award from Illinois State University, and in 2005 she was initiated into their Hall of Fame. In 1999, she received the Distinguished Nurse Research Award from the Illinois Nurses Association. She also received the SAGE award for mentoring nurse leaders in 2001 from the Illinois Leadership Institute. She is a distinguished lecturer for Sigma Theta Tau, International, and was an associate editor of the journal *IMAGE: The Journal of Nursing Scholarship*. She is a member of the board of directors of Robert Wood Johnson University Hospital in New Brunswick, New Jersey, and of the statewide NJ MEDPREP committee. She has been selected as a Woman of Excellence by the New Jersey Women In AIDS Network.

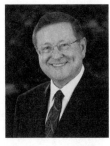

Jerry D. Durham, PhD, RN, FAAN, is a chancellor and professor of nursing at Allen College, Waterloo, Iowa. He previously held the positions of vice-chancellor for academic affairs and professor of nursing at the University of Missouri–St. Louis, where he initially served as dean of the Barnes College of Nursing and Health Studies.

He holds two baccalaureate and four graduate degrees, including master's degrees in medical-surgical nursing and psychiatric mental health nursing, as well as a doctorate in higher education administration. Dr. Durham is also the coeditor of books focusing on the human immunodeficiency virus and acquired immunodeficiency syndrome, tuberculosis, and private practice in psychiatric-mental health nursing. These publications have received five Book of the Year Awards from the *American Journal of Nursing*. He has also served as a reviewer for and member of the editorial boards of several nursing journals.

Emerging Infectious Diseases

Trends and Issues

Second Edition

Edited by

Felissa R. Lashley, RN, PhD, ACRN,
FACMG, FAAN
and
Jerry D. Durham, PhD, RN, FAAN

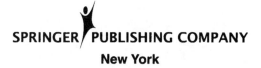

SPRINGER PUBLISHING COMPANY

New York

Springer Publishing Company, LLC
11 West 42nd Street
New York, NY 10036-8002
www.springerpub.com

Acquisitions Editor: James Costello
Managing Editor: Mary Ann McLaughlin
Production Editor: Tenea Johnson
Cover Design: Mimi Flow
Composition: Aptara, Inc.

07 08 09 10/ 5 4 3 2 1

Library of Congress Cataloging-in-Publication Data

Emerging infectious diseases : trends and issues / [edited by] Felissa R. Lashley, Jerry D. Durham. – 2nd ed.
     p. ; cm.
   Includes bibliographical references and index.
   ISBN 978-0-8261-0250-8 (hardback)
   1. Emerging infectious diseases.   2. Drug resistance in microorganisms.
3. Epidemiology.   I. Lashley, Felissa R., 1941–   II. Durham, Jerry D.
[DNLM: 1. Communicable Diseases, Emerging–epidemiology. WA 110 E5356 2007]

RA643.E465   2007
616.9–dc22

                                                              2006102115

Printed in the United States of America by Bang Printing.

To my very special and loving family: My children and grandchildren, Peter and Julie, Ben, Hannah and Lydia; Heather and Chris; Neal and Anne, Jacob and Grace; and my mother, Ruth Lashley, and the memory of my father, Jack Lashley. May all the infectious diseases you encounter be mild and curable.

Felissa R. Lashley

To my wife, Kathy Durham, for her dedication to providing the highest quality of care to her patients and for her support of me during our lives together.

Jerry D. Durham

Contents

Contributors

Daniel G. Bausch, MD, MPH&TM, is an associate professor in the Department of Tropical Medicine, Tulane School of Public Health and Tropical Medicine, Tulane University, Health Sciences Center, New Orleans, Louisiana.

L. Scott Chavers, MPH, PhD, is director of Global Pharmacovigilance, Pharmacoepidemiology Department, Schering Plough Research Institute, Springfield, New Jersey.

James E. Cheek, MD, MPH, is the director of the Division of Epidemiology and Disease Prevention, Indian Health Service, Albuquerque, New Mexico.

Miriam Cohen, RN, MSN, is a consultant in Hillsborough, New Jersey.

Inge B. Corless, RN, PhD, FAAN, is a professor in the graduate program in nursing at the MGH Institute of Health Professions, Boston, Massachusetts.

Victoria Davey, RN, MPH, is the deputy chief officer of Public Health and Environmental Hazards, Department of Veterans Affairs, Washington, DC.

Barbara Jeanne Fahey, RN, BSN, MPH, is a nurse consultant liaison in the Materials Management Department, Clinical Center, National Institutes of Health, Bethesda, Maryland.

Ron A. M. Fouchier, PhD, is in the Department of Virology, Erasmus Medical Center, Rotterdam, The Netherlands.

Barbara A. Goldrick, RN, MPH, PhD, CIC, is a consultant in Chatham, Massachusetts.

Amy V. Groom, MPH, is chief, Immunization Section, Infectious Diseases Branch, Division of Epidemiology and Disease Prevention, Indian Health Service, Albuquerque, New Mexico.

Bart L. Haagmans, PhD, is in the Department of Virology, Erasmus Medical Center, Rotterdam, The Netherlands.

Stephan Harbarth, MD, MS, is a hospital epidemiologist and senior research scientist at the Infection Control Program and Division of Infectious Diseases, Geneva University Hospitals, Geneva, Switzerland.

Jeanne Beauchamp Hewitt, RN, PhD, is an associate professor in the School of Nursing, University of Wisconsin, Milwaukee, Wisconsin.

Barbara J. Holtzclaw, RN, PhD, FAAN, is a professor, nurse scientist, and research liaison at the University of Oklahoma College of Nursing and the University of Minnesota School of Nursing Bridges to the Doctorate for Native American and Alaskan Native Nurses and a professor emeritus in the School of Nursing, University of Texas Health Science Center at San Antonio, Texas.

Matthew R. Moore, MD, MPH, is a commander with the United States Public Health Service and a medical epidemiologist with the Centers for Disease Control and Prevention, Atlanta, Georgia.

Albert D. M. E. Osterhaus, DVM, PhD, is a professor in the Department of Virology, Erasmus Medical Center, Rotterdam, The Netherlands.

David S. Perlin, PhD, is director of the Public Health Research Institute Center and professor of microbiology and molecular genetics, NJMS-UMDNJ at the International Center for Public Health, Newark, New Jersey.

C. J. Peters, MD, was formerly head of the Special Pathogens Branch at the Centers for Disease Control and Prevention and is professor of microbiology and immunology and of pathology at the University of Texas Medical Branch in Galveston, Texas.

Christina R. Phares, PhD, is an epidemiologist in the Division of Global Migration and Quarantine, Centers for Disease Control and Prevention, Atlanta, Georgia.

Kurt D. Reed, MD, is a senior research scientist at the Marshfield Clinic Research Foundation, Marshfield, Wisconsin.

Neil W. Schluger, MD, is the chief of clinical pulmonary medicine and an associate professor of medicine and public health at the Columbia University College of Physicians and Surgeons and the Columbia University School of Public Health, New York, New York.

James Mark Simmerman, RN, FNP, PhD, is an epidemiologist with the Influenza Branch, Division of Viral and Rickettsial Diseases, National Center for Infectious Diseases, Centers for Disease Control and Prevention, Atlanta, Georgia.

Laurie J. Singel, RN, MSN, BC, is a clinical assistant professor at the School of Nursing, University of Texas Health Science Center at San Antonio, San Antonio, Texas.

Donna Tartasky, RN, PhD, is a health consultant in Elkins Park, Pennsylvania.

Timothy M. Uyeki, MD, MPH, is acting chief, Epidemiology Section, Influenza Branch, Division of Viral and Rickettsial Diseases, National Center for Infectious Diseases, Centers for Disease Control and Prevention, Atlanta, Georgia.

Bernadette G. van den Hoogen, PhD, is in the Department of Virology, Erasmus Medical Center, Rotterdam, The Netherlands.

Sten H. Vermund, MD, PhD, holds the Amos Christie Chair in Global Health and is a professor in the Departments of Pediatrics, Medicine, Preventive Medicine, Obstetrics, and Gynecology and director of the Vanderbilt University School of Medicine Institute for Global Health, Vanderbilt University, Nashville, Tennessee.

Preface

Since the publication of the first edition of this book, emerging and reemerging infectious diseases continue to appear. Interest in emerging and reemerging infectious diseases remains high, both within the scientific, public health, and medical communities and in the general public. This interest followed decades of complacency as a result of the antibiotic era, successful vaccination programs, vector control initiatives, and a trust in the ability of medical science to conquer infectious diseases. Indeed, in 1962, Sir MacFarlane Burnet, the famous Nobel laureate immunologist, wrote in the preface to his well-known book *Natural History of Infectious Disease* that "at times one feels that to write about infectious disease is almost to write of something that has passed into history" (Burnet, 1962, p. 3). In the past 5 years, accelerating interest in emerging infectious diseases among the public, especially in developed nations, is largely a result of concerns about outbreaks that have captured headlines in the world's newspapers including severe acute respiratory syndrome (SARS), avian influenza, increasing community-acquired antimicrobial-resistant infections such as *Clostridium difficile*, monkeypox, metapneumovirus, increasing fungal infections, widespread *Escherichia coli* O157:H7 infections, and others.

The 1992 Institute of Medicine report, followed by reports from the Centers for Disease Control and Prevention, called attention to the increasing emergence of infectious diseases resulting from newly recognized diseases caused by known microorganisms, newly recognized microorganisms causing diseases, diseases and microorganisms found in new geographic areas, microorganisms resistant to antimicrobial agents, microorganisms of animals that have extended their host range to newly infect humans, new reservoirs for microorganisms, microorganisms that have become more virulent, as well as diseases that have markedly increased in incidence. These reports were followed by a 2003 report from the Institute of Medicine further delineating the scope of emerging infectious diseases and their root causes as well as looking further at surveillance, treatment, and prevention approaches.

Many reasons exist for the emergence and reemergence of infectious diseases and agents including changes in hosts, microorganisms, and the environment resulting from changes in social and cultural behaviors; the relative ease and rapidity of global travel for people and goods; changes in traditional natural boundaries; demand for exotic foods and fast foods; the effects of civil unrest and wars; deliberate release of biological agents; advances in diagnostic techniques to identify microbes undetectable previously; advances in agricultural practices, deforestation, irrigation, and dam building, which change ecology; weather and climate effects as well as natural disasters; decline in funding of the public health infrastructure in many countries; increasing contact of humans and animals through recreation and living proximity; and advances in medical science changing host immunity, increasing organ transplantation, or increasing the use of new devices. Broad efforts to reduce the inappropriate use of antimicrobial therapy in both animals and humans, especially in light of the emergence of microbes that are resistant to treatment (e.g., vancomycin-resistant enterococci), reflect growing concerns.

Also contributing to the growing interest in emerging infectious diseases is a mounting fear that microorganisms hold the potential to serve as an instrument of war among terrorists, individuals, and rogue nations. In the face of such threats, public health scientists have worked diligently to develop local, regional, and national plans aimed at combating bioterrorism. These plans, which focus on early detection and response to bioterrorism threats, require coordination of multidisciplinary efforts of clinicians, behavioral and biological scientists, and law enforcement personnel. Such efforts are likely to grow appreciably as a result of the September 11, 2001, attacks by terrorists on the World Trade Center and the Pentagon, and the October 2001 delivery of anthrax spores through the U.S. mail, causing anthrax that was thought to be either a biocrime or bioterrorism but for which perpetrators were never revealed. These instances have jarred public awareness that terrorists and individuals are capable of employing weapons of mass destruction, including infectious agents, to achieve their goals. It is no longer unthinkable that terrorists might consider unleashing smallpox, anthrax, botulism, or plague on an unsuspecting population. These realistic concerns about bioterrorism will loom large in the arena of public opinion and public policy in the future.

Health professionals and the general public now understand that, with respect to infectious diseases, we live in a global community in which the health of developed and developing nations is intertwined. In this global community, infectious diseases can spread rapidly around the world, making global surveillance and control of emerging infections vital to world health. These organisms may migrate from one part of the world to another on wind currents, among migratory fowl, or among travelers. Exotic infectious diseases on distant continents, once seen as posing little threat to the developed world, are now viewed with growing concern among scientists worldwide. Ecological changes and changes wrought by peoples of the world have contributed to the emergence of infectious diseases. These "advances of mankind" include movement of humans and domestic animals into new habitats, deforestation, irrigation, urbanization, and increased air travel. Moreover, public policy and politics—for example, decisions influencing poverty, economic development, population movements, refugees and migrants, and cooperation among governments that can exert enormous influence on the detection, surveillance, treatment, and prevention of emerging infectious diseases—also shape patterns of emerging and reemerging infectious diseases. Individual and group behaviors heavily influence transmission of infectious diseases. In addition, the global decline of public health systems serves to render the world more susceptible to infectious diseases of all kinds.

Important health organizations with a national or worldview of disease (e.g., the Centers for Disease Control and Prevention and the World Health Organization) have restructured themselves to place greater emphasis on infectious diseases and rapid responses to epidemics, wherever they emerge. Developed nations, recognizing the threat to their economic welfare and social stability, have poured increasing resources into prevention, detection, surveillance, and treatment of emerging infectious diseases and pledged to fight infectious diseases around the world in various cooperative efforts. Funds to support research aimed at understanding and controlling emerging infectious diseases have increased significantly over the past decade as governments have recognized the importance of this threat.

This book provides readers the knowledge to better understand the factors contributing to the emergence and reemergence of infectious diseases and microbial resistance in a broad context. In addition, multiple chapters focus on specific emerging infectious diseases of increasing interest to both the scientific community and the general public. These disease-specific chapters examine the epidemiology, microbiology, clinical picture, treatment, and prevention of these diseases. A chapter on bioterrorism explores this topic and potential agents for such use. In the final section, emerging infectious diseases are viewed in broader contexts, such as their contribution to chronic diseases and cancer, their connection to travel and recreation, and the behavioral and cultural influences contributing to the spread of emerging infectious diseases, followed by a look into the future. The future is upon us, and how we prevent and respond to outbreaks of emerging infectious diseases will influence our social, political, and economic status as well as our security for the coming decades.

FELISSA R. LASHLEY
JERRY D. DURHAM

REFERENCE

Burnet, F. M. (1962). *Natural history of infectious disease* (3rd ed.). Cambridge: Cambridge University Press.

EMERGING INFECTIOUS DISEASES

TRENDS AND ISSUES

Second Edition

PART I

Background

CHAPTER ONE

An Introduction to Emerging and Reemerging Infectious Diseases

L. Scott Chavers and Sten H. Vermund

Great strides have been and are being made in the prevention and control of infectious diseases. The eradication of smallpox demonstrated that the world had hope against historic scourges. The lessons from the eradication of smallpox have inspired and informed the near eradication of poliomyelitis and dracunculiasis (guinea worm), events that the world hopes to celebrate within the first decade of the 21st century (Aylward, 2006; Centers for Disease Control and Prevention [CDC], 2006a; Ruiz-Tiben & Hopkins, 2006). Oral rehydration salts have led to the diminution of mortality from infant diarrhea at modest global cost (Edejer et al., 2005). From these successes, a popular misconception emerged among health professionals and policy makers in industrialized nations that infectious diseases had been largely conquered and chronic diseases were the principal new frontier (Fauci, Touchette, & Folkers, 2005). Of course, this was untrue unless one took a highly ethnocentric point of view, ignored the developing world, and was naively optimistic that no new pathogens would emerge or reemerge.

Indeed, since the publication of the first edition of this book, strides continue to be made in the prevention and control of infectious diseases. The first vaccine shown to be effective in the prevention of human papillomavirus (HPV) strains linked to genital warts has recently been approved for use in the United States (Villa et al., 2005; see chapter 24); a new rotavirus vaccine is now available (Parashar, Alexander, Glass, Advisory

Committee on Immunization Practices, & CDC, 2006); and progress has been reported in the development of a vaccine against Ebola and Marburg viruses (Jones et al., 2005; see chapter 8). However, during this same time period, the first pandemic of the 21st century occurred when more than 8,400 cases and greater than 800 deaths from severe acute respiratory syndrome (SARS) were reported in 32 countries within 5 months (LeDuc & Barry, 2004; see chapter 22). Subsequently, the SARS coronavirus remains quiescent, but there are continuing fears of another pandemic from influenza type A spurred by the emergence of H5N1 avian influenza in Asia (see chapter 14). The United States witnessed the largest encephalitis epidemic in its history from June 10 to December 31, 2002, due to West Nile virus (CDC, 2003; see chapter 23). This time period also saw the emergence of the first inhalational anthrax cases in the United States from an intentional act of bioterrorism that remains of mysterious origin 5 years later (Jernigan et al., 2001).

Many infectious diseases continue to emerge as international threats. The prevalence rates of tuberculosis and malaria resistance, both major killers, are increasing, and the treatment of these diseases has become more difficult with the emergence of drug-resistant strains. In 2005 the global distribution of dengue viruses became comparable to malaria, with 2.5 billion people living in areas at risk for epidemic transmission (see chapter 7). The prevalence of the human immunodeficiency virus (HIV) continues to increase worldwide. Duration of survival among those infected with HIV has increased substantially in the last 10 years with the advent of new treatments (Vermund, 2006; Walensky et al., 2006). However, HIV has decimated many developing countries to the point that the stability of many nations is in question (chapter 13). Why are we seeing such a wide assortment of emerging and reemerging infectious diseases? This book seeks to illuminate this key question.

Among the factors that contribute to emerging and reemerging infectious diseases are the following:

1. demographic factors including population growth, migration, housing density, and distribution of population within a region;
2. social and behavioral changes such as the increased use of child care, liberalized sexual behavior, outdoor recreational pursuits, alcohol and drug use, patterns and styles of the transportation of goods, and widespread business and leisure travel;
3. advances in health care technology including modern chemotherapies, styles and institutions of health care delivery, iatrogenic immunosuppression, health care-associated antibiosis and antisepsis with consequent selective pressure and development of drug resistance, and invasive catheter techniques that introduce foreign objects either through natural orifices or parenteral routes;

4. changes in the treatment and handling of foodstuff, including mass production of nearly all food products, water processing, and use of adjunct agricultural practices such as antibiotics in animal feed;
5. climatologic changes and environmental alterations such as those associated with the El Niño ocean current centered off the coast of Peru, global warming, natural disasters such as volcanic eruptions, deforestation, and land use development (including dams, farming, irrigation, and mining) with attendant expansion of vector–reservoir–human contacts;
6. microbial evolution including natural variation, mutation, and cross-species zoonotic transmission;
7. war and/or natural disasters with the consequent breakdown of public health measures, including disease control activities, with or without economic collapse; and
8. deliberate release of microorganisms as a component of war or terrorism as with the 2001 intentional release of *Bacillus anthracis* through the U.S. mail in 2001.

These factors will be addressed here, alerting the reader to the relationships between social or behavioral phenomena and the risk of emerging pathogens (Lederberg, Shope, & Oaks, 1992). These factors have been more finely subdivided by a subsequent Institute of Medicine Report (Smolinski, Hamburg, & Lederberg, 2003) into the following categories: microbial adaptation and change, human susceptibility to infection, climate and weather, changing ecosystems, human demographics and behavior, economic development and land use, international travel and commerce, technology and industry, breakdown of public health measures, poverty and social inequality, war and famine, lack of political will, and intent to harm. Further discussion may also be found in Lashley (2006).

Factors that contribute immediately to the emergence of a given agent are often conceptualized as an ecological triangle, framing the emergence of an infectious disease via interactions of (a) the causal agent, (b) the human host, and (c) the social and biological environment, often mediated through an animal reservoir and/or an insect vector. The agents involved in emerging infectious diseases are as diverse as the agents in nature: viruses, bacteria, fungi, protozoa, helminths, and even prions, which are communicable proteins that do not meet conventional definitions of a microorganism but are nonetheless infectious from person to person or from animal to person (see chapter 21). Host characteristics include biological and genetic predictors of susceptibility and infectiousness, often mediated by the complex behavioral, social, economic, political, religious, and technological features of a host environment. Environmental influences increase or diminish the degree to which an infectious agent and vulnerable humans come into contact or the likelihood with which humans become infected with the given agent. For example, higher temperature and humidity are obvious influences on insect vectors of disease and also are associated with wearing loose, light clothing that facilitates insect biting. Environmental pollution that changes vector breeding patterns, natural disasters, water use patterns, human waste and garbage sanitation, and social conditions that influence behavior all are critical contributors to disease incidence. The all-important political response that can temper or exacerbate disease is a variable often overlooked except in extremes of war or famine (Garfield, Frieden, & Vermund, 1987; Roberts, Lafta, Garfield, Khudhairi, & Burnham, 2004). It is a misconception that natural balance between the infectious agent, the host, and the environment results in stability by keeping emerging diseases in check. Rather, recurrent epidemics and plagues, along with high endemic rates of many infectious diseases, are dynamic and evolving contributors to human history that continue into contemporary times.

The interaction between humans and the environment is a dynamic process both in their behaviors with each other and in their interactions with the environment (see Table 1.1). How we interact socially, sexually, politically, and economically can often be linked to migrant labor and urbanization, which are related, in turn, to the influences of technology and population growth. Of course, diseases can emerge from nature without human influences. A prevalent mammalian hantavirus emerged in humans when a drought drove deer mice into proximity with human dwellings. Ebola virus emerged mysteriously and disappeared just as inexplicably. Yet many modern aspects mediate disease transmission. For example, HIV entered human populations through traditional means of hunting and bush meat preparation yet became pandemic through modern travel, use of dirty medical injection needles, and sexual promiscuity (Stoneburner & Low-Beer, 2004a, 2004b; Vermund, Tabereaux, & Kaslow, 1999).

While our environment is manipulated in order to facilitate a higher quality of life, the very act of manipulation can carry new infectious risks. Construction of dams may create new vectors and intermediate host environments conducive to malaria, onchocerciasis (river blindness), schistosomiasis, or filariasis (Oladejo & Ofoezie, 2006). Great advances in technology may diminish many historic infectious risks, yet these same advances create new problems sometimes unforeseen at the time of implementation. Both drug-resistant microbes and insecticide-resistant vectors are examples (Breman, Alilio, & Mills, 2004). Infectious diseases are emerging also due to our ability to detect them; some were always present but hitherto unrecognized due to technical limitations and/or due to low numbers of afflicted persons in previous years. Cryptosporidiosis, cyclosporiasis, Legionnaire disease, hantavirus pulmonary syndrome, and Lyme disease all emerged without specific diagnostic techniques optimized

Table 1.1. Factors Contributing to Emerging and Reemerging Infectious Diseases

Contributing Factor	Specific Examples	Selected Related Diseases
Demographic factors	Population growth, migration, housing density, population distribution, aging	Dengue, tuberculosis, influenza, HIV, malaria, tropical parasitic diseases such as filariasis and leishmaniasis
Social and behavioral changes	Increased use of child care, liberalized sexual behavior, outdoor recreational pursuits, alcohol and drug use, transportation and distribution of goods, changes in travel frequency	HIV and other STDs, hepatitis A-B-C, pelvic inflammatory disease, measles, diphtheria, pertussis, Lyme disease
Advances in health care technology	Modern chemotherapies, styles and institutions of health care delivery, iatrogenic immunosuppression, health care-associated antibiosis and antisepsis, invasive catheter techniques	Multidrug-resistant TB, MRSA, VRE, opportunistic infections in immunosuppressed persons
Changes in treatment and handling of water/foodstuff	Mass production of nearly all food products, water processing, use of adjunct agricultural practices such as antibiotic supplementation of feed	Cryptosporidiosis, guinea worm, schistosomiasis, diarrheal diseases, hookworm, listeriosis, hemolytic uremic syndrome, cyclosporiasis, salmonellosis, Creutzfeldt–Jakob disease, VRE, leptospirosis
Climatologic changes and environmental alterations	El Niño, global warming, natural disasters, deforestation, land use development	Tickborne diseases, highland malaria, hantavirus pulmonary syndrome, plague
Microbial evolution	Natural variation, mutation, cross-species zoonotic transmission	Influenza, HIV, leptospirosis, plague, trichinellosis, African sleeping sickness, antibiotic-resistant bacteria
War and/or natural disasters	Breakdown of public health measures	Vaccine preventable diseases, cholera, STDs, TB
Deliberate release of pathogens	Bioterrorism, biowarfare	Anthrax, smallpox, plague, tularemia, botulism, salmonellosis, others

HIV = human immunodeficiency virus; MRSA = methicillin-resistant *Staphylococcus aureus*; STD = sexually transmitted disease; TB = tuberculosis; VRE = vancomycin-resistant enterococci.

to detect them. It is notable how quickly diagnostic approaches were developed for these particular emerging pathogens. We also can foretell the incidence of such infectious diseases as hantavirus through remote sensing and predicting environmental conditions for its rodent reservoirs (Glass et al., 2000). Yet how many other organisms that might cause diabetes, multiple sclerosis, Alzheimer disease, certain cancers, cardiovascular disease, or autoimmune diseases remain undiagnosed due perhaps to our technological limitations?

As many popular books now highlight, changes in dynamics of human activity within the context of nature, mediated by new technologies, may help explain the emerging and reemerging of infectious diseases (Laxminarayan et al., 2006). Emerging infectious diseases can be considered in several categories:

1. truly new diseases that emerge in humans from zoonotic environmental sources;
2. newly recognized diseases that may have been prevalent or may have been uncommon, but that only now are appreciated;
3. reemerging diseases that represent well-known infections that are now increasing in frequency, often after decades or centuries of declining rates, frequently due to failures in disease control strategies and the emergence of coinfections (like HIV) that facilitate spread; and
4. unexplained syndromes whose definitive diagnosis awaits new technical or scientific insights.

These factors do not exist in a vacuum; social, behavioral, and biological origins of the change in the agent–host–environment–vector relationship contribute to the emergence of infectious diseases.

DEMOGRAPHIC FACTORS

Population pressures in a world with over 6.5 billion inhabitants in 2006 contribute dramatically to infectious diseases; it is estimated that the world population will reach approximately 9.5 billion by 2050 (U.S. Census Bureau, 2006). Population demographics are altered by population growth, migration, and differential mortality. Redistribution of rural populations to urban environments, especially in the developing world, increases crowding and person-to-person contact. In addition, personal behavior is no longer subject to the scrutiny of a tight-knit community with an intact cultural identity.

Overcrowding, poverty, poor hygiene and sanitation, and unsafe water typically accompany urbanization due to the emergence of shanty-towns and other unplanned living quarters. Close quarters may increase tuberculosis and other diseases that exploit increased host susceptibility, especially among the very young, the elderly, or persons who are immunocompromised (Lederberg et al., 1992). The redistribution of migrating populations exposes susceptible individuals to infectious diseases that may be more endemic in their new environment. Microbial traffic accompanies the migration of their human hosts. The influx of new individuals may overwhelm public health infrastructures and disrupt natural reservoirs by deforestation and other environmental interference such as the building of roads, dams, irrigation schemes, agricultural development, and housing settlements in order to accommodate the influx of immigrants or refugees from more rural settings (Cohen & Larson, 1996; Committee on International Science, Engineering, and Technology, 1995; Krause, 1998; Lederberg et al., 1992; Morse, 1993; World Health Organization [WHO], 1999).

Urbanization and environmental disruption allow arthropod vector-borne viral infectious diseases to thrive in areas where they have not previously been a risk to humans. An especially important emerging vector-borne viral infection is dengue and dengue hemorrhagic fever. The global prevalence of dengue has grown dramatically in the last few decades, with two fifths of the world population now at risk (WHO, 2002). The WHO estimates that there may be up to 50 million cases of dengue infection worldwide each year (WHO, 2002). The public health impact of dengue is being increasingly noted in the Americas, with more than 600,000 cases reported in 2001 alone, of which 15,000 were dengue hemorrhagic fever. The number of cases has more than doubled since 1995 (WHO, 2002). The increasing frequency of dengue in the Americas corresponds to the deterioration of mosquito control programs that were extensively promulgated in the 1950s and 1960s (Gubler, 1998). Furthermore, there are large geographic areas of concern such as the southeastern United States where ecological conditions and endemic mosquito vectors favor future dengue transmission.

The impact of demographic changes can be seen in other infectious diseases. Tuberculosis is a disease of crowding and limited resources (Castro, 1998). Influenza thrives when population density rises and when humans live in proximity to pigs or fowl (Snacken, 1999; Snacken, Kendal, Haaheim, & Wood, 1999). Housing density correlates with risk for a number of other respiratory and vaccine-preventable diseases. Demographic shifts result when an increase in mean life expectancy occurs in a population, resulting in more immunosuppression related to chronic disease or old age, an increasing age of hospitalized patients, and consequent health care-associated infections. Economic development may result in migration-related disease or in expanding vector breeding. For example, irrigation programs may result in expanded vector breeding for tropical parasitic and viral diseases that now infect hundreds of millions of people worldwide. Migration can result in persons moving from a zone of high endemicity, introducing infections to other hospitable zones.

SOCIAL CHANGE AND HUMAN BEHAVIOR

Industrialized societies have experienced profound changes in the ways that they conduct day-to-day business. Child care often occurs within a social setting, rather than a family setting, facilitating more social mixing than before. In rural societies, hunting and food gathering, and in industrialized nations, certain occupations or recreations, often result in contact with natural disease vectors (such as ticks or mosquitoes) or infected animals (such as rodents or birds). Plague disproportionately affects Native Americans in the United States due to risk derived from hunting and preparing small feral animals that are plague reservoirs, like squirrels, for food. The recent SARS pandemic has been linked to a number of wildlife species consumed as delicacies in southern China, including the Himalayan masked palm civet, the Chinese ferret badger, and the raccoon dog (WHO, 2004). After several years of hunting for even more plausible sources, Chinese investigators have implicated bats as coronavirus reservoirs (Li et al., 2005). Increased illicit drug and alcohol abuse may result in expansion of previously exotic needle-related diseases or in familiar infections of the "street" lifestyle such as tuberculosis and hepatitis C virus (HCV)-associated liver disease. Central China experienced an HIV-HCV coepidemic due to illegal blood banking practices involving the reinfusion of pooled red cells into donors, an inconceivable practice that was nonetheless promulgated in order to bleed donors more frequently for plasma without precipitating anemia (Qian et al., 2006; Qian, Vermund, & Wang, 2005; Qian, Yang et al., 2005). Transportation of goods and people can itself become a vehicle for infectious spread, as noted with truck drivers and HIV. Immigration, business or leisure travel, and humanitarian missions can all result in appearance of previously distant organisms in local environments.

Changes in modern reproductive technology have led to changes in personal health behaviors and have helped reduce unwanted pregnancies. Greater personal freedom and social standing for women have accompanied lower pregnancy-related mortality. Current research is assessing what part, if any, these technologies may have played in the spread of infectious diseases. Oral contraceptive pill use may augment the risk of chlamydial and gonococcal cervicitis. They may be associated with increased cervical ectopy, which may, in turn, be associated with increased risk of sexually transmitted infections including HIV (Clemetson et al., 1993). Vaginal douching has been linked with increased risk of pelvic inflammatory disease, presumably from disruption of the normal vaginal ecology ideally dominated by hydrogen peroxide-producing lactobacilli (Martino & Vermund, 2002). If the oral contraceptive pill and the intrauterine device are used as sole methods of birth control, rather than combined with condom use, then risk of sexually transmitted infections may be increased due to the absence of a barrier to sexually acquired microbes.

The HIV pandemic captures many elements of social and behavioral contributions to infectious disease spread. HIV is more common where men are away from their families for long periods of time. It spreads rapidly when sexual partners or needle-sharing partners are exchanged more freely. Travelers spread HIV worldwide. Ineffective political responses are the norm, facilitating further spread. Poverty and crowding are relevant, but sociocultural norms governing sexual behavior and prevention of sexually transmitted infections are even more important in predicting HIV spread (Stoneburner & Low-Beer, 2004a, 2004b; Vermund, Kristensen, & Bhatta, 2000).

One of the greatest technological advances in the 20th century has been the increase in the speed and volume of international travel. As travel technology has changed, our ability to journey to previously inaccessible areas has increased. In the age of flight, we can now circumnavigate the globe in less than 2 days, compared to over a year in the clipper ship era of prior centuries. Along with this increase in travel and migration is an efficient pathway for the rapid spread of infectious diseases around the globe. Just as smallpox, measles, and tuberculosis devastated susceptible indigenous populations in the Americas after Columbus's arrival, modern travel carries the potential to introduce microbes and their vectors into previously unexposed populations. Returning soldiers from World War I contributed to the rapidity and magnitude of the Spanish flu pandemic of 1918 and 1919. Without intermediate animal hosts, diseases such as HIV, tuberculosis, chlamydia, influenza, measles, diphtheria, pertussis, hepatitis A, B, and C, and now SARS have spread throughout the globe entirely through human contact. Each year, over 1,000 cases of malaria are diagnosed in the United States among returning travelers and immigrants. Autochthonous cases from local vectorborne transmission are reported every few years in such locations as Long Island, New York, and southern California. Vigilance is needed to avoid the vector-breeding conditions that might sustain expanded disease transmission.

MODERN MEDICAL TECHNOLOGIES

Advances in health care technology have clashed with aging populations, especially in those industrialized societies that can afford higher technology care. Cancer, rheumatologic disease, and infectious diseases can be treated, but the therapies themselves may induce immunosuppression and risk from other infectious agents. In-patient care typically involves catheters, indwelling lines, and other physical facilitators of infectious inoculation. Hospitals and other health care settings often harbor multiresistant organisms that emerge due to the use, often inappropriately, of antibiotics. Intensive care settings may be foci for the most virulent of organisms. Health care-associated exposures to organisms that have been subjected to selective antibiotic pressure and development of resistant bacteria are common sources of serious complications around the world (Tenover & Hughes, 1996).

The dynamics of a hospital setting are more complex than one might imagine. Persons with serious infections may expose visitors and especially hospital staff. Visitors and hospital staff may, in turn, expose patients to infections from outside the hospital. This is particularly hazardous among patients whose immunologic and other host defenses have been impaired by modern medical treatments. Medical treatments that decrease the capacities of the immune system are numerous, including bone marrow or solid organ transplants, chemotherapy, chronic corticosteroid therapy, renal dialysis, and indwelling medical devices. The use of such medical devices and the invasive procedures that incorporate them facilitate the transmission of health care-associated infections. Devices help circumvent the normal integumentary and mucosal defenses against microbial invasion by allowing normal bacteria as well hospital pathogens direct entrance into the body. The antibiotic era dates from the late 1930s. Since that time, bacteria have emerged that are resistant to all known antibiotics. The multiple drug-resistant *Mycobacterium tuberculosis* that has been associated with the HIV epidemic has generated tuberculosis strains that have proven fatal despite rapid diagnosis and the highest sophistication in therapy. We stay barely one step ahead of resistant microorganisms in our biomedical research, at increasingly higher costs for drug discovery and antibiotic purchases.

FOODBORNE AND WATERBORNE DISEASES

Urbanization necessitates food production, storage, transport, and distribution. Food production, especially of meats, often involves antibiotic treatment of animal feed designed to improve animal growth or productivity. Such therapies have been associated directly with human disease from antibiotic-resistant bacteria (Holmberg, Osterholm, Senger, & Cohen, 1984; Witte, 2000; Witte, Tschape, Klare, & Werner, 2000). Improper storage or transport can introduce or help multiply microorganisms

(Keene, 1999). Distribution can introduce agents from food handlers, even at the most distal arm of the food handling process. Waterborne diseases are more common in tropical and resource-poor nations. Yet deteriorating infrastructures for water and sewage treatment in older industrialized cities can result in surprising outbreaks, as with the lethal Milwaukee, Wisconsin, cryptosporidiosis epidemic in 1993, possibly the largest point source waterborne outbreak in history (Eisenberg, Lei, Hubbard, Brookhart, & Colford, 2005). Water can result in disease transmission by harboring the organism, by being in short supply such that water washing for human hygiene is not feasible, by being the source of insect vector breeding, or by being the source of organisms that harbor intermediate hosts of infectious agents, as with the invertebrate cyclops for guinea worm or the snail for schistosomiasis (White, Bradley, & White, 1972). Poor sanitation alone can result in disease transmission from diarrheal diseases or hookworm. Hence, food, sanitation, and water, staples of human existence, are all vehicles for infectious agents.

In the early 20th century, changes in food processing technology including sanitation improvements, refrigeration, improved food storage, and governmental regulations and monitoring greatly reduced the incidence of foodborne diseases in industrialized countries. The role of muckraking journalists like Upton Sinclair was substantial in raising public awareness of the dangers within the food processing industry. At the same time, these new technologies were integrated with changes in agricultural practices that sowed the seeds for new hazards. Farmers moved away from growing multiple crops for local needs and began growing single cash crops for sale and regional or even international export. The cultivation of fruits and vegetables and animal husbandry moved from small private farms to large industrialized farms where massive amounts of vegetables and animals are subjected to the same environmental agents. These modern methods have increased the efficiency and reduced the cost of food products by centralizing the processing of food products, but this centralization increases the chances of accidental contamination of large volumes of food products all at once. When combined with the global economy of many food manufacturers, the contamination of food at any stage in delivery may result in contaminated food products being distributed across the world (Keene, 1999).

Foodborne illnesses are responsible for an estimated 6 to 80 million illnesses and up to 9,000 deaths in the United States each year (Mead et al., 1999). The huge range in these estimates indicates our ignorance about the actual burden of such illness, which may be responsible for US$5 billion in economic losses yearly. In more than half the investigations of foodborne illnesses in the United States, the pathogen is not identified; in fact, most cases of foodborne illnesses are never specifically diagnosed or reported.

While foodborne illnesses often cause diarrhea, *Listeria monocytogenes* can cause abortion in pregnancy or meningitis/sepsis in individuals with reduced immune system responses. *Escherichia coli* strain O157:H7 is a leading cause of hemolytic uremic syndrome and kidney failure, typically from eating undercooked, contaminated meat products. In 2006, the United States found itself coping with an *E. coli* epidemic from spinach, hitherto an improbable source of this organism (CDC, 2006b). Preferences for any raw or lightly cooked foods can also place people at increased risk for foodborne illness. Consumption of raw foods of animal origin, including raw shellfish, unpasteurized milk or fruit beverages, and ground beef, is particularly hazardous.

As consumers have increased their consumption of fresh produce, the number of recognized outbreaks associated with produce has increased. Seasonally, greater than 75% of fresh fruits and vegetables are imported and consumed within days of harvest. The surfaces of fruits and vegetables may become contaminated by soil or feces/manure from humans or animals. Cyclosporiasis has been associated with the consumption of raspberries and lettuce imported to the United States (Herwaldt & Beach, 1999). Use of unclean water supplies can lead to the contamination of produce because water is used to irrigate and wash produce and to make ice used to keep produce cool during trucking. Pathogens identified in fruit- and vegetable-associated illnesses in North America in the 1990s and 2000s included viruses, bacteria, fungi, and parasites such as hepatitis A, *Salmonella* spp., *E. coli* O157:H7, *Shigella flexneri*, aflatoxins, and *Cyclospora cayetanensis*.

Foodborne and waterborne outbreaks have the potential to afflict thousands of persons from a single contamination. In 1985, a salmonellosis associated with contaminated milk from a large dairy resulted in approximately 250,000 illnesses (Cook et al., 1998; Keene, 1999; van den Bogaard & Stobberingh, 2000). In 1994, a nationwide outbreak of *Salmonella* enteritis occurred when ice cream premix was hauled in tanker trucks that had not been thoroughly sanitized after transporting raw liquid egg, leading to an estimated 224,000 cases of salmonellosis. Epidemiologic techniques traced an outbreak of *Salmonella enteritidis* to a single egg-producing farm that housed greater than 400,000 egg-laying hens in five henhouses. Two large multistate outbreaks of enterohemorrhagic *E. coli* disease have resulted from the consumption of undercooked beef hamburgers served by large fast-food chains. Epidemic investigations have shown that the restaurants' cooking practices were insufficient to kill the bacteria, an observation that has now transformed the fast-food industry's technical approaches and safety precautions.

The use of antibiotics to enhance growth and prevent illnesses in domesticated animals has been implicated in the development of antibiotic resistance and the emergence of new, drug-resistant strains of bacterial disease in humans. Supplementing animal feed with antimicrobial agents to enhance growth has been common practice for more than 30 years and is estimated to constitute more than half the total antimicrobial use worldwide. Accumulating evidence now indicates that the use of the glycopeptide avoparcin as a growth promoter has created in food animals a major reservoir of *Enterococcus faecium* resistant to the standard drug treatment with vancomycin (van den Bogaard & Stobberingh, 2000; Witte et al., 2000).

Animal feed production practices have also been implicated in the development of new pathogens (Tan, Williams, Khan, Champion, & Nielsen, 1999). Over 170,000 cases of bovine spongiform encephalopathy have been confirmed in more than 34,000 herds in Britain through 1999, and extension of the epidemic of mad cow disease to mainland Europe occurred in 2000. Supplementation of the diets of calves and dairy cattle with meat and bone meal produced by commercial rendering plants may have been the source of the disease, probably due to contamination with infected neural tissue; cows fed diets containing material from scrapie-infected sheep may have initiated the outbreak. After the disease had been transmitted to cows, it was spread further by the addition of material from infected cows to cattle feed. The onset of the epidemic followed changes in the rendering process in the 1970s, including the use of continuous heating instead of batch heating and the inclusion of more tallow in the bone meal; both changes were likely to increase infection. North America was not spared, with well-documented bovine cases in both the United States and Canada epidemiologically linked and causing huge economic losses in beef sales (CDC, 2004). The human disease, variant Creutzfeldt–Jakob, is an incurable and devastating neurological condition now rising in incidence in Europe.

Agricultural development can lead to infection independent of the food supply per se. Hantavirus causes more than 100,000 infections per year in China. The virus is an infection of the field mouse *Apodemus agarius* that flourishes in rice fields. People usually contract the disease during the rice harvest through contact with infected rodents. Bacterial leptospirosis can be acquired the same way and has even been reported among participants in an international Eco-Challenge sporting event in Malaysia that involved swimming across a river (CDC, 2001).

CLIMATE AND ECOLOGICAL CHANGES

Global warming, a consequence of high energy utilization in resource-ample countries combined with deforestation and environmental degradation in resource-poor nations, is contributing to higher disease rates from such conditions as malaria and arboviruses whose insect vectors are nurtured in such a warming climate (Haines, McMichael, Kovats, & Saunders, 1998; McMichael, Patz, & Kovats, 1998). Environmental alterations such as land development can expand water for insect or snail breeding with dams or irrigation. While farming can be nurtured in environmentally benign ways, slash and burn technologies are often practiced, bringing humans in direct contact with remote jungle organisms. Natural phenomena like the El Niño ocean current off the Peruvian coast, volcanic eruptions, earthquakes, hurricanes, and tsunamis often result in disease-related alterations of the environment and the human condition. Expansion of vector–reservoir–human contacts are the most critical elements of the climatologic threat to human health through emerging and reemerging infectious diseases.

Climate has affected the timing and intensity of disease outbreaks throughout history. Yet modern technologies, particularly the high-volume burning of fossil fuels like gas, oil, and coal, are likely responsible for changes in the global climate of historic proportions (McMichael, Woodruff, & Hales, 2006). The average global temperature has increased by 0.6° C since the industrial revolution; 9 of the 11 hottest years of the 20th century occurred after 1985. Scientists from the Intergovernmental Panel on Climate Change forecast a 1° C to 3.5° C increase in average global temperature by the year 2100. Such temperature increases expand the niche for insect vectors that depend on higher temperature and humidity for their breeding and sustenance. Sweden has experienced a northern expansion in the distribution of tick vectors probably due to increasing temperatures in the North. During the 1980s and 1990s, there was a resurgence of highland malaria in Latin America, central and east Africa, and Asia corresponding to warming and to increases in insect populations. Global warming is implicated in these disease shifts. A widespread and accelerating retreat of tropical summit glaciers, the growth of plants at higher altitudes, a diminution of the freezing zone by 150 meters, and the acceleration of global warming since 1970 all bode ill for further climate change that will facilitate disease expansion.

MICROBIAL EVOLUTION

Inherent in the microbial world is the natural variation and mutation of organisms. Influenza mutates within its porcine or avian primary hosts and quickly spreads to humans with new pandemic viral types each and every year. Cross-species zoonotic transmission can happen precipitously with cataclysmic consequences, as with HIV in the 20th century (Gao et al., 1999). Alternatively, it can occur periodically and routinely as with influenza and with many zoonoses that afflict persons in endemic locales such as leptospirosis, plague, and trichinellosis. Some organisms continually reinvent their surface antigen profiles in order to evade the host immune responses, such as trypanosomiasis, the parasitic cause of African sleeping sickness. In 2000, poliomyelitis reemerged in both the Dominican Republic and Haiti after vaccine coverage rates dropped (Kew et al., 2002). This occurred nearly a decade after the Americas were declared polio free, a dramatic event that presaged hoped-for global eradication in the early 21st century. The Hispaniola outbreak may have resulted from circulating mutant vaccine-strain poliovirus in a nonimmune population; there is no substitute for vigilance and persistence in eradication efforts.

Pandemic influenza and other zoonotic diseases have agricultural origins so intimate with human society as to defy intervention. In China, farmers raise pigs and ducks together. Population density is high and land is scarce. Waterfowl are a major reservoir of influenza viruses; pigs can serve as recombinant mixing vessels for new mammalian influenza strains. Integrated pig–duck agriculture puts these two species in contact with each other and with man, enabling efficient reproduction of recombinant mutant viruses and transfer to humankind. It is common for fowl, pigs, and humans to live in close proximity in China, and the potential implications of these interactions can be seen in the current concerns around the H5N1 subtype.

This inherent variability and adaptability of microorganisms guarantee that they will never be eliminated as sources of human disease. Our public health strategy must be one of control and containment. Furthermore, we must not be lulled into the false promises of elimination of infectious diseases as important contributors to human disease; the inherent variability of these organisms alone will be enough to guarantee future emerging and reemerging infectious diseases.

WAR AND/OR NATURAL DISASTERS

Humankind has learned much about the control of infectious diseases. Soap, water, personal hygiene, clean water, safe fecal disposal, uncrowded housing, basic medical care, and rodent control can all prevent infection and disease. Such basic sanitation is taken for granted in many parts of the world. Yet in areas of chronic poverty, war, or in conditions of natural disaster, all these may fail with tragic results. The breakdown of public health measures, including disease control activities, can occur even in relatively prosperous countries in conditions of war or disaster. In poorer nations, war, civil strife, or natural disaster often is accompanied with economic collapse, famine, and homelessness; the decline in public health control measures is exacerbated by the general economic decline. Few conditions are more conducive to infectious disease spread or emergence of novel pathogens than wars or disasters. Makeshift refugee camps are associated with attendant miseries consequent to privation and violence; rape, sexually transmitted diseases, burn injuries, vaccine-preventable diseases, and water/sanitation/rodent-related diseases are all too common.

Even in conditions of improving government services to control infectious diseases, war and natural disasters can undermine control strategies when health care workers, representing the government, are targeted by rebel forces or are dislocated in the aftermath of natural disaster. The breakdown in public health control measures was responsible for malaria expansions in Nicaraguan war zones after the U.S.-sponsored Contra rebels began attacking government health workers and clinics (Garfield et al., 1987). This is especially tragic in settings where progress is being made in public health but is interrupted or reversed by the civil unrest. Crises in the early 21st century have included Congo, Angola, Sierra Leone, Liberia, Bosnia, Kosova, Chechnya, Iraq, Afghanistan, several central Asian nations, and Haiti, among others (Roberts et al., 2004). Public infrastructure was utterly decimated after Hurricane Katrina struck the U.S. Gulf Coast in 2005 and after the December 2004 tsunami struck Indonesia, Sri Lanka, and other south Asian nations (CDC, 2005; Lim, Yoon, Jung, Joo Kim, & Lee, 2005). Although neither of these natural disasters resulted in widespread infectious diseases, these episodes call into question the ability of even developed nations to respond to widespread disease outbreaks when infrastructure is decimated.

DELIBERATE RELEASE OF ORGANISMS

Early in the 21st century, a long-anticipated and feared deliberate use of infectious agents as biological weapons was seen in the United States with the intentional spread of anthrax via the postal system (CDC, 2001). The use of biological agents as weapons is a significant threat to the general public physical, social, and psychological well-being. The 1984 inoculation of salad bars with *Salmonella typhimurium* in an area of Oregon (described in chapter 27) was seen as more of an oddity than a true threat to the public health (Török et al., 1997). Both outbreaks resulted in considerable mental health, economic, and societal burdens, salmonellosis on a local scale, and anthrax on an international scale. The most recent episode and additional fears have galvanized the United States and world communities to address these concerns with initiatives as diverse as vaccinia vaccine production for smallpox to education of health care workers for disease recognition. The reality of biological weapons has resulted in a renewed emphasis on the importance of our prevention infrastructure; coping with biological agents depends on the integrity of the public health system (CDC, 2000).

SUMMARY

Technologies can expand infectious diseases. Technologies can also help control infectious diseases. Some interventions are daunting in their complexity, such as how to slow global warming by reducing energy consumption; nations with high fossil fuel energy consumption are unmotivated to change their comparatively luxurious lifestyles. Other interventions, feasible in a shorter time frame, include increased coverage with vaccinations, oral rehydration fluids, and HIV prevention strategies. Some interventions are of intermediate complexity, such as the provision of clean water and sanitation, the reform of food processing, improved antibiotic practices in hospital settings, and expanded primary health care with essential drugs. International political response in times of natural disaster to prevent the spread of infectious disease is an intervention that proved successful in the weeks and months after the tsunami disaster in South and Southeast Asia. This book seeks to articulate both the problems we face and the solutions we must exploit to address the challenge of emerging and reemerging diseases.

REFERENCES

Aylward, R. B. (2006). Eradicating polio: Today's challenges and tomorrow's legacy. *Annals of Tropical Medicine & Parasitology, 100,* 401–413.

Breman, J. G., Alilio, M. S., & Mills, A. (2004). Conquering the intolerable burden of malaria: What's new, what's needed: A summary. *American Journal of Tropical Medicine and Hygiene, 71,* 1–15.

Castro, K. G. (1998). Global tuberculosis challenges. *Emerging Infectious Diseases, 4,* 408–409.

Centers for Disease Control and Prevention. (2000). Biological and chemical terrorism: Strategic Plan for Preparedness and Response-Recommendations of the CDC Strategic Planning Workgroup. *Morbidity and Mortality Weekly Report, 49*(RR-4).

Centers for Disease Control and Prevention. (2001). Update: Outbreak of acute febrile illness among athletes participating in Eco-Challenge-Sabah 2000— Borneo, Malaysia, 2000. *Morbidity and Mortality Weekly Report, 50,* 21–4.

Centers for Disease Control and Prevention. (2003). *Epidemic/epizootic West Nile virus in the United States: Guidelines for surveillance, prevention, and control.* Retrieved August 27, 2006, from http://www.cdc.gov/ncidod/dvbid/ westnile/resources/wnv-guidelines-aug-2003.pdf

Centers for Disease Control and Prevention. (2004). Bovine spongiform encephalopathy in a dairy cow—Washington state, 2003. *Morbidity and Mortality Weekly Report, 52,* 1280–1285.

Centers for Disease Control and Prevention. (2005). Infectious disease and dermatologic conditions in evacuees and rescue workers after Hurricane Katrina—Multiple states, August–September, 2005. *Morbidity and Mortality Weekly Report, 54,* 961–964.

Centers for Disease Control and Prevention. (2006a). Progress toward poliomyelitis eradication—India, January 2005–June 2006. *Morbidity and Mortality Weekly Report, 55,* 772–776.

Centers for Disease Control and Prevention. (2006b). Ongoing multistate outbreak of *Escherichia coli* serotype O157:H7 infections associated with consumption of fresh spinach—United States, September 2006. *Morbidity and Mortality Weekly Report, 55,* 1045–1046.

Clemetson, D. B., Moss, G. B., Willerford, D. M., Hensel, M., Emony, W., Holmes, K. K., et al. (1993). Detection of HIV DNA in cervical and vaginal secretions. Prevalence and correlates among women in Nairobi, Kenya. *Journal of the American Medical Association, 269,* 2860–2864.

Cohen, F., & Larson, E. (1996). Emerging infectious diseases: Nursing responses. *Nursing Outlook, 44,* 164–168.

Committee on International Science, Engineering, and Technology. (1995). *Report of the National Science and Technology Council Committee on International Science. Engineering and Technology Working Group on emerging and re-emerging infectiousdisease.* Washington, DC: National Science and Technology Council.

Cook, K. A., Dobbs, T. E., Hlady, W. G., Wells, J. G., Barrett, J. J., Puhr, N. D., et al. (1998). Outbreak of *Salmonella* serotype Hartford infections associated with unpasteurized orange juice. *Journal of the American Medical Association, 280,* 1504–1509.

Edejer, T. T., Aikins, M., Black, R., Wolfson, L., Hutubessy, R., & Evans, D. B. (2005). Cost effectiveness analysis of strategies for child health in developing countries. *British Medical Journal, 331,* 1177 (online: doi:10.1136/bmj.38652.550278.7C).

Eisenberg, J. N., Lei, X., Hubbard, A. H., Brookhart, M. A., & Colford, J. M., Jr. (2005). The role of disease transmission and conferred immunity in outbreaks: Analysis of the 1993 *Cryptosporidium* outbreak in Milwaukee, Wisconsin. *American Journal of Epidemiology, 161,* 62–72.

Fauci, A. S., Touchette, N. A., & Folkers, G. K. (2005). Emerging infectious diseases: A 10-year perspective from the National Institute of Allergy and Infectious Diseases. *Emerging Infectious Diseases, 11,* 519–525.

Gao, F., Bailes, E., Robertson, D. L., Chen, Y., Rodenburg, C. M., Michael, S. F., et al. (1999). Origin of HIV-1 in the chimpanzee *Pan troglodytes troglodytes. Nature, 397*(6718), 436–441.

Garfield, R. M., Frieden, T., & Vermund, S. H. (1987). Health related outcomes of war in Nicaragua. *American Journal of Public Health, 77,* 615–618.

Glass, G. E., Cheek, J. E., Patz, J. A., Shields, T. M., Doyle, T. J., Thorough-man, D. A., et al. (2000). Using remotely sensed data to identify areas at risk for hantavirus pulmonary syndrome. *Emerging Infectious Diseases, 6,* 238–247.

Gubler, D. J. (1998). Resurgent vector-borne diseases as a global health problem. *Emerging Infectious Diseases, 4,* 442–450.

Haines, A., McMichael, A. J., Kovats, S., & Saunders, M. (1998). Majority view of climate scientists is that global warming is indeed happening. *British Medical Journal, 316,* 1530.

Herwaldt, B. L., & Beach, M. J. (1999). The return of *Cyclospora* in 1997: Another outbreak of cyclosporiasis in North America associated with imported raspberries. Cyclospora Working Group. *Annals of Internal Medicine, 130,* 210–220.

Holmberg, S. D., Osterholm, M. T., Senger, K. A., & Cohen, M. L. (1984). Drug-resistant *Salmonella* from animals fed antimicrobials. *New England Journal of Medicine, 311,* 617–622.

Jernigan, J. A., Stephens, D. S., Ashford, D. A., Omenaca, C., Topiel, M. S., Galbraith, M., et al. (2001). Bioterrorism-related inhalational anthrax: The first 10 cases reported in the United States. *Emerging Infectious Diseases, 7,* 933–944.

Jones, S. M., Feldmann, H., Stroher, U., Geisbert, J. M., Fernando, L., Grolla, A., et al. (2005). Live attenuated recombinant vaccine protects nonhu-man primates against Ebola and Marburg viruses. *Nature Medicine, 11,* 786–790.

Keene, W. E. (1999). Lessons from investigations of foodborne disease outbreaks. *Journal of the American Medical Association, 281,* 1845–1847.

Kew, O., Morris-Glasgow, V., Landaverde, M., Burns, C., Shaw, J., Garib, Z., et al. (2002). Outbreak of poliomyelitis in Hispaniola associated with circulating type 1 vaccine-derived poliovirus. *Science, 296,* 356–359.

Krause, R. M. (1998). Emerging Infections. In R. M. Krause (Ed.), *Emerging infections* (pp. 6–7). San Diego: Academic Press.

Lashley, F. R. (2006). Emerging infectious diseases at the beginning of the 21st century. *Online Journal of Issues in Nursing, 11*(1), 2–16.

Laxminarayan, R., Mills, A. J., Breman, J. G., Measham, A. R., Alleyne, G., Claeson, M., et al. (2006). Advancement of global health: Key messages from the Disease Control Priorities Project. *Lancet, 367,* 1193–1208.

Lederberg, J., Shope, R. E., & Oaks, Jr., S. C. (1992). *Emerging infection: Microbial threats to health in the United States.* Washington, DC: Institute of Medicine, National Academy Press.

LeDuc, J. W., & Barry, M. A. (2004, November). SARS, the first pandemic of the 21st century [Electronic version]. *Emerging infectious diseases, 10*(11). Retrieved August 15, 2006, from http://www.cdc.gov/ncidod/EID/vol10no11/04-0797_02.htm

Li, W., Shi, Z., Yu, M., Ren, W., Smith, C., Epstein, J. H., et al. (2005). Bats are natural reservoirs of SARS-like coronaviruses. *Science, 310,* 676–679.

Lim, J. H., Yoon, D., Jung, G., Joo Kim, W., & Lee, H.C. (2005). Medical needs of tsunami disaster refugee camps. *Family Medicine, 37,* 422–428.

Martino, J. L., & Vermund, S. H. (2002). Vaginal douching: Evidence for risks or benefits to women's health. *Epidemiologic Reviews, 24,* 109–124.

McMichael, A. J., Patz, J., & Kovats, R. S. (1998). Impacts of global environmental change on future health and health care in tropical countries. *British Medical Bulletin, 54,* 475–488.

McMichael, A. J., Woodruff, R. E., & Hales, S. (2006). Climate change and human health: Present and future risks. *Lancet, 367,* 859–869.

Mead, P. S., Slutsker, S., Dietz, V., McCaig, L. F., Bresee, J. S., Shapiro, C., et al. (1999). Food-related illness and death in the United States. *Emerging Infectious Diseases, 5,* 607–625.

Morse, S. S. (1993). Examining the origins of emerging virus. In S. S. Morse (Ed.), *Emerging viruses* (pp. 10–28). New York: Oxford University Press.

Oladejo S. O., & Ofoezie I. E. (2006). Unabated schistosomiasis transmission in Erinle River Dam, Osun State, Nigeria: Evidence of neglect of environmental effects of development projects. *Tropical Medicine and International Health, 11,* 843–850.

Parashar, U. D., Alexander, J. P., Glass, R. I., Advisory Committee on Immunization Practices, & Centers for Disease Control and Prevention. (2006). Prevention of rotavirus gastroenteritis among infants and children. Recommendations of the Advisory Committee on Immunization Practices (ACIP). *Morbidity and Mortality Weekly Reports, 55*(RR-12), 1–13.

Qian, H. Z., Vermund, S. H., Kaslow, R. A., Coffey, C. S., Chamot, E., Yang, Z., et al. (2006). Coinfection with HIV and hepatitis C virus in former plasma/blood donors: Challenge for patient care in rural China. *AIDS, 20,* 1429–1435.

Qian, H. Z., Vermund, S. H., & Wang, N. (2005). Risk of HIV/AIDS in China: Sub-populations of special importance. *Sexually Transmitted Infections, 81,* 442–447.

Qian, H. Z., Yang, Z., Shi, X., Gao, J., Xu, C., Warg, L., et al. (2005). Hepatitis C virus in communities with former commercial plasma donors in rural Shanxi Province, China: The China-CIPRA Project. *Journal of Infectious Diseases, 192,* 1694–1700.

Roberts, L., Lafta, R., Garfield, R., Khudhairi, J., & Burnham, G. (2004). Mortality before and after the 2003 invasion of Iraq: Cluster sample survey. *Lancet, 364,* 1857–1864.

Ruiz-Tiben, E., & Hopkins, D. R. (2006). Dracunculiasis (Guinea worm disease) eradication. *Advances in Parasitology, 61,* 275–309.

Smolinski, M. S., Hamburg, M. A., & Lederberg, J. (Eds.). (2003). *Microbial threats to health: Emergence, detection and response.* Washington, DC: Institute of Medcine, National Academy Press.

Snacken, R. (1999). Control of influenza. Public health policies. *Vaccine, 17*(Suppl. 3), S61–63.

Snacken, R., Kendal, A. P., Haaheim, L. R., & Wood, J. M. (1999). The next influenza pandemic: Lessons from Hong Kong, 1997. *Emerging Infectious Diseases, 5,* 195–203.

Stoneburner, R. L., & Low-Beer, D. (2004a). Population-level HIV declines and behavioral risk avoidance in Uganda. *Science, 304,* 714–718.

Stoneburner, R. L., & Low-Beer, D. (2004b). Sexual partner reductions explain human immunodeficiency virus declines in Uganda: Comparative analyses of HIV and behavioural data in Uganda, Kenya, Malawi, and Zambia. *International Journal of Epidemiology, 33,* 624.

Tan, L., Williams, M. A., Khan, M. K., Champion, H. C., & Nielsen, N. H. (1999). Risk of transmission of bovine spongiform encephalopathy to humans in the United States: Report of the Council on Scientific Affairs. American Medical Association. *Journal of the American Medical Association, 281,* 2330–2339.

Tenover, F. C., & Hughes, J. M. (1996). The challenges of emerging infectious diseases. Development and spread of multiply-resistant bacterial pathogens. *Journal of the American Medical Association, 275,* 300–304.

Török, T. J., Tauxe, R. V., Wise, R. P., Livengood, J. R., Sokolow, R. Mauvais S., et al. (1997). A large community outbreak of salmonellosis caused by intentional contamination of restaurant salad bars. *Journal of the American Medical Association, 278,* 389–95.

U.S. Census Bureau. (2006). *World population information.* Retrieved August 15, 2006, from http://www.census.gov/ipc/www/world.htm

van den Bogaard, A. E., & Stobberingh, E. E. (2000). Epidemiology of resistance to antibiotics. Links between animals and humans. *International Journal of Antimicrobial Agents, 14,* 327–335.

Vermund, S. H. (2006). Millions of life-years saved with potent antiretroviral drugs in the United States: A celebration, with challenges. *Journal of Infectious Diseases, 194,* 1–5.

Vermund, S. H., Kristensen, S., & Bhatta, M. P. (2000). HIV as an STD. In K. H. Mayer & H. F. Pizer (Eds.), *The emergence of AIDS: The impact on immunology, microbiology and public health* (pp. 121–128). Washington, DC: United Brook Press.

Vermund, S. H., Tabereaux, P. B., & Kaslow, R. A. (1999). Epidemiology of HIV infection. In T. Merigan, D. Bolognesi, & J. Bartlett (Eds.), *Textbook of AIDS medicine* (2nd ed., pp. 101–109). Baltimore: Williams & Wilkins.

Villa, L. L., Costa, R. L., Petta, C. A., Andrade, R. P., Ault, K. A., Guiliano, A. R., et al. (2005). Prophylactic quadrivalent human papillomavirus (types 6, 11, 16, and 18) L1 virus-like particle vaccine in young women: A randomised double-blind placebo-controlled multicentre phase II efficacy trial. *Lancet Oncology, 6,* 271–278.

Walensky, R. P., Paltiel, A. D., Losina, E., Mercincavage, L. M., Schackman, B. R., Sax, P. E., et al. (2006). The survival benefits of AIDS treatment in the United States. *Journal of Infectious Diseases, 194,* 1–5.

White, G. F., Bradley, D. J., & White, A. U. (1972). *Drawers of water: Domestic water use in East Africa.* Chicago, IL: University of Chicago Press.

Witte, W. (2000). Ecological impact of antibiotic use in animals on different complex microflora: Environment. *International Journal of Antimicrobial Agents, 14,* 321–325.

Witte, W., Tschape, H., Klare, I., & Werner, G. (2000). Antibiotics in animal feed. *Acta Veterinaria Scandinavica Supplementum, 93,* 37–44.

World Health Organization. (1999). *Removing obstacles to healthy development.* Geneva: World Health Organization.

World Health Organization. (2002). *Dengue and dengue hemorrhagic fever.* Retrieved August 15, 2006, from http://www.who.int/mediacentre/factsheets/fs117/en/

World Health Organization. (2004, October). *WHO guidelines for the global surveillance of severe acute respiratory syndrome (SARS). Updated recommendations, October 2004.* Retrieved August 15, 2006, from http://www.who.int/csr/resources/publications/WHO_CDS_CSR_ARO_2004_1/en/

CHAPTER TWO

Microbial Resistance to Antibiotics

Stephan Harbarth

Sixty years after the introduction of the first antimicrobial agents, microbial resistance to antibiotics has emerged in most bacterial, viral, and fungal species that cause disease in man, except a few particular drug-pathogen combinations (e.g., absence of penicillin resistance in *Streptococcus pyogenes*). Today, antibiotic resistance is an important health and economic problem throughout the world. Resistant bacteria reduce the options for treating infections effectively and increase the risk of complications and fatal outcome for patients with severe infections.

This chapter provides an overview of issues related to antibiotic resistance and presents information about emerging trends. The chapter is organized into three main sections, the first addressing general issues, the second focusing on three specific pathogens of high interest, and the third summarizing promising approaches for control of resistance. The chapter, while selective of topics and brief, serves as a starting point for readers interested in antibiotic resistance.

SECTION 1: GENERAL ISSUES

What Is Microbial Resistance to Antibiotics?

Antimicrobial resistance describes the ability of a microorganism to resist the growth-suppressing or microbicidal effects of particular antimicrobial agents. This ability can reflect a naturally occurring property of an organism (e.g., having a thick cell wall) or might develop through alteration of the organism's genes. In some cases, genes and mobile elements conferring resistance to a particular antimicrobial can be transferred between different strains of microorganisms, the recipient organisms thus becoming resistant.

In a clinical context, antibiotic resistance refers to a reduction in clinical efficacy so that either the benefits for the individual patient receiving a specific antibiotic agent or the benefits to general public health are compromised (Simonsen, Tapsall, Allegranzi, Talbot, & Lazzari, 2004). Thus, antimicrobial drug resistance jeopardizes the effectiveness of antimicrobial treatment for many types of common infections.

Is Antibiotic Resistance Only a Man-Made Phenomenon?

Antibiotic resistance not only represents a man-made phenomenon, but also occurs in natural environments. For instance, the soil may harbor bacteria resistant to many bactericidal substances (D'Costa, McGrann, Hughes, & Wright, 2006). Several landmark investigations performed in the 1960s have shown that indigenous populations never previously exposed to antibiotic agents may already harbor low-level resistant bacteria that can be traced back to naturally occurring resistance mechanisms (Gardner, Smith, Beer, & Möellering, 1969). More recent studies (Bartoloni et al., 2004) have shown that antibiotic resistance caused by human or veterinary use of antibiotics may spread and persist in remote areas of our planet, without the need of sustained antibiotic selection pressure.

Many classes of antibiotics that are used today are derived from substances that have first been isolated in nature. Typical examples include the penicillins, cephalosporins, and aminoglycosides. Only a few antibiotic classes, such as the fluoroquinolones (e.g., ciprofloxacin), are a product of modern biochemical engineering.

How Do Bacteria Become Resistant to Antibiotics?

Bacterial clones with natural or acquired resistance have been continuously selected as an evolutionary response to the human or veterinarian use of antibiotics. Resistance can be acquired as a result of genetic events causing alterations in the preexisting bacterial genome, such as point mutations or gene amplifications. The other major mechanism is horizontal gene transfer between bacteria both within and between species, where transposons, integrons, or plasmids are introduced into an organism (Livermore, 2004).

Alterations in bacteria cause resistance to antibiotics in one or more of four ways (Weber & Courvalin, 2005): (1) The target molecules are structurally altered to prevent antibiotic binding; (2) antibiotics are inactivated, for example, through enzymatic degradation; (3) antibiotics are excluded from cell entry; or (4) they are or pumped out of the cell (efflux). Typical examples of the four mechanisms are (a) *Staphylococcus aureus* resistant to synthetic penicillins and cephalosporins; (b) extended-spectrum beta-lactamase-producing *Escherichia coli*; (c) vancomycin-resistant *S. aureus*; and (d) *Pseudomonas aeruginosa* resistant to imipenem.

When Was Antibiotic Resistance First Described in the Medical Literature?

The sulfonamides were the first class of antibiotics to see widespread clinical use in the mid-1930s, showing early efficacy against common infections. However, life-threatening infections responded less robustly, and staphylococcal drug resistance arose rapidly within a few years after their introduction. In the early 1940s, the introduction of penicillin temporarily solved the problem of staphylococcal and streptococcal infections. However, as early as 1941, investigators demonstrated the in vitro induction of staphylococcal resistance by serially passing staphylococci through increasing concentrations of penicillin. Nosocomial *S. aureus* infections became resistant to virtually all available systemic antibiotics by the end of the 1950s. From 1947 to 1957, while the mortality from pneumococcal bacteremia was falling, the mortality associated with staphylococcal bacteremia increased almost fivefold in one Boston hospital due to spread of antibiotic resistance (Finland, Jones, & Barnes, 1959).

Why Should We Worry About Antibiotic Resistance?

Infections caused by antibiotic-resistant organisms are thought to result in increased morbidity, longer length of hospital stay, and higher treatment costs when compared to infections caused by susceptible strains (Cosgrove & Carmeli, 2003). Under certain circumstances, antibiotic resistance may even contribute to excess mortality. However, the magnitude of effect may vary based on the pathogen, adequacy of treatment, and patient population studied. In particular, microbiologically inappropriate therapy of severe infections caused by antibiotic-resistant pathogens may increase the likelihood of death in critically ill patients (Harbarth et al., 2003). Table 2.1 summarizes important adverse outcomes related to antibiotic resistance.

Although most experts would agree that antibiotic resistance constitutes a long-term threat to public health, the overall disease burden of antibiotic resistance remains unclear. Limited data are available to quantify the total burden of antibiotic-resistant infections. In a report intended

Table 2.1. Clinical Implications, Adverse Outcomes, and Disease Burden Related to Antibiotic Resistance

Adverse Outcome	Example	References
Treatment failure due to wrong choice	Prolonged illness and need for additional antibiotic therapy due to pyelonephritis caused by antibiotic-resistant gram-negative bacteria	Talan et al., 2000
Increased in-hospital mortality	Infections caused by multiresistant *Enterococcus faecium* and *Pseudomonas aeruginosa*	Carmeli, Eliopoulos, Mozaffari, & Samore, 2002; Carmeli, Troillet, Karchmer, & Samore, 1999
Increased direct costs and length of hospital stay	Emergence of multiresistant *Enterobacter* spp. during antibiotic therapy	Cosgrove, Kaye, Eliopoulous, & Carmeli, 2002
Indirect costs, diminished quality of life, and lost productivity	Severe *Acinetobacter* spp. infections in veterans of the Gulf War or Tsunami survivors	Davis, Moran, McAllister, & Gray, 2005; Maegele et al., 2005
Use of more toxic, less efficacious, and more expensive alternatives	Treatment of MRSA infections with vancomycin or linezolid	Bishop, Melvani, Howden, Charles, & Grayson, 2006; Nathwani & Tillotson, 2003
Increased antibiotic costs due to the need to cover empirically potential antibiotic-resistant infections	Empiric coverage of severe infections due to antibiotic-resistant pathogens in the critical care setting	Harbarth et al., 2003
Added burden of nosocomial infections	MRSA infections do not replace MSSA infections, but add on to the already existing burden of staphylococcal infections	Office for National Statistics, 2006
Infrastructure costs of surveillance programs	Excess costs related to contact isolation of MRSA carriers	Herr, Heckrodt, Hofmann, Schnettler, & Eikmann, 2003

MRSA = methicillin-resistant *Staphylococcus aureus*; MSSA = methicillin-susceptible *S. aureus*.

for policy makers in the U.S. Congress, the General Accounting Office stated in 1999 that "No systematic information is available about deaths from diseases caused by resistant bacteria or about the costs of treating resistant disease. Consequently, the overall extent of disease, death, and treatment costs resulting from resistant bacteria is unknown" (p. 7). In 2006, the situation remains unchanged since no well-conducted studies are available to assess the overall public health burden of antibiotic resistance. The few valid studies relating antibiotic-resistant infections to specific patient outcomes (increased length of stay, direct costs, excess deaths) have been conducted in U.S. tertiary care centers and may not be generalizable to other settings, countries with fewer resources, or other types of health care systems.

What Contributes to the Emergence and Spread of Antibiotic Resistance?

Emergence of antimicrobial resistance in infectious organisms at a population level is dependent on the survival and further spread of resistant organisms. The extensive use of antimicrobial agents sustains this process by eliminating sensitive microorganisms, which in turn allows the resistant ones a greater opportunity to spread.

When analyzing changes in prevalence of antibiotic resistance at a hospital level, several factors may contribute to the increase of antibiotic-resistant bacteria. First, mutation of resistance genes and introduction of mobile elements can alter the genetic material and the resistance pattern of susceptible bacteria present in the hospital. Second, transfer of patients or heath care workers colonized with already resistant bacteria may become the source for further spread. Third, once introduced, bacteria can be transferred because of low compliance in hand hygiene and breaks in infection control. Finally, antibiotic selection pressure may further enhance the survival advantage of resistant bacteria in the hospital environment.

In the community, similar processes contribute to the spread of antibiotic resistance. Once resistant clones are selected, their spread is promoted by factors such as overcrowding and poor hygiene. One example is day care centers, which provide ample opportunities for the transmission of infectious diseases and, in particular, the spread of resistant *Streptococcus pneumoniae*. The combination of the presence of susceptible children suffering from recurrent infections and the use of broad-spectrum antibiotics makes such environments ideal for the carriage and transmission of these bacteria (Samore et al., 2001). Another example is the spread of multidrug-resistant tuberculosis or community-acquired, methicillin-resistant *S. aureus* (MRSA) in the prison setting (Pan et al., 2003).

What Is the Relation Between Antibiotic Use and Resistance?

The causal relationship between antibiotic consumption and antimicrobial resistance is not as straightforward as one might think. A simple observation is that resistant organisms have been found for every antibiotic introduced, and the amount of resistance is, in general, increasing with the volume of antibiotic use. The circumstantial nature of these findings, however, prompts cautious interpretation. Although the appearance of resistance has been well established in vitro, many more variables come into play *in vivo* (e.g., dosage, duration and route of antibiotic administration, type of microorganism, interaction between microorganisms, and mechanisms of resistance). For instance, use of oxacillin or nafcillin does not increase the likelihood of emergence or transmission of MRSA.

Different types of epidemiological studies have been used to quantify the association between antibiotic exposure and resistance. These studies included outbreak reports, laboratory-based surveys, randomized trials, and prospective or retrospective cohort studies based on analyses of individual patient-level data or aggregated data. Notwithstanding these methodological differences, many studies have shown a correlation between antibiotic use and resistance. For instance, the prevalence of penicillin-nonsusceptible pneumococci is clearly associated with the use of lactams and with total antibiotic use as measured on a national or regional scale (Albrich, Monnet, & Harbarth, 2004; Goossens, Ferech, Vander Stichele, & Elseviers, 2005). Resistance occurs not only in pathogenic microorganisms against which antibiotic therapy was instituted in patients treated for an infection, but also in the endogenous flora of the host. Conversely, concerns raised that the use of vancomycin is associated with an increase in the prevalence of patients colonized with vancomycin-resistant enterococci (VRE) may not be justified based on studies using adequate epidemiologic methods (Carmeli, Samore, & Huskins, 1999). Indeed, in patients previously free of VRE, intravenous vancomycin use may have a limited role in facilitating new acquisition of VRE, while broad-spectrum cephalosporins or antianaerobic agents may have a more pronounced effect (Harbarth, Cosgrove, & Carmeli, 2002).

Can Antibiotic Resistance Be Reversible?

The potential reversibility of resistance is subject to ongoing controversy. The rationale for reversibility is that resistant bacteria will have a disadvantage over susceptible strains in environments without antibiotics, as most resistance mechanisms will confer a reduction in bacterial fitness, that is, a slower growth rate, reduced virulence, or decreased transmission rate. Thus, a decreased volume of antibiotic use should lead to lower selection pressure and a reduction in the proportion of bacteria resistant to a certain antibiotic. Thereby resistant organisms will be replaced by susceptible ones (Nordberg, Monnet, & Cars, 2005).

This picture is complicated, however, by the fact that bacteria may reduce the biological costs associated with resistance through compensatory evolution. The role of compensatory mutations that maintain the fitness of resistant strains is now well established. Increasing levels of biologically competitive resistant bacteria are detected in the community, with no decrease in survival fitness compared to nonresistant strains. Thus, resistance levels may be slow to reverse and sometimes appear to be irreversible. In addition, genetic linkage between resistance genes will result in coselection of the genes. Consequently, when bacteria have developed resistance toward several antibiotics, even a substantial reduction of one drug may be ineffective in reducing overall resistance (Nordberg et al., 2005).

Trends in antibiotic resistance follow an S-shaped curve with a quick ascent, a plateau, and, sometimes, a slow decline. More than one report has demonstrated that the decline in resistance after reduction in the volume or pattern of antibiotic use is much slower than its emergence. In addition to antibiotic-selection pressure, the persistence of resistance is favored by inadequate treatment, case-mix factors, and ineffective infection control.

Is Antibiotic Resistance a Global Problem?

There is no region anywhere in the world that has been excluded from the inexorable spread of increasingly resistant bacteria. A number of phenomena of modern society have enhanced the opportunities for resistant clones to spread globally, including increasing international trade, travel and migration, ecosystem disturbances, urbanization, and the increasing number of immunocompromised people (Harbarth & Samore, 2005). As global travel and economic exchange increase, more antibiotic-resistant bacteria are transferred from one country to another, thereby making antibiotic resistance a global problem. Once introduced into a country, these bacteria can become established, and the resistance genes can move into new strains or even new species.

Molecular epidemiological studies have shown numerous examples of the rapid spread of resistant strains between countries and continents (e.g., global spread of multiple antibiotic-resistant pneumococci; Nuermberger & Bishai, 2004). The export and import of food products may also contribute to the global spread of antibiotic resistance. International outbreaks of salmonellosis due to resistant strains have occurred because of the sale of contaminated food products in several countries

(Nordberg et al., 2005). The importance of trading live animals for breeding purposes may also be a cause of the worldwide spread of resistant bacteria. In 2003, for example, a boar imported for breeding purposes from Canada to Denmark was found to harbor multiresistant *Salmonella enterica* (Aarestrup, Hasman, Olsen, & Sorensen, 2004).

What Are Current Resistance Trends in the United States of Clinically Important Bacteria?

The continuing increase in antibiotic resistance in the U.S. health care system remains a serious concern, as demonstrated by recent data from the National Nosocomial Infections Surveillance (NNIS) system (Centers for Disease Control and Prevention [CDC], 2004). This voluntary surveillance system receives monthly reports of nosocomial infections and also microbiological data from a nonrandom sample of more than 300 hospitals in 42 U.S. states. The microbiological data include antimicrobial-susceptibility test results on all nonduplicate clinical isolates processed by the microbiology laboratories during each month, stratified by patients' hospital locations. A recent NNIS report (CDC, 2004) showed that in 2003, 60% of all *S. aureus* isolates in the participating U.S. intensive care units (ICUs) were methicillin resistant, 29% of all enterococci were vancomycin resistant, and 89% of all coagulase-negative staphylococci were methicillin resistant. More than 30% of all *P. aeruginosa* isolates from ICU patients were resistant to fluoroquinolones or ceftazidime. Of note, there has been a nearly 50% increase in nonsusceptible *Klebsiella pneumoniae* isolates to third-generation cephalosporins between 2002 and 2003.

Another nosocomial pathogen that is increasingly colonizing and infecting patients in the hospital environment is *Acinetobacter baumannii*. Patients with debilitating conditions are at especially high risk of acquiring pneumonia or bacteremia with this pathogen (Van Looveren & Goossens, 2004). The wide use of broad-spectrum antibiotics is one of the most important risk factors for colonization and infection with *A. baumannii*. Villers et al. (1998) illustrated the complex relation between use of fluoroquinolones and the occurrence of *A. baumannii* infections in critically ill patients. They showed that epidemic infections coexisted with endemic infections favored by the selection pressure of intravenous fluoroquinolones.

Antibiotic resistance in the U.S. community shows several noteworthy trends. Pneumococcal drug resistance has decreased in young children and older persons due to the introduction of new conjugate vaccines (Kyaw et al., 2006). Fluoroquinolone resistance in gram-negative bacilli, especially in *E. coli* and *P. aeruginosa*, is steadily growing (MacDougall, Powell, Johnson, Edmond, & Polk, 2005; Polk, Johnson, McClish, Wenzel, & Edmond, 2004). Community MRSA (C-MRSA) has become an increasing problem in the United States with several alarming outbreaks in the last years (Young et al., 2004). Deaths in children have been reported in cases where they were admitted to hospitals with C-MRSA infections that were treated empirically with cephalosporin antibiotics, ineffective in such cases. Overall, the United States has the unenviable position of being one of the world leaders in the prevalence of methicillin resistance among *S. aureus* isolates, both within and outside the health care setting (Styers, Sheehan, Hogan, & Sahm, 2006).

Why Are There Such Differences Between Resistance Rates in Different Parts of the World?

Why do resistance rates vary so much across countries? First, different practices in detection and laboratory identification of resistant pathogens may lead to detection and misclassification bias. Second, prescribers of antibiotics may differ in their use of antibiotic agents. Third, characteristics of patient populations and case mix may lead to different transmission patterns. Fourth, socioeconomic factors and consumer attitudes may influence the demand for antibiotics. Fifth, macrolevel factors related to the health care environment may differ. Examples of these include legal issues as well as regulatory health care policies that may influence antibiotic prescribing practices. Last, infection control practices such as use of alcohol-based hand disinfection and barrier precautions may also have an effect on the transmission of resistant organisms (Harbarth, Albrich, Goldmann, & Huebner, 2001).

Overall, cultural and economic factors pervade all aspects of antibiotic use and resistance. In the community, factors that influence antibiotic use and resistance include cultural conceptions, patient demands, economic incentives, the level of training among health staff and pharmacists, and marketing pressure on prescribers (Harbarth, Albrich, & Brun-Buisson, 2002). Consequently, the patterns of antibiotic use differ substantially between and within countries. In Europe, for example, antibiotic consumption is four times higher in France than in the Netherlands, although there is no reason to believe that the burden of disease differs between the two countries (Goossens et al., 2005).

The most extreme example is illustrated by health care providers in several Asian countries who can earn a significant proportion of their income from dispensing drugs. Traditionally, those physicians have compensated for relatively low medical service revenue by prescribing a high volume of broad-spectrum antimicrobial agents. Thus, financial incentives linked to the pharmaceutical reimbursement system and physician— industry interactions strongly influence antibiotic prescribing and increase antibiotic resistance problems in certain parts of the world.

SECTION 2: SPECIAL PATHOGENS OF INTEREST

While resistance to antimicrobial agents is becoming a problem with regard to many pathogens, a few have become especially problematic and widespread. MRSA, VRE, *S. pneumoniae*, and *Clostridium difficile* will be discussed below.

Methicillin-Resistant *Staphylococcus aureus*

Methicillin-resistance in *S. aureus* is the clinically most relevant, chromosomally encoded antibiotic resistance mechanism. The responsible resistance gene *mecA* codes for the low-affinity penicillin-binding protein PBP2' and is located on a variable mobile genetic element called staphylococcal chromosomal cassette (SCC) *mec*. To date, five major SCC*mec* types (I to V) have been described, with Types I, II, III, and IVb widespread in nosocomial strains and Types IVa and V most commonly present in C-MRSA.

The altered penicillin binding protein causes resistance to all beta-lactam agents (including penicillinase-resistant penicillins, cephalosporins, and carbapenems). Nosocomial strains are frequently multiresistant, expressing resistance to aminoglycosides, macrolides, fluoroquinolones, or trimethoprim–sulfamethoxazole. In contrast to health care-associated MRSA, C-MRSA strains are often susceptible to many non-beta-lactam antibiotics such as trimethoprim—sulfamethoxazole, fluoroquinolones, and clindamycin, antibiotic agents that can be administered orally.

Health Care-Associated MRSA

Methicillin resistance in a clinical isolate of *S. aureus* was first reported in 1961. The prevalence of methicillin resistance in U.S. hospitals remained low for two decades despite sporadic outbreaks. The MRSA lull ended in the early 1980s, however, as the organism resurfaced in clinical isolates in Australia, the United States, and the Irish Republic. In the United States, the prevalence of MRSA more than doubled from 2.4% nationwide in 1975 to 6% in 1981. The prevalence of MRSA rose to 20–50% in some teaching hospitals during this period. By the year 2006, most hospitals in the United States had hyperendemic MRSA, with an MRSA prevalence of at least 40% among all nonduplicate *S. aureus* isolates.

Vancomycin-Resistant MRSA

Since the emergence of strains that are insensitive or have reduced sensitivity to glycopeptides, there is real danger of the spread of pan-resistant MRSA. As of March 2006, five cases of vancomycin-resistant *S. aureus*

(VRSA) had been reported from the United States. All patients had several comorbidities and were exposed to multiple antibiotics prior to isolation of VRSA. Strikingly, cocolonization with VRE and MRSA was present in all patients, demonstrating the danger of these common nosocomial pathogens.

The last case reported from Michigan serves as a a recent example of VRSA acquisition. The patient was a 58-year-old female with multiple comorbidities who developed a postoperative wound infection 2 weeks after hernia repair in June 2005. While the patient was recovering in a rehabilitation facility from July through November, cultures taken from the abdominal wound in August and September each grew a variety of organisms, including MRSA. The patient received vancomycin for a total of 4 weeks. Subsequently, an abdominal wound culture grew *P. aeruginosa*, VRE, and VRSA. The VRSA isolate was susceptible to gentamicin, linezolid, rifampin, tetracycline, and trimethoprim—sulfamethoxazole. The patient did not receive antimicrobial therapy for the VRSA-positive wound culture, as there was no longer an apparent infection. VRSA was recovered from a surveillance culture of the groin in close proximity to the wound site. Five days of chlorhexidine showers were used to decolonize the patient, and follow-up cultures were negative for VRSA (Sievert et al., 2006).

Community MRSA

As mentioned above, C-MRSA strains are genetically distinct from health care-associated MRSA, since they contain the Type IVa SCC*mec* element and share unique virulence factors such as the Panton—Valentine leukocidin toxin (Naimi et al., 2003). C-MRSA are frequently involved in recurrent skin infections in otherwise healthy young people. In North America, outbreaks of C-MRSA have already been reported in prisons, military camps, and health care institutions involving children and health care personnel (Zinderman et al., 2004). Control of this emerging pathogen is difficult and will require innovative approaches including new antistaphylococcal vaccines, since classic approaches used for nosocomial MRSA control are only of limited usefulness.

Control of Hospital MRSA

Successful control of nosocomial MRSA depends on the use of several complementary control strategies (Figure 2.1). Clearly, there is no level of MRSA prevalence where control measures are not warranted any more.

First, early detection of MRSA carriage may allow rapid contact isolation of identified MRSA carriers and improve the adequacy of antibiotic

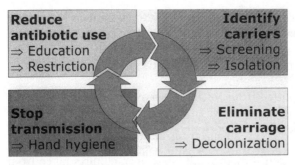

Figure 2.1. Complementary strategies for control of nosocomial methicillin-resistant *Staphylococcus aureus*.

prophylaxis and treatment (e.g., vancomycin). Several recent studies have shown the importance of surveillance cultures in order to prevent MRSA transmission and infection (Harbarth et al., 2006; Lucet et al., 2005). Although the most efficient MRSA screening strategy depends on the local situation and is still a matter of debate, most affected acute care hospitals should install a screening policy for patient groups at high risk for MRSA carriage (e.g., roommates of newly identified MRSA carriers) and apply specific preventive measures (contact isolation) to all identified carriers, especially in the ICU setting (Cooper et al., 2004).

Second, eradicating MRSA carriage may reduce the rates of MRSA infection. In particular, mupirocin nasal ointment has been used to eradicate carriage because of its effectiveness, safety, and relatively low cost. Although some data suggest that mupirocin is effective at reducing nasal carriage of *S. aureus*, a recent systematic review concluded that there is insufficient evidence to support widespread use of topical or systemic antimicrobial therapy for eradicating extranasal MRSA carriage, beyond well-defined outbreak settings (Loeb, Main, Walker-Dilks, & Eady, 2003).

Third, strict compliance with standard precautions and hand hygiene could prevent most cases of cross-transmission, even without the need for recognition of individual MRSA carriers. Unfortunately, many studies have shown that compliance of health care workers with hand hygiene recommendations remains low. Implementing alcohol-based hand rinses can improve compliance and decrease MRSA infection rates (Johnson et al., 2005; Pittet et al., 2000).

Finally, antibiotic selection pressure contributes to the increase in MRSA prevalence (MacDougall et al., 2005). Data from two recently published studies suggest that restriction of fluoroquinolone use may decrease MRSA rates (Charbonneau et al., 2006; Madaras-Kelly, Remington, Lewis, & Stevens, 2006). Other well-designed investigations are needed to confirm that reduction in antimicrobial overuse has a favorable effect on MRSA infection rates.

Vancomycin-Resistant Enterococci

Enterococci are among the most common causes of nosocomial infections. Their reservoir is usually the patient's bowel. As with many other antimicrobial-resistant organisms, VRE colonization is more frequent than true infection. The emergence of VRE is mainly the result of the appearance and spread of transposons encoding *vanA* and *vanB* genes. This usually occurs within environments where there is heavy usage of cephalosporins and other broad-spectrum antibiotics, for example, in renal, hematology, oncology, and transplant units. A recent NNIS report noted that the percentage of VRE implicated in nosocomial infections in ICUs increased from 0.4% in 1989 to 29% in 2003 (CDC, 2004). This increase probably reflects a convergence of risk factors including severe illness and preceding antibiotic therapy with broad-spectrum agents active against anaerobes.

Since de novo emergence of vancomycin resistance in enterococci through genetic mutations induced by vancomycin exposure in an individual patient is extremely unlikely, the inexorable increase in the prevalence of VRE in many U.S. hospitals during the last decade was accelerated by cross-transmission via the hands of health care workers, contaminated equipment, and environmental surfaces (Martinez, Ruthazer, Hansjosten, Barefoot, & Snydman, 2003). Therefore, the presence of VRE within a hospital environment raises important issues in order to prevent VRE transmission. First, improved hand hygiene practices and reliable cleaning techniques are warranted to decrease the spread of VRE. Second, the fact that many seriously ill patients may be asymptomatically colonized requires screening policies for early detection and special isolation precautions for patients carrying VRE. Finally, excessive antibiotic usage has been identified as one of the most important modifiable risk factors for VRE occurrence within the hospital setting (Harbarth, Cosgrove, et al., 2002).

In summary, screening patients identifies colonization, elucidates the epidemiology, and permits introduction of appropriate preventative measures, including contact isolation. Other VRE control measures should include improved antibiotic prescribing, hand hygiene, surveillance, adequate environmental cleaning, and cohorting of patients with designated staff.

Drug-Resistant Pneumococci

S. pneumoniae is the single most important cause of infections of the lower respiratory tract, some of which are potentially life threatening (pneumonia, meningitis). It is also the main cause of otitis media in children. Penicillin and other beta-lactam antibiotics have been the drugs of choice since the 1940s. Within the past two decades, however, increasingly resistant *S. pneumoniae* have complicated antibiotic treatment of pneumococcal infections. A steady decrease of penicillin susceptibility has been reported from many countries worldwide. There is a clear relationship between increased antibiotic consumption and increased levels of resistance in pneumococci (Albrich et al., 2004).

By early 2000, at least 30% of pneumococci in the Unites States were intermediately susceptible or resistant to penicillin. Historically, penicillin-resistant pneumococci have been recovered more frequently from children 5 years old or younger. Since 1995, however, an increased frequency of resistant bacteria has been demonstrated in adults. Since many of these isolates are cross-resistant to other non-beta-lactam antibiotics, the agents available for use are limited. Often, more expensive or less efficacious antibiotics are required for therapy. In the case of pneumococcal meningitis, vancomycin remains the only drug available to treat highly penicillin- and cephalosporin-resistant infections.

Recently, good news about slowing or decreasing dissemination of antibiotic-resistant pneumococci has been reported. In several high-antibiotic-usage countries like France, Spain, and the United States, a decrease in pneumococcal resistance rates among invasive isolates has been noted, coinciding with a decrease in antibiotic consumption after nationwide campaigns and the introduction of the conjugate pneumococcal vaccine (Guillemot et al., 2005; Kyaw et al., 2006; Oteo, Lazaro, de Abajo, Baquero, & Campos, 2004). Nevertheless, uncertainty persists about possible replacement by infections caused by serotypes not covered in currently available vaccines.

Clostridium difficile

Diarrhea caused by *C. difficile* strikes up to 1% of all hospitalized patients. While infection rates vary depending on geography and across institutions and seasons, *C. difficile* is a common nosocomial pathogen in institutions with widespread use of broad-spectrum antibiotics. Recent surveillance studies in Europe, Canada, and the Unites States suggest that the incidence of *C. difficile*-associated diarrhea (CDAD) is rising (Archibald, Banerjee, & Jarvis, 2004; Warny et al., 2005). Some regions have experienced alarming outbreaks associated with higher than expected morbidity and mortality rates (Pepin, Valiquette, & Cossette, 2005).

CDAD was classically described following clindamycin administration but has subsequently been correlated with virtually all antibiotics (except aminoglycosides, glycopeptides, and metronidazol) and is now most frequently associated with the widespread use of broad-spectrum cephalosporins and fluoroquinolones (Loo et al., 2005). A previously uncommon but virulent strain of *C. difficile* has become more resistant to fluoroquinolones and has emerged as a cause of several large-scale outbreaks of CDAD in North America (McDonald et al., 2005). Thus, resistance of specific *C. difficile* strains to certain antimicrobial agents may contribute to their hospital dissemination and explain, in part, their propensity to trigger nosocomial outbreaks (Samore et al., 2006). Overall, these recently published studies support the perspective that nosocomial CDAD is appropriately framed as an antimicrobial resistance problem.

Given that the two major risk factors for CDAD are exposure to the organism and exposure to antibiotics, prevention strategies should aim at reducing these risk factors. *C. difficile* persists in the hospital environment as spores for many months. Thus, appropriate cleaning and disinfection procedures are essential to decrease *C. difficile* contamination in the close patient environment and to minimize the likelihood of cross-infection. Antibiotic stewardship may further decrease the risk of nosocomial CDAD acquisition. For instance, a study from Australia has shown the effectiveness of an antibiotic policy restricting cephalosporin use on the incidence of CDAD (Thomas, Stevenson, Williamson, & Riley, 2002).

SECTION 3: CONTROL OF ANTIBIOTIC RESISTANCE

Future Determinants of Spread of Antibiotic Resistance

Pessimistic viewpoints about the low chances of success to stop the development of antibiotic resistance have repeatedly been reported (Livermore, 2004). From an evolutionary perspective, the emergence of antibiotic-resistant bacteria is unavoidable (Courvalin, 2005). Nevertheless, it remains unclear whether the current epidemic of antibiotic resistance will lead to a "postantibiotic era" or will finally succumb to current efforts to limit its spread.

The drivers of uncertainty regarding the long-term trends of antibiotic resistance are numerous. These potential determinants can be grouped into four categories (Table 2.2; Harbarth & Samore, 2005). The first group is related to the molecular characteristics of the discussed pathogens, their virulence, transmissibility, and survival fitness. Progress in microbiologic detection and identification of infectious pathogens is likely to influence diagnostic uncertainty and antibiotic prescribing patterns. The second group of determinants is linked to the prescribing physicians, who may change their prescription patterns of antibiotic agents. Recent antibiotic consumption data from different parts of the world show promise in this area. The third group is related to host factors

Table 2.2. Determinants Potentially Influencing Future Dissemination and Control of Antibiotic Resistance

Dimension	Determinants
Pathogen and bacterial ecology	Evolution Survival fitness Virulence Laboratory detection and identification
Physician's prescribing practice	Antibiotic usage pattern Diversity of antibiotic prescribing Training and knowledge
Population characteristics	Migration, travel, and globalization Case mix and host susceptibility to infections Antibiotic demand and health beliefs Transmission and infection rates
Politics and health care policy	Health care policy Promotional activities by industry Technological development

Source: Harbarth & Samore, 2005.

and infection rates of patient populations, as well as consumer attitudes and migration patterns related to globalization. Certainly, an increase in immunocompromised patients, the growing life expectancy, and the susceptibility of very aged people to infections will indirectly contribute to greater antibiotic use and dissemination of resistant bacteria. A fourth group of determinants is linked to macrolevel factors, including regulatory policies that may influence antibiotic prescribing, infection control practices, technological development, and drug discovery. For instance, modern vaccinology is likely to contribute to the decreased transmission and impact of antibiotic-resistant bacteria in the near future.

Core Strategies to Control Antibiotic Resistance

The World Health Organization has published a global strategy to contain antibiotic resistance, but few countries have started to implement it. There is an urgent need to implement the following core strategies to improve the control of antibiotic resistance throughout the world (Simonsen et al., 2004).

1. Public education about preventing infection and reducing transmission. It is essential that people have the knowledge to make informed decisions about how to prevent infection and reduce transmission of infectious diseases though simple and effective measures.

2. Provider education about accurate diagnosis and management of common infections, antimicrobial use, containment of antibiotic resistance, disease prevention, and infection control. Teaching providers about all the issues surrounding antibiotic resistance is important for containing antibiotic resistance. Unfortunately, relevant topics are often not covered in education programs. Furthermore, continuing education activities are often heavily dependent upon pharmaceutical companies, which may be more interested in promoting their own antimicrobial sales.

3. Development, updating, and use of essential medicines lists, guidelines, and treatment algorithms. Evidence-based, regularly updated essential medicines lists and clinical guidelines, for each level of care, are essential for promoting rational use of medicines. Antimicrobial guidelines and treatment algorithms for infectious diseases may further aid rational use of antimicrobials. Provided there is reliable data, local resistance trends should be taken into account. Governments can facilitate compliance with essential medicines lists and clinical guidelines by ensuring that public sector reimbursement policies are based on the national essential medicines list or clinical guidelines.

4. Restriction of availability of antimicrobials. In many low- and middle-income countries, antibiotics are freely available over the counter without prescription. Unlicensed dispensing leads to serious antibiotic misuse. Such misuse may be reduced by enforcing regulations to limit the availability of antimicrobials to licensed dispensing outlets upon receipt of a prescription written by an authorized prescriber.

5. Active infection prevention programs in hospitals. Hospitals are hotbeds for the development and spread of antibiotic resistance due to the close proximity of patients colonized with resistant bacteria and receiving antibiotic agents (Lipsitch & Samore, 2002). An active infection control program should be implemented in all hospitals, undertaking active surveillance, interventions to prevent infections, and the development and implementation of policies and procedures to prevent the transmission of resistant bacteria.

6. Controlling nonhuman use of antimicrobials. Only about half of all antimicrobials are consumed by humans. Most of the rest is added to animal feed (particularly pigs and poultry) for mass treatment against infectious diseases or for growth promotion. Although the majority of human antibiotic resistance results from human use, there is evidence of spread of certain resistant bacteria (e.g., *Campylobacter* spp.) from animals to humans.

7. International cooperation in research, surveillance, and technological development. New modalities for prevention and treatment of infection should be enhanced, including behavioral change programs to increase health care workers' compliance with basic infection control. Continued support for research into new drugs, diagnostic tests, and alternatives to conventional antibiotics (e.g., bacteriophage therapy) should be ensured.

SUMMARY

At the beginning of the 21st century, antibiotic resistance is common, has developed against every class of antibiotics, and appears to be spreading into new clinical niches. It will continue to cause much concern. MRSA in particular presents a tremendous challenge, since this virulent pathogen is now spreading within the community. Stringent MRSA control will remain difficult to implement worldwide and will require intensive efforts and substantial resources. To achieve this goal may not be impossible, as shown by several examples, where successful action against MRSA has been endorsed by strong policy support.

Hopefully, adding infection control and antimicrobial stewardship to new drug development will help avert the realization of pessimistic predictions about the future of antibiotic resistance. International collective action is essential to tackle the global resistance problem. Yet, as responsibility for health remains predominantly national, there remains a significant disparity between the problems and potential solutions associated with antibiotic resistance and the institutions and mechanisms available to deal with them. Clearly, the discrepancy between the growth of the resistance problem and the pace at which new drugs, vaccines, and diagnostic tests are being developed justify more concerted actions on an international level.

REFERENCES

Aarestrup, F. M., Hasman, H., Olsen, I., & Sorensen, G. (2004). International spread of bla(cmy-2)-mediated cephalosporin resistance in a multiresistant *Salmonella enterica* serovar Heidelberg isolate stemming from the importation of a boar by Denmark from Canada. *Antimicrobial Agents and Chemotherapy, 48,* 1916–1917.

Albrich, W. C., Monnet, D. L., & Harbarth, S. (2004). Antibiotic selection pressure and resistance in *Streptococcus pneumoniae* and *streptococcus pyogenes. Emerging Infectious Diseases, 10,* 514–517.

Archibald, L. K., Banerjee, S. N., & Jarvis, W. R. (2004). Secular trends in hospital-acquired *Clostridium difficile* disease in the United States, 1987–2001. *Journal of Infectious Diseases, 189,* 1585–1589.

Bartoloni, A., Bartalesi, F., Mantella, A., Dell'Amico, E., Roselli, M., Strohmeyer, M., et al. (2004). High prevalence of acquired antimicrobial resistance unrelated to heavy antimicrobial consumption. *Journal of Infectious Diseases, 189*(7), 1291–1294.

Bishop, E., Melvani, S., Howden, B. P., Charles, P. G., & Grayson, M. L. (2006). Good clinical outcomes but high rates of adverse reactions during linezolid therapy for serious infections: A proposed protocol for monitoring therapy in complex patients. *Antimicrobial Agents and Chemotherapy, 50,* 1599–1602.

Carmeli, Y., Eliopoulos, G., Mozaffari, E., & Samore, M. (2002). Health and economic outcomes of vancomycin-resistant enterococci. *Archives of Internal Medicine, 162,* 2223–2228.

Carmeli, Y., Samore, M. H., & Huskins, C. (1999). The association between antecedent vancomycin treatment and hospital-acquired vancomycin-resistant enterococci: A meta-analysis. *Archives of Internal Medicine, 159,* 2461–2468.

Carmeli, Y., Troillet, N., Karchmer, A. W., & Samore, M. H. (1999). Health and economic outcomes of antibiotic resistance in *Pseudomonas aeruginosa. Archives of Internal Medicine, 159,* 1127–1132.

Centers for Disease Control and Prevention. (2004). National Nosocomial Infections Surveillance system report, data summary from January 1992 through June 2004. *American Journal of Infection Control, 32,* 470–485.

Charbonneau, P., Parienti, J. J., Thibon, P., Ramakers, M., Daubin, C., du Cheyron, D., et al. (2006). Fluoroquinolone use and methicillin-resistant *Staphylococcus aureus* isolation rates in hospitalized patients: A quasi experimental study. *Clinical Infectious Diseases, 42,* 778–784.

Cooper, B. S., Stone, S. P., Kibbler, C. C., Cookson, B. D., Roberts, J. A., Medley, G. F., et al. (2004). Isolation measures in the hospital management of methicillin resistant *Staphylococcus aureus*: Systematic review of the literature. *British Medical Journal, 329,* 533.

Cosgrove, S. E., & Carmeli, Y. (2003). The impact of antimicrobial resistance on health and economic outcomes. *Clinical Infectious Diseases, 36,* 1433–1437.

Cosgrove, S. E., Kaye, K. S., Eliopoulous, G. M., & Carmeli, Y. (2002). Health and economic outcomes of the emergence of third-generation cephalosporin resistance in *Enterobacter* species. *Archives of Internal Medicine, 162,* 185–190.

Courvalin, P. (2005). Antimicrobial drug resistance: "Prediction is very difficult, especially about the future." *Emerging Infectious Diseases, 11,* 1503–1506.

Davis, K. A., Moran, K. A., McAllister, C. K., & Gray, P. J. (2005). Multidrug-resistant *Acinetobacter* extremity infections in soldiers. *Emerging Infectious Diseases, 11,* 1218–1224.

D'Costa, V. M., McGrann, K. M., Hughes, D. W., & Wright, G. D. (2006). Sampling the antibiotic resistome. *Science, 311*(5759), 374–377.

Finland, M., Jones, W. F., Jr., & Barnes, M. W. (1959). Occurrence of serious bacterial infections since the introduction of antibacterial agents. *Journal of the American Medical Association, 170*, 2188–2197.

Gardner, P., Smith, D. H., Beer, H., & Moellering, R. C., Jr. (1969). Recovery of resistance (r) factors from a drug-free community. *Lancet, 2*, 774–776.

General Accounting Office. (1999). *Antimicrobial resistance—Data to assess public health threat from resistant bacteria are limited.* Washington: Author.

Goossens, H., Ferech, M., Vander Stichele, R., & Elseviers, M. (2005). Outpatient antibiotic use in Europe and association with resistance: A cross-national database study. *Lancet, 365*, 579–587.

Guillemot, D., Varon, E., Bernede, C., Weber, P., Henriet, L., Simon, S., et al. (2005). Reduction of antibiotic use in the community reduces the rate of colonization with penicillin g-nonsusceptible *Streptococcus pneumoniae. Clinical Infectious Diseases, 41*, 930–938.

Harbarth, S., Albrich, W., & Brun-Buisson, C. (2002). Outpatient antibiotic use and prevalence of antibiotic-resistant pneumococci in France and Germany: A sociocultural perspective. *Emerging Infectious Diseases, 8*, 1460–1467.

Harbarth, S., Albrich, W., Goldmann, D. A., & Huebner, J. (2001). Control of multiply resistant cocci: Do international comparisons help? *Lancet Infectious Diseases, 1*, 251–261.

Harbarth, S., Cosgrove, S., & Carmeli, Y. (2002). Effects of antibiotics on nosocomial epidemiology of vancomycin-resistant enterococci. *Antimicrobial Agents and Chemotherapy, 46*, 1619–1628.

Harbarth, S., Garbino, J., Pugin, J., Romand, J. A., Lew, D., & Pittet, D. (2003). Inappropriate initial antimicrobial therapy and its effect on survival in a clinical trial of immunomodulating therapy for severe sepsis. *American Journal of Medicine, 115*, 529–535.

Harbarth, S., Masuet-Aumatell, C., Schrenzel, J., Francois, P., Akakpo, C., Renzi, G., et al. (2006). Evaluation of rapid screening and pre-emptive contact isolation for detecting and controlling methicillin-resistant *Staphylococcus aureus* in critical care: An interventional cohort study. *Critical Care, 10*, R25.

Harbarth, S., & Samore, M. H. (2005). Antimicrobial resistance determinants and future control. *Emerging Infectious Diseases, 11*, 794–801.

Herr, C. E., Heckrodt, T. H., Hofmann, F. A., Schnettler, R., & Eikmann, T. F. (2003). Additional costs for preventing the spread of methicillin-resistant *Staphylococcus aureus* and a strategy for reducing these costs on a surgical ward. *Infection Control and Hospital Epidemiology, 24*, 673–678.

Johnson, P. D., Martin, R., Burrell, L. J., Grabsch, E. A., Kirsa, S. W., O'Keeffe, J., et al. (2005). Efficacy of an alcohol/chlorhexidine hand hygiene program in a hospital with high rates of nosocomial MRSA infection. *Medical Journal of Australia, 183*, 509–514.

Kyaw, M. H., Lynfield, R., Schaffner, W., Craig, A. S., Hadler, J., Reingold, A., et al. (2006). Effect of introduction of the pneumococcal conjugate vaccine on drug-resistant *Streptococcus pneumoniae*. *New England Journal of Medicine, 354,* 1455–1463.

Lipsitch, M., & Samore, M. H. (2002). Antimicrobial use and antimicrobial resistance: A population perspective. *Emerging Infectious Diseases, 8,* 347–354.

Livermore, D. (2004). Can better prescribing turn the tide of resistance? *Nature Reviews: Microbiology, 2,* 73–78.

Loeb, M., Main, C., Walker-Dilks, C., & Eady, A. (2003). Antimicrobial drugs for treating methicillin-resistant *Staphylococcus aureus* colonization. *Cochrane Database of Systematic Reviews, 4,* CD003340.

Loo, V. G., Poirier, L., Miller, M. A., Oughton, M., Libman, M. D., Michaud, S., et al. (2005). A predominantly clonal multi-institutional outbreak of *Clostridium difficile*-associated diarrhea with high morbidity and mortality. *New England Journal of Medicine, 353,* 2442–2449.

Lucet, J. C., Paoletti, X., Lolom, I., Paugam-Burtz, C., Trouillet, J. L., Timsit, J. F., et al. (2005). Successful long-term program for controlling methicillin-resistant *Staphylococcus aureus* in intensive care units. *Intensive Care Medicine, 31,* 1051–1057.

MacDougall, C., Powell, J. P., Johnson, C. K., Edmond, M. B., & Polk, R. E. (2005). Hospital and community fluoroquinolone use and resistance in *Staphylococcus aureus* and *Escherichia coli* in 17 US hospitals. *Clinical Infectious Diseases, 41,* 435–440.

Madaras-Kelly, K. J., Remington, R. E., Lewis, P. G., & Stevens, D. L. (2006). Evaluation of an intervention designed to decrease the rate of nosocomial methicillin-resistant *Staphylococcus aureus* infection by encouraging decreased fluoroquinolone use. *Infection Control and Hospital Epidemiology, 27,* 155–169.

Maegele, M., Gregor, S., Steinhausen, E., Bouillon, B., Heiss, M. M., Perbix, W., et al. (2005). The long-distance tertiary air transfer and care of tsunami victims: Injury pattern and microbiological and psychological aspects. *Critical Care Medicine, 33*(5), 1136–1140.

Mare, I. J. (1968). Incidence of R factors among gram negative bacteria in drug-free human and animal communities. *Nature, 220*(171), 1046–1047.

Martinez, J. A., Ruthazer, R., Hansjosten, K., Barefoot, L., & Snydman, D. R. (2003). Role of environmental contamination as a risk factor for acquisition of vancomycin-resistant enterococci in patients treated in a medical intensive care unit. *Archives of Internal Medicine, 163,* 1905–1912.

McDonald, L. C., Killgore, G. E., Thompson, A., Owens, R. C., Jr., Kazakova, S. V., Sambo, S. P., et al. (2005). An epidemic, toxin gene-variant strain of *Clostridium difficile*. *New England Journal of Medicine, 353,* 2433–2441.

Naimi, T. S., LeDell, K. H., Como-Sabetti, K., Borchardt, S. M., Boxrud, D. J., Etienne, J., et al. (2003). Comparison of community- and health care-associated methicillin-resistant *Staphylococcus aureus* infection. *Journal of the American Medical Association, 290,* 2976–2984.

Nathwani, D., & Tillotson, G. S. (2003). Vancomycin for *Staphylococcus aureus* therapy of respiratory tract infections: The end of an era? *International Journal of Antimicrobial Agents, 21,* 521–524.

Nordberg, P., Monnet, D. L., & Cars, O. (2005). *Antibacterial drug resistance: Options for concerted action.* Geneva: WHO.

Nuermberger, E. L., & Bishai, W. R. (2004). Antibiotic resistance in *Streptococcus pneumoniae*: What does the future hold? *Clinical Infectious Diseases, 38*(Suppl. 4), S363–371.

Office for National Statistics (UK). (2006). Deaths involving MRSA: England and Wales, 2000–2004. *Health Statistics Quarterly, 29,* 63–68.

Oteo, J., Lazaro, E., de Abajo, F. J., Baquero, F., & Campos, J. (2004). Trends in antimicrobial resistance in 1,968 invasive *Streptococcus pneumoniae* strains isolated in Spanish hospitals (2001 to 2003): Decreasing penicillin resistance in children's isolates. *Journal of Clinical Microbiology, 42,* 5571–5577.

Pan, E. S., Diep, B. A., Carleton, H. A., Charlebois, E. D., Sensabaugh, G. F., Haller, B. L., et al. (2003). Increasing prevalence of methicillin-resistant *Staphylococcus aureus* infection in California jails. *Clinical Infectious Diseases, 37,* 1384–1388.

Pepin, J., Valiquette, L., & Cossette, B. (2005). Mortality attributable to nosocomial *Clostridium difficile*-associated disease during an epidemic caused by a hypervirulent strain in Quebec. *Canadian Medical Association Journal, 173,* 1037–1042.

Pittet, D., Hugonnet, S., Harbarth, S., Mourouga, P., Sauvan, V., Touveneau, S., et al. (2000). Effectiveness of a hospital-wide programme to improve compliance with hand hygiene. *Lancet, 356,* 1307–1312.

Polk, R. E., Johnson, C. K., McClish, D., Wenzel, R. P., & Edmond, M. B. (2004). Predicting hospital rates of fluoroquinolone-resistant *Pseudomonas aeruginosa* from fluoroquinolone use in US hospitals and their surrounding communities. *Clinical Infectious Diseases, 39,* 497–503.

Samore, M. H., Magill, M. K., Alder, S. C., Severina, E., Morrison-De Boer, L., Lyon, J. L., et al. (2001). High rates of multiple antibiotic resistance in *Streptococcus pneumoniae* from healthy children living in isolated rural communities: Association with cephalosporin use and intrafamilial transmission. *Pediatrics, 108,* 856–865.

Samore, M. H., Venkataraman, L., DeGirolami, P. C., Merrigan, M. M., Johnson, S., Gerding, D. N., et al. (2006). Genotypic and phenotypic analysis of *Clostridium difficile* correlated with previous antibiotic exposure. *Microbial Drug Resistance, 12*(1), 23–28.

Sievert, D., Dyke, T. L., Bies, S., Robinson-Dunn, B., Hageman, J., Patel, J., et al. (2006). *Fifth case of vancomycin-resistant* Staphylococcus aureus *in United States and third for Michigan.* Paper presented at the 16th Annual Meeting of the Society for Healthcare Epidemiology of America, Chicago, IL.

Simonsen, G. S., Tapsall, J. W., Allegranzi, B., Talbot, E. A., & Lazzari, S. (2004). The antimicrobial resistance containment and surveillance approach—A public health tool. *Bulletin of the World Health Organization, 82,* 928–934.

Styers, D., Sheehan, D. J., Hogan, P., & Sahm, D. F. (2006). Laboratory-based surveillance of current antimicrobial resistance patterns and trends among *Staphylococcus aureus*: 2005 status in the United States. *Annals of Clinical Microbiology Antimicrobials, 5,* 2.

Talan, D. A., Stamm, W. E., Hooton, T. M., Moran, G. J., Burke, T., Iravani, A., et al. (2000). Comparison of ciprofloxacin (7 days) and trimethoprim-sulfamethoxazole (14 days) for acute uncomplicated pyelonephritis pyelonephritis in women: A randomized trial. *Journal of the American Medical Association, 283,* 1583–1590.

Thomas, C., Stevenson, M., Williamson, D. J., & Riley, T. V. (2002). *Clostridium difficile*-associated diarrhea: Epidemiological data from Western Australia associated with a modified antibiotic policy. *Clinical Infectious Diseases, 35,* 1457–1462.

Van Looveren, M., & Goossens, H. (2004). Antimicrobial resistance of *Acinetobacter* spp. in Europe. *Clinical Microbiology Infection, 10,* 684–704.

Villers, D., Espaze, E., Coste-Burel, M., Giauffret, F., Ninin, E., Nicolas, F., et al. (1998). Nosocomial *Acinetobacter baumannii* infections: Microbiological and clinical epidemiology. *Annals of Internal Medicine, 129,* 182–189.

Warny, M., Pepin, J., Fang, A., Killgore, G., Thompson, A., Brazier, J., et al. (2005). Toxin production by an emerging strain of *Clostridium difficile* associated with outbreaks of severe disease in North America and Europe. *Lancet, 366,* 1079–1084.

Weber, J. T., & Courvalin, P. (2005). An emptying quiver: Antimicrobial drugs and resistance. *Emerging Infectious Diseases, 11,* 791–793.

Young, D. M., Harris, H. W., Charlebois, E. D., Chambers, H., Campbell, A., Perdreau-Remington, F., et al. (2004). An epidemic of methicillin-resistant *Staphylococcus aureus* soft tissue infections among medically underserved patients. *Archives of Surgery, 139,* 947–951.

Zinderman, C. E., Conner, B., Malakooti, M. A., LaMar, J. E., Armstrong, A., & Bohnker, B. K. (2004). Community-acquired methicillin-resistant *Staphylococcus aureus* among military recruits. *Emerging Infectious Diseases, 10,* 941–944.

CHAPTER THREE

Categories and Highlights of Significant Current Emerging Infectious Diseases

Felissa R. Lashley

Emerging infectious diseases (EIDs) may be thought of in various ways: by the category of the organism, the routes of transmission, the most prevalent methods of spread, or geographic distribution. Emerging infectious diseases will be discussed below in terms of the classification of the infectious agent (bacterial, viral, parasitic, fungal, and prion) and in terms of their chief mode of dissemination to humans—limited here to those agents that are food- and/or waterborne, zoonotic, or vectorborne and those that are transmissible by blood transfusion or transplant. Some of the latter categories overlap. For example, babesiosis is a parasitic, vectorborne disease that is also transmissible by blood transfusion. Another important aspect of infectious disease transmission and acquisition has to do with animal and human behavior and culture which are considered in detail in chapter 28. After this general discussion, chapters follow highlighting specific EIDs that are of special interest or importance. Numerous tables providing information about a large number of EIDs appear in Appendices A and B.

Some EIDs are transmitted to humans from their usual animal hosts and are known as zoonoses. About 75% of EIDs in humans are caused by zoonotic pathogens (Wolfe, Daszak, Kilpatrick, & Burke, 2005). In addition to microorganism, vector or vehicle, and host characteristics that may facilitate the transmission of emerging zoonotic diseases to humans, situations that bring humans and animals, especially wildlife, into increased close contact amplify the risk of zoonotic infectious disease emergence. This includes human behavior such as choice of travel or recreational pursuit, examples of which are the acquisition of leptospirosis by a vacationer from California exploring a cave in Malaysia (Mortimer, 2005) and *Escherichia coli* O157:H7 acquired by children at a petting zoo (Centers for Disease Control and Prevention [CDC], 2005). Other human factors include agricultural encroachment, for example, clearing the land in Venezuela for agricultural use, creating a more favorable environment for the cane mouse leading to an outbreak of Venezuelan hemorrhagic fever due to the Guanarito virus; and through weather and climate changes that may increase the population or range of vectors or wildlife reservoirs so that they are more apt to be in a higher density ratio with humans. An example of this is the 1993 hantavirus pulmonary syndrome outbreak in the southwestern United States due to the Sin Nombre virus. When increased rainfall resulted in increased vegetation, and increased food and shelter, for small rodents, their population grew and brought them closer to humans (Engelthaler et al., 1999; Lashley, 2004; Smolinsky, Hamburg, & Lederberg, 2003; Wolfe et al., 2005). In instances of drought and scarce food, rodents may be driven into human dwellings in search of food.

Recent literature has speculated on the potential infectious disease consequences of close contact between humans and nonhuman primates at temples throughout South and Southeast Asia where the temple monkeys have a role in Buddhist and Hindu culture (Jones-Engel et al., 2006). Molecular advances have resulted in increased recognition of certain diseases as zoonotic in origin as well as the discovery of new organisms that were not previously recognized. Emerging infectious diseases of zoonotic origin may appear as human infections in an episodic way, such as happens with Lassa fever (see chapter 8), or may more permanently jump the species barrier, often through a mutation in the organism as is believed to have occurred in the case of the human immunodeficiency virus (HIV) infection. It is believed that HIV-1 originated as the simian immunodeficiency virus from the *Pan troglodytes troglodytes* (Gao et al., 1999) and HIV-2 from the sooty mangabey (Hahn, Shaw, De Cock, & Sharp, 2000; see chapter 13). Some zoonoses are relatively benign, others cause limited disease, and still others result in more serious and extensive outbreaks.

As in other chapters, the definition of EIDs includes newly identified diseases caused by previously known organisms; newly identified diseases caused by previously unknown organisms; the recognition of a new organism; or a familiar organism whose geographic range has extended, whose host has changed, whose incidence has increased, or that has changed to become more virulent or antibiotic resistant. In many cases, identification of new microorganisms has occurred because of the recent availability of new molecular diagnostic techniques.

EMERGING INFECTIONS BY MICROORGANISM CLASSIFICATION

Emerging Bacterial Diseases

Bacteria were the first disease-causing microbes to yield to modern pharmacologic interventions. Morbidity from "old" bacterial illnesses such as tuberculosis (TB) and cholera, however, continues to be a problem. While fewer significant "new" bacteria and bacterial diseases have been identified in the last 35 years (e.g., legionellosis, discussed further in chapter 15; newer rickettsial diseases such as *Rickettsia honei* causing Flinders Island spotted fever, with further data available in Appendix A, Table A.4; and *Bartonella henselae*, the agent of cat scratch disease, discussed further below) when compared with newly identified viruses and viral diseases, other problems are seen. Bacteria have been identified as emerging or reemerging due to the spread to new geographic areas; infection of new hosts or populations, such as with cholera; and the emergence of antimicrobial-resistant forms or increasing virulence of certain strains. This may include multidrug-resistant TB (MDR-TB) and extensively drug-resistant TB (XDR-TB); vancomycin-resistant enterococci (VRE) infections caused by *Enterococcus faecalis* or *Enterococcus faecium*, resulting in significant problems from nosocomial infections; resistant forms of *Streptococcus pneumoniae*, the major bacterial cause of meningitis, pneumonia, and otitis media; or *Clostridium difficile*. Outbreaks of a new strain of *E. coli*, a familiar bacteria, known as O157:H7 fit this pattern causing diarrhea and hemolytic uremic syndrome (see chapter 9). Likewise, although cholera is an ancient disease, new virulent strains such as the El Tor strain of *Vibrio cholerae* have emerged, and there is an endemic focus of infection in the United States as well as increased cases due to imported foods or travelers (see chapter 4). *Staphylococcus aureus*, a frequent cause of infection in nosocomial settings and the immunosuppressed, has become resistant to various antibiotics, especially methicillin (methicillin-resistant *S. aureus*, or MRSA) and, more recently, to vancomycin, probably due to horizontal resistance transfer from VRE organisms (see chapter 2).

Other microorganisms are defined as resurgent due to changes in their geographic distribution or increased incidence of infection, often following the decline of the public health system. An example of the latter is the resurgence of diphtheria (caused by *Corynebacterium diphtheriae*) and pertussis (whooping cough; caused by *Bordetella pertussis*), both vaccine-preventable diseases, in former states of the Soviet Union. Pertussis is also being increasingly seen in adolescents and adults in the United States, and due to travel and migration unusual forms of diphtheria such as cutaneous lesions are being seen in developed countries (Crowcroft & Pebody, 2006; Halperin, 2007; Raguckas, Vandenbussche, Jacobs & Klepser, 2007; Sing & Heesemann, 2005). In another example, both *Clostridium novyi* and *Clostridium histolyticum* were considered emerging when they were responsible for illness outbreaks in injection-drug users via contaminated heroin in Great Britain, the former in 2000 and the latter in 2003 and 2004 (Brazier, Gal, Hall, & Morris, 2004). Also, mild cases of botulism from the toxin produced by *Clostridium botulinum* have resulted from inhalation of adulterated cocaine (Roblot et al., 2006). Another unusual way to develop botulism has been iatrogenic. Four persons developed botulism after injection of a concentrated unlicensed preparation of botulinum toxin A for cosmetic reasons (Chertow et al., 2006). New bacterial diseases such as Lyme disease, ehrlichiosis, anaplasmosis, and various rickettsial fevers have been identified (see chapter 16). Emerging bacterial diseases are summarized in Appendix A, Table A.1. Some of these diseases will be briefly discussed below or in individual chapters.

Toxic shock syndrome (TSS), a febrile illness associated with shock, multiorgan dysfunction, and high death rates, was first described in association with staphylococci in 1978 (Todd, Fishaut, Kapral, & Welch, 1978) but came to national attention in 1979–1980 when a new and initially puzzling entity was affecting young healthy women. The connection with menstruation, tampon use (especially the tampon absorbency), and TSS from *S. aureus* led to some misperceptions that TSS occurred only in association with these variables. Although TSS did initially appear to occur disproportionately in menstruating women, there has been an increasing proportion of nonmenstrual cases, with many reported subsequent to surgical procedures (Hajjeh et al., 1999; Reingold, 1998). *S. aureus* is a gram-positive, nonmotile, non-spore-forming cocci that can cause a wide spectrum of diseases such as skin conditions and abscesses, cellulitis, pneumonia, endocarditis, and osteomyelitis. It can produce toxins directly by the bacteria, for example, on the skin, and cause staphylococcal scalded skin syndrome or TSS, or it can produce toxin when present in food or drink and lead to gastroenteritis in the person who ingests it (M. Lorber, 2005; Moreillon, Que, & Glauser, 2005). Beginning in the 1960s, strains of *S. aureus* that were methicillin-resistant (as well as resistant to many other antibiotics) began to emerge (Fridkin et al., 2005). Infections due to MRSA have increased in prevalence worldwide, but until relatively recently they were considered nosocomial and were essentially endemic in hospitals, especially in intensive care units. It was noted that spread from patient to patient was largely via the hands of health care workers

(Henderson, 2006). The organism has also developed strains resistant to vancomycin, which were first reported in the United States in 2002 (CDC, 2002).

Beginning in 1993 with reports from Western Australia, community-associated (CA) MRSA strains began to emerge and have been isolated from both children and adults with skin and soft tissue infections, septicemia, TSS, necrotizing fasciitis, necrotizing pneumonia, and septic arthritis. CA-MRSA appears more prevalent among the homeless, men who have sex with men, prisoners, military recruits, children in day care centers, tattoo recipients, and others (CDC, 2006b; Grundmann, Aires-de-Sousa, Boyce, & Tiemersma, 2006). Community-associated strains are now finding their way into hospitals (Grundmann et al., 2006). Nosocomial MRSA is associated with persons having dialysis, organ transplantation, catheters, and surgical procedures; persons who have immune defects such as diabetes, HIV infection, alcoholism, older age, and so on; as well as those who are chronic nasal or skin carriers of *S. aureus* (Moreillon et al., 2005). Bahrain, Vasiliades, Wolff, and Younus (2006) consider bacterial endocarditis after CA-MRSA furunculosis an emerging infectious entity. Finding an effective antibiotic and implementing guidelines to reduce transmission are vital.

In the mid-1980s, a resurgence of severe, invasive group A streptococcal (GAS) infections was seen, leading to TSS and necrotizing fasciitis. Group A streptococcal infections had been known previously but had appeared to be declining prior to this resurgence, which was attributed to an increased virulence of the organism. It is also known that host susceptibility plays a vital role in predisposition of persons to GAS. Any illness caused by *Streptococcus pyogenes* can result in streptococcal TSS, which is an acute febrile illness often with tissue infection that can progress to shock, multiorgan failure, and death. The death rate is high—reported as 30% to 80% (Chuang, Huang, & Lin, 2005). GAS infection resulting in necrotizing fasciitis with or without TSS has emerged becoming known in the popular press as "flesh-eating" bacteria. Mortality is high with this condition, and survivors often need major debridement and/or amputation of limbs. About half of these cases are associated with TSS (Hasham, Matteucci, Stanley, & Hart, 2005). Necrotizing fasciitis due to CA-MRSA is also considered an emerging entity (Miller et al., 2005).

C. difficile infection increased 26% as a discharge diagnosis from hospitals between 2000 and 2001 in the United States. *C. difficile* is a gram-positive spore-forming bacteria capable of producing exotoxins (CDC, 2005). Its range of infection is from uncomplicated diarrhea to sepsis and death (Sunenshine & McDonald, 2006). It is a major component of antibiotic-associated diarrhea (Fordtran, 2006). Typically, it has affected older or severely ill patients in the hospital or long-term care settings but is now being found affecting previously healthy people in the community

(CDC, 2005). It is increasing in incidence and severity of disease due to increased virulence and multidrug resistance of some strains (Oldfield, 2006; Sebaihia et al., 2006). Transmission is by the fecal–oral route through hand and patient environment contamination (Fordtran, 2006; Sunenshine & McDonald, 2006).

Bartonella (formerly called *Rochalimaea*) *quintana* was recognized as the cause of trench fever during World War I, and another species, *B. bacilliformis*, was recognized as the cause of Oroya fever. Many new species have been identified, some of which resulted from renaming and some from phylogenetic studies resulting in reclassification of *Grahamella* species to *Bartonella* in 1995 (Slater & Welch, 2005). The number of species known to cause disease in humans is increasing and includes *B. bacilliformis*, *B. henselae*, *B. quintana*, *B. elizabethae*, *B. clarridgeiae*, *B. vinsonii*, *B. grahamii*, *B. washoensis*, and *B. koehlerae* (Boulouis, Chang, Henn, Kasten, & Chomel, 2005). The major diseases caused are trench fever, Oroya fever, cat scratch fever, bacillary angiomatosis (BA), bacillary peliosis (BP), endocarditis, and bacteremia, depending on the species. *Bartonella* are aerobic, fastidious, gram-negative bacteria, some of which have flagella such as *B. bacilliformis* and *B. clarridgeiae*. Some *Bartonella* may be transmitted by a vector such as the body louse, which transmit *B. quintana* and result in trench fever (Boulouis et al., 2005; Slater & Welch, 2005; Walker, Maguiña, & Minnick, 2006), and ticks and cat fleas are considered as possible vectors (Chomel, Boulouis, Maruyama, & Breitschwerdt, 2006).

B. henselae has been identified as the major cause of cat scratch disease. Cat scratch disease is the most commonly recognized *Bartonella* infection. In the United States, it is estimated that 25,000 cases occur each year. The cat flea is believed to be involved in transmission. Typically, in about 90% of cases there is a history of a cat bite, scratch, or lick, and one risk factor is having a cat in the home, especially with children under 1 year of age. Typically, children between 2 and 14 years of age are affected. The disease is usually self-limiting in the immunocompetent, in whom it usually occurs, with one or more papules, vesicles, or pustules occurring 3 to 10 days after the bite or scratch. Lymphadenopathy then develops, commonly axillary, cervical, or inguinal. These can take several months to resolve. Sometimes low-grade fever and malaise may be seen. Antibiotic therapy does not usually alter the course of infection. Complicated or atypical cat scratch disease can include neurologic, ophthalmologic, and systemic manifestations and is more likely in persons who are immunosuppressed (Boulouis et al., 2005; Slater & Welch, 2005; Walker et al., 2006).

In 1983, Stoler, Bonfiglio, Steigbigel, and Pereira described atypical skin lesions that became known as bacillary angiomatosis (BA) in persons with acquired immunodeficiency syndrome (AIDS). Bacillary angiomatosis is a vascular, proliferative lesion that occurs most frequently subcutaneously as nodules, or more superficially as papules, warts, or hyperkeratotic plaques that are typically reddish purple with a diameter of about 1 cm. Histologically, lobular proliferation of blood vessels is seen, and the lesions may bleed easily. Lesions may occur in other sites such as the gastrointestinal tract, the larynx, and bones and may also occur in the immunocompetent (Slater & Welch, 2005). Bacillary peliosis (BP) is a vasculoproliferative lesion resulting in the development of cystic blood-filled spaces that occurs most frequently in the liver parenchyma, spleen, and sometimes lymph nodes, nearly always in persons with AIDS (Slater & Welch, 2005). Bacillary angiomatosis and BP can result from both *B. quintana* and *B. henselae*. Bacteremia and endocarditis may occur in both the immunocompetent and the immunocompromised, often from *B. quintana*, *B. elizabethae*, and *B. henselae* (Walker et al., 2006).

Emerging Viral Diseases

The greatest number of significant emerging infectious agents and diseases are viral. Many of these are hemorrhagic fevers whose agents have been recognized relatively recently and tend to be seen in certain geographic distributions in North America (such as hantavirus pulmonary syndrome), Asia (such as hemorrhagic fever with renal syndrome), Africa (such as Ebola fever), and South America (such as Bolivian hemorrhagic fever), often with high mortality rates (see chapters 11 and 8). The arbovirus causing dengue has extended its range. In addition, metapneumovirus, monkeypox, severe acute respiratory syndrome (SARS), West Nile virus (see chapters 18, 19, 22, and 23), Nipah virus (see below), human bocavirus (see Appendix A, Table A.4), and others were recognized. The most notorious new viral EID was HIV infection/AIDS, which has had a considerable clinical, social, and political impact (see chapter 13). Less exotic, but nevertheless a very important viral disease, is influenza or the flu (see chapter 14), in which new strains have evolved. Also, further newly identified viruses cause hepatitis and other liver diseases such as hepatitis C (see chapter 12) and the TT virus. Chikungunya virus has been known since the 1950s in Africa but has extended its range not only to Asia but to islands in the Indian Ocean and affects more than 260,000 persons (Parola et al., 2006). As of fall 2006, this mosquito-borne virus has infected more than 25% of the inhabitants of the Reunion Islands and has characteristics and severity previously undescribed (Bessaud et al., 2006). Specific emerging viral infections are discussed in individual chapters and in Appendix A, Table A.4. Two are considered briefly below.

Influenza itself is not a true emerging infectious disease; however, the virus strains causing influenza mutate frequently, resulting in lack of

resistance in human populations. Influenza has caused pandemics leading to the deaths of millions. Some flu strains have crossed species. For
example, in 1997, in Hong Kong, a child died of viral pneumonia and
multiorgan failure after an outbreak of H5N1 avian influenza occurred
in fowl such as ducks and chickens. It was the first time that an avian
influenza virus was isolated from a human with respiratory infection, and
this led to fears of a new pandemic (Shortridge et al., 2000).

Currently, there is concern worldwide about the possibility of a new
pandemic due to the avian influenza A strain H5N1. Despite the fact
that human-to-human transmission has not been effective, by February 6,
2007, 272 confirmed human cases and 166 reported deaths had been identified by the World Health Organization (2007). As well as for human
cases, surveillance is being maintained worldwide for cases in poultry,
migratory birds, waterfowl, and the like, and depending on infection,
various steps have been taken that include bans on imports, culling, restricting live markets and restrictions on movement of animals. Guidelines
for pharmacological management of sporadic avian influenza A (H5N1)
virus infection have been issued by WHO and would not apply to a pandemic situation (Schünemann et al., 2007). Other strains of influenza virus
such as H9N2 have been isolated from poultry. This strain has also been
isolated from pigs, other animals, and persons with influenza-like illness,
and it is also a candidate for causing a pandemic (Shortridge et al., 2000).
Because fowl are a reservoir for the influenza virus, the practice of raising
pigs and ducks together as is done in China, where crowding is also a
factor, allows viruses to recombine, with pigs as a vessel, and enables the
virus to potentially cross the species barrier to humans. Altered viral genes
can result not only in cross-species transfer but also in altered virulence
(Hatta, Gao, Halfmann, & Kawaoka, 2001). This is also an example of
how cultural practices and social conditions influence infectious disease
spread. Avian influenza is discussed in depth in chapter 14. Another example of close contact of various food animals and their microorganisms
with each other and with humans comes in the so-called "wet markets"
featuring a wide variety of exotic animals including civet cats and bats that
are sold as delicacies (Cheng, 2007; Chomel, Belotto, & Meslin, 2007;
Woo et al., 2006). These markets are popular in Asia, and also in urban
areas with large Asian populations such as San Francisco. Woo, Lau and
Yuen (2006) discuss the role of the Chinese wet markets in the emergence,
amplification, and dissemination of EIDs.

Both Nipah and Hendra viruses have been recently identified and are
in the Henipavirus family (Eaton, Broder, Middleton, & Wang, 2006).
Hendra virus was identified in Australia as follows. An outbreak of an
acute, lethal respiratory disease in Hendra, a suburb of Brisbane, occurred
in a group of thoroughbred horses in September 1994. A trainer and a
stable hand became ill, and the trainer died of respiratory disease (Selvey

et al., 1995). The next reported incident involved a sugarcane farmer in Mackay, near Hendra, who had assisted at autopsies of horses that had died of an acute illness in August 1994. He was subsequently diagnosed with a viral infection in 1995 that was then called equine morbillivirus (the earlier name for Hendra virus). The farmer died later of meningoencephalitis, which was believed to have been in a latent phase for a year before reactivating to result in his fatal illness. A search for a reservoir of the infection resulted in the isolation of the virus from fruit bats, known also as flying foxes, that was shown to be identical to the virus from the lung of one of the horses that had died. Presumably, in both cases the humans were infected by close contact with the horses that had been infected by the fruit bats (Mackenzie, 1999; Murray et al., 1998). Since that time, a few other human cases have been identified, most recently in 2004. Nipah virus, on the other hand, has caused larger, more serious outbreaks. It was first identified in humans in 1998 in Malaysia, where it caused mainly neurological illness including encephalitis, and was associated with infected pigs that acquired the disease from flying foxes (bats) carrying the organism. The most recent outbreaks have occurred in Bangladesh from 2001 to 2004, with a case fatality rate of approximately 75% and documented person-to-person transmission (Eaton et al., 2006; Eaton, Broder, & Wang, 2005). Both of these viruses have biosafety levels of 4, and Nipah virus is considered a potential agent for bioterrorism.

Emerging Fungal Diseases

In comparison with the other categories of microbes, fewer known emerging fungal diseases affect humans. Invasive fungi have increased in incidence. In many cases, they appear as opportunistic infections threatening patients who are immunosuppressed because of such conditions as HIV infection, malignancy, organ transplantation, prematurity, or even aging, and there is also a connection with medical interventions such as medical devices (Pfaller, Pappas, & Wingard, 2006). In immunocompromised persons, the opportunistic infection seen may depend on the infection endemic in the geographic area or on where the patient has traveled. *Penicillium marneffei*, for example, is most commonly seen in Southeast Asia, where it is a relatively frequent opportunistic infection in persons with HIV infection. It has also been seen in AIDS patients outside of this region (Vanittanakom, Cooper, Fisher, & Sirisanthana, 2006). Other endemic fungi such as *Coccidioides immitis* in the southwestern United States cause respiratory disease and are increasing in incidence in both the immunologically compromised and in those who have relocated to endemic areas, many of whom are elderly and have some degree of immunosuppression. Another problematic area is the recognition of some infections due to fungi originally thought to be nonpathogenic, and the finding that some species are becoming resistant to treatment with the standard antifungal agents (Kauffman, 2006; Pfaller, et al., 2006). Furthermore, there has been a change in etiology of these infections, with non-albicans *Candida* species and non-*fumigatus Aspergillus* species becoming more frequent as are other invasive moulds such as Zygomycetes (e.g., *Mucor* spp., *Rhizopus* spp.), *Fusarium* spp., and *Scedosporium* spp. and other yeasts such as *Trichosporon* spp. and *Cryptococcus gattii* (Kauffman, 2006; Nucci & Anaissie, 2005; Nucci & Marr, 2005).

C. *gattii* is an emerging yeast infection that was known to cause illness in immunocompetent people and was largely restricted to Australia, where it was believed to have an ecologic niche related to eucalyptus. It is also known to affect persons with AIDS in the United States, Australia, Southeast Asia, Africa, and more rarely in Europe. Since 1999, it has been recognized as the cause of an outbreak on Vancouver Island in Canada that affected more than 100 persons (Chaturvedi, Dyavaiah, Larsen, & Chaturvedi, 2005; Kidd et al., 2004; Nucci & Marr, 2005). Infections have been also identified on the British Columbia mainland and in the states of Washington and Oregon in persons who have not traveled elsewhere. Infection is through inhalation, and both pulmonary and central nervous system disease can occur. C. *gattii* has been isolated in vehicle wheel wells and on footwear, and dispersal may also occur during forestry activities. Dispersal of the organism might also occur through bird and animal migration but the environmental conditions responsible for this emergence are not yet known (Kidd et al., 2007; MacDougall et al., 2007; Nucci & Marr, 2005). *Fusarium* spp. are ubiquitous in soil and plants but are increasingly associated with systemic and localized infections in humans (Zhang et al., 2006). As of May 18, 2006, the CDC (2006g) identified 130 confirmed cases from 26 states of *Fusarium* keratitis. Most of the people affected were contact lens wearers, and infection was severe enough that about one third required corneal transplantation. An association was made between use of Bausch & Lomb's ReNu with MoistureLoc contact lens solution and the infection. The product was voluntarily removed from the market on May 15, 2006. Emerging fungal infections are considered in depth in Chapter 10 and are summarized in Appendix A, Table A.2.

Emerging Parasitic Diseases

Many of the emerging parasitic diseases were thought of as affecting relatively few people in developed countries. This view began to change when an increased prevalence of what were thought of as rare or exotic infections began to be seen more commonly in connection with the immunosuppression of HIV disease. This view also had to be quickly reevaluated when the outbreak of cryptosporidiosis, resulting from contamination of the municipal water supply, affecting over 400,000 persons occurred in Milwaukee, Wisconsin, in 1993. Many of the parasitic diseases are already known, but parasites that have emerged relatively recently are *Cyclospora cayetanensis* (see chapter 6), *Cryptosporidium hominis* and *Cryptosporidium parvum* (see chapter 5), *Babesia microti* (see chapter 16), and microsporidia. Most are protozoal parasites, but increased helminth infections are also being seen. Many are food- or waterborne (see Appendix B, Table B.1) and are discussed later in this chapter. Malaria, an important parasitic disease worldwide, is increasingly changing its geographic range and becoming resistant to the usual agents used in treatment (see chapter 17).

A familiar parasite, *Trichinella*, usually acquired through ingestion of undercooked pork, is now emerging as a result of infected horsemeat in countries in Europe where eating horsemeat is popular. Acquiring the parasite may also result from eating bear meat and other exotic meats as the demand for variety and the unusual expands (Pozio, 2000; Slifko, Smith, & Rose, 2000). Likewise, *Taenia solium*, the pork tapeworm, was recognized in the 1980s as causing neurocysticercosis or infection of the central nervous system. Recognition of neurocysticercosis as a major cause of neurologic disease including epilepsy resulted from improved diagnostic examinations such as computed axial tomography and magnetic resonance imaging scanning; from large numbers of immigrants to the United States from developing countries who were diagnosed with neurocysticercosis (for example, in Los Angeles, the diagnosis increased fourfold between 1977 and 1981); and from improved serological assays for diagnosis that allowed accurate prevalence estimates. In the United States, most cases appear in immigrants or in persons born in this country who have traveled to rural areas in endemic countries such as parts of Africa, Asia, and Latin America (Garcia, Wittner, Coyle, Tanowitz, & White, 2006). In the United States, there are more prevalent foci of infection in the New York City area, Texas, and parts of California near the Mexican border. However, it may be an unrecognized problem in other areas, especially those with a high concentration of Hispanic immigrants ("Cyticercosis" 2007; Townes, Hoffmann, & Kohn, 2004). Seizures are the presenting symptom in the majority of cases, but some learning disabilities in children have been found to be indicators of neurocysticercosis (Garcia et al., 2006). Locally acquired cases are known in the United States. In one well-known instance, orthodox Jews in one New York community, who would not have themselves been in contact with pork, acquired neurocysticercosis through eating food prepared by immigrant domestic workers who carried *Taenia* (Schantz et al., 1992).

While malaria is no longer considered endemic in the United States, it once was, and its range and resistance patterns are extending. Conditions are met in the United States for the potential transmission of malaria, including people who have malarial parasites in their blood and the presence of the appropriate vector. While cases of malaria have been diagnosed in the United States subsequent to travel to endemic regions (see chapter 17), outbreaks of mosquito-borne transmission in New York, New Jersey, California, Texas, and other areas in the United States have been described. These are usually due to *Plasmodium vivax*, but some are also due to the more severe *Plasmodium falciparum*. In 2004, the last year data were available, the CDC (Skarbinski et al., 2006) reported 8 cases of malaria that were acquired in the United States.

Microsporidia are a group of obligate intracellular parasites that have been considered as protozoa but that may be reclassified to fungi because of the results of molecular phylogenetic analysis (Weiss & Schwartz, 2006). The first human case of microsporidiosis was reported in 1959 in a 9-year-old child with neurological symptoms (Matsubayashi, Koike, Mikata, Takei, & Hagiwara, 1959). Various genera and species infect humans, and the *Encephalitozoon* particularly affect immunosuppressed populations (Walker et al., 2006). In 1985, there were reports of diarrhea in patients with AIDS due to *Enterocytozoon bieneusi*, thus beginning the recognition of their importance in persons with AIDS (Desportes et al., 1985). At present, the following genera are known to cause human infection: *Vittaforma, Nosema, Pleistophora, Encephalitozoon, Enterocytozoon, Trachipleistophora, Anncaliia* (formerly *Brachiola*), and *Microsporidium* (Didier & Weiss, 2006; Franzen, Nassonova, Scholmerich, & Issi, 2006; Mathis, Weber, & Deplazes, 2005; Weiss & Schwartz, 2006). While immunocompromised persons are most susceptible to microsporidiosis, those who are immunocompetent may also develop infection. The microsporidia can cause a wide range of infection including the digestive, reproductive, muscle, respiratory, excretory, and nervous systems as well as eye infections, sinusitis, and disseminated infections (Weiss & Schwartz, 2006). Person-to-person transmission through the fecal–oral and oral–oral pathways, inhalation of air droplets, ingestion of contaminated water or food, and, in the *Encephalitozoon* species, sexual transmission are all possible (Mathis et al., 2005; Walker et al., 2006). Transplacental transmission occurs among some nonhuman species (Didier & Weiss, 2006).The microsporidia and other emerging parasitic diseases are summarized in Appendix A, Table A.3.

Emerging Prion Diseases

In the past, there have been debates over the nature of prions, a type of protein particle that is devoid of nucleic acids. Prion proteins that are altered usually through conformational changes such as misfolding are considered to be the etiologic agents of a group of fatal neurodegenerative diseases known as the transmissible spongiform encephalopathies (TSEs), also called the prion diseases (Collinge, 2005). Animal diseases include bovine spongiform encephalopathy (BSE), scrapie, and others. In humans, TSEs include inherited (also called genetic or familial), sporadic, and acquired forms. The human TSEs that have attracted the most attention are Creutzfeldt–Jakob disease, especially that acquired through iatrogenic means such as growth hormone injections and corneal transplants; variant Creutzfeldt–Jakob disease (vCJD), a human form of BSE, commonly referred to as "mad cow" disease; and kuru, acquired through formerly practiced ritualistic cannibalism in the Fore tribe in Papua New Guinea. The current BSE epidemic in the United Kingdom emerged in the 1980s and has been reported in other countries as well. Linkage to vCJD was first noted in a 1996 report (Will et al., 1996). It was not until March 2006 that the European Union lifted the ban on British beef imports. North America has not been immune to BSE. In Canada, a BSE-infected cow was discovered in Alberta in May 2003, and two more were confirmed in 2005. The United States confirmed BSE in a dairy cow in Washington that had been imported from Canada, and in June 2005, BSE was confirmed in a cow in Texas born in the United States. In March 2006, another case was confirmed in a native-born cow in Alabama. All were born before the 1997 feed regulations were put in place. The trade repercussions varied in severity and time (Mathews, Vandeveer, & Gustafson, 2006). Prion diseases can be transmitted via stainless steel surgical instruments; because infective prions have shown resistance to the usual sterilization procedures, there are recommendations for sterilization (Belay & Schonberger, 2005). Continued concern about transmission from infected meats, meat products such as gelatin, or even products such as bone meal has led to various bans of imported products. Effects and reactions are political, social, and economic. Prion diseases are considered in depth in chapter 21.

SELECTED TRANSMISSION MODES OF EIDS

Vectorborne Diseases

Vectors usually are arthropods, especially insects, that are capable of transmitting microorganisms to vertebrate hosts. Arthropods are vectors for viral, bacterial, and parasitic agents. Arthropod-borne viral diseases called arboviruses are more common than bacterial or parasitic diseases spread in this way. More than 40% of viruses that infect mammals move from host to host by arthropod vectors (van den Heuvel, Hogenhout, & van der Wilk, 1999). Vectors such as mosquitoes can also be dispersed by air travel and by container ships, allowing the possible establishment of new foci, depending on whether other conditions such as climate are favorable (Tatem, Hay, & Rogers, 2006). There are about 100 known arboviruses that are pathogenic for humans—some of which are emerging or reemerging and others that do not fit this classification. Among bacteria, the group known as rickettsiae is often arthropod associated. Rickettsial diseases include many of the "spotted" and tick-bite fevers (Parola, Paddock, & Raoult, 2005). Examples of emerging vectorborne diseases are listed in Appendix B, Table B.3. Selected important vectorborne EIDs are further discussed in relation to recreational activities and travel in chapter 25 as well as in relation to specific diseases such as Lyme disease, ehrlichiosis, anaplasmosis, babesiosis, and malaria in chapters 16 and 17.

Primary vectors are the major species involved in transmission of a specific disease, while secondary vectors include species involved in transmission of a specific disease only under certain conditions (Goddard, 1999). Thus, not every mosquito can transmit *Plasmodium vivax*, one of the parasites causing malaria. Rather, *P. vivax* is mainly transmitted by the *Anopheles* mosquito, species of which are distributed throughout the United States. Arthropods may transmit microorganisms mechanically (e.g., when flies feed on excrement and then walk on food) or biologically (e.g., when the organism multiplies or develops in the arthropod, as in the multiplication of *Plasmodium* in mosquitoes transmitting malaria) (Ribeiro & Valenzuela, 2006). Mosquitoes are the major vector of infectious diseases in humans, followed by ticks (Parola & Raoult, 2001). Arthropods known to transmit microorganisms leading to disease are listed with a disease example:

- mosquitoes (*Culex pipiens*, West Nile virus, and West Nile fever),
- lice (the body louse, *Rickettsia prowazekii*, and epidemic typhus),
- ticks (the deer tick, *Borrelia burgdorferi*, and Lyme disease),
- mites (mouse mite, *Rickettsia akari*, and rickettsialpox),
- midges (biting midges, Oropouche virus, and Oropouche fever),
- fleas (the oriental rat flea, *Yersinia pestis*, and plague), and
- flies (tsetse fly, *Trypanosoma brucei gambiense*, and sleeping sickness or human African trypanosomiasis, Gambian type) (Guerrant, Walker, & Weller, 2006; Mandell, Bennett, & Dolin, 2005).

Of interest in understanding, managing, and ultimately preventing and controlling the vectorborne EIDs is knowledge about (a) the contributions of ecologic, meteorologic, and climactic conditions in influencing environmental, vector, and reservoir variables; (b) the biology of the vector and the host reservoir; and (c) the human characteristics that contribute to emergence including behavior and culture (see chapter 28). Vectorborne diseases are particularly affected by environmental factors, including climate and weather conditions such as temperature increase, rainfall amounts, and other factors such as carbon dioxide concentrations, urbanization, deforestation, irrigation, agricultural techniques, increased global trade, and travel (Sutherst, 2004). For example, the emergence of the Sin Nombre virus resulting in hantavirus pulmonary syndrome initially in the southwestern United States was said to occur following specific weather conditions that led to an increase in prevalence of the piñon nuts that fed deer mice carrying the hantavirus as well as promoting the growth of the vegetation providing shelter for them (Engelthaler et al., 1999). A concern with vectorborne diseases is the potential for an organism to adapt to a new vector and thus expand its geographic range. An example is the outbreak in eastern Arizona from 2002 to 2004 of Rocky Mountain spotted fever outside its usual range via the common dog tick, *Rhipicephalus sanguineus*, as a vector for the causative rickettsia, *Rickettsia rickettsii* (Demma et al., 2005). In another instance, the Lone Star ticks usually found in the Southeast have been increasing in number in New England. They are more aggressive and are known to be able to transmit such diseases as ehrlichiosis, Rocky Mountain spotted fever, and tularemia but are not yet known to transmit Lyme disease, which is endemic in the area ("Lone Star tick," 2006).

Foodborne and Waterborne Diseases

Overlap exists to some extent between foodborne and waterborne infectious diseases. Those organisms that are ingested and then cause illness (usually gastrointestinal) are usually transmissible through food, water, or both. In addition, food may be contaminated by water sources during activities such as planting, growing, harvesting, processing, preparation, and handling. The fecal–oral and person–person modes are the major routes of transmission of foodborne and waterborne EIDs. Causes of emerging foodborne illness include viruses, bacteria, parasites, altered prions, toxins that may or may not be of microbial origin, and other nonmicrobial substances. Each year approximately 76 million cases of foodborne illness and about 5,000 deaths occur in the United States (CDC, 2006d). In many countries, particularly developing ones, true global estimates are lacking for many reasons including the inability to link most outbreaks with a given food, lack of organization and funds to conduct surveillance, and other reasons (Flint et al., 2005). In the United States, the Foodborne Diseases Active Surveillance Network (FoodNet) of the CDC's Emerging

Infections Program collects data from 10 states across the country to compare infections due to specific bacterial and parasitic infections as does the Division of Foodborne Disease Outbreak Surveillance System of CDC. Not all are included in surveillance. In the most recent report of FoodNet for 2005, the highest number of cases in descending order of frequency were from *Salmonella*, *Campylobacter*, *Shigella*, *Cryptosporidium*, *Listeria*, *Vibrio*, and *Cyclospora* species as well as *E. coli* O157:H7.

Viruses are a frequent cause of gastroenteritis from food but are not easily monitored due to laboratory requirements. For example, norovirus is not routinely monitored in this surveillance, yet it is considered that noroviruses cause a large proportion of foodborne gastroenteritis in the United States, causing more than 23 million infections each year (Estes, Prasad, & Atmar, 2006). Noroviruses (formerly Norwalk viruses) were recognized in 1972 in connection with a gastroenteritis outbreak in Norwalk, Ohio, that occurred in 1968. In a recent outbreak due to norovirus infection at a fast-food restaurant in Michigan in 2005, gastroenteritis affecting over 100 people resulted from a food handler who returned to work within a few hours of his own gastrointestinal illness, which he had acquired from his child (CDC, 2006c). Rotavirus diarrhea, occurring primarily in children, was first identified in 1973 in Australia. In another instance, several hepatitis A virus outbreaks, including one in 2003 in Pennsylvania, were due to green onions imported from Mexico and served in a salsa (Wheeler et al., 2005). Raw fruits and vegetables are increasingly a source for foodborne disease. *Cryptosporidium*, usually thought of as a waterborne infection, can also be transmitted directly from food and was transmitted to 88 people in Washington, DC, through raw produce prepared by an infected food handler (Quiroz et al., 2000).

Several factors are thought to be responsible for the increase in the number and type of foodborne diseases. These include:

- demographic changes resulting in growing numbers of the population with immune compromise such as in chronic illness, HIV infection, aging, or posttransplant;
- breakdown in surveillance;
- demand for organic foods;
- demand for exotic food, in some cases resulting in smuggled trade of delicacies such as bushmeat that may be infected and in travel to eat exotic meats such as civet cats which are considered a delicacy but which have been implicated as a source of the 2003 SARS outbreak in southern China (Cheng, 2007);
- demand for more and out-of-season produce leading to importation from some developing countries where agricultural practices result in compromised food safety;

- increased consumption of internationally distributed foods, such as when a cholera outbreak in Maryland resulted from ingestion of coconut milk imported from Southeast Asia and an incident of staphylococcal food poisoning in the United States was associated with eating mushrooms canned in China;
- cultural food practices and habits such as eating undercooked pork leading to trichinosis in Laotians in the United States and eating raw or lightly cooked foods of animal origin such as shellfish, fish (as sushi or sashimi), or ground beef (as in steak tartare or served very rare);
- decrease in knowledge of food safety practices in the home such as washing hands thoroughly after handling raw poultry;
- reliance on convenience foods with a higher consumption of food not prepared in the home (this includes food from both eat-in restaurants and take-out facilities such as fast-food restaurants and supermarkets; it also includes partial preparation of foods such as melons sliced in the produce section of supermarkets, allowing contamination of the inner surface by microbes on the outer surface);
- greater prevalence of food served in a salad bar or buffet setting, allowing contamination or varying temperature controls; and
- economic development changes (e.g., shifting from a cold season oyster harvest to year round harvests in the Gulf of Mexico has been associated with the emergence of *Vibrio vulnificans* in oysters [Slutsker, Altekruse, & Swerdlow, 1998], which could be prevented if raw and undercooked oysters were not eaten).

Another contributing factor is rising temperatures of ocean water. In one instance, gastroenteritis occurred among passengers on a cruise ship. The source was raw oysters contaminated with *Vibrio parahaemolyticus*, a gram-negative bacterium that inhabits warm waters. In this instance, they were harvested from Alaskan waters, formerly thought to be too cold to support high enough levels of the organism to cause disease (McLaughlin et al., 2005). In 2006, a large outbreak occurred connected to eating raw or undercooked oysters from Washington ("*Vibrio parahaemolyticus*, Shellfish," 2006).

Contamination of foods can occur at multiple points from planting, growing, harvesting, and initial processing through transporting, distributing, later processing, preparing, and serving. Contamination can arise from contaminated irrigation water; use of manure or human fertilizer; poor sanitary practices in the fields, in handling areas, and during preparation, and serving; contaminated wash water; use of unclean vehicles for transportation and/or distribution; and cross contamination. In a graphic illustration, observers have described Guatemalan raspberries in open containers waiting for shipment being contaminated by bird droppings until they were coated in white. The first identified outbreaks of *C. cayetanensis* in the United States resulted from eating contaminated Guatemalan raspberries (see chapter 6). Outbreaks arise from newly recognized pathogens and also from known pathogens contaminating foods not previously known to support their growth such as lettuce, green onions, spinach, and apple cider (*E. coli* O157:H7).

Because of changes in food distribution, outbreaks may now be widespread and harder to recognize. For example, an outbreak of *Salmonella* serotype Enteritidis infection was noticed because of an increase of gastroenteritis in southern Minnesota. An ice cream premix that was pasteurized at a plant on-site had to be transported to another plant to be made into a nationally distributed brand of ice cream. The tanker trucks had previously been used to haul raw eggs. Postpasteurization contamination of the premix resulted in about 250,000 illnesses from eating the ice cream prepared from the premix that became contaminated during transport (Hennessy et al., 1996). *Salmonella* serotype Enteritidis is decreasing after being the most commonly implicated *Salmonella* serotype contaminating eggs, many of which were contaminated by the transovarian route. The decrease is attributed to programs to prevent the organism from infecting flocks, early refrigeration of eggs, and education about the risk of eating raw or undercooked eggs (Braden, 2006). In 2006, two outbreaks involving 29 persons of *Salmonella enterica* serotype Enteritidis were traced to certain frozen stuffed chicken entrees that were prepared in the microwave. It is believed that the microwave cooking may have resulted in not evenly heating the entrees to the required temperature for full cooking ("Salmonellosis, frozen chicken," 2006).

The consumption of fish, often raw or undercooked, has increased due to several factors: improvements in transport of fish, greater accessibility, awareness of health benefits, cultural influences, and increased per capita income. Sushi bars serving raw fish have multiplied. A new disease, metorchiasis, is caused by the North American liver fluke, *Metorchis conjunctus*, a helminth that is considered to have emerged in 1993. In Montreal, Canada, 27 persons became ill after eating sashimi (raw fish) infected with this organism at a picnic. The long-term oncogenic potential of this infection is unknown (MacLean, 1998). Another popular way of eating fish raw, as ceviche, prepared with lemon or lime juice to "cook" it, has resulted in foodborne infection. Gnathostomosis (gnathostomiasis), caused by a nematode, is another parasitic disease contracted from undercooked fish (Rojas-Molina, Pedraza-Sanchez, Torres-Bibiano, Meza-Martinez, & Escobar-Gutierrez, 1999). Other foodborne trematodes such as liver, intestinal, and lung flukes are considered emerging, in part because of the expansion of aquaculture and greater ease in bringing freshwater fish and crustaceans to both local and international markets (Keiser & Utzinger, 2005). For example, in California, a small number of cases of *Paragonimus* (a lung fluke) infection occurred in California after eating raw or undercooked freshwater imported crab ("Paragonimus," 2006). In China, an outbreak beginning in August 2006 involved imported partly cooked Amazonian black snails, which are considered a delicacy. This resulted in more than 130 cases of *Angiostrongylus* meningitis (*"Angiostrongylus* meningitis," 2006).

Foodborne illnesses have a public health impact beyond the discomfort of acute gastroenteritis. Many can cause disability and chronic sequelae, particularly in those who are immunologically compromised to some degree such as the elderly, children, transplant recipients, and persons with HIV infection. An example is Guillain–Barré syndrome and reactive arthritis secondary to *Campylobacter* infection (Leirisalo-Repo, 2005; Tam et al., 2006). Foodborne illness is often underreported, particularly when milder or nonspecific in nature. Some foodborne pathogens are also spread through water or from person to person, and some of these pathogens are probably not yet identified.

Among well-publicized outbreaks of food-related emerging infections have been those of *E. coli* O157:H7 through contaminated ground beef, unpasteurized apple cider, spinach, lettuce, and alfalfa sprouts (see chapter 9); *Cyclospora* contamination of Guatemalan raspberries, mesclun lettuce, fresh snow peas, and fresh basil leaves (see chapter 6); vCJD and contaminated beef (see chapter 21); *Listeria monocytogenes* and hot dogs, soft cheeses, and deli meats (Gottlieb et al., 2006); and strains of *Salmonella enterica* serotype Newport contaminating alfalfa sprouts (CDC, 2001a). Increasingly, fresh produce such as lettuce has been a vehicle for more foodborne illnesses than previously known, such as outbreaks of *Yersinia pseudotuberculosis* linked to fresh lettuce. Research is revealing more about methods of contamination. For example, in the case of *E. coli* O157:H7, lettuce plants irrigated with contaminated water can take up the organism, ultimately resulting in distribution throughout the leaves of the plant. Warm tomatoes that are put into cold water can take up *Salmonella*. Thus, protection must be tailored to these sources of infection because consumer washing of the produce in these cases would not be protective (Tauxe, 2004).

L. monocytogenes is an anaerobic nonsporulating gram-positive bacterium capable of causing various illness in both humans and animals. In the past, it has been mostly associated with disease in those who are immunocompromised, including the elderly and pregnant women, their fetuses, and newborns (Gottlieb et al., 2006; B. Lorber, 2005). Transmission is foodborne or occurs vertically from the infected mother to child transplacentally or at birth, although less commonly there can be cross-infection in nurseries (B. Lorber, 2005). Epidemic illnesses have been largely linked to refrigerated ready-to-eat foods such as coleslaw, hot dogs, deli meats, milk, soft low-acid cheeses such as Brie and feta, pâté, and, in one instance, to contaminated corn in a salad (Aureli et al., 2000; CDC, 2001a). In a recent outbreak, in 2002, turkey deli meat was the source of infection, and the investigation led to new regulations for control (Gottlieb et al., 2006). The usual clinical picture includes diarrhea, nausea, vomiting, and fever, which commonly progresses or presents as bacteremia or meningitis. The case fatality rate is high, being about 25%. Pregnant women are particularly vulnerable, with manifestations of an acute febrile illness often with headache, backache, and myalgias along with bacteremia. There is a high risk of spontaneous abortion, stillbirth, or neonatal death, and among women with listeriosis in pregnancy, about two thirds of surviving newborns develop neonatal listeriosis (B. Lorber, 2005).

Waterborne emerging infections may result from ingestion of contaminated drinking water or from contact with contaminated recreational water. Such infections may originate in the community in which the person resides or may occur in the course of recreational pursuits in developed areas, during travel to foreign locales, or in wilderness areas (see chapter 25 for a discussion of EIDs in relation to travel and recreation). Conditions such as flooding may provide temporary favorable conditions for outbreaks of emerging infectious diseases through a variety of mechanisms including runoff from contaminated fields. Contaminated water may contaminate food such as in grocery store spray systems, or contamination may result from direct exposure to organisms in these sprays such as *Legionella pneumophila*. Waterborne infections can also occur from showering. In an outbreak of legionellosis in a children's hospital, showering was implicated as the means of exposure to contaminated potable water (Campins et al., 2000). Hospital water supplies and water used for therapeutic purposes can unwittingly become the source for emerging infections such as *Legionella* and atypical mycobacteria (Emmerson, 2001). *L. pneumophila* infections can be acquired through exposure to sprays from whirlpools, hot tubs, spas, and the like and have even been associated with visiting an aquarium (Greig et al., 2004). *Legionella* is discussed in depth in chapter 15. Noroviruses have increasingly been associated with drinking water outbreaks, often causing gastroenteritis. They are often difficult to recognize because of the difficulty in growing them prior to newer technology that uses genome-based methods, because an outbreak may not be recognized, and because the number of organisms may be low. Noroviruses have been implicated in both waterborne and foodborne outbreaks on cruise ships, hospitals, nursing homes, and other closed environments. Infection is widespread and common. In developed countries, more than 50% show antibodies to norovirus. Incubation periods are typically 24 to 48 hours and result in gastroenteritis. There is a high secondary attack rate. Typically, resolution occurs spontaneously, but sometimes there are recurrent outbreaks; for example, in one instance 12 recurrent outbreaks were reported despite attempts to determine the source and to disinfect the ship between sailings (Maunula, Miettinen, & von Bonsdorff, 2005; Treanor & Dolin, 2005).

The CDC defines recreational water settings as swimming pools, wading pools, whirlpools, hot tubs, spas, water parks, interactive fountains, and fresh and marine surface waters such as lakes, beaches, and springs (CDC, 2006f). The most frequent illnesses resulting from recreational waterborne infections are gastrointestinal illness, dermatitis, respiratory, and meningoencephalitis, the latter resulting from infection by free-living amoeba such as *Naegleria fowleri* when warm fresh water or heated swimming pool water is forced up the nose of a person engaging in water activities including swimming or diving, usually during the summer when conditions are favorable for such infection (CDC, 2004, 2006f; Visvesvara & Maguire, 2006). In an outbreak in 2003, multiple members of a college football team developed MRSA after using a spa treated with an unapproved disinfectant (CDC, 2006f). In one outbreak in Maine, involving a toddler wading pool in July 2002, 9 persons were affected. The cause was *E. coli* O157:H7. Tap water was used to fill the pool, and it is believed that high density and a fecal accident were contributing factors (CDC, 2004).

Drinking water systems may be community or noncommunity systems. The latter may be transient or nontransient. Millions of people per year use noncommunity water systems while traveling or working, usually without being aware of this. For example, transient noncommunity systems include highway rest stations, restaurants, and parks with their own water systems. Treatment, standards, and regulations vary according to the type of system (CDC, 2006e). Contamination of drinking water may occur through surface or groundwater source contamination, breaks in the integrity of well and/or distribution systems, and breaks in disinfection or water treatment. Waterborne disease outbreaks associated with both drinking water and recreational water are discussed below.

During 2003 and 2004, the most recent data available, 19 states reported 36 outbreaks of waterborne infection associated with drinking water, 30 of which were associated with water intended for drinking, causing illness in about 2,760 persons. Of the outbreaks where a cause was identified, 17 or 68.0% were of known infectious etiology: 76.5% were bacterial including 61.5% that were caused by *Legionella* spp., and others such as *Campylobacter* spp. and *E. coli* O157:H7; 11.8% were mixed etiology, 5.9% were caused by a parasite, and 5.9% were caused by norovirus. Included in mixed etiology were *Helicobacter* spp., *Campylobacter* spp., *Cryptosporidium* spp., *Entamoeba* spp., and *Giardia* spp. (CDC, 2006e). In 1997, in one of the cryptosporidiosis outbreaks in Texas, about 1,400 persons became ill after a lightening storm caused a spill of raw sewage that resulted in contamination of municipal utility district wells, illustrating how weather conditions can play a role, even indirectly, in the emergence of infectious diseases (CDC, 2000). Earlier, *Cryptosporidium* was responsible for the largest known outbreak of emerging infectious disease, an occurrence of contamination of drinking water in the United States, when about 403,000 persons became ill in Milwaukee, Wisconsin, in 1993 (MacKenzie et al., 1994; see chapter 5).

Regarding recreational waterborne outbreaks during the same period, 26 states reported 62 outbreaks associated with recreational water (about 30% were fresh water and about 70% were treated water), causing illness in about 2,698 persons. About two-thirds were infectious in origin. The etiology was 32.3% bacterial, 29.0% unidentified, 24.2% parasitic, 9.7% viral, and 4.8% due to a chemical or toxin. Clinically, the most frequent outcomes seen were gastroenteritis, followed by dermatitis, meningoencephalitis, and acute respiratory illness. The most frequent bacterial pathogens were *Pseudomonas aeruginosa* (usually causing dermatitis), *Legionella* spp., *Plesiomonas shigelloides*, MRSA, *Shigella sonnei*, *Leptospira* spp., and others. The most frequent parasite was *Cryptosporidium*, followed by *Giardia intestinalis*, and *Naegleria fowleri*. Norovirus was identified in most of the outbreaks due to viral etiology, and there was one outbreak in which echovirus 9 was responsible for causing meningitis (CDC, 2006f). Prevention of food and waterborne infections is discussed in Appendix C, Tables C.1, C.2, and C.3.

Transfusion- and Transplant-Transmitted Emerging and Reemerging Infections

With the knowledge that HIV infection could be acquired via transfusion of blood or blood products came extensive political pressure to ensure the absolute safety of the transfusion of blood and blood products, especially in the United States. The ability to transmit infection by transfusion depends on a variety of elements including the pathogenicity of the agent, its prevalence in the blood donor population, the ability to persist in a host and if so in which cell type, recipient immunity, whether an asymptomatic phase is present, and if the infectious agent can persist in stored blood.

Changes in approaches to blood donation and screening have resulted in minimal risk for transfusion-transmitted diseases in the United States but not in zero risk. Elsewhere, the picture is different. The majority of countries do not have policies in place that would ensure safe blood donations, and many of these countries have a heavy burden of emerging infectious agents (Dodd & Leiby, 2004; Klein, 2000).

At times, pockets of specific risk occur that need to be immediately addressed such as the 1997 deferral of blood donations of members of the National Guard who had been exposed to ticks during a training exercise. Several later developed ehrlichiosis or Rocky Mountain spotted fever (Klein, 2000; McQuiston, Childs, Chamberland, & Tabor, for the Working Group on Transfusion Transmission of Tick-borne Diseases, 2000). Other examples of specific deferrals in response to potential emerging or reemerging infectious-disease risk include the decision in the United States to restrict donations as described in chapter 21 for those at risk for acquisition of the agent (altered prions) responsible for bovine spongiform encephalopathy and vCJD, including deferral for relatives of persons with Creutzfeldt–Jakob disease, and deferral of Desert Storm veterans because of exposure to *Leishmania donovani*, the parasitic agent of leishmaniasis (Klein, 2000). In light of the wider than realized spread of vCJD, most notably in Britain and western Europe, more stringent blood donation restrictions have been put in place to exclude persons who may have become infected with vCJD but who are not symptomatic. Donors of other tissues might also be considered for exclusion (Roos, 2001).

The HIV epidemic focused attention on transfusion and transplant safety issues in regard to emerging infections. Even in the last 20 years, a variety of viral agents with the potential to be transmitted via blood transfusion have emerged. In addition to HIV-1 and -2, they include human T-cell lymphotropic virus 1 (HTLV-1); HTLV-2; hepatitis C; Kaposi's sarcoma-associated virus, or human herpesvirus 8; the hepatitis G virus, or GB virus C; human herpesvirus 6; the putative hepatitis-linked TT virus, and West Nile virus (Alter, 2005; Dodd & Leiby, 2004). The potential for other nonemerging agents to be transmitted in this way also occurs. These agents include cytomegalovirus, dengue virus, *Trypanosoma cruzi*, *Plasmodium* spp., Epstein–Barr virus, and others, some of which pose particular risk to subsets of recipients such as those who are immunosuppressed. It is also believed that the SARS coronavirus may be transmissible in this way (Dodd & Leiby, 2004). Other microorganisms such as *B. microti*, and the prions responsible for variant Creutzfeldt-Jakob disease are transfusion transmissible (Alter, Stramer, & Dodd, 2007; Dietz et al., 2007; Leiby, 2006). Some agents pose a greater risk in areas with a high density of persons who have emigrated from countries where these agents are prevalent. They may also pose a risk to travelers needing a blood transfusion in countries where screening of the blood supply does not occur and where there are high concentrations of persons who have been infected (some chronically) with infectious agents such as those that cause malaria, HIV infection, hepatitis, dengue, trypanosomiasis, and others. For example, in Latin America, Chagas disease, caused by *T. cruzi*, is endemic. In the United States, persons who acquired the disease in childhood and who have immigrated to this country may be chronically infected, even if they are currently asymptomatic. Thus, the frequency of the organism in human blood varies across the population, being higher in areas of high concentration of immigrants from endemic countries. It has been suggested that prospective Latin American donors in the United States should be screened for *T. cruzi*, but this is a very sensitive area (Kirchhoff et al., 2006). Chagas disease has also been transmitted by transplantation (CDC, 2006a). In the United States in 2003 and 2004, one case and no cases, respectively, of transfusion-transmitted malaria in the United States were reported (Eliades et al., 2005; Skarbinski et al., 2006). Appendix B, Table B.3, provides information on transfusion-transmitted emerging/reemerging infectious diseases.

The current system used in the United States to ensure blood safety includes sensitive screening tests; education and stringent screening, questionnaires, selection, and deferral procedures for donors; postdonation product quarantine; a safety surveillance system; and donor tracing and notification when needed. Newer methods of testing donated blood such as nucleic acid testing increase blood safety (Chamberland, Alter, Busch, Nemo, & Ricketts, 2001). Xenotransplantation, the use of tissues and organs for animal to human transplantation, poses a potential risk of the transfer of zoonoses from the animal donor not only to the human recipient but also to persons who come into professional or personal contact with him or her. Of particular concern are viruses, especially those that can cross species barriers. The porcine endogenous retroviruses have been noted as particularly worrisome since pigs are thought to be a major potential future source of tissues and organs for transplant for infants and children (Cox & Zhong, 2005). These issues are discussed in the U.S. Public Health Service guideline on infectious disease issues in xenotransplantation (CDC, 2001b). Human-to-human transplantation has been a method of spread for CJD (see chapter 21), and rabies has also been transmitted by transplantation (Srinivasan et al., 2005). Parvovirus B19 has been transmitted by transplantation of both solid organs and stem cells. Since it is not screened for, the incidence is probably underestimated. It can manifest as refractory anemia posttransplant (Eid, Brown, Patel, & Razonable, 2006). There has been a reported case of lymphocytic choriomeningitis virus, causing meningitis, being transmitted by organ transplantation (Foster et al., 2006).

CONCLUSION

Emerging infectious diseases may belong to any of the classifications of infectious agents and are transmitted to humans by a variety of mechanisms. The reasons for their emergence may be complex and are delineated in chapter 1. Often, several factors converge so that conditions become favorable for an organism to emerge. The best ways to protect against the major consequences of such outbreaks is by having a good public health infrastructure with appropriate surveillance mechanisms and response plans and by educating health care practitioners to be alert when encountering a patient with unusual symptoms. The chapters in part II highlight specific emerging infectious diseases that have affected or have the potential to impact health care significantly.

REFERENCES

Alter, H. J. (2005). Hepatitis G virus and TT virus. In G. L. Mandell, J. E. Bennett, & R. Dolin (Eds), *Mandell, Douglas, and Bennett's principles and practice of infectious diseases* (6th ed., pp. 1981–1989). Philadelphia: Churchill Livingstone Elsevier.

Alter, H. J., Stramer, S. L., & Dodd, R. Y. (2007). Emerging infectious diseases that threaten the blood supply. *Seminars in Hematology, 44*, 32–41.

Angiostrongylus meningitis—China (02). (2006, August 22). *ProMED Digest, 376*, unpaginated.

Aureli, P., Fiorucci, G. C., Caroli, D., Marchiaro, G., Novara, O., Leone, L., et al. (2000). An outbreak of febrile gastroenteritis associated with corn contaminated by *Listeria monocytogenes*. *New England Journal of Medicine, 342*, 1236–1241.

Bahrain, M., Vasiliades, M., Wolff, M., & Younus, F. (2006). Five cases of bacterial endocarditis after furunculosis and the ongoing saga of community-acquired methicillin-resistant *Staphylococcus aureus* infections. *Scandinavian Journal of Infectious Diseases, 38*, 702–707.

Belay, E. D., & Schonberger, L. B. (2005). The public health impact of prion diseases. *Annual Review of Public Health, 26*, 191–212.

Bessaud, M., Peyrefitte, C. N., Pastorino, B. A. M., Tock, F., Merle, O., Colpart, J.-J., et al. (2006). Chikungunya virus strains, Reunion Island outbreak. *Emerging Infectious Diseases, 12*, 1604–1606.

Boulouis, H.-J., Chang, C.-C., Henn, J. B., Kasten, R. W., & Chomel, B. B. (2005). Factors associated with the rapid emergence of zoonotic *Bartonella* infections. *Veterinary Research, 36*, 383–410.

Braden, C. R. (2006). *Salmonella enterica* serotype Enteritidis and eggs: A national epidemic in the United States. *Clinical Infectious Diseases, 43,* 512–517.

Brazier, J. S., Gal, M., Hall, V., & Morris, T. E. (2004). Outbreak of *Clostridium histolyticum* infections in injecting drug users in England and Scotland. *European Surveillance, 9*(9), 15–16.

Campins, M., Ferrer, A., Callis, L., Pelaz, C., Cortes, P. J., Pinart, N., et al. (2000). Nosocomial Legionnaires' disease in a children's hospital. *Pediatric Infectious Disease Journal, 19,* 228–234.

Centers for Disease Control and Prevention. (2000). Probable locally acquired mosquito-transmitted *Plasmodium vivax* infection—Suffolk county, New York, 1999. *Morbidity and Mortality Weekly Report, 49,* 495–498.

Centers for Disease Control and Prevention. (2001a). Diagnosis and management of foodborne illnesses: A primer for physicians. *Morbidity and Mortality Weekly Report, 50*(RR-02), 1–69.

Centers for Disease Control and Prevention. (2001b). U.S. Public Health Service guideline on infectious disease issues in xenotransplantation. *Morbidity and Mortality Weekly Report, 50*(RR-15), 1–50.

Centers for Disease Control and Prevention. (2002). *Staphylococcus aureus* resistant to vancomycin—United States, 2002. *Morbidity and Mortality Weekly Report, 51,* 566–567.

Centers for Disease Control and Prevention. (2004). Surveillance for waterborne-disease outbreaks associated with recreational water—United States, 2001–2002. *Morbidity and Mortality Weekly Report, 53*(SS-8), 1–22.

Centers for Disease Control and Prevention. (2005). Severe *Clostridium difficile*-associated disease in populations previously at low risk—Four states, 2005. *Morbidity and Mortality Weekly Report, 54,* 1201–1205.

Centers for Disease Control and Prevention. (2006a). Chagas disease after organ transplantation—Los Angeles, California, 2006. *Morbidity & Mortality Weekly Report, 55,* 798–800.

Centers for Disease Control and Prevention. (2006b). Methicillin-resistant *Staphylococcus aureus* skin infections among tattoo recipients—Ohio, Kentucky, and Vermont, 2004–2006. *Morbidity and Mortality Weekly Report, 55,* 677–679.

Centers for Disease Control and Prevention. (2006c). Multisite outbreak of norovirus associated with a franchise restaurant—Kent County, Michigan, May, 2005. *Morbidity and Mortality Weekly Report, 55,* 395–397.

Centers for Disease Control and Prevention. (2006d). Surveillance for foodborne-disease outbreaks—United States, 1998-2002. *Morbidity and Mortality Weekly Report, 55*(SS-10), 1–42.

Centers for Disease Control and Prevention. (2006e). Surveillance for waterborne-disease outbreaks associated with drinking water—United States, 2001–2002. *Morbidity and Mortality Weekly Report, 55*(SS-12), 31–66.

Centers for Disease Control and Prevention. (2006f). Surveillance for waterborne-disease outbreaks associated with recreational water—United States, 2001–2002. *Morbidity and Mortality Weekly Report, 55*(SS-12), 1–30.

Centers for Disease Control and Prevention. (2006g). Update: *Fusarium* keratitis—United States, 2005–2006. *Morbidity and Mortality Weekly Report, 55,* 563–564.

Didier, E. S., & Weiss, L. M. (2006). Microsporidiosis: Current status. *Current Opinion in Infectious Diseases, 19,* 485–492.

Chamberland, M. E., Alter, H. J., Busch, M. P., Nemo, G., & Ricketts, M. (2001). Emerging infectious disease issues in blood safety. *Emerging Infectious Diseases, 7*(3, Suppl.), 552–553.

Chaturvedi, S., Dyavaiah, M., Larsen, R. A., & Chaturvedi, V. (2005). *Cryptococcus gattii* in AIDS patients, southern California. *Emerging Infectious Diseases, 11,* 1686–1692.

Cheng, M. H. (2007). SARS source back on the menu. *Lancet Infectious Diseases, 7,* 14.

Chertow, D. S., Tan, E. T., Maslanka, S. E., Schulte, J., Bresnitz, E. A., Weisman, R. S. et al. (2006). Botulism in 4 adults following cosmetic injections with an unlicensed, highly concentrated botulinum preparation. *Journal of the American Medical Association, 296,* 2476–2479.

Chomel, B. B., Belotto, A., & Meslin, F.-X. (2007). Wildlife, exotic pets, and emerging zoonoses. *Emerging Infectious Diseases, 13,* 6–11.

Chomel, B. B., Boulouis, H.-J., Maruyama, S., & Breitschwerdt, E. B. (2006). *Bartonella* spp. in pets and effect on human health. *Emerging Infectious Diseases, 12,* 389–394.

Chuang, Y. Y., Huang, Y. C., & Lin, T. Y. (2005). Toxic shock syndrome in children: Epidemiology, pathogenesis, and management. *Paediatric Drugs, 7,* 11–25.

Collinge, J. (2005). Molecular neurology of prion disease. *Journal of Neurology, Neurosurgery and Psychiatry, 76,* 906–919.

Cox, A., & Zhong, R. (2005). Current advances in xenotransplantation. *Hepatobiliary Pancreatic Disease International, 4,* 490–494.

Crowcroft, N. S., & Peabody, R. G. (2006). Recent developments in pertussis. *Lancet, 367,* 1926–1936.

Cysticercosis—US. (2007, February12). *ProMed Digest, 2007* (077), unpaginated.

Demma, L. J., Traeger, M. S., Nicholson, W. L., Paddock, C. D., Blau, D. M., Eremeeva, M. E., et al. (2005). Rocky Mountain spotted fever from an unexpected tick vector in Arizona. *New England Journal of Medicine, 353,* 551–553.

Desportes, I., Le Charpentier, Y., Galian, A., Bernard, F., Cochand-Priollet, B., Lavergne, A. et al. (1985). Occurrence of a new microsporidan: *Enterocytozoon bieneusi* n.g., n. sp., in the enterocytes of a human patient with AIDS. *Journal of Protozoology, 32,* 250–254.

Didier, E. S., & Weiss, L. M. (2006). Microsporidiosis: Current status. *Current Opinion in Infectious Diseases, 19,* 485–492.

Dietz, K., Raddatz, G., Wallis, J., Müller, N., Zerr, I., Duerr, H.-P., et al. (2007). Blood transfusion and spread of variant Creutzfeldt-Jakob disease. *Emerging Infectious Diseases, 13,* 89–95.

Dodd, R. Y., & Leiby, D. A. (2004). Emerging infectious threats to the blood supply. *Annual Review of Medicine, 55,* 191–207.

Eaton, B. T., Broder, C. C., Middleton, D., & Wang, L. F. (2006). Hendra and Nipah viruses: Different and dangerous. *Nature Reviews Microbiology, 4*, 23–35.

Eaton, B. T., Broder, C. C., & Wang, L. F. (2005). Hendra and Nipah viruses: Pathogenesis and therapeutics. *Current Molecular Medicine, 5*, 805–816.

Eid, A. J., Brown, R. A., Patel, R., & Razonable, R. R. (2006). Parvovirus B19 after transplantation: A review of 98 cases. *Clinical Infectious Diseases, 43*, 40–48.

Eliades, M. J., Shah, S., Nguyen-Dinh, P., Newman, R. D., Barber, A. M., Nguyen-Dinh, P., et al. (2005). Malaria surveillance—United States, 2003. *Morbidity and Mortality Weekly Report, 54*(SS-02), 25–40.

Emmerson, A. M. (2001). Emerging waterborne infections in health-care settings. *Emerging Infectious Diseases, 7*, 272–276.

Engelthaler, D. M., Mosley, D. G., Cheek, J. E., Levy, C. E., Komatsu, K. K., Ettestad, P., et al. (1999). Climatic and environmental patterns associated with hantavirus pulmonary syndrome, Four Corners region, United States. *Emerging Infectious Diseases, 5*, 87–94.

Estes, M. K., Prasad, B. V. V., & Atmar, R. L. (2006). Noroviruses everywhere: Has something changed? *Current Opinion in Infectious Diseases, 19*, 467–474.

Flint, J. A., Van Duynhoven, Y. T., Angulo, F. J., DeLong, S. M., Braun, P., Kirk, M., et al. (2005). Estimating the burden of acute gastroenteritis, foodborne disease, and pathogens commonly transmitted by food: An international review. *Clinical Infectious Diseases, 41*, 698–704.

Fordtran, J. S. (2006). Colitis due to *Clostridium difficile* toxins: Underdiagnosed, highly virulent, and nosocomial. *Proceedings (Baylor University Medical Center), 19*(1), 3–12.

Foster, E. S., Signs, K. A., Marks, D. R., Kapoor, H., Casey, M., Stobierskim M. G., et al. (2006). Lymphocytic choriomeningitis in Michigan. *Emerging Infectious Diseases, 12*, 851–853.

Franzen, C., Nassonova, E. S., Scholmerich, J., & Issi, I. V. (2006). Transfer of the members of the genus *Brachiola* (microsporidia) to the genus *Anncaliia* based on ultrastructural and molecular data. *Journal of Eukaryotic Microbiology, 53*, 26–35.

Fridkin, S. K., Hageman, J. C., Morrison, M., Sanza, L. T., Como-Sabetti, K., Jernigan, J. A., et al. (2005). Methicillin-resistant *Staphylococcus aureus* disease in three communities. *New England Journal of Medicine, 352*, 1436–1444.

Gao, F., Bailes, E., Robertson, D. L., Chen, Y., Rodenburg, C. M., Michael, S. F., Cummins, L. B., et al. (1999). Origin of HIV-1 in the chimpanzee *Pan troglodytes* troglodytes. *Nature, 397*, 436–441.

Garcia, H. H., Wittner, M., Coyle, C. M., Tanowitz, H. B., & White, A. C., Jr. (2006). Cysticercosis. In R. L. Guerrant, D. H. Walker, & P. F. Weller (Eds.), *Tropical infectious diseases* (2nd ed., pp. 1289–1303). Philadelphia: Churchill Livingstone Elsevier.

Goddard, J. (1999). Arthropods, tongue worms, leeches, and arthropod-borne diseases. In R. L. Guerrant, D. H. Walker, & P. F. Weller (Eds.), *Tropical infectious diseases: Principles, pathogens, & practice* (pp. 1325–1342). Philadelphia: Churchill Livingstone.

Gottlieb, S. L., Newbern, E. C., Griffin, P. M., Graves, L. M., Hoekstra, R. M., Baker, N. L., et al. (2006). Multistate outbreak of listeriosis linked to turkey deli meat and subsequent changes in US regulatory policy. *Clinical Infectious Diseases, 42,* 29–36.

Greig, J. E., Carnie, J. A., Tallis, G. F., Ryan, N. J., Tan, A. G., Gordon, I. R., et al. (2004). An outbreak of Legionnaires' disease at the Melbourne Aquarium, April, 2000: Investigation and case-control studies. *Medical Journal of Australia, 180,* 566–572.

Grundmann, H., Aires-de-Sousa, M., Boyce, J., & Tiemersma, E. (2006). Emergence and resurgence of methicillin-resistant *Staphylococcus aureus* as a public-health threat. *Lancet, 368,* 874–885.

Guerrant, R. L., Walker, D. H., & Weller, P. F. (Eds.). (2006). *Tropical infectious diseases* (2nd ed.). Philadelphia: Churchill Livingstone Elsevier.

Hahn, B., Shaw, G., De Cock, K., & Sharp, P. (2000). AIDS as a zoonosis: Scientific and public health implications. *Science, 287,* 607–614.

Hajjeh, R. A., Reingold, A., Weil, A., Shutt, K., Schuchat, A., & Perkins, B. A. (1999). Toxic shock syndrome in the United States: Surveillance update, 1979–1996. *Emerging Infectious Diseases, 5,* 807–810.

Halperin, S. A. (2007). The control of pertussis—2007 and beyond. *New England Journal of Medicine, 356,* 110–113.

Hasham, S., Matteucci, P., Stanley, P. R. W., & Hart, N. B. (2005). Necrotising fasciitis. *BMJ, 330,* 830–833.

Hatta, M., Gao, P., Halfmann, P., & Kawaoka, Y. (2001). Molecular basis for high virulence of Hong Kong H5N1 influenza A viruses. *Science, 293,* 1840–1842.

Henderson, D. K. (2006). Managing methicillin-resistant staphylococci: A paradigm for preventing nosocomial transmission of resistant organisms. *American Journal of Infection Control, 34,* S46–54, S64–73.

Hennessey, T. W., Hedberg, C. W., Slutsker, L., White, K. E., Besser-Wiek, J. M., Moen, M. E., et al. (1996). A national outbreak of *Salmonella enteritidis* infections from ice cream. *New England Journal of Medicine, 334,* 1281–1286.

Jones-Engel, L., Engel, G. A., Heidrich, J., Chalise, M., Poudel, N., Viscidi, R., et al. (2006). Temple monkeys and health implications of commensalism, Kathmandu, Nepal. *Emerging Infectious Diseases, 12,* 900–906.

Kauffman, C. A. (2006). The changing landscape of invasive fungal infections: Epidemiology, diagnosis, and pharmacologic options. *Clinical Infectious Diseases, 43*(Suppl. 1), S1–2.

Keiser, J., & Utzinger, J. (2005). Emerging foodborne trematodiasis. *Emerging Infectious Diseases, 11,* 1507–1514.

Kidd, S. E., Bach, P. J., Hingston, A. O., Mak, S., Chow, Y., MacDougall, L., et al. (2007). *Cryptococcus gattii* dispersal mechanisms, British Columbia, Canada. *Emerging Infectious Diseases, 13,* 51–57.

Kidd, S. E., Hagen, F., Tscharke, R. L., Huynh, M., Bartlett, K. H., Fyfe, M., et al. (2004). A rare genotype of *Cryptococcus gattii* caused the cryptococcosis outbreak on Vancouver Island (British Columbia, Canada). *Proceedings of the National Academy of Sciences, USA, 101,* 17258–17263.

Kirchhoff, L. V., Paredes, P., Lomelí-Guerrero, A., Paredes-Espinoza, M., Ron-Guerrero, C. S., Delgado-Mejía, M., et al. (2006). Transfusion-associated Chagas disease (American trypanosomiasis) in Mexico: Implications for transfusion medicine in the United States. *Transfusion, 46,* 298–304.

Klein, H. G. (2000). Will blood transfusion ever be safe enough? *Journal of the American Medical Association, 284*(2), 238–240.

Lashley, F. R. (2004). Emerging infectious diseases: Vulnerabilities, contributing factors, and approaches. *Expert Reviews of Anti-infective Therapy, 2,* 299–316.

Leiby, D. A. (2006). Babesiosis and blood transfusion: Flying under the radar. *Vox Sanguinis, 90,* 157–165.

Leirisalo-Repo, M. (2005). Reactive arthritis. *Scandinavian Journal of Rheumatology, 34,* 251–259.

Lone star tick—USA: New England. (2006, July 24). *ProMED Digest, 328,* unpaginated.

Lorber, B. (2005). *Listeria monocytogenes.* In G. L. Mandell, J. E. Bennett, & R. Dolin (Eds), *Mandell, Douglas, and Bennett's principles and practice of infectious diseases* (6th ed., pp. 2478–2484). Philadelphia: Churchill Livingstone Elsevier.

Lorber, M. (2005). Endocarditis from *Staphylococcus aureus. Journal of the American Medical Association, 294,* 2972–2973.

MacDougall, L., Kidd, S. E., Galanis, E., Mak, S., Ljeslie, M. J., Cieslak, P. R., et al. (2007). Spread of *Cryptococcus gattii* in British Columbia, Canada, and detection in the Pacific Northwest, USA. *Emerging Infectious Diseases, 13,* 42–50.

Mackenzie, J. S. (1999). Emerging viral diseases: An Australian perspective. *Emerging Infectious Diseases, 5,* 1–8.

MacKenzie, W. R., Hoxie, N. J., Proctor, M. E., Gradus, M. S., Blair, K. A., Peterson, D. E., et al. (1994). A massive outbreak in Milwaukee of *Cryptosporidium* infection transmitted through the public water supply. *New England Journal of Medicine, 331,* 161–167.

MacLean, J. D. (1998). The North American liver fluke, *Metorchis conjunctus.* In W. M. Scheld, W. A. Craig, & J. M. Hughes (Eds.), *Emerging infections 2* (pp. 243–256). Washington, DC: ASM Press.

Mathews, K. H. Jr., Vandeveer, M., & Gustafson, R. A. (2006, June 6). An economic chronology of bovine spongiform encephalopathy in North America. Economic Research Service, U. S. Department of Agriculture, Report No. LDPM-14301, 1–18.

Mathis, A., Weber, R., & Deplazes, P. (2005). Zoonotic potential of the microsporidia. *Clinical Microbiology Reviews, 18,* 423–445.

Matsubayashi, N., Koike, T., Mikata, I., Takei, N., & Hagiwara, S. (1959). A case of Encephalitozoon-like body infection in man. *Archives of Pathology, 67,* 181–187.

Maunula, L., Miettinen, I. T., & von Bonsdorff, C. H. (2005). Norovirus outbreaks from drinking water. *Emerging Infectious Diseases, 11,* 1716–1721.

McLaughlin, J. B., DePaola, A., Bopp, C. A., Martinek, K. A., Napolilli, N. P., Allison, C. G., et al. (2005). Outbreak of *Vibrio parahaemolyticus* gastroenteritis associated with Alaskan oysters. *New England Journal of Medicine, 353,* 1463–1470.

McQuiston, J. H., Childs, J. E., Chamberland, M. E., & Tabor, E., for the Working Group on Transfusion Transmission of Tick-borne Diseases. (2000). Transmission of tick-borne agents of disease by blood transfusion: A review of known and potential risks in the United States. *Transfusion, 40,* 274–284.

Miller, L. G., Perdreau-Remington, F., Rieg, G., Mehdi, S., Perlroth, J., Bayer, A. S., et al. (2005). Necrotizing fasciitis caused by community-associated methicillin-resistant *Staphylococcus aureus* in Los Angeles. *New England Journal of Medicine, 352,* 1445–1453.

Moreillon, P., Que, Y.-A., & Glauser, M. P. (2005). In G. L. Mandell, J. E. Bennett, & R. Dolin (Eds), *Mandell, Douglas, and Bennett's principles and practice of infectious diseases* (6th ed., pp. 2321–2351). Philadelphia: Churchill Livingstone Elsevier.

Mortimer, R. B. (2005). Leptospirosis in a caver returned from Sarawak, Malaysia. *Wilderness and Environmental Medicine, 16,* 129–131.

Murray, K., Eaton, B., Hooper, P., Wang, L., Williamson, M., & Young, P. (1998). Flying foxes, horses, and humans: A zoonosis caused by a new member of the Paramyxoviridae. In W. M. Scheld, D. Armstrong, & J. M. Hughes (Eds.), *Emerging infections I* (pp. 43–38). Washington, DC: ASM Press.

Nucci, M., & Marr, K. A. (2005). Emerging fungal diseases. *Clinical Infectious Diseases, 41,* 521–526.

Oldfield, E. C., III. (2006). *Clostridium difficile*-associated diarrhea: Resurgence with a vengeance. *Reviews of Gastroenterological Disorders, 6*(2), 79–96.

Paragonimus—US (California). (2006, August 20). *ProMED Digest, 372,* unpaginated.

Parola, P., de Lamballerie, X., Jourdan, J., Rovery, C., Vaillant, V., Minodier, P., et al. (2006). Novel Chikungunya virus variant in revelers returning from Indian Ocean islands. *Emerging Infectious Diseases, 12,* 1493–1499.

Parola, P., Paddock, C. D., & Raoult, D. (2005). Tick-borne rickettsioses around the world: Emerging diseases challenging old concepts. *Clinical Microbiology Reviews, 18,* 719–756.

Parola, P., & Raoult, D. (2001). Ticks and tickborne bacterial diseases in humans: An emerging infectious threat. *Clinical Infectious Diseases, 32,* 897–928.

Pfaller, M. A., Pappas, P. G., & Wingard, J. R. (2006). Invasive fungal pathogens: Current epidemiological trends. *Clinical Infectious Diseases, 43*(Suppl. 1), S3–14.

Pozio, E. (2000). Is horsemeat trichinellosis an emerging disease in the EU? *Parasitology Today, 16,* 266.

Quiroz, E. S., Bern, C., MacArthur, J. R., Xiao, L., Fletcher, M., Arrowood, M. J., et al. (2000). An outbreak of cryptosporidiosis linked to a foodhandler. *Journal of Infectious Diseases, 181,* 695–700.

Raguckas, S. E., Vandenbussche, H. L., Jacobs, C., & Klepser, M. E. (2007). Pertussis resurgence: Diagnosis, treatment, prevention, and beyond. *Pharmacotherapy, 27,* 41–52.

Ribeiro, J. M. C., & Valenzuela, J. G. (2006). In Guerrant, R. L., Walker, D. H., & Weller, P. F. (Eds.), *Tropical infectious diseases* (2nd ed., pp. 73–82). Philadelphia: Churchill Livingstone Elsevier.

Reingold, A. L. (1998). Toxic shock syndrome (staphylococcal). In A. S. Evans & P. S. Brachman (Eds.), *Bacterial infections of humans* (3rd ed., pp. 759–775). New York: Plenum Medical.

Roblot, F., Popoff, M., Carlier, J. P., Godet, C., Abbadie, P., Matthis, S., et al. (2006). Botulism in patients who inhale cocaine: The first cases in France. *Clinical Infectious Diseases, 43*, e51–e52.

Rojas-Molina, N., Pedraza-Sanchez, S., Torres-Bibiano, B., Meza-Martinez, H., & Escobar-Gutierrez, A. (1999). Gnathostomosis, an emerging foodborne zoonotic disease in Acapulco, Mexico. *Emerging Infectious Diseases, 5*, 264–266.

Roos, R. P. (2001). Controlling new prion diseases. *New England Journal of Medicine, 344*, 1548–1551.

Salmonellosis, frozen chicken—USA (Minnesota) (02). (2006, July 24). *ProMED Digest, 328*, unpaginated.

Schantz, P. M., Moore, A. C., Munoz, J. L., Hartman, B. J., Schaefer, J. A., Aron, A. M., et al. (1992). Neurocysticercosis in an orthodox Jewish community. *New England Journal of Medicine, 327*, 692–695.

Schünemann, H. J., Hill, S. R., Kakad, M., Bellamy, R., Uyeki, T. M., Hayden, F. G., et al. (2007). WHO rpaid advice guidelines for pharmacological management of sporadic human infection with avian influenza A (H5N1) virus. *Lancet Infection, 7*, 21–31.

Sebaihia, M., Wren, B. W., Mullaney, P., Fairweather, N. F., Minton, N., Stabler, R., et al. (2006). The mulidrug-resistant human pathogen *Clostridium difficile* has a highly mobile, mosaic genome. *Nature Genetics, 38*, 779–786.

Selvey, L. A. R. M., Wells, J. G., McCormack, A. J., Ansford, K., Murray, R. J., Rogers, R. J., et al. (1995). Infection of humans and horses by a newly described morbillivirus. *Medical Journal of Australia, 162*, 642–645.

Shortridge, K. F., Gao, P., Guan, Y., Ito, T., Kawaoka, Y., Markwell, D., et al. (2000). Interspecies transmission of influenza viruses: H5N1 virus and a Hong Kong SAR perspective. *Veterinary Microbiology, 74*, 141–147.

Sing, A., & Heesemann, J. (2005). Imported cutaneous diphtheria, Germany, 1997–2003. *Emerging Infectious Diseases, 11*, 343–344.

Skarbinski, J., Eliades, M. J., Causer, L. M., Barber, A. M., Mali, S., Nguyen-Dinh, P., et al. (2006). Malaria surveillance—United States, 2004. *Morbidity and Mortality Weekly Report, 55*(SS-04), 23–40.

Slater, L. N., & Welch, D. F. (2005). *Bartonella* including cat-scratch disease. In G. L. Mandell, J. E. Bennett, & R. Dolin (Eds), *Mandell, Douglas, and Bennett's principles and practice of infectious diseases* (6th ed., pp. 2733–2748). Philadelphia: Churchill Livingstone Elsevier.

Slifko, T. R., Smith, H. V., & Rose, J. B. (2000). Emerging parasite zoonoses associated with water and food. *International Journal of Parasitology, 30*, 1379–1393.

Slutsker, L., Altekruse, S. F., & Swerdlow, D. L. (1998). Foodborne diseases: Emerging pathogens and trends. *Infectious Disease Clinics of North America, 12*, 199–214.

Smolinski, M. S., Hamburg, M. A., & Lederberg, J. (Eds.). (2003). *Microbial threats to health: Emergence, detection and response.* Washington, DC: Institute of Medcine, National Academy Press.

Srinivasan, A., Burton, E. C., Kuehnert, M. J., Rupprecht, C., Sutker, W. L., Ksiazek, T. G., et al. (2005). Transmission of rabies virus from an organ donor to four transplant recipients. *New England Journal of Medicine, 352*, 1103–1111.

Stevens, D. L. (2006). Streptococcal and staphylococcal infections. In R. L. Guerrant, D. H. Walker, & P. F. Weller (Eds.), *Tropical infectious diseases* (2nd ed., pp. 356–368). Philadelphia: Churchill Livingstone Elsevier.

Stoler, M. H., Bonfiglio, T. A., Steigbigel, R. T., & Pereira, M. (1983). An atypical subcutaneous infection associated with acquired immune deficiency syndrome. *American Journal of Clinical Pathology, 80*, 714–718.

Sunenshine, R. H., & McDonald, L. C. (2006). *Clostridium difficile*-associated disease: New challenges from an established pathogen. *Cleveland Clinic Journal of Medicine, 73*, 187–197.

Sutherst, R. W. (2004). Global change and human vulnerability to vector-borne diseases. *Clinical Microbiology Review, 17*, 136–173.

Tam, C. C., Rodrigues, L. C., Petersen, I., Islam, A., Hayward, A., & O'Brien, S. J. (2006). Incidence of Guillain-Barre syndrome among patients with *Campylobacter* infection; a general practice research database study. *Journal of Infectious Diseases, 194*, 95–97.

Tatem, A. J., Hay, S. I., & Rogers, D. J. (2006). Global traffic and disease vector dispersal. *Proceedings of the National Academy of Sciences USA, 103*, 6242–6247.

Tauxe, R. V. (2004). Salad and pseudoappendicitis: *Yersinia pseudotuberculosis* as a foodborne pathogen. *Journal of Infectious Diseases, 189*, 761–763.

Todd, J., Fishaut, M., Kapral, F., & Welch, T. (1978). Toxic-shock syndrome associated with phage-group-I *Staphylococci*. *Lancet, 2*, 1116–1118.

Townes, J. M., Hoffmann, C. J., & Kohn, M. A. (2004). Neurocysticercosis in Oregon, 1995–2000. *Emerging Infectious Diseases, 10*, 508–510.

Treanor, J. J., & Dolin, R. (2005). Noroviruses and other caliciviruses. In G. L. Mandell, J. E. Bennett, & R. Dolin (Eds), *Mandell, Douglas, and Bennett's principles and practice of infectious diseases* (6th ed., pp. 2194–2200). Philadelphia: Churchill Livingstone Elsevier.

van den Heuvel, J. F. J. M., Hogenhout, S. A., & van der Wilk, F. (1999). Recognition and receptors in virus transmission by arthropods. *Trends in Microbiology, 7*, 71–76.

Vanittanakom, N., Cooper, C. R., Jr., Fisher, M. C., & Sirisanthana, T. (2006). *Penicillium marneffei* infection and recent advances in the epidemiology and molecular biology aspects. *Clinical Microbiology Reviews, 19*, 95–110.

Vibrio parahaemoliticus, shellfish—USA (multistate). (2006, August 5). *ProMED Digest (352)*, unpaginated.

Visvesvara, G. S., & Maguire, J. H. (2006). Pathogenic and opportunistic free-living amebas: *Acanthamoeba* spp., *Balamuthia mandrillaris*, *Naegleria fowleri*, and *Sappina diploidia*. In R. L. Guerrant, D. H. Walker, & P. F. Weller (Eds.), *Tropical infectious diseases* (2nd ed., pp. 1114–1125). Philadelphia: Churchill Livingstone Elsevier.

Walker, D. H., Maguiña, C., & Minnick, M. (2006). Bartonelloses. In R. L. Guerrant, D. H. Walker, & P. F. Weller (Eds.), *Tropical infectious diseases* (2nd ed., pp. 454–462). Philadelphia: Churchill Livingstone Elsevier.

Weiss, L. M., & Schwartz, D. A. (2006). Microsporidiosis. In R. L. Guerrant, D. H. Walker, & P. F. Weller (Eds.), *Tropical infectious diseases* (2nd ed., pp. 1126–1140). Philadelphia: Churchill Livingstone Elsevier.

Wheeler, C., Vogt, T. M., Armstrong, G. L., Vaughan, G., Weltman, A., Nainan, O. V., et al. (2005). An outbreak of hepatitis A associated with green onions. *New England Journal of Medicine, 353,* 890–897.

Will, R. G., Ironside, J. W., Zeidler, M., Cousens, S. N., Estibeiro, K., Alperovitch, A., et al. (1996). A new variant of Creutzfeldt-Jakob disease in the U.K. *Lancet, 347,* 921–925.

Wolfe, N. D., Daszak, P., Kilpatrick, A. M., & Burke, D. S. (2005). Bushmeat hunting, deforestation, and prediction of zoonoses emergence. *Emerging Infectious Diseases, 11,* 1822–1827.

Woo, P. C. Y., Lau, S. K. P., & Yuen, K. Y. (2006). Infectious diseases emerging from Chinese wet-markets: Zoonotic origins of severe respiratory viral infections. *Current Opinion in Infectious Diseases, 19,* 401–407.

World Health Organization. (2007). Cumulative number of confirmed human cases of avian influenza A (H5N1) reported to WHO. Retrieved February 11, 2007, from http://www.who.int.csr/disease/avian_influenza/country/cases_table_2007_02_06/en/index.html

Zhang, N., O'Donnell, K., Sutton, D. A., Nalim, F. A., Summerbell, R. C., Padhye, A. A., et al. (2006). Members of the *Fusarium solani* species complex that cause infections in both humans and plants are common in the environment. *Journal of Clinical Microbiolgy, 44,* 2186–2190.

PART II

Specific Diseases

CHAPTER FOUR

Cholera

Laurie J. Singel and Felissa R. Lashley

The devastation caused by the 2004 tsunami that hit 8 countries including Indonesia, Sri Lanka, South India, and Thailand left about 225,000 people dead and thousands more stranded without food, water, sanitation, or shelter. The images of those stranded families caused a worldwide outpouring of sympathy and support. Public health officials were very concerned that the combination of overcrowded conditions, lack of water and facilities, and tropical climate would lead to an epidemic of communicable diseases such as cholera, diphtheria, dysentery, and typhoid (Centers for Disease Control and Prevention [CDC], 2005a). Epidemics following natural disasters include risk of disease due to lack of clean water, inadequate sanitation, the presence of dead bodies, displacement of people, exposure to animals and vectors, and crowding among other factors, and often involve food and waterborne disease (Watson, Gayer, & Connolly, 2007; see chapters 1 and 3). Americans watched the news stories on television, but because of their distance from the disaster area, the tsunami did not seem a viable threat. Less than a year later, the Gulf Coast of the United States was struck by two major hurricanes, Hurricane Katrina in August, followed by Hurricane Rita in September. These storms' high winds and storm surges caused unprecedented damage along the Louisiana Gulf Coast. When the levees along New Orleans broke, large residential areas were flooded (CDC, 2006). Health and Human Services Secretary Mike Leavitt stated at a news conference that he was "gravely concerned about the potential for cholera, typhoid, and dehydrating diseases that can come as a result of the stagnant water and conditions ("150 Years," 2005, p. 957). This new disaster, on American homeland, prompted new fears of widespread diseases among evacuees, health care workers, and the general public.

Cholera, the acute diarrheal disease caused by the bacterium *Vibrio cholerae*, is no longer restricted to developing countries but is considered to have a worldwide distribution and is endemic in much of the world. In 2005, 52 countries officially reported cholera to the World Health Organization (WHO), for a total of 131,943 cases worldwide, an increase from the previous year. The majority of the global cases were from Africa (94%), especially Senegal, Guinea-Bissau, the Democratic Republic of the Congo, Nigeria, Mauritania, Mozambique, Uganda, Equatorial Guinea, Mali, Cameroon, Burundi, South Africa, and Tanzania, followed by Asia (WHO, 2006b). In spring 2006, a severe outbreak occurred in Angola, and as of June 6, 2006, 43,076 cases had been reported (WHO, 2006a). Since underreporting is common in developing countries, there are probably many more affected people.

V. cholerae are highly motile, gram-negative anerobic bacteria with long, unipolar flagella that propel them through water. They prefer an alkaline environment. These bacteria thrive in brackish water that contains elevated sodium levels and organic matter, but they can also survive in fresh water. They can survive freezing. *V. cholerae* are classified into groups based on the O antigen of the organism (Albert & Morris, 2000; Levine, Gotuzzo, & Sow, 2006). There are at least 200 serogroups of *V. cholerae* that are now recognized, but there are two serogroups of *V. cholerae* known to cause cholera, O1 and O139 (also called Bengal after the site of its origin). *V. cholerae* O1 has two serotypes, Inaba and Ogawa, which are divided into biotypes, the classic and El Tor (Butler & Camilli, 2005). *V. cholerae* has the ability to essentially hibernate in less favorable environmental conditions, and while it is viable in this state, it may not be able to be cultured. It can survive up to 14 days in foods and can be shed by humans for months or even years (Seas & Gotuzzo, 2005). *V. cholerae* has a natural reservoir in warm estuarine waters, where it may attach to plankton and other plant life as well as invade shellfish or be free living (Albert & Morris, 2000; Colwell, 2004). Once humans are infected, pathogenic strains of *V. cholerae* that cause cholera produce a toxin that results in the typical severe diarrhea and fluid and electrolyte loss described below (Sack, Sack, Nair & Siddique, 2004).

Descriptions of what some historians believe was cholera were first noted in the writings of Hindu physicians about 400 B.C. (Cartwright, 1972), but there has been much debate among medical historians whether cholera is a disease of ancient populations or whether it emerged in the early 19th century as a new infectious disease of humans (Levine et al., 2006). Cholera outbreaks were historically associated with the industrial civilization of developing countries. Rapidly growing cities attracted large numbers of workers, who flooded into crowded slums and overwhelmed the public health services available. Breaks in sanitation led to contamination of food and water supplies, with resultant epidemics. During the cholera epidemics in London in the 1850s, the classic work of John Snow regarding the Broad Street pump as the source of infection, and ultimately in establishing the importance of clean water in preventing cholera, is well known (Newsom, 2006). The establishment of European empires in Asia helped cholera spread from its homeland in the Bengal basin, at the delta of the Ganges and Brahmaputra Rivers, to other parts of the world in repeated pandemic waves that affected virtually all of the inhabited world. Of the seven pandemics of cholera since the first was recorded in 1817, six have originated in the Ganges delta of India, an estuarine environment with ideal conditions for *V. cholerae*, where it is endemic (Sack et al., 2004; Tauxe, 1998).

Cholera then went into an unexplained 50-year lull after the sixth pandemic but emerged again in 1961 on the Celebes island of Sulawesi, Indonesia, and moved to Asia, parts of Europe, and Africa by the 1970s largely through trade, tourism, and religious pilgrimage routes (Albert & Morris, 2000; Levine et al., 2006). This seventh pandemic, caused by the *V. cholerae* O1 El Tor strain, has continued since then. At this time, cases of cholera were identified in the southern United States and in northeastern Australia, but these cases were determined not to be part of the pandemic (Tauxe & Barrett, 1998). In 1991, cholera outbreaks began in Peru, and by 1992, most of Central and South America had been affected. This was believed to result from a ship carrying contaminated water from Asia in its ballast tanks to the coast of Peru, where the tanks were discharged and contaminated shellfish beds. The contamination can occur because oysters feed by using their gills to filter water. If the water is contaminated with parasites, they can harbor the parasites in their gills. When humans eat the oysters raw or without adequate cooking, infection can result. In 1992, the then new strain of *V. cholerae*, O139, emerged in Madras, India, and spread quickly through Asia. Some refer to this as a possible eighth pandemic while others do not (Levine et al., 2006; Tauxe & Barrett, 1998). In many countries, cholera has become endemic after the pandemic has passed through the area. In addition to the Ganges delta in India, cholera is now endemic in the Philippines, a number of countries in Southeast Asia, sub-Saharan Africa, and several Latin American countries including Peru and Ecuador (Levine et al., 2006; Sack et al., 2004).

Cholera cases are relatively rare in the United States, and most cases have been sporadic, with a few small outbreaks and an association with foreign travel. There is a small endemic focus of toxigenic *V. cholerae* O1 that exists in the Gulf of Mexico (CDC, 2005). In the period 1996–2005, 64 cases of cholera were reported to the CDC. While 35 were acquired during foreign travel, 29 were acquired in the United States, and 7 were linked to eating Gulf Coast seafood. Two cases of toxigenic *V. cholerae* infection in a husband and wife occurred in October 2005 following Hurricane Rita and were thought to have resulted from eating shrimp that were not properly handled or cooked according to recommendations. The shrimp were cooked for less than the recommended 10 minutes, and some of the cooked shrimp were returned to a cooler that also contained uncooked shrimp, and these cooked shrimp were eaten later. Stool specimens from the couple confirmed toxigenic *V. cholerae* O1, serotype Inaba, biotype El Tor; they were treated with rehydration therapy and antibiotics and recovered (CDC, 2006).

The majority of cholera cases in the United States have been travel associated—either U.S. residents who returned to their country of origin to visit, or non-U.S. residents who visited the United States from cholera-affected countries. In 1992, an Aerolineas Argentina flight originating in Buenos Aires with a stop in Lima, Peru, arrived in Los Angeles. One week later, 31 people, most dispersed to California or Nevada, were found to have culture-confirmed *V. cholerae* infection, while 54 others had diarrheal illness (CDC, 1992a). In another example, a man boarded a flight in the Philippines bound for Hawaii. While on board, he developed severe diarrhea that was later determined to be *V. cholerae* O1, biotype El Tor (CDC, 1992b). Other United States cases have been acquired through contaminated foods, often imported ones, including the following examples.

In August 1991, 3 cases of cholera resulted when people attended a party that included eating a homemade rice pudding with a topping containing frozen coconut milk that was produced in Thailand and exported to the United States and was the source of the outbreak (CDC, 1991a). In two separate instances in 1991, visits by two persons to Ecuador included buying crab meat there, which was frozen and brought back to the United States. It was then served cooked at their respective dinner parties and resulted in 8 cases of cholera in New Jersey and 4 in New York (CDC, 1991b, 1991c). In March 1994, a woman in California developed cholera after eating raw seaweed that a friend had brought back from the Philippines (Vugia et al., 1997).

Turning to cases not associated with travel, in 1973, one case of cholera was reported from Texas—that of a fisherman who had the *V. cholerae* O1 El Tor strain—and 5 years later, an outbreak of the identical strain occurred in about 24 persons resulting from undercooked, contaminated seafood from the Gulf of Mexico and leading to identification of a focus of infection in the brackish Gulf waters that affected persons in Louisiana and Texas (Blake et al., 1980; Sack et al., 2004; Weissman et al., 1974). Cases of cholera in the United States not associated with travel are most often due to eating contaminated shellfish such as crabs, shrimp, or oysters from the Gulf of Mexico, which hosts a persistent strain of *V. cholerae*. Mobile Bay oyster beds were found contaminated with the El Tor biotype of *V. cholerae* during a routine check in 1991 and were closed for a time. About 8 months after reopening, they were again found contaminated and were closed until August 1992 (CDC, 1993).

The major source for the transmission of cholera is contaminated water, especially when a common source is used for washing, bathing, and drinking. The fecal–oral route of transmission is the major one. Food that has been in contact with contaminated water is another major source, and foods known to have transmitted cholera have included shellfish, coconut milk, raw vegetables, and cooked rice, lentils, and other grains, especially when these are reheated. Acidifying condiments such as lemons, limes, tomatoes, or yogurt can help prevent the growth of the organism on grains. Nosocomial transmission is possible but is not a major source of infection. Cholera is not usually spread through person-to-person contact, but in some instances this does occur (Albert & Morris, 2000). Transmission coincidental with sharing food with an infected person and eating food at a funeral feast in Africa for deceased cholera victims have been described. Methods of geographic spread have included travel-associated cases involving an asymptomatic infected person (Tauxe & Barrett, 1998). In one case, such an individual who became infected abroad transmitted *V. cholerae* to others via a dish of sliced fresh fruit she prepared in the United States (Ackers et al., 1997). Other methods of spread have been through commercial and recreational travel, and the Muslim pilgrimage to Mecca (the Hajj) has played a role in several of the pandemics (Tauxe & Barrett, 1998). Other ways in which cholera enters a new geographic site include through contaminated foods from another country and from the ballast waters of ships. In these cases, ships had taken on ballast water in countries with cholera infections. They then exchanged the water in ports where cholera was not present previously, contaminating shellfish beds and washing to shore. It has been recommended that ships exchange ballast waters on the high seas before entry into U.S. ports (McCarthy & Khambaty, 1994).

Susceptibility and severity of illness are determined by many factors, including size of the inoculum, the biotype, any preexisting immunity, and other host and organism factors. Persons with blood group O (Harris et al., 2004) and those with hypochlorhydria from most causes such as malnutrition, medications that reduce acid in the stomach, atrophic gastritis, and chronic *Helicobacter pylori* infection appear to be particularly vulnerable. In regard to age, in endemic areas, a peak incidence is observed in children aged 2 to 9 years, while it is rare in children below 1 year (Albert & Morris, 2000). The elderly may be susceptible because of decreased immunity or less gastric acid (Tauxe, 1998). In nonendemic areas, cases may be distributed across age groups (Albert & Morris, 2000). Women of childbearing age may be particularly susceptible. Cases are rare among health staff caring for cholera patients, microbiologists, and undertakers preparing the bodies of cholera victims for burial, which highlights the effectiveness of simple hygienic measures in the prevention of cholera transmission (Tauxe & Barrett, 1998).

Seasonality is observed in endemic areas that are related in India and other parts of Asia to the monsoon onset and to warm weather (Albert & Morris, 2000). A role has been postulated for a relationship between cholera and the El Niño–Southern Oscillation that is a source of inter-annual variation in climate in Bangladesh (Anyamba, Chretier, Small, Tucker, & Linthicum, 2006). Elevated ocean surface temperatures off the coast of Peru, due in part to El Niño, correlated with cholera incidence in Peru (Colwell, 2004). Global warming is associated with floods and droughts, both of which can promote waterborne diseases such as cholera. Excess rains from warmed seas has resulted in thousands of cases of cholera such as occurred in Honduras after Hurricane Mitch (Epstein, 2000).

In developing countries, a presumptive diagnosis of cholera is made when a report is received of two or more adults with severe watery diarrhea or an adult dying of watery diarrhea (Tauxe & Barrett, 1998). In the United States, anyone with a severe diarrheal illness who has recently traveled to a developing country is suspected to have been infected with V. *cholerae* and appropriate stool cultures are done. While the symptoms may be presumptively diagnostic, particularly during an epidemic, several commercial rapid tests are available that are based on immunoassay, and rapid tests such as dark-field microscopy are available. Polymerase chain reaction and DNA probe testing can be used (Albert & Morris, 2000; Sack et al., 2004). The incubation period for cholera may range from 12 to 72 hours, with 18 to 40 hours being the average, depending on the inoculum ingested and the susceptibility of the host (Levine et al., 2006). After ingestion, the bacteria pass through the stomach to the small intestine, where they produce the cholera toxin that binds to receptors in the mucosa of the small intestine; affects a variety of functions; and, ultimately, causes the intestines to fill with an alkaline, salty fluid, greatly facilitating the growth of V. *cholerae* (Sack et al., 2004; Tauxe & Barrett, 1998).

Although the majority of cholera infections are either asymptomatic or mildly symptomatic, in the full clinically manifested cases, the first symptom is usually diarrhea that begins when the diarrheal fluid accumulates in the small intestine and causes distention, increased intestinal motility, and decreased transit time (Albert & Morris, 2000). This diarrhea (which may have a "fishy" odor) progresses over several hours to assume a translucent rice-water appearance that is typical of cholera. The fluid loss through diarrhea can be as much as 1 liter per hour, leading rapidly to dehydration, tachycardia, hypotension, and vascular collapse. Patients may develop acidosis with Kussmaul breathing and signs of severe dehydration such as lack of urine production, sunken eyes, raspy voices, and poor skin turgor. Vomiting, generally a clear watery fluid, may occur even before the diarrhea. As the severity of the illness increases, patients can become obtunded although they are usually conscious (Albert & Morris, 2000; Sack et al., 2004). Severe muscular cramping may occur, particularly in the legs. Rehydration is the cornerstone of treatment.

If dehydration is not severe, oral rehydration using oral rehydration solution (ORS) can be accomplished and is relatively inexpensive with excellent results in most cases. In severe dehydration, intravenous fluid therapy, such as with Ringer solution, may be needed to restore fluid volume quickly and correct metabolic acidosis and electrolyte deficits; this treatment is then followed by ORS (Albert & Morris, 2000; Sack et al., 2004; Sack, Sack, & Chaignant, 2006). Intravenous therapy may not always be available. Antibiotic therapy is generally secondary to the fluid replacement. The choice of antibiotic depends on the sensitivity patterns of the organism if known. Increasingly, *V. cholerae* strains are resistant to tetracyclines, and other antibiotics such as erythromycin, ciprofloxacin, and azithromycin are used. Recommendations by the WHO had been for adults to receive a single dose of doxycycline or ciprofloxacin while the recommendations for children were for a 3-day course of either tetracycline or erythromycin ("150 Years," 2005). In a study by Saha et al. (2006), a single dose of azithromycin resulted in cessation of diarrhea in 73% of the patients within 48 hours and was inexpensive. One of the potential problems in widespread use of antimicrobial therapy in cholera is the potential for increasing antimicrobial resistance (Guerrant, 2006). Cholera cots have been used for patients with severe diarrhea to facilitate stool collection and disposal. Often both diagnosis and treatment must take place under field conditions in developing countries during epidemics, and procedures for such conditions have been developed by the WHO. Fortunately, "the disease is reversible to the moment of death" (Tauxe, 1998, p. 235). With rapid and appropriate rehydration and therapy, mortality commonly thought to be 25% to 50% if untreated becomes uncommon (Sack et al., 2004).

Groups such as the WHO and the CDC have developed simple strategies for use in developing countries with increased potential for cholera outbreaks. Prevention of cholera transmission appears to be relatively clear-cut for an individual: basic hygienic procedures such good hand washing; clean, chlorinated water sources with good pressure; avoidance of raw or undercooked shellfish; thorough cooking of all foods;

avoidance of shellfish from potentially contaminated waters; avoidance of food and beverages sold by street vendors; use of narrow-necked containers to store water so that the water is not contaminated by hands scooping water from them; and appropriate disposal of human waste. As *V. cholerae* are exquisitely sensitive to acid, simple modifications in food preparation including the use of lemons, limes, tomatoes, tamarinds, and yogurt can acidify foods so that *V. cholerae* cannot survive (Levine et al., 2006; Rodrigues et al., 2000). Training of street vendors in appropriate sanitation and educating consumers regarding food vendors are also important (Tauxe, 1998). Industrialized countries such as the United States have the resources to provide these basic services and a network of surveillance agencies to monitor public health concerns. In developing countries, building infrastructures to support delivery of clean water and proper elimination of waste products is often considered too expensive and complicated to implement but is necessary for long-term prevention.

Although oral cholera vaccines are available in countries outside the United States, they provide only short-term protection and varying effects, and U.S. public health authorities have not been eager to recommend widespread use of such vaccines although WHO is more liberal about use recommendations. An oral cholera vaccine has been licensed for use in the European Union and is believed to protect 61% to 86% of persons against cholera serotype O1 for 4 to 6 months (Hill, Ford, & Lalloo, 2006). Of particular concern is evidence from several studies of *V. cholerae* that have shown a continued emergence of new clones of the bacteria in areas where epidemic cholera occurs due to such means as natural selection, host population immunity, and genetic reassortment (Basu et al., 2000). In the initial phases of the seventh pandemic, most of the organisms were susceptible to the common antibiotics, but resistance is increasingly seen. Cholera, an ancient disease, is still not conquered throughout the world. However, the knowledge is present for prevention through sanitation and hygiene. It is imperative that all people in the world have adequate sanitation and access to clean water.

REFERENCES

150 years of cholera epidemiology. (2005). *Lancet, 366,* 957.

Ackers, M., Pagaduan, R., Hart, G., Greene, K. D., Abbott, S., Mintz, E., et al. (1997). Cholera and sliced fruit: Probable transmission from an asymptomatic carrier in the United States. *International Journal of Infectious Diseases, 1,* 212–214.

Albert, M. J., & Morris, J. G., Jr. (2000). Cholera and other vibrioses. In G. T. Strickland (Ed.). *Hunter's tropical medicine and emerging infectious diseases* (pp. 323–331). Philadelphia: WB Saunders.

Anyamba, A., Chretier, J. P., Small, J., Tucker, C. J., & Linthicum, K. J. (2006). Developing global climate anomalies suggest potential disease risks for 2006–2007. *International Journal of Health Geography, 5,* 60.

Basu, A., Garg, P., Datta, S., Chakraborty, S., Bhattacharya, T., Khan, A., et al. (2000). *Vibrio cholerae* O139 in Calcutta, 1992–1998: Incidence, antibiograms and genotypes. *Emerging Infectious Diseases, 6,* 139–147.

Blake, P. A., Allegra, D. T., Snyder, J. D., Barrett, T. J., McFarland, L., Caraway, C. T., et al. (1980). Cholera—a possible endemic focus in the United States. *New England Journal of Medicine, 302,* 305–309.

Butler, S. M., & Camilli, A. (2005). Going against the grain: Chemotaxis and infection in *Vibrio cholerae. Nature Reviews Microbiology, 3,* 611–620.

Cartwright, F. (1972). *Disease and history.* New York: Dorset Press.

Centers for Disease Control. (1991a). Cholera associated with imported frozen coconut milk—Maryland, 1991. *Morbidity and Mortality Weekly Report, 40,* 844–845.

Centers for Disease Control. (1991b). Cholera—New Jersey and Florida. *Morbidity and Mortality Weekly Report, 40,* 287–289.

Centers for Disease Control. (1991c). Cholera—New York. *Morbidity and Mortality Weekly Report, 40,* 516–518.

Centers for Disease Control. (1992a). Cholera associated with an international airline flight, 1992. *Morbidity and Mortality Weekly Report, 41,* 134–135.

Centers for Disease Control. (1992b). Cholera associated with international travel, 1992. *Morbidity and Mortality Weekly Report, 41,* 664–667.

Centers for Disease Control and Prevention. (1993). Isolation of *Vibrio cholerae* O1 from oysters—Mobile Bay, 1991–1992. *Morbidity and Mortality Weekly Report, 42,* 91–93.

Centers for Disease Control and Prevention. (2004). Cholera epidemic associated with raw vegetable—Lusaka, Zambia, 2003–2004. *Morbidity and Mortality Weekly Report, 53,* 783–786.

Centers for Disease Control and Prevention. (2005a). Rapid health response, assessment, and surveillance after a tsunami—Thailand, 2004–2005. *Morbidity and Mortality Weekly Report, 54,* 61–64.

Centers for Disease Control and Prevention. (2005b). *Vibrio* illnesses after Hurricane Katrina—Multiple states, August–September 2005. *Morbidity and Mortality Weekly Report, 54,* 928–931.

Centers for Disease Control and Prevention. (2006). Two cases of toxigenic *Vibrio cholerae* O1 infection after Hurricanes Katrina and Rita—Louisiana, October 2005. *Morbidity and Mortality Weekly Report, 55,* 31–32.

Colwell, R. R. (2004). Infectious disease and environment: Cholera as a paradigm for waterborne disease. *International Microbiology, 7,* 285–289.

Epstein, P. R. (2000). Is global warming harmful to health? *Scientific American, 283*(2), 50–57.

Guerrant, R. L. (2006). Cholera—Still teaching hard lessons. *New England Journal of Medicine, 354,* 2500–2502.

Harris, J. B., Khan, A. I., LaRocque, R. C., Dorer, D. J., Chowdhury, F., Faruque, A. S., et al. (2005). Blood group, immunity, and risk of infection with *Vibrio cholerae* in an area of endemicity. *Infection and Immunity, 73,* 7422–7427.

Hill, D. R., Ford, L., & Lalloo, D. G. (2006). Oral cholera vaccines: Use in clinical practice. *Lancet Infectious Diseases, 6,* 361–373.

Levine, M. M., Gotuzzo, E., & Sow, S. O. (2006). In R. L. Guerrant, D. H. Walker, & P. F. Weller (Eds.), *Tropical infectious diseases: Principles, pathogens and practice* (2nd ed., pp. 273–282). Philadelphia: Churchill Livingstone Elsevier.

McCarthy, S. A., & Khambaty, F. M. (1994). International dissemination of epidemic *Vibrio cholerae* by cargo ship ballast and other nonpotable waters. *Applied Environmental Microbology, 60,* 2597–2601.

Newsom, S. W. (2006). Pioneers in infection control: John Snow, Henry Whitehead, the Broad Street pump, and the beginnings of geographical epidemiology. *Journal of Hospital Infection, 64*(3), 210–216.

Sack, D. A., Sack, R. B., & Chaignant, C.-L. (2006). Getting serious about cholera. *New England Journal of Medicine, 355,* 649–651.

Sack, D. A., Sack, R. B., Nair, G. B., & Siddique, A. K. (2004). Cholera. *Lancet, 363,* 223–233.

Saha, D., Karim, M., Khan, W. A., Ahmed, S., Salam, M. A., & Bennish, M. L. (2006). Single-dose azithromycin for the treatment of cholera in adults. *New England Journal of Medicine, 354,* 2452–2462.

Seas, C., & Gotuzzo, E. (2005). *Vibrio cholerae.* In G. L. Mandell, J. E. Bennett, & R. Dolin (Eds.), *Mandell, Douglas, and Bennett's principles and practice of infectious diseases* (6th ed., pp. 2536–2550). Philadelphia: Elsevier Churchill Livingstone.

Tauxe, R. V. (1998). Cholera. In A. S. Evans & P. S. Brachman (Eds.), *Bacterial infections of humans: Epidemiology and control* (3rd ed., pp. 223–242). New York: Plenum Medical Book Company.

Tauxe, R. V., & Barrett, T. J. (1998). Cholera and *Vibrio cholerae*: New challenges from a once and future pathogen. In W. M. Scheld, W. A. Craig, & J. M. Hughes (Eds.), *Emerging infections 2* (pp. 125–144). Washington, DC: ASM Press.

Vugia, D., Shefer, A., Douglas, J., Greene, K., Bryant, R., & Werner, S. (1997). Cholera from raw seaweed transported from the Philippines to California. *Journal of Clinical Microbiology, 35,* 284–285.

Watson, J. T., Gayer, M., & Connolly, M. A. (2007). Epidemics after natural disasters. *Emerging Infectious Diseases, 13,* 1–5.

Weissman, J. B., DeWitt, W. E., Thompson, J., Muchnick, C. M., Portnoy, B. L., Feeley, J. C., et al. (1974). A case of cholera in Texas, 1973. *American Journal of Epidemiology, 100,* 487–498.

World Health Organization. (2006a). Cholera, Angola—Update. *Weekly Epidemiological Record, 81,* 237–238.

World Health Organization. (2006b). Cholera 2005. *Weekly Epidemiological Record, 80,* 261–268.

CHAPTER FIVE

Cryptosporidiosis

Jeanne Beauchamp Hewitt

The largest known cryptosporidiosis outbreak occurred when an estimated 403,000 people were affected during a waterborne outbreak in late March and early April 1993 in Milwaukee, Wisconsin (MacKenzie et al., 1994). Officials at the Milwaukee Health Department noticed widespread absenteeism among students, teachers, and hospital personnel, which prompted them to notify the Wisconsin Division of Health on April 5. Subsequently, two laboratories confirmed the presence of *Cryptosporidium* oocysts in stool samples from seven adult residents of the Milwaukee area.

Two water treatment plants supplied 800,000 Milwaukee residents and 10 other municipalities (MacKenzie et al., 1994). Water quality records showed an increased turbidity at the south plant beginning around March 21, with much higher levels of turbidity noted from March 23 through April 5. A boil-water advisory was issued the evening of April 7, and the south plant was temporarily closed on April 9. The 14 local clinical laboratories were requested to report positive *Cryptosporidium* tests from March 1 through May 15. From March 1 through April 6, 12 of 42 (29%) specimens tested positive for *Cryptosporidium*; from April 8 through April 16, 331 of 1,009 (33%) specimens tested positive.

The Milwaukee cryptosporidiosis outbreak continues to serve as a model for understanding this parasitic disease. A seroprevalence study of blood from lead-tested children 6 months to 12 years of age in 1993 showed a marked increase in antigen response 3 weeks after gastrointestinal symptoms peaked (McDonald et al., 2001). The proportion of children served by the South and North treatment plants who had cryptosporidiosis was estimated to be 70% and 37%, respectively. In a study of elderly residents, Naumova, Egorov, Morris, & Griffiths (2003) found elders to have an increased risk of cryptosporidiosis both before and during the Milwaukee outbreak, to have a shorter latency period, and to experience a higher rate of person-to-person transmission than adults in general. Medical record audits for the 4 months during and after the Milwaukee outbreak showed that an estimated 88% of the population infected with *Cryptosporidium* did not seek medical care, 11% sought outpatient care, and 1% were hospitalized for an average of 8 days (Corso et al., 2003). Cost estimates for mild, moderate, and severe cases averaged $116, $475, and $7,808, respectively, for self- or medical treatment and lost work time for personal illness or to provide care for affected family members. In total, the Milwaukee outbreak cost approximately $96.2 million, with 67% of that figure attributed to lost productivity. In a 2-year follow-up study, 54 death records in the Milwaukee area listed cryptosporidiosis as a contributing or underlying cause of death; 85% of these cases were associated with acquired immunodeficiency syndrome (AIDS; Hoxie, Davis, Vergeront, Hashold, & Blair, 1997).

Although the gastrointestinal protozoan *Cryptosporidium* was first described in 1907, the first human cases of cryptosporidiosis were reported only in 1976 (Fayer, 2004). Recent advances in diagnostic testing and genotyping have led to changes in the taxonomy of *Cryptosporidium*. *Cryptosporidium hominis*, formerly referred to as *Cryptosporidium parvum*, Type 1, is associated with human reservoirs, while *C. parvum*, formerly called Type 2, is associated with bovine and human reservoirs (Bushen, Lima, & Guerrant, 2006). *C. hominis* and/or *C. parvum* are the most frequently implicated species in human infection when genotyping is done. Other *Cryptosporidium* species such as *Cryptosporidium felis*, *Cryptosporidium meleagridis*, and a new cervine (deer) genotype that is still unnamed, although uncommon causes of human infection, may be responsible for illness in human immunodeficiency virus (HIV)-infected persons more than in the immunocompetent host (Bushen et al., 2006; Coupe, Sarfati, Hamane, & Derouin, 2005; Matos, Alves, Xiao, Cama, & Antunes, 2004; Ong et al., 2002); however, they do occur, especially in children (Caccio, Pinto, Fantini, Mezzaroma, & Pozio, 2002; Xiao et al., 2001).

Cryptosporidium has been found in a variety of biological hosts: fish; amphibians; reptiles including snakes, lizards, and tortoises; wild and domesticated birds including chickens, turkeys, ducks, canaries, and cockatiels; and mammals including rodents, cats, dogs, sheep, goats, pigs, deer, cows, and humans (Fayer, 2004). *Cryptosporidium* spp. may be transmitted via the fecal–oral route through oocyst-contaminated drinking or recreational water, food, or close contact with humans or other species infected with the organism such as animals in petting zoos as well as contaminated surfaces (Fayer, 2004; Hellard, Hocking, Willis, Dore, & Fairley, 2003; Roy et al., 2004). Based on mathematical modeling of Milwaukee outbreak data, Eisenberg, Lei, Hubbard, Brookhart, & Colford (2005) estimated that person-to-person transmission accounted for 10% of the cases in the Milwaukee outbreak, whereas the majority of cases resulted from human–environment–human transmission. The incubation period for *Cryptosporidium* infection is estimated to range from 2 to 14 days with a median incubation period of 7 days (Fayer, 2004), with shorter incubation periods (median of 5 days) for children (Insulander, Lebbad, Stenstrom, & Svenungsson, 2005) and the elderly (Naumova et al., 2003). Food sources implicated in outbreaks have included a variety of raw vegetables, basil, cilantro, fresh-pressed and even ozone-treated apple cider, chicken salad, and shellfish (Blackburn et al., 2006; Centers for Disease Control and Prevention [CDC], 2001; White, 2005). In one outbreak in Minnesota, a caterer changed an infant's diaper and later prepared chicken salad for a social event, resulting in the infection of 50 people (CDC, 1996).

Environmental contamination with *Cryptosporidium* spp. is common and worldwide (Fayer, 2004). Of 179 wastewater samples tested in Milwaukee between 2000 and 2002, 50 specimens were positive (Zhou, Singh, Jiang, & Xiao, 2003). The most prevalent species were *C. hominis* (13.4%), *Cryptosporidium andersoni* (12.8%), *Cryptosporidium cervid* (3.3%), *C. parvum* (2.8%), *Cryptosporidium muris* (2.2%), and the mouse genotype (0.6%). Zoonotic transmission of cryptosporidiosis has been documented in the community (Goh et al., 2004; Howe et al., 2002) and among veterinary science students (Preiser, Preiser, & Madeo, 2003). Surveillance data on cryptosporidiosis in the United Kingdom showed that an epidemic of foot and mouth disease among livestock was associated with a significant decline (35%) in cryptosporidiosis incidence in humans (Smerdon, Nichols, Chalmers, Heine, & Reacher, 2003). The serendipitous decline in cryptosporidiosis was attributed to the culling of livestock, as well as restriction of access to the countryside and movement of farm animals to halt the foot and mouth disease outbreak (Goh et al., 2005; Hunter, Chalmers et al., 2004; Smerdon et al., 2003).

National surveillance for cryptosporidiosis from 1999 to 2002 reported 12,700 laboratory-confirmed cases in the United States (Hlavsa, Watson, & Beach, 2005). Although underreporting of cryptosporidiosis is a major problem, Mead and colleagues (1999) used multiple data sources to estimate that 300,000 cases of cryptosporidiosis occur annually in the United States, of which 10% were foodborne. Across the United States, cryptosporidiosis affects persons of all ages, but with greater numbers in the 1–9 and 30–39 age groups (Hlavsa et al., 2005). Although cryptosporidiosis is geographically widespread, the highest incidence in 2002 occurred in the upper Midwest (Wisconsin, Minnesota, North Dakota, South Dakota) and Vermont. Cryptosporidiosis peaks between June and October, and this seasonal pattern is greatest for children 1–9 years of age. Widespread use of protease inhibitors to treat HIV infection has decreased the prevalence of cryptosporidiosis in HIV-infected persons. In addition to HIV-infected persons, others who have some degree of immunosuppression such as those with malignancies or on immunosuppressive medications, the elderly, and, to some degree, those who are transplant recipients are vulnerable to cryptosporidiosis, which may be harder to treat in them than in the immunocompetent person and may result in more severe sequelae (Fayer, 2004; Mofenson et al., 2004; Zardi, Picardi, & Afeltra, 2005). In young children, cryptosporidiosis has been associated with failure to thrive and impaired cognitive function (Savioli, Smith, & Thompson, 2006).

Cryptosporidiosis may be a greater problem in developed countries than commonly recognized. Morris, Naumova, and Griffiths (1998) found that cryptosporidiosis may have been affecting Milwaukee residents for more than 1 year prior to the recognized outbreak. In the San Francisco Bay area, drinking tap water was associated with significantly increased risks for cryptosporidiosis in immunocompromised persons (Aragon et al., 2003). In immunocompetent persons, travel more than 100 miles from home (Khalakdina, Vugia, Nadle, Rothrock, & Colford, 2003) and international travel (Khalakdina et al., 2003; Roy et al., 2004), but not drinking local tap water (Khalakdina et al., 2003), was associated with a significantly increased risk of laboratory-confirmed cryptosporidiosis. Current laboratory-based surveillance of cryptosporidiosis in the United States indicates that about 3,000 cases are reported annually, but this is likely to be a significant underreporting due to the presence of asymptomatic disease, failure to seek medical care by many who are symptomatic, failure of some health care providers to order specific tests to detect cryptosporidiosis, and underreporting of positive laboratory findings to the public health surveillance system (Hlavsa et al., 2005). Better estimates of the prevalence of cryptosporidiosis should be forthcoming because seroprevalence data have been collected as part of the National Health and Nutrition Examination Survey since 1999. Similarly, there is an international effort to improve the tracking and prevention of foodborne illnesses (Flint et al., 2005).

The major symptom of cryptosporidiosis is diarrhea. In the 1993 Milwaukee outbreak, 100% of laboratory-confirmed cases had diarrhea (MacKenzie et al., 1994). The median duration of diarrhea was 9 days (range 1–53 days) with a median of 12 stools per day. Cryptosporidial diarrhea commonly is accompanied by copious loss of fluids (Fayer, 2004). Symptoms reported by persons with laboratory-confirmed cryptosporidiosis included diarrhea (91.3%), loss of appetite (87.0%), abdominal cramps (86.4%), and nausea (75.6%; Mathieu et al., 2004). In the United Kingdom, sequelae of infection with *C. hominis* or *C. parvum* in immunocompetent hosts included recurrent gastroenteritis symptoms (40%), whereas infection with *C. hominis*, but not *C. parvum*, was associated with increased risk of joint pain, eye pains, recurrent headaches, dizzy spells, and fatigue (Hunter, Hughes, et al., 2004). In immunocompromised hosts, in whom CD4$^+$ cells exceed 200/mm^3, cryptosporidiosis is more likely to be acute and resolve (Chen, Keithly, Paya, & LaRusso, 2002). Fewer than 100 CD4$^+$ cells/mm^3 are associated with chronic (potentially lifelong) and extraintestinal forms of the disease, while fewer than 50 CD4$^+$ cells/mm^3 are associated with a fulminant, life-threatening form of cryptosporidiosis.

Extraintestinal infections occur (Chen et al., 2002; Fayer, 2004; White, 2005). In young persons (ages 7–27 years), presenting symptoms associated with *Cryptosporidium* infection not confined to the intestinal tract included arthritis, tenosynovitis, conjunctivitis, urethritis, plantar fasciitis, and/or erythema of the oral mucosa (Fayer, 1997). Extraintestinal infections also have been associated with site-specific symptoms such as conjunctivitis, cholangitis, pancreatitis, hepatitis, and pulmonary infections (Chen et al., 2002). Additional symptoms associated with pulmonary cryptosporidiosis include coughing, wheezing, croup, hoarseness, and shortness of breath.

During the acute phase of cryptosporidiosis, the number of oocysts excreted daily can vary widely (Fayer, 2004) up to 10^9 oocysts per day (Hlavsa et al., 2005). In immunocompetent persons, *Cryptosporidium* oocysts may be excreted for 1 to several weeks (Fayer, 2004). In persons with AIDS, cryptosporidiosis can range from being asymptomatic to a fulminant form of the disease in which watery diarrhea of 2 liters or more is lost daily (Chen et al., 2002). *Cryptosporidium* oocysts may be excreted for 1 to several weeks or longer after gastroenteritis symptoms subside (Fayer, 2004). In both symptomatic and asymptomatic individuals, excretion of oocysts is intermittent. As a result, three independent stool samples (obtained on different days) should be evaluated to reduce the chance of false negatives (Bushen et al., 2006). Newer diagnostic methods, which are highly sensitive and specific, are now available and used in clinical laboratories and offer the additional advantage of being cost effective since they require less time and skill (Coupe et al., 2005). These include immunofluorescent assays using specific monoclonal antibodies and antigen detection assays for rapid testing as well as polymerase chain reaction (White, 2005). Genotyping, which was not available during the Milwaukee outbreak, has advanced our knowledge of routes of transmission (Fayer, 2004; McLauchlin, Amar, Pedraza-Diaz, & Nichols, 2000;

Pedraza-Diaz, Amar, Nichols, & McLauchlin, 2001) and therefore is a means to achieve primary prevention.

Primary prevention of cryptosporidiosis focuses on environmental controls, including the handling of animal waste and the prevention of human infection through contaminated water, food, and fomites (Fayer, 2004). The best overall strategy to control this infection in domestic animal populations is to move the animals to uninfected areas because desiccation renders the oocysts noninfective (Fayer, 2004). Flood control measures help prevent runoff from contaminated soil, often from animals who may be asymptomatic but excrete *Cryptosporidium* oocysts to surface water and wells (Thurston-Enriquez, Gilley, & Eghball, 2005; Trask, Kalita, Kuhlenschmidt, Smith, & Funk, 2004). Sewage is also a source of human infection when water treatment fails to remove *Cryptosporidium* oocysts adequately or when the drinking water distribution system is infiltrated with sewage (Carnicer-Pont et al., 2005; Dalle et al., 2003; Goh et al., 2004; Goh et al., 2005; Howe et al., 2002; Smerdon et al., 2003). Primary prevention by means of environmental controls, therefore, depends on maintaining the integrity of sewage wastewater distribution systems and isolation from treated drinking water distribution systems, as well as the effective removal of *Cryptosporidium* oocysts in drinking water through such means as filtration (Goh et al., 2005), ozonation, and ultraviolet (UV) light (Johnson et al., 2005; Keegan, Fanok, Monis, & Saint, 2003; Mendez-Hermida, Castro-Hermida, Ares-Mazas, Kehoe, & McGuigan, 2005; Peeters, Mazas, Masschelein, Martinez de Maturana, & DeBacker, 1989). Recreational water, including swimming pools, water parks, lakes, rivers, and streams, are major sources of outbreaks (Causer et al., 2006; Insulander et al., 2005; Lim, Varkey, Giesen, & Edmonson, 2004; Mathieu et al., 2004; Yokoi et al., 2005). After an outbreak attributed to a pool, closure and special cleaning procedures should be followed before the pool is reopened (CDC, 2001; Insulander et al., 2005; Yokio et al., 2005). Further ways to prevent waterborne and foodborne infections are listed in Appendix C.

For individuals, the best strategies are to use good personal hygiene such as hand washing, institute procedures using appropriate disinfectants, and effectively decontaminate recreational and drinking water (Fayer, 2004). Additional measures recommended for HIV-infected persons (and possibly other immunocompromised persons) are provided by the CDC (Kaplan, Masur, Holmes, U.S. Public Health Service, & Infectious Disease Society of America, 2002).

Secondary prevention measures consist of early diagnosis and management of cryptosporidiosis. In immunocompetent persons, cryptosporidiosis is usually self-limited and symptoms can be managed with oral rehydration and antidiarrheal medication (Bushen et al., 2006).

Current chemotherapy is suboptimal, but if symptoms are severe, suggested chemotherapy consists of paromycin for 7 days or, in children 1–11 years, nitazoxanide for 3 days (CDC, 2004). In persons with AIDS, highly active antiretroviral therapy (HAART) to improve the immune system is the optimal strategy (Chen et al., 2002; Kaplan et al., 2002); however, when HAART is not an option or is ineffective, paramomycin, azithromycin, and nitazoxanide may be used with antidiarrheal agents to treat cryptosporidiosis (Chen et al., 2002; Palmieri et al., 2005; Smith & Corcoran, 2004).

Laboratory studies reviewed by Fayer (1997) showed that *Cryptosporidium* oocysts are resistant to many chemical disinfectants, including chlorine, CIDEX, and Lysol. Effective chemical disinfectants include formol saline (10% for 18 hours), ammonia (5% for 18 hours or 100% gas for 24 hours), and ethylene oxide gas (100% for 24 hours). Fayer concluded that high temperature (45° C for 20 minutes, 64.2° C for 5 minutes, or 72.4° C for 1 minute), low temperature (−20° C for 3 days), and desiccation (air-dried feces, 1–4 days) were the most effective and practical methods of environmental decontamination. Subsequently, Barbee, Weber, Sobsey, and Rutala (1999) demonstrated that, of seven disinfectants tested, only 6% and 7.5% hydrogen peroxide inactivated *C. parvum*, but that sterilization procedures using steam, ethylene oxide, and STERRAD 100 (a form steam autoclave system that uses hydrogen peroxide vapor) effectively inactivated this organism at 3 logs or greater (the level of detection of the cell culture assay). For the treatment of water, low-pressure UV light at 20 mJ/cm^2 (>2 $\log_{10}$) and solar disinfection (830 W/m^{2-} at 40° C for 12 hours) were effective at inactivating oocysts (Keegan et al., 2003; Mendez-Hermida et al., 2005), and UV light was found to be equally effective against *C. hominis* and *C. parvum* (Johnson et al., 2005). The chemical disinfection of soil, housing, and tools was examined using hydrogen peroxide-based disinfectants, which were effective at concentrations of 10% for Ox-Virin (H_2O_2 with peracetic acid for 60 minutes) and 3% Ox-Agua (H_2O_2 with silver nitrate for 30 minutes; Quilez, Sanchez-Acedo, Avendano, del Cacho, & Lopez-Bernad, 2005). Regarding food, the practice of washing beef carcasses with hot water (60° C for 45 seconds or 75° C for 20 seconds) was found to render oocysts noninfective (Moriarty et al., 2005).

Heat-sensitive medical equipment, such as endoscopes, can serve as fomites for nosocomial transmission of *Cryptosporidium*. Endoscopic equipment can be disinfected using hydrogen peroxide gas plasma sterilization (Barbee et al., 1999; Vassal, Favennec, Ballet, & Brasseur, 1998), or ammonia, ethylene oxide, or methyl bromide gases (Fayer, Graczyk, Cranfield, & Trout, 1996). Glutaraldehyde solution (i.e., CIDEX) is ineffective as a disinfectant in the presence of organic material

(Wilson & Margolin, 2003). Nosocomial infections can be prevented by the prompt mechanical cleaning of endoscopes after use to remove organic material followed by disinfection and drying of endoscopes (Nelson et al., 2004).

Water filtration systems that meet or exceed regulatory requirements do not entirely prevent cryptosporidiosis outbreaks (Goldstein et al., 1996; Haas, 2000) or *Cryptosporidium* oocysts from entering drinking water supplies (LeChevallier, Norton, & Lee, 1991). These are discussed in detail in " Proactive Detection of Cryptosporidiosis by Clinical Laboratories" (Working Group on Waterborne Cryptosporidiosis, 1997). Other measures to avoid cryptosporidiosis, particularly in high-risk individuals, include using reverse osmosis water filter systems (Addiss et al., 1996; CDC, n.d.; Roy et al., 2004) or drinking bottled water (Aragon et al., 2003; Kaplan et al., 2002). When the drinking water supply may be contaminated with bacteria, protozoa, or hepatitis A, the CDC and the Environmental Protection Agency recommend boiling water at a rolling boil for 1 minute and/or filtration through a submicron filter (Kaplan et al., 2002). Haas (2000) notes that protecting the drinking water of the general public may not protect those who are more vulnerable because of immunosuppression.

Although the 1993 cryptosporidiosis outbreak in Milwaukee is the largest and most well known, a number of outbreaks have been reported. Examples of outbreaks attributed to cryptosporidiosis are summarized in the Table 5.1. Waterborne outbreaks predominate (Hlavsa et al., 2005).

Nosocomial transmission, such as through the use of inadequately disinfected endoscopes, has not been addressed widely in the literature but is a concern due to the resistance of C. *parvum* oocysts to many disinfectants (Fayer, 2004) and the lack of adherence to evidence-based guidelines (Nelson et al., 2004). Standard precautions can be used for most hospitalized patients with cryptosporidiosis. Contact precautions are recommended for children under age 6 who are in diapers or incontinent. Infection control procedures suggest that immunocompromised persons such as those with HIV infection should not share a room with someone infected with *Cryptosporidium* (Garner & the Hospital Infection Control Practices Advisory Committee, 1996). Additional environmental control procedures should be used to reduce the risk of cryptosporidiosis acquired in healthcare settings (CDC, 2003).

Cryptosporidiosis has only been recognized as an infection in humans since 1976. Since that time it has been identified as the responsible agent in a number of large outbreaks of severe diarrheal illness in communities (Table 5.1). In immunocompetent persons, however, illness is usually self-limited, requiring only symptomatic relief. In HIV-infected persons and others who are immunosuppressed, including the elderly, illness may

Table 5.1. Examples of Cryptosporidiosis Outbreaks Reported in the Literature

Publication	No. of Cases	Year of Outbreak	Location(s)	Attribution of Cause
McAnulty, Fleming, & Gonzalez, 1994	55	1992	Lane County, OR	Local wave pool and secondary transmission
MacKenzie et al., 1994	~403,000	1993	Milwaukee, WI	Municipal drinking water
Moss, Bennett, Arrowood, Wahlquist, & Lammie, 1998	64	1993	U.S. Coast Guard cutter	Municipal water obtained while docked in Milwaukee during the 1993 outbreak
CDC, 1994	35	1993	Dane County, WI	Two swimming pools
Millard et al., 1994	160	1993	Maine	Fresh-pressed apple cider consumed at a fair
Goldstein et al., 1996	78	1994	Las Vegas, NV	Municipal drinking water
Kramer et al., 1998	~2,070	1994	New Jersey	Recreational lake water
CDC, 1996	~50	1995	Blue Earth County, MN	Consumption of chicken salad prepared by person who operated a licensed home day care and changed diapers before preparing the salad reportedly after washing her hands
CDC, 1998	369	1997	Minnesota	Water sprinkler at a zoo
Lim, Varkey, Giesen, & Edmonson, 2004	26	1998	Olmstead County, MN	Swimming
CDC, 2001	~1,000	2000	Ohio and Nebraska	Swimming pools
Mathieu et al., 2004	~700	2000	Ohio	Swimming pool
Howe et al., 2002	58	2000	Clitheroe, Lancashire, England	Tap water contaminated with animal feces

Table 5.1. (*Continued*)

Publication	No. of Cases	Year of Outbreak	Location(s)	Attribution of Cause
Glaberman et al., 2002	476	2000–2001	3 areas near Belfast, Northern Ireland	Drinking water
Smith & Corcoran, 2004	17	2000–2001	Minnesota	Day farm
Ashbolt, Coleman, Misrachi, Conti, & Kirk, 2003	47	2001	Tasmania, Australia	Animal nursery at an agricultural show
Causer et al., 2006	358	2001	Illinois	Recreational water park
Insulander, Lebbad, Stenstrom, & Svenungsson, 2005	~800–1,000	2002	Stockholm, Sweden	Municipal swimming pools and secondary transmission
Preiser, Preiser, & Madeo, 2003	7	Unknown	New York, NY	Veterinary science students who had contact with calves in college-operated barn
Carnicer-Pont et al., 2005	100	2005	Gwynedd and Anglesey, Wales	Drinking water

Note: CDC = Centers for Disease Control and Prevention.

be long lasting and result in fatality. While three antiparasitic drugs are available, they are at best only moderately effective. Ensuring the safety of drinking water and recreational water are two major preventive measures to reduce morbidity and mortality associated with *Cryptosporidium* (see Appendix C).

REFERENCES

Addiss, D. G., Pond, R. S., Remshak, M., Juranek, D. D., Stokes, S., & Davis, J. P. (1996). Reduction of risk of watery diarrhea with point-of-use water filters during a massive outbreak of waterborne *Cryptosporidium* infection in Milwaukee, Wisconsin, 1993. *American Journal of Tropical Medicine and Hygiene, 54,* 549–553.

Aragon, T. J., Novotny, S., Enanoria, W., Vugia, D. J., Khalakdina, A., & Katz, M. H. (2003). Endemic cryptosporidiosis and exposure to municipal tap water in persons with acquired immunodeficiency syndrome (AIDS): A case-control study. *BMC Public Health, 3,* 2.

Ashbolt, R. H., Coleman, D. J., Misrachi, A., Conti, J. M., & Kirk, M. D. (2003). An outbreak of cryptosporidiosis associated with an animal nursery at a regional fair. *Communicable Diseases Intelligence, 27,* 244–249.

Barbee, S. L., Weber, D. J., Sobsey, M. D., & Rutala, W. A. (1999). Inactivation of *Cryptosporidium parvum* oocysts infectivity by disinfection and sterilization processes. *Gastrointestinal Endoscopy, 49,* 605–611.

Blackburn, B. G., Mazurek, J. M., Hlavsa, M., Park, J., Tillapaw, M., Parrish, M., et al. (2006). Cryptosporidiosis associated with ozonated apple cider. *Emerging Infectious Diseases, 12,* 684–686.

Bushen, O. Y., Lima, A. A. M., & Guerrant, R. L. (2006). In R. L. Guerrant, D. H. Walker, & P. F. Weller (Eds.), *Tropical infectious diseases* (2nd ed., pp. 1003–1014). Philadelphia: Churchill Livingstone Elsevier.

Caccio, S., Pinter, E., Fantini, R., Mezzaroma, I., & Pozio, E. (2002). Human infection with *Cryptosporidium felis*: Case report and literature review. *Emerging Infectious Diseases, 8,* 85–86.

Carnicer-Pont, D., Atenstaedt, R., Walker, M., Chalmers, R., Rees, A., Rowlands, K., et al. (2005). An outbreak of cryptosporidiosis in Wales, November 2005. *European Surveillance, 10*(12), E051208.4.

Causer, L. M., Handzel, T., Welch, P., Carr, M., Culp, D., Lucht, R., et al. (2006). An outbreak of *Cryptosporidium hominis* infection at an Illinois recreational waterpark. *Epidemiology of Infections, 134,* 147–156.

Centers for Disease Control and Prevention. (n.d.). *Preventing cryptosporidiosis: A guide to water filters and bottled water.* Retrieved August 25, 2006, from http://www.cdc.gov/ncidod/dpd/parasites/cryptosporidiosis/factsht_crypto_prevent_water.htm

Centers for Disease Control and Prevention. (1994). *Cryptosporidium* infections associated with swimming pools—Dane county, Wisconsin. *Morbidity and Mortality Weekly Report, 43,* 561–563.

Centers for Disease Control and Prevention. (1996). Foodborne outbreak of diarrheal illness associated with *Cryptosporidium parvum* Minnesota, 1995. *Morbidity and Mortality Weekly Report, 45,* 783–784.

Centers for Disease Control and Prevention. (1998). Outbreak of cryptosporidiosis associated with a water sprinkler fountain—Minnesota, 1997. *Morbidity and Mortality Weekly Report, 45,* 783–784.

Centers for Disease Control and Prevention. (2001). Protracted outbreaks of cryptosporidiosis associated with swimming pool use—Ohio and Nebraska, 2000. *Morbidity and Mortality Weekly Report, 50,* 406–410.

Centers for Disease Control and Prevention. (2003). Guidelines for environmental infection control in health-care facilities. Recommendations of the CDC and the Healthcare Infection Control Practices Advisory Committee (HICPAC). *Morbidity and Mortality Weekly Report, 52*(RR-10), 1–42.

Centers for Disease Control and Prevention. (2004). Diagnosis and management of foodborne illnesses: A primer for physicians and other health care professionals. *Morbidity and Mortality Weekly Report, 53*(RR-4), 1–40.

Chen, X. M., Keithly, J. S., Paya, C. V., & LaRusso, N. F. (2002). Cryptosporidiosis. *New England Journal of Medicine, 346*, 1723–1731.

Corso, P. S., Kramer, M. H., Blair, K. A., Addiss, D. G., Davis, J. P., & Haddix, A. C. (2003). Cost of illness in the 1993 waterborne *Cryptosporidium* outbreak, Milwaukee, Wisconsin. *Emerging Infectious Diseases, 9*, 426–431.

Coupe, S., Sarfati, C., Hamane, S., & Derouin, F. (2005). Detection of cryptosporidium and identification to the species level by nested PCR and restriction fragment length polymorphism. *Journal of Clinical Microbiology, 43*, 1017–1023.

Dalle, F., Roz, P., Dautin, G., Di-Palma, M., Kohli, E., Sire-Bidault, C., et al. (2003). Molecular characterization of isolates of waterborne *Cryptosporidium* spp. collected during an outbreak of gastroenteritis in South Burgundy, France. *Journal of Clinical Microbiology, 41*, 2690–2693.

Eisenberg, J. N., Lei, X., Hubbard, A. H., Brookhart, M. A., & Colford, J. M., Jr. (2005). The role of disease transmission and conferred immunity in outbreaks: Analysis of the 1993 *Cryptosporidium* outbreak in Milwaukee, Wisconsin. *American Journal of Epidemiology, 161*, 62–72.

Fayer, R. (1997). The general biology of *Cryptosporidium*. In R. Fayer (Ed.), *Cryptosporidium and cryptosporidiosis* (pp. 2–42). Boca Raton, FL: CRC Press.

Fayer R. (2004). *Cryptosporidium*: A water-borne zoonotic parasite. *Veterinary Parasitology, 126*(1/2), 37–56.

Fayer, R., Graczyk, T. K., Cranfield, M. R., & Trout, J. M. (1996). Gaseous disinfection of *Cryptosporidium parvum* oocysts. *Applied Environmental Microbiology, 62*, 3908–3909.

Flint, J. A., Van Duynhoven, Y. T., Angulo, F. J., DeLong, S. M., Braun, P., Kirk, M., et al. (2005). Estimating the burden of acute gastroenteritis, foodborne disease, and pathogens commonly transmitted by food: An international review. *Clinical Infectious Diseases, 41*, 698–704.

Garner, J. S., & the Hospital Infection Control Practices Advisory Committee. (1996). Guideline for isolation precautions in hospitals. Part II. Recommendations for isolation precautions in hospitals. *Infection Control and Hospital Epidemiology, 17*, 53–80.

Glaberman, S., Moore, J. E., Lowery, C. J., Chalmers, R. M., Sulaiman, I., Elwin, K., et al. (2002). Three drinking-water-associated cryptosporidiosis outbreaks, Northern Ireland. *Emerging Infectious Diseases, 8*, 631–633.

Goh, S., Reacher, M., Casemore, D. P., Verlander, N. Q., Chalmers, R., Knowles, M., et al. (2004). Sporadic cryptosporidiosis, North Cumbria, England, 1996–2000. *Emerging Infectious Diseases, 10*, 1007–1015.

Goh, S., Reacher, M., Casemore, D. P., Verlander, N. Q., Charlett, A., Chalmers, R. M., et al. (2005). Sporadic cryptosporidiosis decline after membrane filtration of public water supplies, England, 1996–2002. *Emerging Infectious Diseases, 11*, 251–259.

Goldstein, S. T., Juranek, D. D., Ravenholt, O., Hightower, A. W., Martin, D. G., Mesnik, J. L., et al. (1996). Cryptosporidiosis: An outbreak associated with drinking water despite state-of-the-art water treatment. *Annals of Internal Medicine, 124*, 459–468.

Haas, C. N. (2000). Epidemiology, microbiology, and risk assessment of water-borne pathogens including *Cryptosporidium*. *Journal of Food Protection, 63,* 827–831.

Hellard, M., Hocking, J., Willis, J., Dore, G., & Fairley, C. (2003). Risk factors leading to *Cryptosporidium* infection in men who have sex with men. *Sexually Transmitted Infections, 79,* 412–414.

Hlavsa, M. C., Watson, J. C., & Beach, M. J. (2005). Cryptosporidiosis surveillance in the United States 1999–2002. *Morbidity and Mortality Weekly Report, 54*(SS-01), 1–8.

Howe, A. D., Forster, S., Morton, S., Marshall, R., Osborn, K. S., Wright, P., et al. (2002). *Cryptosporidium* oocysts in a water supply associated with a cryptosporidiosis outbreak. *Emerging Infectious Diseases, 8,* 619–624.

Hoxie, N. J., Davis, J. P., Vergeront, J. M., Nashold, R. D., & Blair, K. A. (1997). Cryptosporidiosis-associated mortality following a massive waterborne outbreak in Milwaukee, Wisconsin. *American Journal of Public Health, 87,* 2032–2035.

Hunter, P. R., Chalmers, R. M., Syed, Q., Verlander, N. Q., Chalmers, R. M., et al. (2004). Sporadic cryptosporidiosis case-control study with genotyping. *Emerging Infectious Diseases, 10,* 1241–1249.

Hunter, P. R., Hughes, S., Woodhouse, S., Raj, N., Syed, Q., Chalmers, R. M., et al. (2004). Health sequelae of human cryptosporidiosis in immunocompetent patients. *Clinical Infectious Disease, 39,* 504–510.

Insulander, M., Lebbad, M., Stenström, T. A., & Svenungsson, B. (2005). An outbreak of cryptosporidiosis associated with exposure to swimming pool water. *Scandinavian Journal of Infectious Diseases, 37,* 354–360.

Johnson, A., Linden, K., Ciociola, K. M., De Leon, R., Widmer, G., & Rochelle, P. A. (2005). UV inactivation of *Cryptosporidium hominis* as measured in cell culture. *Applied and Environmental Microbiology, 71,* 2800–2802.

Kaplan, J. E., Masur, H., Holmes, K. K., USPHS, & Infectious Disease Society of America. (2002). Guidelines for preventing opportunistic infections among HIV-infected persons—2002. Recommendations of the U.S. Public Health Service and the Infectious Diseases Society of America. *Morbidity and Mortality Weekly Report, 51*(RR-8), 1–52.

Keegan, A., Fanok, S., Monis, P. T., & Saint, C. P. (2003). Cell culture-TaqMan PCR assay for evaluation of *Cryptosporidium parvum* disinfection. *Applied and Environmental Microbiology, 69,* 2505–2511.

Khalakdina, A., Vugia, D. J., Nadle, J., Rothrock, G. A., & Colford, J. M., Jr. (2003). Is drinking water a risk factor for endemic cryptosporidiosis? A case-control study in the immunocompetent general population of the San Francisco Bay area. *BMC Public Health, 3,* 11.

Kramer, M. H., Sorhage, F. E., Goldstein, S. T., Dalley, E., Wahlquist, S. P., & Herwaldt, B. L. (1998). First reported outbreak in the United States of cryptosporidiosis associated with a recreational lake. *Clinical Infectious Disease, 26,* 27–33.

LeChevallier, M. W., Norton, W. D., & Lee, R. G. (1991). *Giardia* and *Cryptosporidium* spp. in filtered drinking water supplies. *Applied and Environmental Microbiology, 57,* 2617–2621.

Lim, L. S., Varkey, P., Giesen, P., & Edmonson, L. (2004). Cryptosporidiosis outbreak in a recreational swimming pool in Minnesota. *Journal of Environmental Health, 67,* 16–20, 2728.

MacKenzie, W. R., Hoxie, N. J., Proctor, M. E., Gradus, M. S., Blair, K. A., Peterson, D. E., et al. (1994). A massive outbreak in Milwaukee of *Cryptosporidium* infection transmitted through the public water supply. *New England Journal of Medicine, 331,* 151–167.

Mathieu, E., Levy, D. A., Veverka, F., Parrish, M. K., Sanisky, J., Shapiro, N., et al. (2004). Epidemiologic and environmental investigation of a recreational water outbreak caused by two genotypes of *Cryptosporidium parvum* in Ohio in 2000. *American Journal of Tropical Medicine and Hygiene, 71,* 582–589.

Matos, O., Alves, M., Xiao, L., Cama, V., & Antunes, F. (2004). *Cryptosporidium felis* and *C. meleagridis* in persons with HIV, Portugal. *Emerging Infectious Disease, 10,* 2256–2257.

McAnulty, J. M., Fleming, D. W., & Gonzalez, A. H. (1994). A community-wide outbreak of cryptosporidiosis associated with swimming at a wave pool. *Journal of the American Medical Association, 272,* 1597–1600.

McDonald, A. C., MacKenzie, W. R., Addiss, D. G., Gradus, M. S., Linke, G., Zembrowski, E., et al. (2001). *Cryptosporidium parvum*-specific antibody responses among children residing in Milwaukee during the 1993 waterborne outbreak. *Journal of Infectious Disease, 183,* 1373–1379.

McLauchlin, J., Amar, C., Pedraza-Diaz, S., & Nichols, G. L. (2000). Molecular epidemiological analysis of *Cryptosporidium* spp. in the United Kingdom: Results of genotyping *Cryptosporidium* spp. in 1,705 fecal samples from humans and 105 fecal samples from livestock animals. *Journal of Clinical Microbiology, 38,* 3984–3990.

Mead, P. S., Slutsker, L., Dietz, V., McCaig, L. F., Bresee, J. S., Shapiro, C., et al. (1999). Food-related illness and death in the United States. *Emerging Infectious Diseases, 5,* 607–625.

Mendez-Hermida, F., Castro-Hermida, J. A., Ares-Mazas, E., Kehoe, S. C., & McGuigan, K. G. (2005). Effect of batch-process solar disinfection on survival of *Cryptosporidium parvum* oocysts in drinking water. *Applied and Environmental Microbiology, 71,* 1653–1654.

Millard, P. S., Gensheimer, K. F., Addiss, D. T., Sosin, D. M., Beckett, G. A., Houck-Jankoski, A., et al. (1994). An outbreak of cryptosporidiosis from fresh-pressed apple cider. *Journal of the American Medical Association, 272,* 1592–1596.

Mofenson, L. M., Oleske, J., Serchuck, L., Van Dyke, R., Wilfert, C., Centers for Disease Control and Prevention, National Institutes of Health, & Infectious Disease Society of America. (2004). Treating opportunistic infections among HIV-exposed and infected children: Recommendations from CDC, the National Institutes of Health, and the Infectious Diseases Society of America. *Morbidity and Mortality Weekly Report, 53*(RR-14), 1–92.

Moriarty, E. M., Duffy, G., McEnvoy, J. M., Caccio, S., Sheridan, J. H., McDowell, D., et al. (2005). The effect of thermal treatments on the viability and infectivity of *Cryptosporidium parvum* on beef surfaces. *Journal of Applied Microbiology, 98,* 618–623.

Morris, R. D., Naumova, E. N., & Griffiths, J. K. (1998). Did Milwaukee experience waterborne cryptosporidiosis before the large documented outbreak in 1993? *Epidemiology, 9,* 264–270.

Moss, D. M., Bennett, S. N., Arrowood, M. J., Wahlquist, S. P., & Lammie, P. J. (1998). Enzyme-linked immunoelectrotransfer blot analysis of a cryptosporidiosis outbreak on a United States Coast Guard cutter. *American Journal of Tropical Medicine & Hygiene, 58*(1), 110–118.

Naumova, E. N., Egorov, A. I., Morris, R. D., & Griffiths, J. K. (2003). The elderly and waterborne *Cryptosporidium* infection: Gastroenteritis hospitalizations before and during the 1993 Milwaukee outbreak. *Emerging Infectious Diseases, 9,* 418–425.

Nelson, D. B., Jarvis, W. R., Rutala, W. A., Foxx-Orenstein, A. E., Isenberg, G., Dash, G. P., et al. (2004). Multi-society guideline for reprocessing flexible gastrointestinal endoscopes. *Diseases of the Colon & Rectum, 47,* 413–421.

Ong, C. S., Eisler, D. L., Alikhani, A., Fung, V. W., Tomblin, J., Bowie, W. R., et al. (2002). Novel *Cryptosporidium* genotypes in sporadic cryptosporidiosis cases: First report of human infections with a cervine genotype. *Emerging Infectious Diseases, 8,* 263–268.

Palmieri, F., Cicalini, S., Froio, N., Rizzi, E. B., Goletti, D., Festa, A., et al. (2005). Pulmonary cryptosporidiosis in an AIDS patient: Successful treatment with paromomycin plus azithromycin. *International Journal of STD and AIDS, 16,* 515–517.

Pedraza-Diaz, S., Amar, C., Nichols, G. L., & McLauchlin, J. (2001). Nested polymerase chain reaction for amplication of the *Cryptosporidium* oocyst wall protein gene. *Emerging Infectious Diseases, 7,* 49–56.

Peeters, J. E., Mazas, E. A., Masschelein, W. J., Martinez de Maturana, I. V., & DeBacker, E. (1989). Effects of disinfection of drinking water with ozone or chlorine dioxide on survival of *Cryptosporidium parvum* oocysts. *Applied Environmental Microbiology, 55,* 1519–1522.

Preiser, G., Preiser, L., & Madeo, L. (2003). An outbreak of cryptosporidiosis among veterinary science students who work with calves. *American Journal of College Health, 51,* 213–215.

Quilez, J., Sanchez-Acedo, C., Avendano, C., del Cacho, E., & Lopez-Bernad, F. (2005). Efficacy of two peroxygen-based disinfectants for inactivation of *Cryptosporidium parvum* oocysts. *Applied and Environmental Microbiology, 71,* 2479–2483.

Roy, S. L., DeLong, S. M., Stenzel, S. A., Shiferaw, B., Roberts, J. M., Khalakdina, A., et al. (2004). Risk factors for sporadic cryptosporidiosis among immunocompetent persons in the United States from 1999 to 2001. *Journal of Clinical Microbiology, 42,* 2944–2951.

Savioli, L., Smith, H., & Thompson, A. (2006). *Giardia* and *Cryptosporidium* join the 'Neglected Diseases Initiative.' *Trends in Parasitology, 22,* 203–208.

Smerdon, W. J., Nichols, T., Chalmers, R. M., Heine, H., & Reacher, M. H. (2003). Foot and mouth disease in livestock and reduced cryptosporidiosis in humans, England and Wales. *Emerging Infectious Diseases, 9,* 22–28.

Smith, H. V., & Corcoran, G. D. (2004). New drugs and treatment for cryptosporidiosis. *Current Opinion in Infectious Diseases, 17,* 557–564.

Smith, K. E., Stenzel, S. A., Bender, J. B., Wagsrom, E., Soderlund, D., Leano, F. T., et al. (2004). Outbreaks of enteric infections caused by multiple pathogens associated with calves at a farm day camp. *Pediatric Infectious Disease Journal, 23,* 1098–1104.

Thurston-Enriquez, J. A., Gilley, J. E., & Eghball, B. (2005). Microbial quality of runoff following land application of cattle manure and swine slurry. *Journal of Water Health, 3,* 157–171.

Trask, J. R., Kalita, P. K., Kuhlenschmidt, M. S., Smith, R. D., & Funk, T. L. (2004). Overland and near-surface transport of *Cryptosporidium parvum* from vegetated and nonvegetated surfaces. *Journal of Environmental Quality, 33,* 984–993.

Vassal, S., Favennec, L., Ballet, J.-J., & Brasseur, P. (1998). Hydrogen peroxide gas plasma sterilization is effective against *Cryptosporidium parvum* oocytes. *American Journal of Infection Control, 26,* 136–138.

White, A. C., Jr. (2005). Cryptosporidiosis (*Cryptosporidium hominis, Cryptosporidium parvum,* and other species). In G. L. Mandell, J. E. Bennett, & R. Dolin (Eds.), *Mandell, Douglas, and Bennett's principles and practice of infectious diseases* (6th ed., pp. 3215–3228). Philadelphia: Elsevier Churchill Livingstone.

Wilson, J. A., & Margolin, A. B. (2003). Efficacy of glutaraldehyde disinfectant against *Cryptosporidium parvum* in the presence of various organic soils. *Journal of AOAC International, 86,* 96–100.

Working Group on Waterborne Cryptosporidiosis. (1997). Proactive detection of cryptosporidiosis by clinical laboratories. *Clinical Laboratory Science, 10*(5):246–249.

Xiao, L., Bern, C., Limor, J., Sulaiman, I., Roberts, J., Checkley, W., et al. (2001). Identification of 5 types of *Cryptosporidium* parasites in children in Lima, Peru. *Journal of Infectious Diseases, 183,* 492–497.

Yokoi, H., Tsuruta, M., Tanaka, T., Tsutake, M., Akiba, Y., Kimura, T., et al. (2005). *Cryptosporidium* outbreak in a sports center. *Japanese Journal of Infectious Disease, 58,* 331–332.

Zardi, E. M., Picardi, A., & Afeltra, A. (2005). Treatment of cryptosporidiosis in immunocompromised hosts. *Chemotherapy, 51,* 193–196.

Zhou, L., Singh, A., Jiang, J., & Xiao, L. (2003). Molecular surveillance of *Cryptosporidium* spp. in raw wastewater in Milwaukee: Implications for understanding outbreak occurrence and transmission dynamics. *Journal of Clinical Microbiology, 41,* 5254–5227.

CHAPTER SIX

Cyclospora cayetanensis
Arriving via Guatemalan Raspberries

Felissa R. Lashley

The guests at the June 2000 wedding reception returned home with more than memories or the bridal bouquet. The bride, groom, and many of the guests at a catered wedding reception in Philadelphia, Pennsylvania, developed diarrhea and other gastrointestinal illness within 1 to 7 days after attendance. Of the 83 attendees, 54 had symptoms that met the case definition for cyclosporiasis. The raspberry cream filling in the wedding cake was found to contain DNA fragments of *Cyclospora cayetanensis*. Subsequent investigation revealed that one Guatemalan farm that might have supplied raspberries used in the cake filling was also one of the potential sources for raspberries served at a bridal brunch in Georgia where cyclosporiasis also occurred, although no definitive source for contamination was found (Ho et al., 2002).

In the spring and summer of 1996, newspaper headlines brought into the public consciousness awareness of a relatively new emerging pathogen causing severe diarrhea known as *C. cayetanensis:* "Forbidding Fruit: How Safe Is Our Produce?" "Red-Letter Berries," "Parasite Search Shifts to Raspberries," and finally, "Florida Officials Link *Cyclospora* to Raspberries" (Boodman, 1997; Cohen, 1996; Criswell, 1998; "Florida Officials," 1996). In that time period, 1,465 cases of cyclosporiasis were reported in North America, followed by more than 1,600 cases in 1997 (Guerrant & Thielman, 1998). Little was known about this organism, and the occurrence of multistate outbreaks in consecutive years emphasized the need to learn more about this parasite so that future outbreaks

could be prevented or treated most effectively. At first, the vehicle for
C. cayetanensis was believed to be strawberries. This belief had a mone-
tary effect on that industry before Guatemalan raspberries were identified
as the major culprit in these outbreaks. Before this time, *C. cayetanensis*
was virtually unknown in North America.

C. *cayetanensis* is a coccidian spore-forming protozoan parasite
(Hoang et al., 2005). The species name was proposed after the Uni-
versidad Peruana Cayetano Heredia in Lima, Peru, where Y. R. Ortega
did work on elucidating characteristics of the organism (Taylor, Davis,
& Soave, 1997). *Cyclospora* share many similarities with *Isospora* and
Cryptosporidium, other protozoan parasites causing diarrhea, and the
clinical illnesses caused by the three are very similar. The oocysts of
Cyclospora are spherical and measure 8–10 μm in diameter, which is
larger than those of *Cryptosporidium* but smaller than those of *Isospora*.
Infection occurs by ingesting sporulated oocysts. During sporulation, each
Cyclospora oocyst has two sporocysts, each containing two sporozoites,
in contrast to *Isospora*, which has four sporozoites in two sporocysts, and
Cryptosporidium, which has four sporozoites per oocyst.

In contrast to *Cryptosporidium*, which is immediately infectious to
another host, it appears that a period of time (weeks or months) outside
the human body is necessary for *Cyclospora* to sporulate and become
infectious; thus, direct transmission from person to person is unlikely,
and secondary household cases have not been noted. Transmission can
occur from sufficiently aged stool or stool-contaminated items (Dillingham, Pape, Herwaldt, & Guerrant, 2006; Mansfield & Gajadhar, 2004).
Many other aspects of its basic biology and related issues are not yet
elucidated. Members of other *Cyclospora* species are found in other animals such as snakes, moles, rodents, and centipedes, but *C. cayetanensis*
is the only species known to date to infect humans (Fisk, Keystone, &
Kozarsky, 2005). It is resistant to chlorine and formalin (Taylor et al.,
1997). Asymptomatic carriers may be reservoirs of infection since they
may excrete oocysts without becoming ill, and natives of endemic areas
frequently are asymptomatic (Fisk et al., 2005). Diagnosis is by identification of oocysts in stool samples using microscopy for measuring and
characterizing oocysts. These exhibit bright blue autofluorescence under
ultraviolet light and are acid fast with variable appearance on staining.
Diagnosis may be by oocyst detection in stool, intestinal fluid, or tissue
specimens or by *C. cayetanensis* DNA detection using polymerase chain
reaction in samples. A specific request for *Cyclospora* testing in persons
with prolonged diarrhea may be necessary in order to make the diagnosis (Mansfield & Gajadhar, 2004). Further information may be found in
Centers for Disease Control and Prevention (CDC; 2006).

Identification of *Cyclospora* began to be made more often after acid-
fast staining was modified for the detection of *Cryptosporidium* in the

mid-1980s. Before *Cyclospora* had been characterized and named, it had been described in the literature in various ways, most commonly as coccidian-like, "big Crypto," *Cryptosporidium*-like, cyanobacterium-like body, a fungal spore, and blue-green alga-like body (Pape, Verdier, Boncy, Boncy, & Johnson, 1994; Soave, Herwaldt, & Relman, 1998). Thus, some cases of diarrheal illness attributed to *Cryptosporidium* may actually have been due to *Cyclospora*. Although first described in moles in 1870 (Ortega, Gilman, & Sterling, 1994), the first description of illness with *Cyclospora* in humans was in a 1979 publication describing it as an "undescribed coccidian" seen in human stool specimens "by chance" in Papua New Guinea in 1977 (Ashford, 1979). Other reports followed, and a worldwide distribution has been recognized across age groups.

Much of the information on *Cyclospora* comes from Nepal, Haiti, and Peru, endemic areas where original research was performed early or in reports about illness in a small number of returning travellers. In 1986, diarrheal illness in returning travellers from Haiti and Mexico was associated with a "new intestinal pathogen" that was thought to be either a coccidian parasite or a fungus (Soave, Dubey, Ramos, & Tummings, 1986). In 1989, what is now known to be *Cyclospora* but that was described then as an "alga-like organism," was identified among 59 patients with prolonged diarrhea who attended a clinic for foreign tourists and foreign-born residents living in Katmandu, Nepal; the sickness occurred mainly during the monsoon season (CDC, 1991). In 1994, diarrhea due to *Cyclospora* was identified in British soldiers and dependants in a military detachment in Nepal due to contaminated chlorinated water, pointing out the need for additional water treatment (Rabold et al., 1994). In Peru, among indigenous populations, 22% of children infected with *Cyclospora* had diarrhea, and the organism was recognized to cause mild disease that was asymptomatic (Madico, McDonald, Gilman, Cabrera, & Sterling, 1997). In Jakarta, Indonesia, *Cyclospora* was found to be the main protozoal cause of diarrhea in adult foreign residents in the wet season but rarely caused illness in the indigenous population (Fryauff et al., 1999). *Cyclospora* was reported as the second most frequent cause of diarrhea among foreigners with less than 2 years of residence in Nepal (Shlim et al., 1999). It is increasingly being recognized as a cause of diarrhea among international travelers (Gascon, 2006). The first reported outbreak of *C. cayetanensis* infection in a disease endemic area among susceptible persons occurred among Dutch attendees at a conference in Indonesia in 2001, but no source was identified (Blans, Ridwan, Verweij, Rozenberg-Arska, & Verhoef, 2005).

The first reported outbreak in North America occurred in Chicago among 21 personnel (physician housestaff and 3 others) who drank chlorinated tap water supplied from an apparently contaminated storage tank in a physician's dormitory (Huang et al., 1995). In the spring of 1993, three isolated cases of diarrhea in immunocompetent persons in Massachusetts who had not traveled outside the country were associated with *C. cayetanensis* (Ooi, Zimmerman, & Needham, 1995). An isolated case of explosive diarrhea due to *C. cayetanensis* in 1992 apparently resulted from exposure to sewage that backed up in the patient's basement in Utah (Hale, Aldeen, & Carroll, 1994). Other reports of infection detected in the United States were usually in returning travelers from countries such as Mexico and Thailand (Berlin et al., 1994). In 1995, an outbreak of cyclosporiasis affecting 33 persons was linked to drinking from a water cooler at a New York golf course (Carter, Guido, Jacquette, & Rapoport, 1996; Herwaldt, 2000). Also in 1995, a laboratory in Florida identified cases of *Cyclospora*-associated diarrhea that were both sporadic and in clusters associated with separate social events. This identification occurred as a result of routine screening for the organism in stool specimens. Imported raspberries were implicated in most cases as the source of the infections, but association with contact with soil such as during gardening could not be excluded as a cause in some instances (Koumans et al., 1998). These events are now considered to have been harbingers of the large-scale events that occurred in 1996 and 1997.

In 1996 and 1997, major outbreaks called attention to *Cyclospora* and the need for considering this organism in the differential diagnosis of diarrhea. In 1996, ultimately 1,465 persons in 20 U.S. states (most east of the Rocky Mountains), the District of Columbia, and two Canadian provinces had cyclosporiasis (CDC, 1997; Soave et al., 1998). Imported Guatemalan raspberries were identified as the major vehicle. Control measures were introduced at the end of 1996, and only those Guatemalan farms meeting certain standards in regard to water quality, employee hygiene, and sanitary conditions were allowed to export berries to the United States in 1997 (CDC, 1997; Herwaldt, Beach, & the *Cyclospora* Working Group, 1999; Soave et al., 1998).

In 1997, U.S. health department surveillance systems were put on alert in anticipation of possible *Cyclospora* outbreaks. In the spring, outbreaks began to be reported in association with imported raspberries. Despite the identification of the association in early April 1997, it was not until the end of May that the importation of raspberries into the United States from Guatemala was suspended (Osterholm, 1999). Epidemiologic investigation of the 1997 outbreaks in 18 states, the District of Columbia, and two Canadian provinces implicated not only Guatemalan raspberries but also mesclun (also known as spring mix, mixed baby lettuce, or field greens) and also was associated with fresh basil, which, in one cluster, was served in a cold basil pesto pasta salad (CDC, 1997, 1998b). How these were contaminated was not determined. Outbreaks of infection were again linked to fresh basil in Missouri in July 1999 and in British Columbia in 2001, basil and mesclun in Illinois and Texas in 2004, and basil in Florida and Toronto, Canada in 2005 (CDC, 2004; "Cyclosporiasis—Canada (Ontario)," 2005; "Cyclosporiasis—USA (Texas, Illinois)," 2004; "Cyclosporiasis—USA (Florida) (03)," 2005; Hoang et al., 2005; Lopez et al., 2001). Fresh mixed salad and herbs appeared to be vehicles of infection in a German outbreak in 2000, and fresh snow peas in a pasta salad were implicated in a 2004 outbreak in Pennsylvania (CDC, 2004; Döller et al., 2002). Major non-travel-related outbreaks are summarized in Table 6.1.

The Food and Drug Administration (FDA) did not permit Guatemalan raspberries to be imported into the United States in the spring of 1998 but worked with the Guatemalan government and business community to allow importation under certain conditions in future years. Canada did not enact such a restriction. In the spring of 1998 in Toronto, Canada, clusters of cyclosporiasis were reported to be linked to fresh raspberries from Guatemala (CDC, 1998a), and over 300 persons were affected ("Cyclosporiasis—Canada," 1999). In 1999, there were several outbreaks, and Guatemalan blackberries were suggested but not proven to be the cause in two. In 2000, other outbreaks occurred, and in two of them Guatemalan raspberries were implicated as the source (Herwaldt, 2000).

How the berries were contaminated is not known. Possibilities investigated included fecal contamination of water used to spray fruit for irrigation or pests, contamination during the sorting and packing process through direct handling, and insect- or bird-dropping contamination occurring before picking (Bern et al., 1999; Osterholm, 1999). Improvements related to sanitary practices and use of better quality water on berry farms in 1996 in Guatemala as a result of the 1996 outbreaks did not prevent the 1997 occurrences (Herwaldt et al., 1999). In developing countries, endemic infections with *Cyclospora* seem to fluctuate with the season, with a greater incidence in warm weather and rainy seasons; to display a higher frequency in children aged 18 months to 9 years; to be associated with certain variables such as fowl ownership, drinking untreated water, and type of sewage and water systems; and to affect children under 2 years of age with exposure to soil more frequently (Bern et al., 1999). An epidemiological survey in Peru detected *Cyclospora* on the surfaces of vegetables sold in the marketplace, and while the numbers were reduced, the organism was not eliminated with washing (Ortega et al., 1997).

Cyclospora is noted as one of the important opportunistic intestinal parasites in human immunodeficiency virus (HIV)-infected patients, especially in developing countries and less so in developed countries (Wiwanitkit, 2006). Pape and colleagues (1994) identified *Cyclospora* as the third

Table 6.1. Selected Non-Travel-Related *Cyclospora* Outbreaks

Year	Food Vehicle	Region/Country of Outbreak	Country of Vehicle Origin
1995	Fresh raspberries (?)	Florida, United States	Guatemala (?)
1996	Fresh raspberries	Multiple U.S. states, Canada	Guatemala
1997	Mesclun lettuce	Florida, United States	Peru
1997	Inconclusive	Ontario, Canada	?
1997	Fresh raspberries	California, Florida, Nevada, New York, Texas, United States	Guatemala, Chile (?)
1997	Fresh basil/pesto sauce	Virginia, Maryland, Washington DC, United States	?
1998	Fresh raspberries	Ontario, Canada	Guatemala (?)
1999	Inconclusive	Florida, United States	?
1999	Fresh basil	Missouri, United States	Mexico, United States (?)
2000	Fresh raspberries	Georgia, United States	Guatemala
2000	Fresh raspberries/ cake filling	Pennsylvania, United States	Guatemala
2000	Fresh herbs/mixed salad	Germany	Italy, France
2001	Fresh Thai basil	British Columbia, Canada	Thailand
2004	Fresh snow peas in pasta salad	Pennsylvania, United States	Guatemala
2004	Fresh basil/mesclun	Illinois, Texas, United States	Peru
2005	Fresh basil	Florida, United States	?
2005	Fresh basil	Ontario, Canada	Peru (?)

Note: ? = suspected but not confirmed.
Sources: Centers for Disease Control and Prevention, 2004; "Cyclosporiasis—Canada (Ontario)," 2005; "Cyclosporiasis—USA (Texas, Illinois)," 2004; "Cyclosporiasis—USA (Florida) (03)," 2005); Döller et al., 2002; Herwaldt, 2000; Ho et al., 2002; Hoang et al., 2005; Lopez et al., 2001.

most frequent enteric protozoan in acquired immunodeficiency syndrome (AIDS) patients with diarrhea in their series of 450 patients in Haiti. In HIV-infected persons, the clinical manifestations are more prolonged and harder to treat (Lashley, 2000).

Clinically, *C. cayetanensis* infects both immunocompetent and immunocompromised hosts. It attacks the upper small intestine, causing inflammation, villous atrophy, and crypt hyperplasia (Berlin et al., 1994). D-Xylose absorption is impaired. Inflammatory changes may persist after *Cyclospora* has been eliminated, and a myelin-like material that is visible on electron microscopy may persist in the small intestine (Cross & Sherchand, 2004). The clinical features are very similar to syndromes caused by other parasitic organisms causing diarrhea. Watery diarrhea, often yellow or khaki green in color, without blood or inflammatory cells is the chief symptom. It may be explosive. Severe fatigue, anorexia, nausea, vomiting, increased flatus, abdominal bloating, weight loss, and stomach cramps often accompany the diarrhea. A small percentage may have fever, chills, and flu-like symptoms. There may be cycles of remission and relapse, and episodes of diarrhea may alternate with constipation. Illness may occur as early as 1 day after exposure through 11 days, with an average of 1 week. In untreated immunocompetent adults, the infection may last from up to 1 or 2 months or longer (Dillingham et al., 2006; Fisk et al., 2005). Reiter syndrome (ocular inflammation, oligoarthritis, and sterile urethritis), known to be a sequelae of other enteric infections, has been described following protracted *Cyclospora* infection (Fisk et al., 2005).

Trimethoprim–sulfamethoxazole (TMP-SMX) is the treatment of choice and is very effective. Ciprofloxacin (500 mg twice a day) may be used for those who cannot tolerate sulfa drugs but may not have the same efficacy. TMP-SMX is recommended in a double-strength oral tablet (in adults, 160 mg TMP plus 800 mg SMX) twice per day for 1 week. HIV-infected persons may require higher doses and longer treatment, but the advent of highly active antiretroviral treatment (HAART) has resulted in more effective treatment (Cross & Sherchand, 2004; Dillingham et al., 2006; Wiwanitkit, 2006). Antidiarrheal agents, peristaltic regulators, and histamine-receptor blockers do not appear effective in controlling symptoms. Oral instead of intravenous rehydration is usually adequate. Precautions against acquiring *Cyclospora* during travel are the same as those for other intestinal parasites. Washing berries imported into the United States may or may not be effective in preventing illness, particularly because of the physical composition of raspberries; however, eating them can be avoided, although it may be that their presence in a served dish such as fruit salad may be enough to allow infection without eating the actual contaminated fruit itself.

In summary, *C. cayetanensis* is a recently recognized emerging parasitic pathogen that is both food- and waterborne. Because it is resistant to chlorine, it may be necessary to boil water or use filters for better protection in endemic areas. Low levels of *C. cayetanensis* are sufficient to cause diarrhea. In the United States it has most often been associated with contaminated raspberries imported from Guatemala, mesclun lettuce, and fresh basil, although contaminated water has also been a source. It will be detected more often in coming years as laboratories develop better diagnostic methods and routinely screen for it. *Cyclospora* occurs in both immunocompetent and immunocompromised persons causing diarrhea, fatigue, anorexia, weight loss, and other symptoms and may be seen in returning travelers and in community outbreaks. It has a worldwide distribution and is endemic in many developing countries. It should be considered in persons with prolonged or unexplained diarrhea, particularly if nonresponsive to therapy. *Cyclospora* responds readily to treatment with TMP-SMX, but other therapies need to be identified, especially for those allergic to sulfa drugs.

REFERENCES

Ashford, R. W. (1979). Occurrence of an undescribed coccidian in man in Papua New Guinea. *Annals of Tropical Medicine and Parasitology, 73,* 497–500.

Berlin, G. G. W., Novak, S. M., Porschen, R. K., Long, E. G., Stelma, G. N., & Schaeffer, F. W., III. (1994). Recovery of *Cyclospora* organisms from patients with prolonged diarrhea. *Clinical Infectious Diseases, 18,* 606–619.

Bern, C., Hernandez, B., Lopez, M. B., Arrowood, M. J., de Mejia, M. A., de Merida, A. M., et al. (1999). Epidemiologic studies of *Cyclospora cayetanensis* in Guatemala. *Emerging Infectious Diseases, 5,* 766–774.

Blans, M. C. A., Ridwan, B. U., Verweij, J. J., Rozenberg-Arska, M., & Verhoef, J. (2005). Cyclosporiasis outbreak, Indonesia. *Emerging Infectious Diseases, 11,* 1453–1455.

Boodman, S. G. (1997, July 8). Forbidding fruit: How safe is our produce? *Washington Post,* p. Z10.

Carter, R. J., Guido, F., Jacquette, G., & Rapoport, M. (1996, April). Outbreak of *Cyclospora* at a country club—New York, 1995 [Abstract]. In *45th Annual Epidemic Intelligence Service (EIS) Conference* (p. 58). Atlanta, GA: U.S. Department of Health and Human Services, Public Health Service.

Centers for Disease Control. (1991). Outbreaks of diarrheal illness associated with cyanobacteria (blue-green algae)-like bodies—Chicago, Nepal, 1989 and 1990. *Morbidity and Mortality Weekly Report, 40,* 325–327.

Centers for Disease Control and Prevention. (1997). Update: Outbreak of cyclosporiasis—United States and Canada 1997. *Morbidity and Mortality Weekly Report, 46,* 521–523.

Centers for Disease Control and Prevention. (1998a). Outbreak of cyclosporiasis—Ontario, Canada, May, 1998. *Morbidity and Mortality Weekly Report, 47,* 806–809.

Centers for Disease Control and Prevention. (1998b). *Preventing emerging infectious diseases: A strategy for the 21st century.* Atlanta, GA: Author.

Centers for Disease Control and Prevention. (2004). Outbreak of cyclosporiasis associated with snow peas—Pennsylvania, 2004. *Morbidity and Mortality Weekly Report, 53,* 876–878.

Centers for Disease Control and Prevention. (2006). Surveillance for foodborne-disease outbreaks—United States, 1998–2002. *Morbidity and Mortality Weekly Report, 55* (SS-10), 1–43.

Cohen, J. S. (1996, July 11). Parasite search shifts to raspberries. *USA Today,* p. D1.

Criswell, A. (1998, March 25). Red-letter berries. *Houston Chronicles,* p. F1.

Cross, J. H., & J. B. Sherchand. (2004). Cyclosporiasis. In J. A. Cotruvo, A. Dufour, G. Rees, J. Bartram, R. Carr, D. O. Cliver, et al. (Eds.), *Waterborne zoonoses.* Geneva, Switzerland: World Health Organization.

Cyclosporiasis—Canada (Ontario). (1999). *ProMED Digest, 99*(157), unpaginated.

Cyclosporiasis—Canada (Ontario). (2005, May 6). Message posted to ProMED-mail electronic mailing list, archived at http://www.promedmail.org, Archive No. 20050506.1257.

Cyclosporiasis—USA (Florida) (03). (2005, June 4). Message posted to ProMED-mail electronic mailing list, archived at http://www.promedmail.org, Archive No. 20050604.1564.

Cyclosporiasis—USA (Texas, Illinois). (2004, May 26). Message posted to ProMED-mail electronic mailing list, archived at http://www.promedmail. org, Archive No. 20040526.1419.

Dillingham, R., Pape, J. W., Herwaldt, B. L., & Guerrant, R. L. (2006). *Cyclospora, Isospora,* and *Sarcocystis* infections. In R. L. Guerrant, D. H. Walker, & P. F. Weller (Eds.), *Tropical infectious diseases. Principles, pathogens, & practice* (2nd ed., pp. 1015–1023). Philadelphia: Churchill Livingstone Elsevier.

Döller, P. C., Dietrich, K., Filipp, N., Brockmann, S., Dreweck, C., Vonthein, R., et al. (2002). Cyclosporiasis outbreak in Germany associated with the consumption of salad, 2002. *Emerging Infectious Disases, 8,* 992–994.

Fisk, T. L., Keystone, J. S., & Kozarsky, P. (2005). *Cyclospora cayetanensis, Isospora belli, Sarcocystis* species, and *Blastocystis hominis.* In G. L. Mandell, J. E. Bennett, & R. Dolin (Eds.), *Mandell, Douglas, and Bennett's principles and practice of infectious diseases* (6th ed., pp. 3328–3337). New York: Elsevier Churchill Livingstone.

Florida officials link *Cyclospora* to raspberries. (1996, July 6). *Washington Post,* p. A3.

Fryauff, D. J., Krippner, R., Prodjodipuro, P., Ewald, C., Kawengian, S., Pegelow, K., et al. (1999). *Cyclospora cayetanensis* among expatriate and indigenous populations of West Java, Indonesia. *Emerging Infectious Diseases, 5,* 585–586.

Gascon, J. (2006). Epidemiology, etiology and pathophysiology of traveler's diarrhea. *Digestion, 73*(Suppl. 1), 102–108.

Guerrant, R. L., & Thielman, N. M. (1998). Emerging enteric protozoa: *Cryptosporidium, Cyclospora*, and microsporidia. In W. M. Schield, D. Armstrong, & J. M. Hughes (Eds.), *Emerging infections I* (pp. 233–245). Washington, DC: ASM Press.

Hale, D., Aldeen, W., & Carroll, K. (1994). Diarrhea associated with cyanobacterialike bodies in an immunocompetent host. *Journal of the American Medical Association, 271*, 144–145.

Herwaldt, B. L. (2000). *Cyclospora cayetanensis*: A review, focusing on the outbreaks of cyclosporiasis in the 1990s. *Clinical Infectious Diseases, 31*, 1040–1057.

Herwaldt, B. L., Beach, M. J., & the *Cyclospora* Working Group. (1999). The return of *Cyclospora* in 1997: Another outbreak of cyclosporiasis in North America associated with imported raspberries. *Annals of Internal Medicine, 130*, 210–220.

Ho, A. Y., Lopez, A. S., Eberhart, M. G., Levenson, R., Finkel, B. S., da Silva, A. J., et al. (2002). Outbreak of cyclosporiasis associated with imported raspberries, Philadelphia, Pennsylvania, 2000. *Emerging Infectious Diseases, 8*, 783–788.

Hoang, L. M. N., Fyfe, M., Ong, C., Harb, J., Champagne, S., Dixon, B., et al. (2005). Outbreak of cyclosporiasis in British Columbia associated with imported Thai basil. *Epidemiology and Infection, 133*, 23–27.

Huang, P., Weber, J. T., Sosin, D. M., Griffin, P. M., Long, E. G., Murphy, J. J., et al. (1995). The first reported outbreak of diarrheal illness associated with *Cyclospora* in the United States. *Annals of Internal Medicine, 123*, 409–414.

Koumans, E. H. A., Katz, D. J., Malecki, J. M., Kumar, S., Wahlquist, S. P., Arrowood, M., et al. (1998). An outbreak of cyclosporiasis in Florida in 1995: A harbinger of multistate outbreaks in 1996 and 1997. *American Journal of Tropical Medicine and Hygiene, 59*, 235–242.

Lashley, F. R. (2000). The clinical spectrum of HIV infection and its treatment. In J. D. Durham & F. R. Lashley (Eds.), *The person with HIV/AIDS: Nursing perspectives* (3rd ed., pp. 167–270). New York: Springer.

López, A. S., Dodson, D. R., Arrowood, M. J., Orlandi, P. A., Jr., da Silva, A. J., Bier, J. W., et al. (2001). Outbreak of cyclosporiasis associated with basil in Missouri in 1999. *Clinical Infectious Diseases, 32*, 1010–1017.

Madico, G., McDonald, J., Gilman, P. H., Cabrera, L., & Sterling, C. R. (1997). Epidemiology and treatment of *Cyclospora cayetanensis* infection in Peruvian children. *Clinical Infectious Diseases, 24*, 977–981.

Mansfield, L. S., & Gajadhar, A. A. (2004). *Cyclospora cayetanensis*, a food- and waterborne coccidian parasite. *Veterinary Parasitology, 126*, 73–90.

Ooi, W. W., Zimmerman, S. K., & Needham, C. A. (1995). *Cyclospora* species as a gastrointestinal pathogen in immunocompetent hosts. *Journal of Clinical Microbiology, 33*, 1267–1269.

Ortega, Y. R., Gilman, R. H., & Sterling, C. R. (1994). A new coccidian parasite (Apicomplexa: Eimeriidae) from humans. *Journal of Parasitology, 80*, 625–629.

Ortega, Y. R., Roxas, R., Gilman, R. H., Miller, N. J., Cabrera, L., Taquiri, C., et al. (1997). Isolation of *Cryptosporidium parvum* and *Cyclospora cayetanensis* from vegetables collected in markets of an endemic region in Peru. *American Journal of Tropical Medicine and Hygiene, 57,* 683–686.

Osterholm, M. T. (1999). Lessons learned again: Cyclosporiasis and raspberries. *Annals of Internal Medicine, 130,* 233–244.

Pape, J. W., Verdier, R.-I., Boncy, M., Boncy, J., & Johnson, W. D., Jr. (1994). *Cyclospora* infection in adults infected with HIV. *Annals of Internal Medicine, 121,* 654–657.

Rabold, J. G., Hoge, C. W., Shlim, D. R., Kefford, C., Rajah, R., & Echeverria, P. (1994). *Cyclospora* outbreak associated with chlorinated drinking water. *Lancet, 344,* 1360–1361.

Shlim, D. R., Hoge, C. W., Rajah, R., Scott, R. M., Pandy, P., & Echeverria, P. (1999). Persistent high risk of diarrhea among foreigners in Nepal during the first two years of residence. *Clinical Infectious Diseases, 29,* 613–616.

Soave, R., Dubey, J. P., Ramos, L. J., & Tummings, M. (1986). A new intestinal pathogen? *Clinical Research, 34*(2), 533A.

Soave, R., Herwaldt, B. L., & Relman, D. A. (1998). *Cyclospora. Infectious Disease Clinics of North America, 12,* 1–12.

Taylor, A. P., Davis, L. J., & Soave, R. (1997). *Cyclospora. Current Clinical Topics In Infectious Diseases, 17,* 256–268.

Wiwanitkit, V. (2006). Intestinal parasite infestation in HIV infected patients. *Current HIV Research, 4,* 87–96.

CHAPTER SEVEN

Dengue Fever

Barbara J. Holtzclaw

Residents of the Hawaiian Islands see many travelers and are well acquainted with a variety of infectious diseases imported to their communities by persons who contract the disease in other countries. In addition, Hawaii had not had a dengue fever outbreak of significant proportions in 56 years. Consequently, the incidence of 27 cases of dengue on Oahu, Maui, Kauai, and the Big Island in the summer of 2001 were initially considered by Health Department officials to be imported by travelers. It was not until laboratory tests were compared to patient histories and travel data that officials learned that 19 confirmed cases in Maui were spread among people who had not left the state. More than 100 suspicious cases were centered in East Maui areas of Hana, Nahiku, and Hamoa, and spread as far west as Haiku. From September 12, 2001, to April 30, 2002, a total of 1,644 persons in Hawaii, with no history of recent foreign travel, were tested for possible dengue infection. Although the initial source for the Maui outbreak occurred on Hana, the investigative follow up suggests that additional separate virus introductions led to cases on other affected islands. In Kauai, only one of four dengue-case patients had any known exposure to persons from Maui. None of the 26 confirmed infections on Oahu could be epidemiologically linked to exposures on Kauai or Maui. A total of 43 cases of imported dengue infection were reported, with all 15 dengue virus isolates related to Pacific Island isolates from recent years.

Entomologic surveys found that the usual dengue vector, *Aedes aegypti*, was an unlikely source because the species is isolated to relatively uninhabited areas of the island of Hawaii. Instead, the vector was a common species, *Aedes albopictus*, ubiquitous on all the affected islands.

Phylogenetic analysis shows similarities of the isolates to those found in Tahiti and Easter Island. The recent Hawaii dengue outbreak is a vivid example of how readily pathogens can cross great expanses of ocean to cause outbreaks in new territory. This outbreak emphasizes to health officials the need to monitor closely, respond to disease developments beyond their borders, and maintain surveillance and control of potential disease vectors when no immediate danger seems imminent (Effler et al., 2005).

Dengue (pronounced "denghee") fever (DF), dengue hemorrhagic fever (DHF), and the complications of dengue shock syndrome (DSS) represent a complex of related conditions that rank high among new and newly emerging infectious diseases. These conditions are mosquito-transmitted, acute viral diseases. Dengue is an ancient disease, with known periodic epidemics as early as 1779; however, these earliest outbreaks were usually infrequent; isolated to areas of endemic infections in Asia, Africa, and North America; and thought to be an unpleasant but "self-limiting" disease (Gubler, 1997). Officially, reports of epidemics were localized to isolated areas, and although several members of a household might include survivors of the disease, there were only a few outbreaks over a decade. Widespread epidemics of the 18th and 19th centuries were products of increased shipping activity that transported infected hosts and vectors from one country to another by sea. In the 20th century, wars and rapid transportation contributed to dengue transmission by returning infected military from the Pacific tropics or Southeast Asia to regions where natural vectors existed. By 2000, the number of dengue epidemics mounted dramatically as human and commercial traffic between countries increased (Isturiz, Gubler, & Brea del Castillo, 2000). By 2004, the Centers for Disease Control and Prevention (CDC) issued urgent warnings, citing the 2001 outbreak of dengue in Hawaii, that travelers must take a more active role in preventing spread of the disease by avoiding mosquito exposure (CDC, 2005b).

The agent causing dengue is an RNA virus belonging to the family *Flaviviridae* and is considered to be an arbovirus (arthropod-borne). Four serotypes are known and designated by the names DEN-1, DEN-2, DEN-3, and DEN-4. The specific serotype is determined serologically by the number of antigens the different viruses have in common. One factor that influences the evolution of the disease in new regions is the ability of the virus to develop new strains. Despite the fact that infection with one dengue serotype confers lifelong immunity to that virus, no cross-protective immunity exists against the other serotypes. All four dengue virus types share a number of features in common related to the way they initiate antibody responses. However, it is possible for two or more virus types to infect one host sequentially (secondary infections) and cause an antibody response in the sequential infection that is significantly different from that caused by primary infection. Therefore, the cocirculation of multiple viruses in a region increases the likelihood of this more severe reaction in a population. Immunization with a flavivirus outside the dengue complex also precipitates a secondary antibody response when the host develops a dengue virus infection.

The *Ae. aegypti* mosquito acquires and transmits the virus while probing and feeding on the blood of its host. Other species known to transmit the disease are *Aedes albopictus, Aedes polynesiensis,* and some forms of *Aedes scutellaris.* Humans are most often the original host, but in some regions monkeys have been found to be infected. An infected mosquito harbors the virus throughout its life, and females are capable of passing the virus by transovarian transmission to offspring. This "vertical" transmission of virus in the mosquito has not been recognized as a significant source of dengue outbreaks but remains a source of potential problems in eradicating the vector. *Ae. aegypti* eggs can remain viable for long periods despite months of dry conditions. Inability to survive cool temperatures has kept *Ae. aegypti* confined to the warmer latitudes and lower altitudes nearest to the equator throughout history. However, changing climatic conditions and unusually long warm seasons have allowed the mosquito to stray as far as 45 degrees north (Gubler, 2006; World Health Organization [WHO], 1997). Besides spread through the bite of an infected mosquito, dengue may be acquired through needlestick, transfusion, or transplant (Nemes et al., 2004).

The National Center for Infectious Diseases estimates there are 50–100 million cases of DF and several hundred thousand cases of DHF each year around the globe (CDC, 2005a). The numbers of cases of DF worldwide have steadily increased in the past three decades, particularly in the Western Hemisphere. Only DEN-2 virus was present in the Americas in 1970, but the introduction of DEN-1 in 1977 caused a 16-year epidemic. Introduction of DEN-4 followed a similar pattern and widespread epidemic in 1981. A new strain of DEN-2 from Southeast Asia, introduced to Cuba in 1981, caused the first major epidemic of DHF in the Americas with cases spreading to Venezuela, Colombia, Brazil, French Guiana, Suriname, and Puerto Rico (CDC, 2005b). By 1995, there were 250,000 cases of DF and 7,000 cases of DHF reported in the Americas, and by 2003 the American region reported 24 countries with confirmed DHF cases.

Transmission of a virulent viral disease such as DF depends on successful interaction of the infectious agent (the virus serotype), susceptible hosts (humans), and environmental conditions that harbor the vector (mosquitoes). Mosquitoes belonging to the tropical and subtropical species *Ae. aegypti* are the most common vectors of dengue virus transmission. *Ae. albopictus* and other mosquito types are capable of carrying the virus, although *Ae. aegypti* is particularly adapted to living easily in proximity of humans. The potential for other species as vectors for dengue was clear in the 2001 outbreak of dengue in Hawaii, where no *Ae. aegypti* were found but *Ae. albopictus* was present (Effler et al., 2005).

Humans contribute to the spread of disease. By leaving discarded equipment, cooking vessels, waste containers, and abandoned automobile tires to collect standing water where mosquitoes lay their larvae, human beings contribute to the spread (Gubler, 2006, Wilder-Smith & Schwartz, 2005). International commerce in recycled goods contributed a source of mosquito transport in 1985 when larvae of the *Ae. albopictus* were found in water-logged used tires sent from Japan to Houston for retreading (Moore & Mitchell, 1997) Within 2 years, the CDC reported the mosquito species had invaded 16 states.

There is also growing concern about the possible spread of diseases from one region to another by autochthonous transmission (Effler et al., 2005). Such infections are termed *autochthonous* if individuals were bitten by local mosquitoes that acquired the virus from another person with a case of dengue. This mode of transmission differs from that where the mosquito itself is infected by the virus. The cocirculation of multiple virus serotypes in a given area, known as *hyperendemicity*, contributes to this serious development and creates pools of more virulent infectious agents (Foster, Bennett, Carrington, Vaughan, & McMillan, 2004; Gubler, 1998). In several countries, serotype circulation has gone from absent, or single forms, to multiple serotypes (Isturiz et al., 2000). As new strains evolve, an ongoing resurgence of epidemics occurs.

Infections with dengue virus serotypes encompass a spectrum of severity from asymptomatic to critical illness. The World Health Organization (WHO) classification ranks these illnesses in increasing order of severity as mild dengue, classic dengue, and DHF (WHO, 1997). This classification has been used since 1974, with periodic updates in 1986, 1994, and 1997. Since the last update, recent challenges to the classification were prompted by the changing way dengue presents clinically (Deen et al., 2006). Pediatric patients with illness progressing to DHF do not always fit the criteria deemed necessary by the WHO for the diagnosis. Considerable overlap in symptoms of petechiae, thrombocytopenia, and the tourniquet test occurred between DF and DHF in one study (Phuong et al., 2004). Experts argue that having a consistent classification system worldwide is essential to accurate surveillance and guideline development. The present WHO classification scheme is limited by being based upon clinical findings primarily from Thailand and does not include newer findings from other regions (Rigau-Pérez, 2006).

Mild and classic dengue types are similar in symptomatology, are usually not fatal, and rarely affect children. Incubation is 3 to 14 days with an average of 4 to 7 days (Gubler, 2006). Duration of the milder dengue is less than 72 hours, while the patient with classic dengue is generally very ill for 7 days. In classic DF, symptoms include fever (rarely exceeding 40.5° C) that may drop and rebound, severe headache, retro-orbital pain, joint pains, weakness, and skin rashes as well as nonspecific symptoms. Typically, it is self-limited, lasting up to 7 days, but can include varying degrees of hemorrhagic manifestations such as purpura. Classic dengue is followed by intense weakness for many weeks. The more severe forms of the disease can affect nearly every organ system, either by direct viral invasion or by secondary sepsis, circulatory impairment, or coagulopathy. The newer emerging forms of severe dengue produce differing manifestations that cause confusion in classification, surveillance, and standard treatment (Foster et al., 2004).

The WHO classification (1997) defines DHF as the most severe form of dengue with the following characteristics: presence of high continuous fever (40–41° C) for 2 to 7 days, platelet count $<100,000/mm^3$, hemorrhagic manifestations, and excessive vascular permeability. Cough, headache, vomiting, and abdominal pain accompany fever and persist for 2 to 4 days. DHF is classified by the WHO into four grades of illnesses, based on severity. Grade I DHF includes fever with mild nonspecific symptoms and a positive tourniquet test (i.e., inflating the blood pressure cuff midway between the systolic and diastolic pressure for 5 minutes causes a shower of petechiae to appear below the cuff). Grade II has more severe symptoms and spontaneous hemorrhagic manifestations that include spontaneous petechiae, epistaxis, bleeding gums, and hematuria. Grade III is marked by circulatory failure with rapid weak pulse, narrowed pulse pressure, and hypotension. Grade IV is the most severe form of the disease and leads to DSS. A major drawback to this definition of severity and the term *hemorrhagic* in DHF is the emphases on bleeding and thrombocytopenia, which may be absent in DHF and present in DF (Deen et al., 2006). The defining pathognomonic feature of severe dengue, according to several experts, is the leakage from vascular permeability that promotes the threat of shock (Chaturvedi, Agarwal, Elbishbishi, & Mustafa, 2000). Because delay in diagnosis and treatment for hypervolemic shock from plasma leakage can increase death rates in persons with dengue illness, this danger sign requires as much emphasis as hemorrhage in heralding severe DHF (Deen et al., 2006). While mild DHF may be treated successfully with fluid and electrolyte therapy, the onset of DSS, without appropriate management, can lead quickly to death.

The exact pathogenesis of DHF remains unclear, although there is growing evidence that proinflammatory cytokines, such as interleukins, may play a role. The pyrogenic response to these chemical messengers explains the patient's shaking chills and high body temperatures that have earned the name "breakbone fever." The pathogenic factors determining progression of dengue infection to DHF and DSS are not clear and may involve viral characteristics, secondary infection with a second viral serotype, and such factors as the host immune response. When these antibodies bind to the new serotype, they increase cellular uptake of the virus and set off a cascade of cytokines and complement activation that alter endothelial surfaces, destroy platelets, and consume coagulation factors (Wilder-Smith & Schwartz, 2005). However, because more recent cases of DHF were reported in persons with primary infections, alternate mechanisms have been proposed, including those related to the organism and host response (Bennett et al., 2006; Foster et al., 2004).

Vascular permeability is a hallmark of DHF and DSS and can lower plasma volume more than 20% in severe cases (Gubler, 2006). Leakage of plasma from capillaries contributes to hepatomegaly, pleural or abdominal effusions, hemoconcentration, or hypoproteinemia. The tendency toward hemorrhage involves vascular fragility, thrombocytopenia, and coagulopathy. Thrombocytopenia leads to abnormal blood clotting and disseminated intravascular coagulopathy. Autopsy on most patients who die from DHF reveals gastrointestinal hemorrhage. Extensive circulatory collapse and internal hemorrhaging may result in death or DSS. DSS typically occurs between the third and seventh day of the disease, concurrent with or shortly after the fall in temperature. Neurologic involvement, from headache and dizziness to severe manifestations of convulsions, paresis, and coma, can occur in both DF and DHF. They are generally more severe when DEN-2 and DEN-3 serotypes are involved (WHO, 1997).

In clinical situations, the diagnosis of dengue is usually made by the presenting features of rash and laboratory findings. Infants and young children may present with undifferentiated febrile illness and maculopapular rash, while older children and adults may demonstrate an abrupt fever onset with a typical "saddleback" or bimodal temperature pattern, accompanied by symptoms of headache; muscle, bone, and joint pain; and more incapacitating illness. Adults and older children may also present with petechiae of the skin. According to the WHO criteria for classification of DHF, all four of the following signs must be present: fever, hemorrhagic tendency, thrombocytopenia, and evidence of plasma leakage (WHO, 1997). Diagnostic laboratory parameters include white cell count, hemoglobin, prothrombin time, creatinine, and bilirubin levels. Findings include low levels of white blood cells (leukopenia) and platelets (thrombocytopenia) and, often, an elevated level of the enzyme serum aminotransferase. In a recent study, the use of physical signs and symptoms and these laboratory tests produced an acceptable differentiation between dengue and other infections (Chadwick, Arch, Wilder-Smith, & Paton, 2006). The definitive diagnosis of dengue infection is dependent on laboratory tests on the serum or tissues of suspected cases that include isolating the virus, detecting viral antigen or RNA, or identifying specific antibodies.

Primary treatment of severe DHF involves fluid replacement of lost plasma with plasma, plasma expanders, or electrolyte solutions. Replacement of fluid must often be done rapidly, but with careful monitoring against overhydration to prevent pulmonary edema. Early replacement of fluid usually reverses DSS and can often prevent coagulopathy. The mortality rate of appropriately managed DHF is as low as 1% while the lack of health resources pushes up mortality rates above 5% (McBride, 1999). Patients with mild DHF can usually be treated with oral fluids and non-salicylate antipyretic drugs. There is no specific drug treatment for dengue. Symptom management for pain, muscle aches, and discomfort are basically those used in treating febrile illness. Aspirin and other salicylates are contraindicated because they may precipitate bleeding, acidosis, or Reye syndrome (Gibbons & Vaughn, 2002). Acetaminophen should be used with caution for temperatures above 39° C (CDC, 2006). There is a surprisingly short recovery period for patients with DHF, even those surviving shock, of 2 to 3 days (Gubler, 2006).

The spread of both vector and virus for dengue has been attributed to humans and is definitely a problem of urbanization. The urban environment is favorable to the breeding and survival of the mosquito. Moreover, the increase of international travel has led to shorter intervals between epidemics and to recurrent epidemics involving multiple serotypes (Gubler, 1998). Return of an infected person to a region where mosquitoes are prevalent can create an outbreak in a fresh region. More serious is the returning traveler who brings a new dengue serotype to a region where others already exist. Vigorous attempts to eradicate the vector by insecticidal sprays may bring about a false sense of security. Most authorities agree that controlling or eliminating the breeding sites are the only effective modes for controlling mosquitoes (Castle, Amador, Rawlins, Figueroa, & Reiter, 1999; Isturiz et al., 2000).

The environment is also significantly influenced by climatic changes that provide a favorable milieu for the vector, such as unusually long warm and rainy seasons. In a study of predictive factors for DF, the annual average vapor pressure was the most important individual predictor (Hales, de Wet, Maindonald, & Woodward, 2002). These factors raise concerns about the effects of even minimal changes brought about by global warming that allow vector mosquito species to survive in latitudes as far north as Tokyo, Rome, and New York (Patz, Martens, Focks, &

Jetten, 1998). The effects of El Niño and periodic changes in the environment continue to stimulate the study and prediction of climatic changes and their influence on arboviral disease by environmentalists (Cazelles, Chavez, McMichael, & Hales, 2005). Computer-based simulation analyses predict higher climate-related disease risks for hemorrhagic dengue by the year 2050 related to an average projected temperature elevation of 1.16° C (Patz et al., 1998). Use of new procedures for climate—dengue modeling with mathematical simulation models may improve the ability to predict future water and temperature conditions that favor dengue vectors (Cheng, Kalkstein, Focks, & Nnaji, 1998).

There is presently no available vaccine against dengue viruses, although considerable progress has been made in its development. Ideally, the vaccine should be effective against all serotypes to prevent the possibility of sequential infection and should confer lifelong immunity. Experts have determined that the ideal vaccine to achieve these goals should be a live, attenuated tetravalent vaccine (Gubler, 2006).

The primary mode of controlling dengue virus spread is through eliminating the mosquito vector in domestic sites where most transmission takes place. Early use of DDT in the late 1940s brought remarkable success, but rapidly developing resistance to this and other insecticides points out the shortcomings of this approach. Neighborhood spraying programs and aerial application of insecticide have failed to reduce the mosquito population. Larval source reduction remains a major effort of officials involved in vector control. There is an ongoing attempt to find organisms that are natural predators for controlling the mosquito *Ae. aegypti*. Metal drums, discarded tires, cemetery flower vases, and bromeliad leaf axils are natural water collectors that serve as breeding sites for the mosquito. Field trials in Vietnam tested use of copepods, microcrustacean predators, which were seeded into jars, wells, and water containers with success in reducing larvae numbers and disease incidence (Vu et al., 2005). Despite the severe effects of drought and dry seasons on survival of the copepods in both study regions, the use of this natural predator reduced larvae and may hold promise for mosquito control. Prevention of mosquito bites is discussed in Appendix C, Table C.5.

Community-wide participation is needed for effective vector control to avoid excessive reliance on insecticides and for help in clearing neighborhoods of receptacles that hold water where mosquitoes breed. Experts in control and prevention are not optimistic about success in keeping dengue vectors from spreading unless surveillance and control are supported by individuals, communities, governments, and worldwide health agencies (Gubler, 2002). Educating and motivating the public to be active participants are important steps, while the cooperation of nations in prevention and control is crucial.

REFERENCES

Bennett, S. N., Holmes, E. C., Chirivella, M., Rodriguez, D. M., Beltran, M., Vorndam, V., et al. (2006). Molecular evolution of dengue 2 virus in Puerto Rico: Positive selection in the viral envelope accompanies clade reintroduction. *Journal of General Virology, 87*, 885–893.

Castle, T., Amador, M., Rawlins, S., Figueroa, J. P., & Reiter, P. (1999). Absence of impact of aerial malathion treatment on *Aedes aegypti* during a dengue outbreak in Kingston, Jamaica. *Pan American Journal of Public Health, 5*, 100–105.

Cazelles, B., Chavez, M., McMichael, A. J., & Hales, S. (2005). Nonstationary influence of El Nino on the synchronous dengue epidemics in Thailand. *PLoS Medicine, 2*, e106.

Centers for Disease Control and Prevention. (2005a). *Fact sheet: Dengue/dengue hemorrhagic fever.* Retrieved July 22, 2006, from http://www.cdc.gov/ncidod/dvbid/dengue/facts.htm

Centers for Disease Control and Prevention. (2005b). Travel-associated dengue infections—United States, 2001–2004. *Morbidity and Mortality Weekly Report, 54,* 556–558.

Centers for Disease Control and Prevention. (2006). *Dengue and dengue hemorrhagic fever: Questions and answers—CDC Division of Vector-Borne Infectious Diseases (DVBID).* Retrieved July 15, 2006, from http://www.cdc.gov/ncidod/dvbid/dengue/dengue-qa.htm

Chadwick, D., Arch, B., Wilder-Smith, A., & Paton, N. (2006). Distinguishing dengue fever from other infections on the basis of simple clinical and laboratory features: Application of logistic regression analysis. *Journal of Clinical Virology, 35,* 147–153.

Chaturvedi, U. C., Agarwal, R., Elbishbishi, E. A., & Mustafa, A. S. (2000). Cytokine cascade in dengue hemorrhagic fever: Implications for pathogenesis. *FEMS Immunology and Medical Microbiology, 28,* 183–188.

Cheng, S., Kalkstein, L. S., Focks, D. A., & Nnaji, A. (1998). New procedures to estimate water temperatures and water depths for application in climate-dengue modeling. *Journal of Medical Entomology, 35,* 646–652.

Deen, J. L., Harris, E., Wills, B., Balmaseda, A., Hammond, S. N., Rocha, C., et al. (2006). The WHO dengue classification and case definitions: Time for a reassessment. *Lancet, 368,* 170–173.

Effler, P. V., Pang, L., Kitsutani, P., Vorndam, V., Nakata, M., Ayers, T., et al. (2005). Dengue fever, Hawaii, 2001–2002. *Emerging Infectious Diseases, 11,* 742–749.

Foster, J. E., Bennett, S. N., Carrington, C. V., Vaughan, H., & McMillan, W. O. (2004). Phylogeography and molecular evolution of dengue 2 in the Caribbean basin, 1981–2000. *Virology, 324,* 48–59.

Gibbons, R. V., & Vaughn, D. W. (2002). Dengue: An escalating problem. *British Medical Journal, 324,* 1563–1566.

Gubler, D. J. (1997). Dengue and dengue hemorrhagic fever: Its history and resurgence as a global public health problem. In D. J. Gubler & G. Kuno (Eds.),

Dengue and dengue hemorrhagic fever (pp. 1–22). New York: CAB International.

Gubler, D. J. (1998). Dengue and dengue hemorrhagic fever. *Clinical Microbiology Reviews, 11,* 480–496.

Gubler, D. J. (2002). Epidemic dengue/dengue hemorrhagic fever as a public health, social and economic problem in the 21st century. *Trends in Microbiology, 10,* 100–103.

Gubler, D. J. (2006). Dengue and dengue hemorrhagic fever. In R. L. Guerrant, D. H. Walker, & P. F. Weller (Eds.), *Tropical infectious diseases: Principles, pathogens & practice* (2nd ed., pp. 813–822). Philadelphia: Churchill Livingstone Elsevier.

Hales, S., de Wet, N., Maindonald, J., & Woodward, A. (2002). Potential effect of population and climate changes on global distribution of dengue fever: An empirical model. *Lancet, 360,* 830–834.

Isturiz, R. E., Gubler, D. J., & Brea del Castillo, J. (2000). Dengue and dengue hemorrhagic fever in Latin America and the Caribbean. *Infectious Disease Clinics of North America, 14,* 121–140.

McBride, J.H. (1999). Dengue fever: An Australian perspective. *Australian Family Physician, 28*(4), 319–323.

Moore, C. G., & Mitchell, C. J. (1997). *Aedes albopictus* in the United States: Ten-year presence and public health implications. *Emerging Infectious Diseases, 3,* 329–334.

Nemes, Z., Kiss, G., Madarassi, E. P., Peterfi, Z., Ferenczi, E., Bakonyi, T., et al. (2004). Nosocomial transmission of dengue. *Emerging Infectious Diseases, 10,* 1880–1881.

Patz, J. A., Martens, W. J., Focks, D. A., & Jetten, T. H. (1998). Dengue fever epidemic potential as projected by general circulation models of global climate change. *Environmental Health Perspectives, 106,* 147–153.

Phuong, C. X. T., Nhan, N. T., Kneen, R., Thuy, P. T. T., Van Thien, C., Nga, N. T. T., et al. (2004). Clinical diagnosis and assessment of severity of confirmed dengue infections in Vietnamese children: Is the World Health Organization classification system helpful? *American Journal of Tropical Medicine and Hygiene, 70,* 172–179.

Rigau-Pérez, J. G. (2006). Severe dengue: The need for case definitions. *Lancet Infectious Diseases, 6,* 297–302.

Vu, S. N., Nguyen, T. Y., Tran, V. P., Truong, U. N., Le, Q. M., Le, V. L., et al. (2005). Elimination of dengue by community programs using Mesocyclops (Copepoda) against *Aedes aegypti* in central Vietnam. *American Journal of Tropical Medicine & Hygiene, 72,* 67–73.

Wilder-Smith, A., & Schwartz, E. (2005). Dengue in travelers. *New England Journal of Medicine, 353,* 924–932.

World Health Organization. (1997). Clinical diagnosis. In *Dengue haemorrhagic fever: Diagnosis, treatment, prevention and control* (2nd ed., pp. 12–23). Geneva: World Health Organization.

CHAPTER EIGHT

Ebola, Marburg, Lassa, and Other Hemorrhagic Fevers

Daniel G. Bausch

A 29-year-old woman presents to her local internist with a 3-day history of fever, general malaise, headache, and myalgia. She returned 10 days earlier from a safari in East Africa that included backpacking in the wilderness, swimming in Lake Victoria, and spelunking, accompanied by her husband and 5-year-old daughter. The physical exam reveals hyperthermia, tachycardia, and diaphoresis. Laboratory tests show mild leucopenia and thrombocytopenia and elevated serum urea nitrogen and creatinine. A rapid test for influenza is negative. Acetaminophen and oral rehydration solution are prescribed, and the patient is discharged with a diagnosis of "viral syndrome." However, the next day she presents to the emergency room with worsening symptoms, including severe epigastric pain, persistent vomiting, and a morbilliform rash over her face and torso. She notes that her "menstruation has begun early." Her husband, who accompanied her to the emergency room, also complains of a headache and feeling feverish since that morning. The emergency room physician is concerned about "exotic diseases" and requests consultation from the infectious disease service, which recommends hospitalizing the woman and her husband, implementing isolation measures, and performing a battery of tests, including malaria smears and tests for various viral hemorrhagic fevers. The malaria smears are negative, but enzyme-linked immunosorbent assay (ELISA) testing at the Centers for Disease Control and Prevention (CDC) is positive for Ebola antigen. Local, state, and federal health authorities are alerted and contact tracing is initiated.

Table 8.1. Principal Viruses Causing Hemorrhagic Fevers

Virus	Disease	Geographic Distribution	Principal Reservoir/Vector	Annual Cases	Case: Infection Ratio	Human-to-Human Transmissibility
Filoviridae						
Ebola	Ebola hemorrhagic fever	Sub-Saharan Africa, Philippines?	Unknown	[a]	1:1	High
Marburg	Marburg hemorrhagic fever	Sub-Saharan Africa	Unknown	[a]	1:1	High
Arenaviridae						
Lassa	Lassa fever	West Africa	Rodent (multimammate rat or *Mastomys* spp.)	100,000–300,000	1:5–10	Moderate
Junin	Argentine hemorrhagic fever	Argentine pampas	Rodent (corn mouse or *Calomys musculinus*)	100–200	1:1.5	Low
Machupo	Bolivian hemorrhagic fever	Beni department, Bolivia	Rodent (large vesper mouse or *Calomys callosus*)	<50	1:1.5	Low
Guanarito	Venezuelan hemorrhagic fever	Portuguesa state, Venezuela	Rodent (cane mouse or *Zygodontomys brevicauda*)	<50	1:1.5	Low
Sabiá[b]	Proposed name: Brazilian hemorrhagic fever	Rural area near São Paulo, Brazil?	Unknown (rodent?)	[b]	1:1.5	Low?

Bunyaviridae Hantaan, Seoul, Puumala, Dobrava, Others	Hemorrhagic fever with renal syndrome	Hantaan: northeast Asia; Seoul: urban areas worldwide; Puumala and Dobrava: Europe	Rodent (Hantaan: the striped field mouse or *Apodemus agrarius*; Seoul: Norway rat or *Rattus norvegicus*; Puumala: bank vole or *Clethrionomys glareolus*; Dobrava: yellow-necked field mouse or *Apodemus flavicollis*)	50,000–150,000	Hantaan: 1:1.5 Others: 1:20	No
Rift Valley fever	Rift Valley fever	Sub-Saharan Africa	Domestic livestock/mosquitoes (*Aedes* and others)	100–100,000[a]	1:100	No
Crimean-Congo hemorrhagic fever	Crimean-Congo hemorrhagic fever	Africa, Middle East, Balkans, southern Russia, western China	Wild and domestic vertebrates/tick (*Hyalomma* spp.)	~100	1:1–2	High
Flaviviridae Yellow fever	Yellow fever	Africa, South America	Monkey/mosquito (*Aedes aegypti*, other *Aedes* and *Haemagogus* spp.)	5,000–200,000[c]	1:2–20	No
Dengue	Dengue fever and dengue hemorrhagic fever	Tropics and subtropics worldwide	Human/mosquito (*Aedes aegypti*)	Dengue fever: 100 million, Dengue hemorrhagic fever: 100,000–200,000[c]	1:10–100 depending on age, previous infection, genetic background, and infecting serotype	No

(continued)

Table 8.1. (continued)

Virus	Disease	Geographic Distribution	Principal Reservoir/Vector	Annual Cases	Case: Infection Ratio	Human-to-Human Transmissibility
Omsk hemorrhagic fever	Omsk hemorrhagic fever	Western Siberia	Rodent/tick (*Ixodes*), maintenance cycle incompletely understood	100–200	Unknown	Not reported
Kyasanur Forest disease	Kyasanur Forest disease	Karnataka state, India	Vertebrate (rodents, bats, birds, monkeys, others)/tick (*Ixodes*)	400–500	Unknown	Not reported, but laboratory infections have occurred
Alkhumra hemorrhagic fever[d]	Proposed name: Alkhumra hemorrhagic fever	Saudi Arabia	Ticks?	<50	Unknown	Not reported

[a] Although some endemic transmission of the filoviruses, especially Ebola virus, likely occurs, these viruses have most often been associated with epidemics. Ebola hemorrhagic fever epidemics typically involve <500 people and Marburg <200. Epidemics have been recognized with increasing frequency during the period 1994–2006.

[b] First discovered in 1990. Only 3 cases (1 fatal) of Sabiá virus infection have been noted, 2 of them related to laboratory infection. Disease from this virus is presumed to be similar to the other South American hemorrhagic fevers.

[c] Based on estimates from the World Health Organization. Significant underreporting occurs. Incidence may fluctuate widely depending on epidemic activity.

[d] Alkhumra hemorrhagic fever is considered by some to be a variant of Kyasanur Forest disease virus. Controversy exists over the proper spelling of the virus, written as "Alkhurma" in some publications.

The term "viral hemorrhagic fever" (HF) refers to an acute febrile systemic illness with a propensity for bleeding. Ebola (EBOV), Marburg (MARV), and Lassa (LASV) are some of the most well-known and feared HF viruses. Over the past decade, increased frequency of viral HF outbreaks and heightened scientific interest, as well as public concern, have led to considerable advances in our understanding of these syndromes; however, key questions remain. Here, a brief overview of the viral HFs is first provided, focusing on EBOV and MARV because of their high case fatalities and unknown reservoir and on LASV because of the perennial problem it poses to large populations in West Africa. Then, a few key issues are discussed relevant to our present understanding of the emergence of the HF viruses. Readers interested in a comprehensive description of all viral HFs are referred to recent reviews (Bausch & Ksiazek, 2002; Peters & Zaki, 2006).

HFs may be caused by more than 25 different viruses from 4 families: *Flaviviridae, Arenaviridae, Bunyaviridae,* and *Filoviridae* (Table 8.1). The viruses are composed of small single-stranded RNA with negative, positive, or ambisense replication strategies and genomes in the range of 10–19 kilobases (kb). The error-prone nature of the RNA-dependent RNA polymerase of negative sense viruses, such as EBOV and MARV, heightens the potential for mutation and emergence of quasi-species. The HF viruses are lipid enveloped, which renders them sensitive to inactivation by a wide variety of methods (Chepurnov, Chuev Iu, P'Iankov O, & Efimova, 1995; Elliott, McCormick, & Johnson, 1982; Logan, Fox, Morgan, Makohon, & Pfau, 1975; Lupton, 1981; Mitchell & McCormick, 1984). Little research has been done on the precise duration of the HF viruses in the environment, but it is probably on the order of days to perhaps 1 week, depending upon the environmental conditions (Belanov et al., 1997).

Viral HFs of various etiologies exist worldwide and are generally maintained in zoonotic cycles involving mammalian reservoirs (Table 8.1). The geographic distribution of any given virus is generally restricted by the distribution of its natural reservoir or arthropod vector, although, for unclear reasons, the distributions of the reservoir and human disease frequently do not completely overlap. EBOV, MARV, and LASV are exclusively endemic to sub-Saharan Africa, with the exception of *Reston ebolavirus*, a species that appears to have originated in the Philippines (Figure 8.1).

Depending upon the specific HF virus, introduction into humans from the reservoir may occur through aerosol exposure to virus-contaminated urine, direct exposure to excreta or blood, or the bite of the arthropod vector (Kenyon et al., 1992; McCormick & Fisher-Hoch, 2002; Stephenson, Larson, & Dominik, 1984; ter Meulen et al., 1996). For many

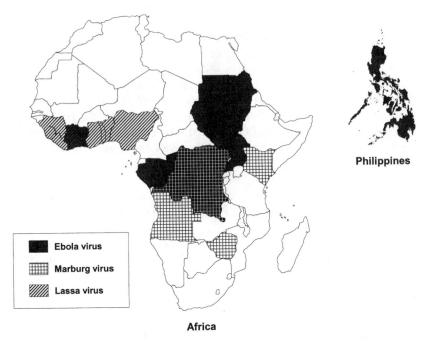

Figure 8.1. Known distributions of Ebola, Marburg, and Lassa viruses.

HF viruses, human infection is rare. The definitive reservoir and mode of introduction of the filoviruses into humans remain unknown, although contact with intermediate nonhuman primate hosts is one path (Formenty, Hatz, et al., 1999; Georges et al., 1999; Martini, Knauff, Schmidt, Mayer, & Baltzer, 1968). LASV transmission occurs through contact with contaminated excreta of its reservoir, *Mastomys* species rodents (Monath, Newhouse, Kemp, Setzer, & Cacciapuoti, 1974).

Secondary human-to-human transmission through direct contact with blood and body fluids may occur with some HF viruses (Table 8.1). Funeral rituals that entail the touching of corpses prior to burial have played a significant role in transmission (CDC, 2001). Epidemiologic as well as limited laboratory-based data do not suggest that aerosol transmission of the HF viruses between humans occurs in natural settings (Baron, McCormick, & Zubeir, 1983; Belanov et al., 1997; Dowell et al., 1999; "Ebola haemorrhagic fever in Sudan," 1978; "Ebola haemorrhagic fever in Zaire," 1978; Ndambi et al., 1999).

Despite intensive field investigation, the identity of the filovirus reservoir remains a mystery (Breman et al., 1999; Leirs et al., 1999). However, a combination of recent epidemiologic, ecologic, and laboratory investigations conspire to make our guesses more educated.

Small clusters of Ebola HF have occurred repeatedly over the last decade in rural forested areas of Gabon and the Republic of the Congo, often linked to contact with wild animals, mostly gorillas and chimps, from which EBOV has been sometimes isolated (Bausch & Rollin, 2004; Boumandouki et al., 2005; Formenty, Boesch, et al., 1999; Georges et al., 1999; Leroy et al., 2004; Nkoghe et al., 2005; Rouquet et al., 2005). All evidence is that filovirus infection in nonhuman primates produces a rapidly fatal disease similar to that seen in humans, suggesting that these animals are also dead-end hosts. In fact, EBOV poses a significant threat to the survival of the great apes (Leroy et al., 2004; Walsh et al., 2003).

The recurrence of EBOV infection in both humans and nonhuman primates in forested regions of West and Central Africa has served to target the search. Fruit bats collected in the Republic of the Congo have been found to be polymerase chain reaction (PCR) and serology positive, a finding consistent with the observation that experimentally infected bats can replicate EBOV and survive infection (Leroy et al., 2005; Swanepoel et al., 1996). Interestingly, a recent seroprevalence study of hunters in southern Cameroon suggested that contact with bats and working as a logger are associated with EBOV seropositivity (Kuniholm et al., 2006). The association with logging may relate to disrupting bat roosts in the process of felling trees.

Cave- or mine-dwelling animals have also been implicated in Marburg HF. Investigation of a large outbreak of MARV (154 cases) in the Democratic Republic of the Congo in 1998–2000 pointed to a gold mine as the site of primary virus introductions into humans (Bausch et al., 2003; Bausch et al., 2006). Bats collected from the mine were PCR and serology positive for MARV, although no virus could be isolated (Swanepoel, 2006). These findings are consistent with two earlier reports of Marburg HF in persons after entering Kitum Cave in Kenya, as well as a third case in which a traveler spent the night in a bat-infested house (Gear et al., 1975a; Johnson et al., 1996; Smith et al., 1982).

Despite the evidence implicating bats, the search for the filovirus reservoir is not concluded. Positive PCR results have also been reported from rodents trapped in the Central African Republic (Morvan et al., 1999). However, although PCR and serological findings are provocative, ultimately, isolation of a filovirus itself from a wild animal will be required to confirm the reservoir. Laboratory studies examining infectibility, virus shedding, and tissue tropism may be necessary to target likely reservoir candidates and specimens before proceeding with more field investigation.

Recent analyses suggest that EBOV outbreaks are closely associated with sharply drier conditions at the end of the rainy season, suggesting unidentified climatic effects on the natural reservoir and/or its interaction with humans (Pinzon et al., 2004). Ecologic niche modeling of filovirus outbreaks and sporadic cases has been used to predict the geographic and ecologic distributions of EBOV and MARV and proved to be correct in placing northern Angola within the range of MARV virus, as evidenced by the large outbreak there in 2005 (CDC, 2005; Peterson, Bauer, & Mills, 2004; Peterson, Lash, Carroll, & Johnson, 2006). Lists of potential reservoir animals inhabiting these ecological niches have also been comprised (Peterson, Carroll, Mills, & Johnson, 2004).

The popular concept of the viral HFs as diseases that occur only in outbreak form is almost certainly a misconception attributable to inadequate surveillance and laboratory capacity in endemic areas of sub-Saharan Africa. In fact, despite some questions regarding the validity of the various diagnostic techniques, studies in forested areas of West and Central Africa consistently show seroprevalence rates for EBOV between 5% and 15% (MARV appears to be much more rare; Kuniholm et al., 2006; Monath, 1999). What accounts for the discrepancy between the highly visible explosive outbreaks typically associated with EBOV and this evidence of relatively silent transmission?

Although cross-reaction with unidentified nonpathogenic filoviruses has been postulated, a more likely explanation can be found through further consideration of the sociopolitical and economic milieu in areas where HF viruses are endemic. In contrast to the explosive high-profile outbreaks usually described, most filovirus transmission probably results in only a few cases initiated via direct inoculation from the primary reservoir or contact with a nonhuman primate for consumption (Bausch & Rollin, 2004). In the rural resource-poor areas where EBOV is endemic, the primary case will usually be cared for at home by family members, typically female, sometimes initiating a few secondary cases. Upon observation of this cluster of severe illness, other villagers will naturally keep their distance for a time, allowing the virus in the particular chain of transmission to extinguish. The ultimate result is a small cluster of deaths with perhaps a survivor or two, who comprise the positive subjects noted in future seroprevalence studies. No laboratory diagnosis is ever made, the usual assumption being that the disease was severe malaria or typhoid fever. Explanations of sorcery are also frequently invoked when illness strikes multiple members of a family (Hewlett, Epelboin, Hewlett, & Formenty, 2005).

What converts the scenario described above, which probably occurs with some frequency, to large outbreaks prompting international responses? Paradoxically enough, the answer is the hospital. In recent decades, well-meaning governments and international aid organizations have promoted the construction of Western-style hospitals and clinics, the use of which has generally been integrated into the long history of traditional medicine in African culture. However, maintenance of sound barrier nursing and the requisite supply of gloves, masks, and clean needles on the planet's poorest continent has proven to be a still greater challenge than the development of the physical infrastructure. Consequently, short supply of personal protective equipment and sterile injection paraphernalia is the norm in many hospitals in sub-Saharan Africa. The EBOV-infected patient admitted to such a hospital, again likely presumed to have malaria, becomes a nidus of infection for health care workers and fellow patients alike through inadequate barrier nursing practices and reuse of needles and multidose vials. Patients who may have been admitted with malaria or other more common ailments become EBOV infected during the course of their care and are discharged, unbeknownst to all at the time, incubating the virus. Their subsequent clinical illness and transmission of EBOV to family caretakers at home, who, in turn, eventually present back to the hospital, begins a dangerous amplification cycle, sometimes compounded by persons fleeing to far away areas out of fear of being admitted to the hospital isolation ward or to seek care at other health centers perceived to offer superior quality.

It is not by chance that large outbreaks occur in countries with deteriorating public health infrastructure, usually as a result of prolonged civil unrest. A brief scan of the sites of large viral HF outbreaks over the last decade reads like a list of the poorest and most conflicted countries mentioned in the news—Angola, the Democratic Republic of the Congo, the Republic of the Congo, Uganda, Sierra Leone, Liberia. Interestingly, the low population density, difficulty of reaching health care centers, and persistent use of traditional medicine in rural Gabon and the Republic of the Congo, where primary transmission of EBOV is most frequent, have likely served as a barrier to amplification and large outbreaks.

Considerable anxiety exists in industrialized countries regarding the risk of imported viral HFs. Nevertheless, based on experience over the last few decades, large outbreaks from sporadic imported human cases appear to be unlikely. Large hospital outbreaks of viral HFs have virtually always been associated with inadequate infection control practices (Fisher-Hoch et al., 1995; Khan et al., 1999; Muyembe-Tamfum, Kipasa, Kiyungu, & Colebunders, 1999; Ndambi et al., 1999). Conversely, when HF cases have been imported into modern hospitals with well-maintained barrier nursing precautions, little secondary transmission has resulted, even when the diagnosis of viral HF appears not to have been considered (Dowell et al., 1999; "Ebola Haemorrhagic Fever in Sudan," 1978; Gear et al., 1975b; Ndambi et al., 1999). Despite over 20 cases of Lassa fever imported from West Africa to various countries in Europe, North America, the Middle East, and Asia, only one putative case of secondary transmission has occurred (Haas et al., 2003). Similarly, although unwitting importation of persons infected with EBOV or MARV, which are probably the most transmissible of all HF viruses, has occasionally resulted in fatalities, extensive secondary spread has not occurred (Formenty, Hatz, et al., 1999; Gear et al., 1975a; Richards et al., 2000).

Nor would large HF outbreaks be likely to result from community contacts with an imported case. Secondary attack rates for EBOV and MARV in poor communities in sub-Saharan Africa with low levels of sanitation (i.e., no running water) and little access to protective materials have been only 16% and 21%, respectively (Borchert et al., 2006; Dowell et al., 1999). This number would likely be even lower in industrialized countries with heightened levels of sanitation and hygiene. A word of caution should be added, however, regarding the potential of HF virus transmission through imported animals, as exemplified through the original MARV outbreak in Europe (32 cases, 7 deaths) traced to monkeys imported from Uganda (Martini et al., 1968; Siegert, Shu, Slenczka, Peters, & Muller, 1968; Todorovitch, Mocitch, & Klasnja, 1971).

Microvascular instability and impaired hemostasis are the pathophysiologic hallmarks of the viral HFs (Bausch & Ksiazek, 2002; Peters & Zaki, 1999). Despite the impaired hemostasis, which may entail endothelial cell, platelet, and/or coagulation factor dysfunction depending on the specific HF virus, frank bleeding is seen in a minority of cases and death from exsanguination is rare. Rather, the severe manifestations of viral HF are usually attributable to insufficient effective circulating intravascular volume, cellular dysfunction, shock, and multiorgan system failure. Dendritic cells and cells of the macrophage–monocyte line appear to be the primary initial sites of virus replication, with subsequent delivery and infection of a wide variety of organ parenchyma, including liver, endothelium, spleen, lymph nodes, kidney, adrenal gland, pancreas, and gonads (Bosio et al., 2004; Schnittler & Feldmann, 1999; Zaki & Goldsmith, 1999). Although cellular necrosis as a direct consequence of virus infection may occur, especially with the filoviruses, it is generally not to a degree sufficient to account for death (Geisbert & Jaax, 1998; Zaki & Goldsmith, 1999). The secretion of various soluble inflammatory mediators and vasoactive substances from infected cells is thought to play a significant role (Feldmann et al., 1996; Ignat'ev, Strel'tsova, Kashentseva, & Patrushev, 1998; Villinger et al., 1999). Filoviruses appear to have an immunosuppressive effect on the host immune system, leaving infected cells hidden from immune surveillance and clearance mechanisms (Chepurnov, Tuzova, Ternovoy, & Chernukhin, 1999; Feldmann & Kiley, 1999; Harcourt, Sanchez, & Offermann, 1998, 1999; Sanchez et al., 2004).

Although classic clinical syndromes are identified for each viral HF, the majority of patients will initially show nonspecific signs and symptoms difficult to distinguish from a host of other febrile illnesses (Table 8.2). There is a spectrum from relatively mild disease to severe vascular

Table 8.2. Differential Diagnosis of the Viral Hemorrhagic Fevers

---

Parasites
Malaria
Amebiasis
Giardiasis
African trypanosomiasis (acute phase)
Bacteria
    Typhoid fever
    Bacillary dysentery (including shigellosis, campylobacteriosis, salmonellosis,
        and enterohemorrhagic *Escherichia coli*)
    Meningococcemia
    Staphylococcemia
    Septicemic plague
    Tularemia
    Anthrax (inhalation or gastrointestinal)
Rickettsia and spirochetes
    Relapsing fever
    Leptospirosis
    Spotted fever group rickettsia (including Rocky Mountain spotted fever,
        Boutonneuse fever, African tick bite fever)
    Typhus group rickettsia (including murineborne and louseborne typhus)
    Q fever
    Ehrlichiosis
    Hemorrhagic or flat smallpox
    Alphavirus infection (including Chikungunya and O'nyong-nyong)
    Other viral hemorrhagic fevers (see Table 8.1)
Noninfectious etiologies
    Thrombotic thrombocytopenic purpura

---

permeability resulting in multiorgan system failure and death. A high index of suspicion, detailed investigation of the travel and exposure history of the patient, and a basic understanding of the incubation periods and distribution of the various reservoirs of the viral HFs are imperative, as are prompt notification and laboratory confirmation.

Viral HF typically begins with fever and constitutional symptoms, which may include chills, headache, myalgia, arthralgia, malaise, anorexia, dizziness, lumbosacral pain, nausea, vomiting, epigastric and abdominal pain, and diarrhea. In severe cases, it then progresses to severe prostration and, depending upon the virus, gastrointestinal, neurologic, and/or pulmonary involvement (Table 8.3). Evidence of vascular permeability includes conjunctival injection/hemorrhage, proteinuria, facial flushing, edema, bleeding, hypotension, and shock. Hemorrhage may manifest as hematemesis, melena, metrorrhagia, petechiae, purpura, epistaxis, and bleeding from the gums and venipuncture sites. The likelihood of clinically discernible hemorrhage varies with the infecting virus. A maculopapular rash or petechial rash is sometimes noted over the thorax, face,

Table 8.3. Clinical Aspects of Viral Hemorrhagic Fevers

Disease	Incubation Period (Days)	Onset	Bleeding	Rash	Jaundice	Heart	Lung	Kidney	CNS	Eye	Case Fatality Ratio
Filoviridae											
Ebola hemorrhagic fever	3–21	Abrupt	++	+++	+	++?	+	+	+	+	50–90%
Marburg hemorrhagic fever	3–21	Abrupt	++	+++	+	++?	+	+	+	+	35–80%
Arenaviridae											
Lassa fever	5–16	Gradual	+	++	0	++	++	0	+	0	2–20%
South American hemorrhagic fevers[a]	7–14	Gradual	+++	0	0	++	++	0	+++	0	15–30%
Bunyaviridae											
Hemorrhagic fever with renal syndrome	9–35	Abrupt	+++	0	0	++	+	+++	+	0	Hantaan: 5–15% Seoul: <1% Puumala: <1%
Rift Valley fever[b]	2–5	Abrupt	+++	+	++	+?	0	+	++	++	50%
Crimean-Congo hemorrhagic fever	3–12	Abrupt	+++	0	++	+?	+	0	++	0	15–30%
Flaviviridae											
Yellow fever	3–6	Abrupt	+++	0	+++	++	++	++	++	0	20–50%
Dengue hemorrhagic fever	3–15	Abrupt	++	+++	+	++	++	0	+	0	Untreated: 10–15% Treated: <1%
Omsk hemorrhagic fever	3–8	Abrupt	++	0	0	+	++	0	+++	+	1–3%
Kyasanur forest disease	3–8	Abrupt	++	0	0	+	++	0	+++	+	3–5%
Alkhumra hemorrhagic fever	3–8	Abrupt	++	+	+	+	+	0	++	+	20–25%

Note: 0 = sign not typically noted/organ not typically affected; + = sign occasionally noted/organ occasionally affected; ++ = sign commonly noted/organ commonly affected; +++ = sign characteristic/organ involvement severe; CNS = central nervous system.

[a] Argentine, Bolivian, Venezuelan, and Brazilian hemorrhagic fevers are grouped as the South American hemorrhagic fevers.

[b] Hemorrhagic fever, encephalitis, and retinitis may be seen in Rift Valley fever independently of each other.

[c] Based on preliminary observations. Less than 100 cases have been reported.

Table 8.4. Clinical Laboratory Findings in the Viral Hemorrhagic Fevers

Disease	Platelets	Leukocyte Count	Clotting Times (PT/PTT)	DIC	Transaminases	Azotemia
Filoviridae						
Ebola and Marburg hemorrhagic fevers	↓↓↓ᵃ	↓/↑	↑↑	↑↑	↑↑	↑↑
Arenaviridae						
Lassa fever	↓ (with impaired aggregation)	→	↑	↑	↑	↑
South American hemorrhagic fevers	↓↓↓ (with impaired aggregation)	↓↓↓	↑↑	↑	↑	↑
Bunyaviridae						
Hemorrhagic fever with renal syndrome	↓↓↓ (with impaired aggregation)	↑↑	↑↑	↑↑	↑	↑↑↑
Rift Valley fever	↓↓	↓↓	↑↑	↑↑	↑↑	↑↑
Crimean-Congo hemorrhagic fever	↓↓↓	↓↓	↑↑↑	↑↑↑	↑↑↑	↑↑↑
Flaviviridae						
Yellow fever	↓↓ (with impaired aggregation)	↓↓	↑↑	↑↑	↑↑↑ (also ↑↑↑ bilirubin)	↑↑
Dengue hemorrhagic fever	↓↓↓ (with impaired aggregation)	↓↓ (neutropenia, atypical lymphocytes)	↑↑	↑↑	↑↑	↑
Omsk hemorrhagic fever	↓↓	↓↓	↑	↑?	↑↑	↑
Kyasanur Forest disease	↓↓	↓↓	↑	↑?	↑↑	↑
Alkhumra hemorrhagic fever	↓↓	↓↓	↑	↑?	↑↑	↑

DIC = disseminated intravascular coagulopathy; PT = prothrombin time; PTT = partial thromboplastin time.
ᵃ The laboratory derangements are estimated by arrows on a 1 to 3 scale, where 1 = *occasional or mild* and 3 = *characteristic and often severe.*

and arms, especially in Whites (Bwaka et al., 1999; Egbring, Slenczka, & Baltzer, 1971; Martini, 1971; McCormick et al., 1987). Cervical lymph nodes become enlarged in Lassa fever. Productive cough, nasal congestion, and jaundice are typically absent in most viral HFs. Common clinical laboratory findings are summarized in Table 8.4. Radiographic and electrocardiogram findings generally correlate with the physical exam (Ketai, Alrahji, Hart, Enria, & Mettler, 2003). Asymptomatic infection is known to occur in EBOV. In Lassa fever, deafness is a sequela in approximately one third of cases.

Assays commonly used in the diagnosis of the viral HFs include ELISA for virus-specific antigen and immunoglobulin (Ig) M and IgG antibodies, the immunofluorescent antibody assay, reverse transcriptase PCR, and virus culture (Bausch et al., 2000; Ksiazek, Rollin, et al., 1999; Ksiazek, West, Rollin, Jahrling, & Peters, 1999; Sanchez et al., 1999). Postmortem diagnosis can be established by pathology examination of formalin-fixed tissues with immunohistochemical staining (Zaki et al., 1999).

The absence of commercially available reagents has severely curtailed research and surveillance, especially in developing countries where they are perhaps most needed (Bausch & Rollin, 2004; Shears, 2000). However, a number of newer diagnostic assays are in development, including ones employing recombinant antigens, real-time PCR, and microarrays (Drosten et al., 2002; Grolla, Lucht, Dick, Strong, & Feldmann, 2005; Palacios et al., 2006; Saijo et al., 2006). These products should eventually allow the detection of viral HFs in remote areas where they are needed, in addition to being of use in surveillance for bioterrorism.

Traditional obstacles to the development of new diagnostic reagents, vaccines, and therapeutics for the viral HFs have included the relatively low incidence of most viral HFs, the remoteness of endemic areas with little capacity for modern clinical or immunological laboratory assessments, and the fact that the populations at risk are typically among the world's poorest, providing little economic incentive in the biomedical industry for product development. Nevertheless, in recent years, industrialized countries' fears of the use of HF viruses as bioweapons have provided an opportunity for product development against the viral HFs not seen since their discovery in the 1960s and 1970s. Major initiatives have been undertaken by the National Institutes of Health to foster research against possible agents of bioterrorism and emerging infectious diseases that are starting to produce results ("NIAID Biodefense Research," 2006).

The treatment of most viral HFs is supportive (Bausch, 2007). Electrolytes and fluid balance should be monitored closely, as third spacing, vomiting, diarrhea, and decreased fluid intake may result in significant derangement. Judicious use of electrolyte and colloid-containing solutions, supplemental oxygen, blood products, vasopressor agents, analgesics, psychoactive or sedative medications, and hemodialysis may all be indicated. Intramuscular and subcutaneous injections and the use of salicylates are contraindicated because of the risk of bleeding. Internal bleeding may be difficult to recognize.

It is reasonable to cover a patient with a suspected viral HF with appropriate antibacterial and/or antiparasitic therapy until the diagnosis can be confirmed or when secondary infection is suspected. Uterine evacuation appears to decrease maternal mortality in pregnant women with viral HF and should be considered given the fetal and neonatal death rates approaching 100%. The antiviral drug ribavirin is effective in the treatment of Lassa fever (McCormick et al., 1986). The main side effect is a mild to moderate anemia, which infrequently necessitates transfusion and disappears with cessation of treatment. The development of therapeutics for the viral HFs lags behind. A recombinant tissue factor inhibitor (rNAPc2) reduced the mortality of EBOV-infected monkeys from 100% to 67%—gains that, while not staggering, still represent a start in a disease where case fatality often approaches 90% (Geisbert et al., 2003). Recombinant human activated protein C, which has been shown to be efficacious in human septic shock, also conferred a modest survival benefit (18% relative to controls) in studies in nonhuman primates (Bernard et al., 2001; Hensley et al., 2006).

All patients suspected to have a viral HF should be presumed infectious and appropriate isolation measures, including strict barrier nursing and disinfection, should be implemented until laboratory results are obtained (Bausch, 2007; CDC & World Health Organization [WHO], 1998). Persons with close contact with the patient during the symptomatic phase of the disease (patients are not infectious before symptom onset), should be monitored daily, including temperature checks, for the duration of the incubation period of the viral HF in question and should be immediately placed in isolation if characteristic signs and symptoms develop. Because secondary attack rates for the viral HFs are generally low and direct contact with infectious blood or body fluids is required for virus transmission, widespread tracing, laboratory testing, or postexposure chemoprophylaxis should not be undertaken for casual contacts.

Community control of Lassa fever is principally based on improving village hygiene to prevent contact with rodents, such as plugging holes that allow rodents entry into houses and eliminating unprotected storage of garbage and foodstuffs (see Appendix C). Rodent trapping is generally not advocated because the rodent reservoir of LASV is so ubiquitous that animals from the surrounding bush will soon repopulate trapped houses. Avoidance of contact with nonhuman primates and other wild animals in endemic areas for the filoviruses is recommended as a control measure but is not always feasible for populations that may rely heavily on these animals as a food source (Bausch & Rollin, 2004). Oral postexposure prophylaxis with ribavirin is sometimes used for persons exposed to LASV, although no data exist regarding its efficacy, and adverse effects, both real and imagined, complicate its use (Hadi, 2007; McCormick et al., 1986).

Vaccines for most viral HFs are at the experimental stages. The most research progress in recent years has been made for vaccines, where protective efficacy has been clearly shown in nonhuman primate studies for EBOV, MARV, and LASV through the use of recombinant virus vectors (Geisbert et al., 2005; Jones et al., 2005; Sullivan et al., 2003). A DNA vaccine for EBOV has been shown to be safe and immunogenic in Phase I clinical trials (Martin et al., 2006).

EMERGING CHALLENGES AND FUTURE DIRECTIONS

Predicting the likelihood of the use of HF viruses as biological weapons is obviously fraught with challenges, given the impossibility of quantifying risk based on deliberately clandestine activities. Even among experts, opinions vary from the alarmist to the dismissive (Cohen, Sidel, & Gould, 2001; Danzig & Berkowsky, 1997; Haas, 2002; Marklund, 2003).

On one hand, the relative rarity and instability of most HF viruses in nature (especially the more virulent ones), low secondary attack rates, lack of natural aerosol transmissibility between humans, high public profile, and relative virulence for those performing unprotected manipulation would seem to make the HF viruses a poor choice for would-be terrorists, at least in the absence of the most sophisticated and well-funded network. The manipulation of HF viruses and delivery mechanisms to invoke large-scale dissemination and fatality would likely require a degree of knowledge and technology presently known to exist in only a handful of sites worldwide. Furthermore, most HF viruses have never been widely disseminated in research laboratories, making them relatively difficult to obtain and clandestinely develop.

On the other hand, the dangers of pathogens generally associated with high case-fatality ratios and rapid disease progression, and the absence of a readily available therapy or vaccine for most viral HFs should not be underestimated. The absence of an endemic presence of most HF viruses in industrialized countries of North America and Europe presumably renders virtually 100% of their populations immunologically naive and thus susceptible. Furthermore, regardless of the actual biological risk, the potential for widespread panic and diversion of resources due to the fear that the HF viruses invoke cannot be overlooked (Slovic, 1987). In the absence of more precise data on which to calculate risk–benefit analyses, the concept of "dual use" (i.e., the development of infrastructure and products of benefit to both military and civil sectors) has been promoted as a strategy to ensure protection against bioterrorism while building a public health system beneficial to all, although the strategy is not without dissenters (Cohen, Gould, & Sidel, 2000).

An increase in frequency of viral HF epidemics in sub-Saharan Africa and industrialized countries' concerns over bioterrorism have spurred a dramatic increase in our understanding of the HF viruses over the past decade. Research advances have rendered novel diagnostics, vaccines, and, to a lesser degree, therapeutics with the potential to diminish drastically the morbidity and mortality of affected populations in endemic areas as well as to protect those potentially vulnerable to the HF viruses as bioweapons. Nevertheless, significant hurdles remain, perhaps paramount among them being navigation of the complex regulatory process required to translate these experimental products into measures that confer real-world benefit to humans in need. The road to licensure and field use is long, often taking years to decades. We can only hope that the sense of urgency presently felt over biodefense will propel these products forward at a swift pace. However, even should Food and Drug Administration approval eventually be obtained, there will be little economic incentive for pharmaceutical companies to produce these products for use in the developing world. A concerted effort from developing country governments and international organizations, including the WHO and international nongovernmental organizations, will be necessary to ensure that these products will benefit all who need them.

And still more scientific research is needed. To date, the research focus has been primarily on the threat to humans from filoviruses, but many other HF viruses, such as Junin and Rift Valley fevers, pose significant threats to both human and animal populations. And there is room for still more discovery. The significance of recently identified putative HF viruses such as Alkhumra and Whitewater Arroyo remains to be determined, and new pathogens, either presently in existence or evolving and readying their emergence, undoubtedly await us. Enhanced investment in public health and research in both industrialized and developing countries alike, and the creation of surveillance and information networks to link them, will be needed if the future challenges are to be met.

ACKNOWLEDGMENTS

The author thanks Kaori Tanaka and Lina Moses for assistance with preparing this chapter.

REFERENCES

Baron, R. C., McCormick, J. B., & Zubeir, O. A. (1983). Ebola virus disease in southern Sudan: Hospital dissemination and intrafamilial spread. *Bulletin of the World Health Organization, 61*, 997–1003.

Bausch, D. G. (2007). Ebola and Marburg viruses. *Physicians' Information and Education Resource.* Retrieved January 5, 2007, from http://pier. acponline.org/physicians/diseases/d891/d891.html

Bausch, D. G., Borchert, M., Grein, T., Roth, C., Swanepoel, R., Libande, M. L., et al. (2003). Risk factors for Marburg hemorrhagic fever, Democratic Republic of the Congo. *Emerging Infectious Diseases, 9*, 1531–1537.

Bausch, D. G., & Ksiazek, T. G. (2002). Viral hemorrhagic fevers including hantavirus pulmonary syndrome in the Americas. *Clinics in Laboratory Medicine, 22*, 981–1020, viii.

Bausch, D. G., Nichol, S. T., Muyembe-Tamfum, J. J., Borchert, M., Rollin, P. E., Sleurs, H., et al. (2006). Marburg hemorrhagic fever associated with multiple genetic lineages of virus. *New England Journal of Medicine, 355*, 909–919.

Bausch, D. G., & Rollin, P. E. (2004). Responding to epidemics of Ebola hemorrhagic fever: Progress and lessons learned from recent outbreaks in Uganda, Gabon, and Congo. In W. M. Scheld, B. E. Murray, & J. M. Hughes (Eds.), *Emerging infections, 6* (pp. 35–57). Washington, DC: ASM Press.

Bausch, D. G., Rollin, P. E., Demby, A. H., Coulibaly, M., Kanu, J., Conteh, A. S., et al. (2000). Diagnosis and clinical virology of Lassa fever as evaluated by enzyme-linked immunosorbent assay, indirect fluorescent-antibody test, and virus isolation. *Journal of Clinical Microbiology, 38*, 2670–2677.

Belanov, E. F., Muntyanov, V. P., Kryuk, D., Sokolov, A. V., Bormotov, N. I., Plyankov, O. V., et al. (1997). Survival of Marburg virus on contaminated surfaces and in aerosol. *Russian Progress in Virology, 1*, 47–50.

Bernard, G. R., Vincent, J. L., Laterre, P. F., LaRosa, S. P., Dhainaut, J. F., Lopez-Rodriguez, A., et al. (2001). Efficacy and safety of recombinant human activated protein C for severe sepsis. *New England Journal of Medicine, 344*(10), 699–709.

Borchert, M., Mulangu, S., Swanepoel, R., Libande, M. L., Tshomba, A., Kulidri, A., et al. (2006). Serosurvey on household contacts of Marburg hemorrhagic fever patients. *Emerging Infectious Diseases, 12*, 433–439.

Bosio, C. M., Moore, B. D., Warfield, K. L., Ruthel, G., Mohamadzadeh, M., Aman, M. J., et al. (2004). Ebola and Marburg virus-like particles activate human myeloid dendritic cells. *Virology, 326*, 280–287.

Boumandouki, P., Formenty, P., Epelboin, A., Campbell, P., Atsangandoko, C., Allarangar, Y., et al. (2005). Prise en charge des malades et des défunts lors de l'épidémie d'Ebola d'octobre-décembre 2003 au Congo [Clinical management of patients and deceased during the Ebola outbreak from October to December 2003 in Republic of Congo]. *Bulletin de la Sociètè de Pathologie Exotique et de ses filiales, 98*(3), 218–223.

Breman, J. G., Johnson, K. M., van der Groen, G., Robbins, C. B., Szczeniowski, M. V., Ruti, K., et al. (1999). A search for Ebola virus in animals in the

Democratic Republic of the Congo and Cameroon: Ecologic, virologic, and serologic surveys, 1979–1980. Ebola Virus Study Teams. *Journal of Infectious Diseases, 179*(Suppl. 1), S139–147.

Bwaka, M. A., Bonnet, M. J., Calain, P., Colebunders, R., De Roo, A., Guimard, Y., et al. (1999). Ebola hemorrhagic fever in Kikwit, Democratic Republic of the Congo: Clinical observations in 103 patients. *Journal of Infectious Diseases, 179*(Suppl. 1), S1–7.

Centers for Disease Control and Prevention. (2001). Outbreak of Ebola hemorrhagic fever Uganda, August 2000–January 2001. *Morbidity and Mortality Weekly Report, 50*, 73–77.

Centers for Disease Control and Prevention. (2005). Outbreak of Marburg virus hemorrhagic fever—Angola, October 1, 2004–March 29, 2005. *Morbidity and Mortality Weekly Report, 54*, 308–309.

Centers for Disease Control and Prevention & World Health Organization. (1998). *Infection control for viral haemorrhagic fevers in the African health care setting.* Atlanta: Centers for Disease Control and Prevention.

Chepurnov, A. A., Chuev Iu, P., P'Iankov O. V., & Efimova, I. V. (1995). The effect of some physical and chemical factors on inactivation of the Ebola virus. *Voprosy Virusologyii, 40*(2), 74–76.

Chepurnov, A. A., Tuzova, M. N., Ternovoy, V. A., & Chernukhin, I. V. (1999). Suppressive effect of Ebola virus on T cell proliferation in vitro is provided by a 125-kDa GP viral protein. *Immunology Letters, 68*, 257–261.

Cohen, H., Sidel, V., & Gould, R. (2001). Preparedness for bioterrorism? *New England Journal of Medicine, 345*, 1423.

Cohen, H. W., Gould, R. M., & Sidel, V. W. (2000). Bioterrorism "preparedness": Dual use or poor excuse? *Public Health Reports, 115*, 403–406.

Danzig, R., & Berkowsky, P. B. (1997). Why should we be concerned about biological warfare? *Journal of the American Medical Association, 278*, 431–432.

Dowell, S. F., Mukunu, R., Ksiazek, T. G., Khan, A. S., Rollin, P. E., & Peters, C. J. (1999). Transmission of Ebola hemorrhagic fever: A study of risk factors in family members, Kikwit, Democratic Republic of the Congo, 1995. Commission de Lutte contre les Epidémies à Kikwit. *Journal of Infectious Diseases, 179*(Suppl. 1), S87–91.

Drosten, C., Gottig, S., Schilling, S., Asper, M., Panning, M., Schmitz, H., et al. (2002). Rapid detection and quantification of RNA of Ebola and Marburg viruses, Lassa virus, Crimean-Congo hemorrhagic fever virus, Rift Valley fever virus, dengue virus, and yellow fever virus by real-time reverse transcription-PCR. *Journal of Clinical Microbiology, 40*, 2323–2330.

Ebola haemorrhagic fever in Sudan, 1976. Report of a WHO/International Study Team. (1978). *Bulletin of the World Health Organization, 56*, 247–270.

Ebola haemorrhagic fever in Zaire, 1976. (1978). *Bulletin of the World Health Organization, 56*, 271–293.

Egbring, R., Slenczka, W., & Baltzer, G. (1971). Clinical manifestations and mechanism of the haemorrhagic diathesis in Marburg virus disease. In G. A. Martini & R. Siegert (Eds.), *Marburg virus disease* (pp. 42–49). Berlin: Springer-Verlag.

Elliott, L. H., McCormick, J. B., & Johnson, K. M. (1982). Inactivation of Lassa, Marburg, and Ebola viruses by gamma irradiation. *Journal of Clinical Microbiology, 16*, 704–708.

Feldmann, H., Bugany, H., Mahner, F., Klenk, H. D., Drenckhahn, D., & Schnittler, H. J. (1996). Filovirus-induced endothelial leakage triggered by infected monocytes/macrophages. *Journal of Virology, 70*, 2208–2214.

Feldmann, H., & Kiley, M. P. (1999). Classification, structure, and replication of filoviruses. *Current Topics in Microbiology Immunology, 235*, 1–21.

Fisher-Hoch, S. P., Tomori, O., Nasidi, A., Perez-Oronoz, G. I., Fakile, Y., Hutwagner, L., et al. (1995). Review of cases of nosocomial Lassa fever in Nigeria: The high price of poor medical practice. *British Medical Journal, 311*, 857–859.

Formenty, P., Boesch, C., Wyers, M., Steiner, C., Donati, F., Dind, F., et al. (1999). Ebola virus outbreak among wild chimpanzees living in a rain forest of Côte d'Ivoire. *Journal of Infectious Diseases, 179*(Suppl. 1), S120–126.

Formenty, P., Hatz, C., Le Guenno, B., Stoll, A., Rogenmoser, P., & Widmer, A. (1999). Human infection due to Ebola virus, subtype Cote d'Ivoire: Clinical and biologic presentation. *Journal of Infectious Diseases, 179*(Suppl. 1), S48–53.

Gear, J. S., Cassel, G. A., Gear, A. J., Trappler, B., Clausen, L., Meyers, A. M., et al. (1975a). Outbreak of Marburg virus disease in Johannesburg. *British Medical Journal, 4*, 489–493.

Gear, J. S., Cassel, G. A., Gear, A. J., Trappler, B., Clausen, L., Meyers, A. M., et al. (1975b). Outbreak of Marburg virus disease in Johannesburg. *British Medical Journal, 4*, 489–493.

Geisbert, T. W., Hensley, L. E., Jahrling, P. B., Larsen, T., Geisbert, J. B., Paragas, J., et al. (2003). Treatment of Ebola virus infection with a recombinant inhibitor of factor VIIa/tissue factor: A study in Rhesus monkeys. *Lancet, 362*, 1953–1958.

Geisbert, T. W., & Jaax, N. K. (1998). Marburg hemorrhagic fever: Report of a case studied by immunohistochemistry and electron microscopy. *Ultrastructural Pathology, 22*, 3–17.

Geisbert, T. W., Jones, S., Fritz, E. A., Shurtleff, A. C., Geisbert, J. B., Liebscher, R., et al. (2005). Development of a new vaccine for the prevention of Lassa fever. *PLoS Medicine, 2*(6), e183.

Georges, A. J., Leroy, E. M., Renaut, A. A., Benissan, C. T., Nabias, R. J., Ngoc, M. T., et al. (1999). Ebola hemorrhagic fever outbreaks in Gabon, 1994–1997: Epidemiologic and health control issues. *Journal of Infectious Diseases, 179*(Suppl. 1), S65–75.

Grolla, A., Lucht, A., Dick, D., Strong, J. E., & Feldmann, H. (2005). Laboratory diagnosis of Ebola and Marburg hemorrhagic fever. *Bulletin de la Sociètè de Pathologie Exotique et de ses filiales, 98*(3), 205–209.

Haas, C. N. (2002). The role of risk analysis in understanding bioterrorism. *Risk Analysis, 22*, 671–677.

Haas, W. H., Breuer, T., Pfaff, G., Schmitz, H., Kohler, P., Asper, M., et al. (2003). Imported Lassa fever in Germany: Surveillance and management of contact persons. *Clinical Infectious Diseases, 36*, 1254–1258.

Harcourt, B. H., Sanchez, A., & Offermann, M. K. (1998). Ebola virus inhibits induction of genes by double-stranded RNA in endothelial cells. *Virology, 252*, 179–188.

Harcourt, B. H., Sanchez, A., & Offermann, M. K. (1999). Ebola virus selectively inhibits responses to interferons, but not to interleukin-1beta, in endothelial cells. *Journal of Virology, 73*, 3491–3496.

Hensley, L. E., Stevens, E. L., Yan, S. B., Geisbert, J. B., Macias, W. L., Larsen, T., et al. (2006, September 17–19). *The role of the anticoagulant protein C system in Ebola hemorrhagic fever: An intervention study in non-human primates.* Paper presented at Filoviruses: Recent Advances and Future Challenges, Winnipeg, Canada.

Hewlett, B. S., Epelboin, A., Hewlett, B. L., & Formenty, P. (2005). Medical anthropology and Ebola in Congo: Cultural models and humanistic care. *Bulletin de la Sociètè de Pathologic Exotique et de ses filiales, 98*, 230–236.

Ignat'ev, G. M., Strel'tsova, M. A., Kashentseva, E. A., & Patrushev, N. A. (1998). Effects of tumor necrosis factor antiserum of the course of Marburg hemorrhagic fever. *Vestnik Rossisko Akademii Meditsinskikh Nauk, 3*, 35–38.

Johnson, E. D., Johnson, B. K., Silverstein, D., Tukei, P., Geisbert, T. W., Sanchez, A. N., et al. (1996). Characterization of a new Marburg virus isolated from a 1987 fatal case in Kenya. *Archives of Virology Supplementum, 11*, 101–114.

Jones, S. M., Feldmann, H., Stroher, U., Geisbert, J. B., Fernando, L., Grolla, A., et al. (2005). Live attenuated recombinant vaccine protects nonhuman primates against Ebola and Marburg viruses. *Nature Medicine, 11*, 786–790.

Kenyon, R. H., McKee, K. T., Jr., Zack, P. M., Rippy, M. K., Vogel, A. P., York, C., et al. (1992). Aerosol infection of rhesus macaques with Junin virus. *Intervirology, 33*(1), 23–31.

Ketai, L., Alrahji, A. A., Hart, B., Enria, D., & Mettler, F., Jr. (2003). Radiologic manifestations of potential bioterrorist agents of infection. *American Journal of Roentgenology, 180*, 565–575.

Khan, A. S., Tshioko, F. K., Heymann, D. L., Le Guenno, B., Nabeth, P., Kerstiens, B., et al. (1999). The reemergence of Ebola hemorrhagic fever, Democratic Republic of the Congo, 1995. Commission de Lutte contre les Epidémies à Kikwit. *Journal of Infectious Diseases, 179*(Suppl. 1), S76–86.

Ksiazek, T. G., Rollin, P. E., Williams, A. J., Bressler, D. S., Martin, M. L., Swanepoel, R., et al. (1999). Clinical virology of Ebola hemorrhagic fever (EHF): Virus, virus antigen, and IgG and IgM antibody findings among EHF patients in Kikwit, Democratic Republic of the Congo, 1995. *Journal of Infectious Diseases, 179*(Suppl. 1), S177–187.

Ksiazek, T. G., West, C. P., Rollin, P. E., Jahrling, P. B., & Peters, C. J. (1999). ELISA for the detection of antibodies to Ebola viruses. *Journal of Infectious Diseases, 179*(Suppl. 1), S192–198.

Kuniholm, M. H., Rossi, C. A., Bausch, D. G., LeBreton, M., Tamoufe, U., Mpoudi-Ngole, E., et al. (2006). *Bat exposure and risk of Ebola virus infection.* Manuscript submitted for publication.

Leirs, H., Mills, J. N., Krebs, J. W., Childs, J. E., Akaibe, D., Woollen, N., et al. (1999). Search for the Ebola virus reservoir in Kikwit, Democratic Republic of the Congo: Reflections on a vertebrate collection. *Journal of Infectious Diseases, 179*(Suppl. 1), S155–163.

Leroy, E. M., Kumulungui, B., Pourrut, X., Rouquet, P., Hassanin, A., Yaba, P., et al. (2005). Fruit bats as reservoirs of Ebola virus. *Nature, 438,* 575–576.

Leroy, E. M., Rouquet, P., Formenty, P., Souquiere, S., Kilbourne, A., Froment, J. M., et al. (2004). Multiple Ebola virus transmission events and rapid decline of central African wildlife. *Science, 303,* 387–390.

Logan, J. C., Fox, M. P., Morgan, J. H., Makohon, A. M., & Pfau, C. J. (1975). Arenavirus inactivation on contact with N-substituted isatin beta-thiosemicarbazones and certain cations. *Journal of General Virology, 28,* 271–283.

Lupton, H. W. (1981). Inactivation of Ebola virus with 60Co irradiation. *Journal of Infectious Diseases, 143,* 291.

Marklund, L. A. (2003). Patient care in a biological safety level-4 (BSL-4) environment. *Critical Care Nursing Clinics of North America, 15,* 245–255.

Martin, J. E., Sullivan, N. J., Enama, M. E., Gordon, I. J., Roederer, M., Koup, R. A., et al. (2006). A DNA vaccine for Ebola virus is safe and immunogenic in a Phase I clinical trial. *Clinical and Vaccine Immunology, 13*(11), 1267–1277.

Martini, G. (1971). Marburg virus disease. Clinical syndrome. In G. Martini & R. Siegert (Eds.), *Marburg virus disease.* New York: Springer-Verlag.

Martini, G. A., Knauff, H. G., Schmidt, H. A., Mayer, G., & Baltzer, G. (1968). A hitherto unknown infectious disease contracted from monkeys. "Marburg-virus" disease. *German Medical Monthly, 13,* 457–470.

McCormick, J. B., & Fisher-Hoch, S. P. (2002). Lassa fever. *Current Topics in Microbiology and Immunology, 262,* 75–109.

McCormick, J. B., King, I. J., Webb, P. A., Johnson, K. M., O'Sullivan, R., Smith, E. S., et al. (1987). A case-control study of the clinical diagnosis and course of Lassa fever. *Journal of Infectious Diseases, 155,* 445–455.

McCormick, J. B., King, I. J., Webb, P. A., Scribner, C. L., Craven, R. B., Johnson, K. M., et al. (1986). Lassa fever. Effective therapy with ribavirin. *New England Journal of Medicine, 314,* 20–26.

Mitchell, S. W., & McCormick, J. B. (1984). Physicochemical inactivation of Lassa, Ebola, and Marburg viruses and effect on clinical laboratory analyses. *Journal of Clinical Microbiology, 20,* 486–489.

Monath, T. P. (1999). Ecology of Marburg and Ebola viruses: Speculations and directions for future research. *Journal of Infectious Diseases, 179*(Suppl. 1), S127–138.

Monath, T. P., Newhouse, V. F., Kemp, G. E., Setzer, H. W., & Cacciapuoti, A. (1974). Lassa virus isolation from *Mastomys natalensis* rodents during an epidemic in Sierra Leone. *Science, 185,* 263–265.

Morvan, J. M., Deubel, V., Gounon, P., Nakoune, E., Barriere, P., Murri, S., et al. (1999). Identification of Ebola virus sequences present as RNA or DNA in organs of terrestrial small mammals of the Central African Republic. *Microbes and Infection, 1,* 1193–1201.

Muyembe-Tamfum, J. J., Kipasa, M., Kiyungu, C., & Colebunders, R. (1999). Ebola outbreak in Kikwit, Democratic Republic of the Congo: Discovery and control measures. *Journal of Infectious Diseases, 179*(Suppl. 1), S259–262.

Ndambi, R., Akamituna, P., Bonnet, M. J., Tukadila, A. M., Muyembe-Tamfum, J. J., & Colebunders, R. (1999). Epidemiologic and clinical aspects of the Ebola virus epidemic in Mosango, Democratic Republic of the Congo, 1995. *Journal of Infectious Diseases, 179*(Suppl. 1), S8–10.

NIAID Biodefense Research. (2006). Retrieved October 6, 2006, from http://www3.niaid.nih.gov/biodefense/

Nkoghe, D., Formenty, P., Leroy, E. M., Nnegue, S., Edou, S. Y., Ba, J. I., et al. (2005). Multiple Ebola virus haemorrhagic fever outbreaks in Gabon, from October 2001 to April 2002. *Bulletin de la Sociètè de Pathologie Exotique et des ses filiales, 98,* 224–229.

Palacios, G., Briese, T., Kapoor, V., Jabado, O., Liu, Z., Venter, M., et al. (2006). MassTag polymerase chain reaction for differential diagnosis of viral hemorrhagic fever. *Emerging Infectious Diseases, 12,* 692–695.

Peters, C. J., & Zaki, S. R. (1999). Viral hemorrhagic fevers: An overview. In R. L. Guerrant, D. H. Walker, & P. F. Weller (Eds.), *Tropical infectious diseases: Principles, pathogens, and practice* (pp. 1182–1190). New York: W. B. Saunders.

Peters, C. J., & Zaki, S. R. (2006). Overview of viral hemorrhagic fevers. In R. L. Guerrant, D. H. Walker, & P. F. Weller (Eds.), *Tropical infectious diseases: Principles, pathogens, and practice* (Vol. 1, pp. 726–733). Philadelphia: Churchill Livingstone.

Peterson, A. T., Bauer, J. T., & Mills, J. N. (2004). Ecologic and geographic distribution of filovirus disease. *Emerging Infectious Diseases, 10,* 40–47.

Peterson, A. T., Carroll, D. S., Mills, J. N., & Johnson, K. M. (2004). Potential mammalian filovirus reservoirs. *Emerging Infectious Diseases, 10,* 2073–2081.

Peterson, A. T., Lash, R. R., Carroll, D. S., & Johnson, K. M. (2006). Geographic potential for outbreaks of Marburg hemorrhagic fever. *American Journal of Tropical Medicine and Hygiene, 75,* 9–15.

Pinzon, J. E., Wilson, J. M., Tucker, C. J., Arthur, R., Jahrling, P. B., & Formenty, P. (2004). Trigger events: Enviroclimatic coupling of Ebola hemorrhagic fever outbreaks. *American Journal of Tropical Medicine Hygiene, 71,* 664–674.

Richards, G. A., Murphy, S., Jobson, R., Mer, M., Zinman, C., Taylor, R., et al. (2000). Unexpected Ebola virus in a tertiary setting: Clinical and epidemiologic aspects. *Critical Care Medicine, 28,* 240–244.

Rouquet, P., Froment, J. M., Bermejo, M., Yaba, P., Delicat, A., Rollin, P. E., et al. (2005). Wild animal mortality monitoring and human Ebola outbreaks, Gabon and Republic of Congo, 2001–2003. *Emerging Infectious Diseases, 11,* 283–290.

Saijo, M., Niikura, M., Ikegami, T., Kurane, I., Kurata, T., & Morikawa, S. (2006). Laboratory diagnostic systems for Ebola and Marburg hemorrhagic fevers developed with recombinant proteins. *Clinical and Vaccine Immunology, 13,* 444–451.

Sanchez, A., Ksiazek, T. G., Rollin, P. E., Miranda, M. E., Trappier, S. G., Khan, A. S., et al. (1999). Detection and molecular characterization of Ebola viruses causing disease in human and nonhuman primates. *Journal of Infectious Diseases, 179*(Suppl.1), S164–169.

Sanchez, A., Lukwiya, M., Bausch, D., Mahanty, S., Sanchez, A. J., Wagoner, K. D., et al. (2004). Analysis of human peripheral blood samples from fatal and nonfatal cases of Ebola (Sudan) hemorrhagic fever: Cellular responses, virus load, and nitric oxide levels. *Journal of Virology, 78*, 10370–10377.

Schnittler, H. J., & Feldmann, H. (1999). Molecular pathogenesis of filovirus infections: Role of macrophages and endothelial cells. *Current Topics in Microbiology and Immunology, 235*, 175–204.

Shears, P. (2000). Emerging and reemerging infections in Africa: The need for improved laboratory services and disease surveillance. *Microbes and Infection, 2*, 489–495.

Siegert, R., Shu, H. L., Slenczka, H. L., Peters, D., & Muller, G. (1968). The aetiology of an unknown human infection transmitted by monkeys (preliminary communication). *German Medical Monthly, 13*, 1–2.

Slovic, P. (1987). Perception of risk. *Science, 236*, 280–285.

Smith, D. H., Johnson, B. K., Isaacson, M., Swanepoel, R., Johnson, K. M., Killey, M., et al. (1982). Marburg-virus disease in Kenya. *Lancet, 1* (8276), 816–820.

Stephenson, E. H., Larson, E. W., & Dominik, J. W. (1984). Effect of environmental factors on aerosol-induced Lassa virus infection. *Journal of Medical Virology, 14*, 295–303.

Sullivan, N. J., Geisbert, T. W., Geisbert, J. B., Xu, L., Yang, Z. Y., Roederer, M., et al. (2003). Accelerated vaccination for Ebola virus haemorrhagic fever in non-human primates. *Nature, 424*, 681–684.

Swanepoel, B. (2006, September 17–19). *Ecological studies on Marburg virus, Northeastern Democratic Republic of Congo.* Paper presented at Filoviruses: Recent Advances and Future Challenges, Winnipeg, Canada.

Swanepoel, R., Leman, P. A., Burt, F. J., Zachariades, N. A., Braack, L. E., Ksiazek, T. G., et al. (1996). Experimental inoculation of plants and animals with Ebola virus. *Emerging Infectious Diseases, 2*, 321–325.

ter Meulen, J., Lukashevich, I., Sidibe, K., Inapogui, A., Marx, M., Dorlemann, A., et al. (1996). Hunting of peridomestic rodents and consumption of their meat as possible risk factors for rodent-to-human transmission of Lassa virus in the Republic of Guinea. *American Journal of Tropical Medicine and Hygiene, 55*, 661–666.

Todorovitch, K., Mocitch, M., & Klasnja, R. (1971). Clinical picture of two patients infected by the Marburg vervet virus. In G. A. Martini & R. Siegert (Eds.), *Marburg virus disease* (pp. 19–23). Berlin: Springer-Verlag.

Villinger, F., Rollin, P. E., Brar, S. S., Chikkala, N. F., Winter, J., Sundstrom, J. B., et al. (1999). Markedly elevated levels of interferon (IFN)-gamma, IFN-alpha, interleukin (IL)-2, IL-10, and tumor necrosis factor-alpha associated with fatal Ebola virus infection. *Journal of Infectious Diseases, 179*(Suppl. 1), S188–191.

Walsh, P. D., Abernethy, K. A., Bermejo, M., Beyers, R., De Wachter, P., Akou, M. E., et al. (2003). Catastrophic ape decline in western equatorial Africa. *Nature, 422*, 611–614.

Zaki, S. R., & Goldsmith, C. S. (1999). Pathologic features of filovirus infections in humans. *Current Topics in Microbiology and Immunology, 235*, 97–116.

Zaki, S. R., Shieh, W. J., Greer, P. W., Goldsmith, C. S., Ferebee, T., Katshitshi, J., et al. (1999). A novel immunohistochemical assay for the detection of Ebola virus in skin: Implications for diagnosis, spread, and surveillance of Ebola hemorrhagic fever. Commission de Lutte contre les Epidémies à Kikwit. *Journal of Infectious Diseases, 179*(Suppl. 1), S36–47.

CHAPTER NINE

Escherichia coli O157:H7

Donna Tartasky

During 2004–2005, three outbreaks of *Escherichia coli* O157:H7 infections occurred among agricultural fair, festival, and petting zoo visitors in Arizona, Florida, and North Carolina (Centers for Disease Control and Prevention [CDC], 2005b). No deaths occurred, and illnesses primarily affected children who visited petting zoos. In North Carolina, 108 people became ill with an *E. coli* O157:H7 infection. Of these, 20 people were hospitalized and 15 were diagnosed with hemolytic uremic syndrome (HUS). Eighty-two people (78%) reported visiting a petting zoo. Risk factors for *E. coli* O157:H7 in children less than 6 years of age were identified as touching or stepping in manure; sitting or falling on the ground; and using a pacifier, "sippy" cup, or sucking one's thumb while in the zoo (CDC, 2005b). Similarly, in Florida, 63 cases of *E. coli* O157:H7 infection were identified after visits to state fairs and festivals. Of these, 17 persons were hospitalized and 7 developed HUS. The median patient age was 4 years. Thirty-four people (54%) were reported to have touched an animal. Likewise, in Arizona, 2 children were hospitalized with *E. coli* O157:H7 infections after visiting a petting zoo. A report of another agricultural fair outbreak has also been described (Durso, Reynolds, Bauer, & Keen, 2005). In this outbreak, both livestock exhibitors and visitors to the fair were affected. After a state fair in Texas, 25 cases of *E. coli* O157:H7 infection were detected. There were 4 cases of HUS and 1 case of thrombotic thrombocytopenic purpura (TTP). A larger outbreak of *E. coli* O157:H7 infection occurred in 1999, at a fair in Albany, New York, where 65 persons were hospitalized, 11 children developed HUS, and 2 persons died—a 3-year-old girl from HUS and a 79-year-old man from

HUS/TTP. All infections were related to water from an unchlorinated well (CDC, 1999). Infections from *E. coli* O157:H7 resulting from contact between animals and humans at agricultural fairs, festivals, and petting zoos are becoming increasingly more common and demonstrate the virulence and pervasive nature of this bacteria.

Recently, two *E. coli* O157:H7 outbreaks have been the focus of national attention. The first outbreak was found to be related to fresh spinach and affected 183 people in 26 states (CDC, 2006). More than half of those affected were hospitalized and 16% developed HUS. Bagged spinach, contaminated with *E. coli* O157:H7 and packaged in California, was identified as the source of this outbreak. In the second outbreak, which involved a fast-food restaurant chain, cases were more limited and were found to be associated with contaminated green onions. Together, these outbreaks suggest that *E. coli* O157:H7 contaminated the soil where the onions and spinach were grown; however, investigations as to the exact source continue.

E. coli are gram-negative, non-spore-forming, rod-shaped bacteria of the Enterobacteriaceae family. They are one of the major organisms in the intestine (Steiner, Thielman, & Guerrant, 2006). They are capable of surviving in the soil and in food for long periods (Weber & Rutala, 2001). Pathogenic strains that can cause diarrhea are categorized in various ways, often as enterovirulent but sometimes also as enterohemorrhagic, enterotoxigenic, enteroinvasive, enteroaggregative, and diffusely adherent based on virulence mechanisms (Steiner et al., 2006). Serotypes are designated on the basis of their O (somatic) and H (flagellar) antigens (Griffin & Boyce, 1998); however, other subtypes of *E. coli* O157:H7, as well as non-O157 serotypes, have been described. Subtypes of O157:H7, based on the *E. coli* flagellar antigen, have been noted (Rutala, Salmenlinna, Eklund, Keskimäki, & Siitonen, 2003). Additional subtypes may be described further in the future because the genetics and serology of *E. coli* O157:H7 are still evolving. Most studies on outbreaks relate predominately to *E. coli* O157:H7, the most common serotype of *E. coli* that causes infection (Tarr, Gordon, & Chandler, 2005).

This chapter will focus on *E. coli* O157:H7, a pathogen that has been responsible for several large outbreaks throughout the world. *E. coli* O157:H7 is responsible for over 73,000 illnesses annually in the United States, with HUS occurring in 3–7% of reported cases (CDC, 2005b). In an analysis of *E. coli* O157:H7 cases ranging from 1982 to 2002, it was reported that the number of reported outbreaks began rising in 1993 and peaked in 2000 (Rangel, Sparling, Crowe, Griffin, & Swerdlow, 2005). While the number of reported cases may have declined, the CDC uses the 1999 data to discuss the incidence of this illness. The pervasiveness of this illness in the United States is demonstrated by an annual cost of $405 million (in 2003 dollars), including $370 million for premature deaths,

$30 in medical care, and $5 million in lost productivity related to *E. coli* O157:H7 infection (Frenzen, Drake, Angulo, & the Emerging Infections Program FoodNet Working Group, 2005).

E. coli O157:H7 has the ability to produce two toxins called Shiga-like or Shiga toxins (known as *stx*1 and *stx*2), because of their similarity to toxins produced by *Shigella dysenteriae*, and referred to as Shiga-toxin *E. coli* (STEC). *E. coli* O157:H7 also has the ability to adhere closely to mucosa and is classified as enterohemorrhagic (EHEC). As a result, both sporadic and epidemic gastrointestinal infections are caused by *E. coli* O157:H7. Transmission is foodborne, waterborne, and through animal-to-human and person-to-person contact, largely through the fecal–oral route. Nosocomial transmission has been described (Bolduc et al., 2004). Relatively few organisms are needed for infection, ranging from as few as 10 to around 100–200 (López, Prado-Jiménez, O'Ryan-Gallardo, & Contrini, 2000; Schubert, 2001). In a 1994 outbreak involving salami, the infectious dose was estimated to be lower than 50 organisms (Tilden et al., 1996). Asymptomatic carriage of *E. coli* O157:H7 can occur and is important in secondary spread of this pathogen (Coia, 1998). Person-to-person transmission is the predominant mode of infection in outbreaks of *E. coli* O157:H7 in group settings such as day care facilities and in nursing homes and institutions (Belongia et al., 1993; Reiss, Kunz, Koin, & Keefe, 2006). Household transmission rates have been estimated at 4% to 15% (Weber & Rutala, 2001).

E. coli O157:H7 was first described as a human pathogen in 1982 when it was implicated as the causative agent in two outbreaks of hemorrhagic colitis, a clinical entity characterized by abdominal cramps, bloody stools, and little or no fever (CDC, 1982). The following year, researchers described an association between *E. coli* and Shiga toxins (*stx*) and HUS, a clinical condition marked by acute renal injury, thrombocytopenia, and microangiopathic hemolytic anemia (Karmali, Steele, Petric, & Lim, 1983). In a multicenter study, the rate of isolation of this pathogen from stool specimens with visible blood was higher that that of any pathogen (Slutsker et al., 1997). While the numbers of infections are relatively small compared with other enteric pathogens, *E. coli* O157:H7 has the potential to produce severe, life-threatening illness. Unfortunately, natural infections with *E. coli* O157:H7 do not confer immunity and no vaccination is available to protect against this pathogen and specific *stx*-producing strains.

The incubation period from time of exposure to *E. coli* O157:H7 to presentation of symptoms is 1–10 days after exposure (Weir & Hay, 2006). The most common clinical presentation is bloody or nonbloody diarrhea accompanied by severe cramping abdominal pain. Fever is uncommon, but vomiting occurs in about half of people who are infected (Coia, 1998). Most people have symptoms that subside in about a week, but sequelae can include HUS, TTP, and even death (Frenzen et al., 2005; Griffin & Boyce, 1998).

Estimates of the rate of HUS, the most significant clinical complication of *E. coli* O157:H7, range from 3% to 7% of all patients (CDC, 2005b). This variability may be due to the presence of the *eae* gene, presence of the *stx*2 gene, being very young, and having bloody diarrhea (Ethelberg et al., 2004). Others speculate the development of HUS is related to the amount of prothrombotic activation early in infection and to the intensity of the subsequent coagulation response (Tarr et al., 2005). *E. coli* O157:H7 infection is the most common cause of HUS in children, especially those under 5 years of age, and in the elderly, but it can occur at any age. Manifestations of HUS include microangiopathic anemia, TTP, acute renal failure, and central nervous system manifestations (CDC, 1999, 2001a; Tarr et al., 2005). Complications related to manifestations of HUS may occur and include stroke, blindness, seizures, coma, and chronic kidney failure. Some patients who regain renal function may develop end-stage kidney disease or other long-term sequelae such as hypertension, neurological complications, diabetes mellitus, and cardiomyopathy (Green, Murphy, & Uttley, 2000; Mead & Griffin, 1998; Tarr et al., 2005). Thrombotic thrombocytopenic purpura, mostly occurring in adults, tends to have fewer renal manifestations and more neurological involvement. Approximately 3–5% of persons who develop HUS die (CDC, 1999, 2005b). Risk factors for HUS have been bloody diarrhea, fever, elevated blood leukocytes, decreased and increased age, antibiotics, and treatment with antimotility agents (Griffin & Boyce, 1998; Tarr et al., 2005).

Antibiotic treatment has been shown to have an association with the development of HUS in children with *E. coli* O157:H7 infection; therefore, such treatment is not recommended (Tarr et al., 2005; Wong, Jelacic, Habeeb, Watkins, & Tarr, 2000). In fact, a retrospective review of *E. coli* O157:H7 from 1992 to 1999 in Spain revealed that 41% of 141 STEC O157:H7 strains showed resistance to antimicrobial agents (Mora et al., 2005). However, others have noted that only trimethoprim–sulfamethoxazole and beta-lactams are associated with the development of HUS (Safdar, Said, Gangnon, & Maki, 2002). As a result, while most researchers report that antibiotics should not be used to treat this illness, there are some who differ in this opinion. Transfusion of packed red blood cells is recommended if the hemoglobin concentration falls below 6.0 g/dL or symptomatic anemia is present. Peritoneal or kidney dialysis may also be indicated with HUS. In general, supportive measures are recommended for the treatment of *E. coli* O157:H7, including correcting and maintaining fluid and electrolyte balance, particularly in children (López et al., 2000).

E. *coli* O157:H7 has been reported primarily in industrialized countries and has been noted in numerous countries in all continents. Recently, however, reports of E. *coli* O157:H7 infection in Kinshasa, the capital of the Democratic Republic of the Congo, confirms the presence of this pathogen in undeveloped countries. Indeed, an outbreak of E. *coli* O157:H7 in Africa in 2003 led to the death of 56 infants (Koyange et al., 2004). While E. *coli* O157:H7 is becoming pandemic, FoodNet data for the United States reported 530 E. *coli* O157:H7 infections and a 22% decline in the incidence of this pathogen from 1996 to 1999 (CDC, 2000). Despite this recent decline in the incidence of new cases, however, any case of E. *coli* O157:H7 is considered reportable (CDC, 2002). In this country during the period from 1982 to 2002, data collected by the CDC demonstrated that 49 states reported 350 E. *coli* O157:H7 outbreaks, representing 8,568 cases. Of these, 17% were hospitalized and 4% developed HUS, with an overall 0.5% mortality rate. The transmission route for 183 cases demonstrated that 52% were foodborne, 21% unknown, 14% person to person, 9% waterborne, 3% due to animal contact, and 0.3% laboratory related. The sources for food outbreaks were due to ground beef (41%) and produce (21%; Rangel et al., 2005). It is important to note that produce can also be infected from a waterborne source. For example, excess rainfall has been implicated in waterborne outbreaks of E. *coli* O157:H7. This has occurred when runoff from water contaminated with E. *coli* O157:H7 came in contact with municipal water supplies (Auld, MacIver, & Klaassen, 2004; Olsen et al., 2002). Other outbreaks have implicated a wide variety of foods such as uncooked ground beef, yogurt, unpasteurized milk, apple cider, fruits, salad vegetables, alfalfa sprouts, and chocolate (Baylis et al., 2004; CDC, 1997, 2001a). In Argentina, where a large number of HUS cases have been reported, STEC has been identified in fecal samples of cattle used for meat and milk production (Lopez et al., 2000).

The largest U.S. outbreak of E. *coli* O157:H7, which affected several hundred persons in Washington, Idaho, California, and Nevada, was due to undercooked hamburgers served at a restaurant chain. Although the outbreak began in November 1992, it came to the attention of the CDC in January 1993 when a physician in Washington recognized a cluster of children with HUS and an increase in bloody diarrhea in the emergency room (CDC, 1993). Similarly, a smaller outbreak of E. *coli* O157:H7 in Japan in 2004 was associated with eating ground beef. As a result, approximately 90,000 pounds of frozen ground beef in the United States and at U.S. military bases in the Far East were recalled (CDC, 2005a). Efforts to quell outbreaks related to ground beef suggest that E. *coli* O157:H7 is more prevalent in restaurants that individually cook hamburgers than in fast food chains (Kassenborg et al., 2004). An investigation of one outbreak among Japanese factory workers linked eating radish sprout salad during lunch to illness (Watanabe et al., 1999). An outbreak of infection in the United States related to eating alfalfa sprouts has also been reported (Lopez et al., 2000). Analysis of another outbreak involving alfalfa sprouts in two states demonstrated that affected alfalfa sprouts came from the same seed distributor (Ferguson et al., 2005). The decontamination of the seeds has been noted to be problematic, and raw alfalfa sprouts are not recommended for young children, the elderly, or those who are immuno-compromised. National surveillance data, as well as continued outbreaks of *E. coli* O157:H7 associated with ground beef consumption, have led to discussion of commercial use of irradiation of meat and poultry as a possible intervention aimed at decreasing the burden of disease (Osterholm, 2004).

Although reports of waterborne *E. coli* O157:H7 are relatively uncommon, they have been noted. In the spring of 2000, a large scale outbreak of *E. coli* O157:H7 occurred in Walkerton, Ontario, following heavy rain that washed bacteria from cattle manure into the shallow town well that was the public water supply. Seven people died and over 2,000 people became ill (Ali, 2004). In another outbreak, unchlorinated municipal water that was contaminated when surface water containing deer and elk feces ran into a town's unconfined aquifer in Wyoming caused several cases of HUS (Olsen et al., 2002). The appearance of *E. coli* O157:H7 has also been documented in unchlorinated swimming water and lakes (Griffin & Boyce, 1998; Wang & Doyle, 1998). An outbreak of swimming-associated transmission of *E. coli* O157:H7 in freshwater was reported in Finland (Paunio et al., 1999). Surveillance of *E. coli* O157:H7 has shown that over 60% of cases occur between May and September. Although the reason for this increased incidence in the summer is unknown, it is speculated that it may be related to increased ambient temperature (Michael et al., 1999). Others have conjectured that the seasonal variation may reflect factors related to farming practices, variations in ground beef consumption, or cooking practices (Griffin & Boyce, 1998).

Studies aimed at variations in farming practices have recently been closely examined. In one study, the effect of sand and sawdust as bedding materials was compared in order to determine the fecal prevalence of *E. coli* O157:H7 in dairy cows (LeJeune & Kauffman, 2005). The use of sawdust was noted to be associated with significantly higher prevalence of *E. coli* O157:H7, which in turn can lead to higher amounts of environmental contamination. Researchers have examined the terminal rectum of cattle and found that the terminal rectum is the main site of *E. coli* O157:H7 carriage in the bovine host (Low et al., 2005). Mucosal carriage at the terminal rectum leads to a high level of fecal excretion, which may be important epidemiologically as it can lead to contamination by other animals as well as spread of the bacteria. *E. coli* O157:H7 has also been noted in other farm animals besides cattle. In one study, 25% of Dutch belted rabbits acquired from a commercial source were positive for EHEC, including the O157:H7 strain (Garcia & Fox, 2003). Another study found *E. coli* O157:H7 in colon fecal samples of pigs (Feder et al., 2003).

The importance of quick and accurate laboratory diagnosis of an *E. coli* O157:H7 outbreak is underscored by the need for case finding to define the extent of the outbreak, investigate the source of contamination, examine specimens from suspected reservoirs of infection, and provide appropriate treatment measures. Isolates of *E. coli* O157:H7 are typically identified using pulsed-field gel electrophoresis (PFGE; Jay et al., 2004). Public health laboratories in the United States routinely subtype all *E. coli* O157:H7 isolates by PFGE as part of a national network (PulseNet). Pulsed-field gel electrophoresis patterns can then be compared using commercial software to determine if patterns are shared by multiple isolates in different states (Gupta et al., 2004). According to PulseNet policy, isolates with indistinguishable patterns that have potential epidemiological significance should also be digested with secondary enzyme (Gupta et al., 2004). The importance of this is underscored by an investigation of a cluster of *E. coli* O157:H7 infections that were found to have originated from two separate sources after a second round of testing with another enzyme (Public Health Agency of Canada, 2005). Another molecular method has been used to detect *E. coli* O157:H7. Specifically, a real-time SYBR Green assay was developed to detect *stx*1 and *stx*2 toxin genes of STEC, in addition to the *E. coli* O157:H7 serotype (Yoshitomi, Jinneman, & Weagant, 2006). Further descriptions of this process are just being described in the literature (Yoshitomi et al., 2006).

Primary prevention of *E. coli* O157:H7 is the most important way to prevent infection and HUS, as well as other complications. Such prevention requires multiple interventions that address cultural, behavioral, and societal factors. Since most preventive measures necessitate behavioral changes, they are often difficult to accomplish. Educating people about the need to cook meat thoroughly and to drink and eat only pasteurized milk, cheese, and juices would help decrease outbreaks from these sources. Of parallel importance, people need not only to be educated about the prevention of *E. coli* O157:H7 but also to be aware of the relationship between their health practices and the health of others. For example, individuals who handle food either in restaurants or the home need to understand how improper food handling can affect the health of others. Measures to prevent *E. coli* and other foodborne infections are given in Appendix C, Table C.1.

REFERENCES

Ali, S. H. (2004). A socio-ecological autopsy of *E. coli* O157:H7 outbreak in Walkerton, Ontario, Canada. *Social Science & Medicine, 58,* 2601–2612.

Auld, H., MacIver, D., & Klaassen, J. (2004). Heavy rainfall and waterborne disease outbreaks: The Walkerton example. *Journal of Toxicology & Environmental Health, Part A, 67,* 1879–1887.

Baylis, C. L., MacPhee, S., Robinson, A. J., Griffiths, R., Lilley, K., & Betts, R. P. (2004). Survival of *Escherichia coli* O157:H7, O111:H- and O26-H11 in artificially contaminated chocolate and confectionary products. *International Journal of Food Microbiology, 96,* 35–48.

Belongia, E. A., Osterholm, M. T., Soler, J. T., Ammend, D. A., Braun, J. E., & MacDonald, K. L. (1993). Transmission of *Escherichia coli* O157:H7 infection in Minnesota child day-care facilities. *Journal of the American Medical Association, 269,* 883–888.

Bolduc, D., Srour, L. F., Sweet, L., Neatbyk, A., Galanis, E., Isaacs, S., et al. (2004). Severe outbreak of *Escherichia coli* O157:H7 in health care institutions in Charlottetown, Prince Edward Island, fall, 2002. *Canadian Communicable Disease Report, 30,* 81–88.

Centers for Disease Control. (1982). Isolation of *E. coli* O157:H7 from sporadic cases of hemorrhagic colitis—United States. *Morbidity and Mortality Weekly Report, 34,* 581–585.

Centers for Disease Control and Prevention. (1993). Update: Multistate outbreak of *Escherichia coli* O157:H7 infections from hamburgers—Western United States, 1992–1993. *Morbidity and Mortality Weekly Report, 42,* 258–263.

Centers for Disease Control and Prevention. (1997). Outbreaks of *Escherichia coli* O157:H7 infection and cryptosporidiosis associated with drinking unpasteurized apple juice—Connecticut and New York, October, 1996. *Morbidity and Mortality Weekly Report, 46,* 4–8.

Centers for Disease Control and Prevention. (1999). Outbreak of *Escherichia coli* O157:H7 and *Campylobacter* among attendees of the Washington County Fair—New York. *Morbidity and Mortality Weekly Report, 48,* 803–805.

Centers for Disease Control and Prevention. (2000). Preliminary FoodNet data on the incidence of foodborne illness—selected sites. United States, 1999. *Morbidity and Mortality Weekly Report, 49,* 201–205.

Centers for Disease Control and Prevention. (2001a). Diagnosis and management of foodborne illnesses. A primer for physicians. *Morbidity and Mortality Weekly Report, 50*(RR-02), 1–69.

Centers for Disease Control and Prevention. (2001b). Outbreaks of *Escherichia coli* O157:H7 infections among children associated with farm visits—Pennsylvania and Washington, 2000. *Morbidity and Mortality Weekly Report, 50,* 293–297.

Centers for Disease Control and Prevention. (2002). Summary of notifiable diseases—United States, 2000. *Morbidity and Mortality Weekly Report, 49*(MM 53), 1–17.

Centers for Disease Control and Prevention. (2005a). *Escherichia coli* O157:H7 infections associated with ground beef from a U.S. military installation—Okinawa, Japan, February 2004. *Morbidity and Mortality Weekly Report, 54*, 40–42.

Centers for Disease Control and Prevention. (2005b). Outbreaks of *Escherichia coli* O157:H7 associated with petting zoos—North Carolina, Florida, and Arizona, 2004 and 2005. *Morbidity and Mortality Weekly Report, 54*, 1277–1280.

Centers for Disease Control and Prevention. (2006). Ongoing multistate outbreak of *Escherichia coli* serotype O157:H7 infections associated with consumption of fresh spinach—United States, September 2006. *Morbidity and Mortality Weekly Report, 55*, 1045–1046.

Coia, J. E. (1998). Clinical, microbiological and epidemiological aspects of *Escherichia coli* O157:H7 infection. *FEMS Immunology and Medical Microbiology, 20*, 1–9.

Durso, L. M., Reynolds, K., Bauer, N., & Keen, J. E. (2005). Shiga-toxigenic *Escherichia coli* O157:H7 infections among livestock exhibitors and visitors at a Texas county fair. *Vector-Borne and Zoonotic Diseases, 5*, 193–201.

Ethelberg, S., Olsen, K. E. P., Scheutz, F., Jensen, C., Schiellerup, P., Enberg, J., et al. (2004). Virulence factors for hemolytic uremic syndrome, Denmark. *Emerging Infectious Diseases, 10*, 842–847.

Feder, I., Wallace, F. M., Gray, J. T., Fratamico, P., Fedorka-Cray, P. J., Pearce, R. A., et al. (2003). Isolation of *Escherichia coli* O157:H7 from intact colon fecal samples of swine. *Emerging Infectious Diseases, 9*, 380–383.

Ferguson, D. D., Scheftel, J., Cronquist, A., Smith, K., Woo-Ming, A., Anderson, E., et al. (2005). *Epidemiology and Infection, 133*, 439–447.

Frenzen, P. D., Drake, A., Angulo, F. J., & the Emerging Infections Program FoodNet Working Group. (2005). Economic cost of illness due to *Escherichia coli* O157:H7 infections in the United States. *Journal of Food Protection, 68*, 2623–2630.

Garcia, A., & Fox, J. G. (2003). The rabbit as a new reservoir host of enterohemorrhagic *Escherichia coli*. *Emerging Infectious Diseases, 9*, 1592–1597.

Green, D. A., Murphy, W. G., & Uttley, W. S. (2000). Haemolytic uraemic syndrome: Prognostic factors. *Clinical Laboratory Hematology, 22*, 11–14.

Griffin, P. M., & Boyce, T. G. (1998). *Escherichia coli* O157:H7. In W. M. Scheld, D. Armstrong, & J. M. Hughes (Eds.), *Emerging infections I* (pp. 137–145). Washington, DC: ASM Press.

Gupta, A., Hunter, S. B., Bidol, S. A., Dietrich, S., Kincaid, J., & Salehi, E., et al. (2004). *Escherichia coli* O157 cluster evaluation. *Emerging Infectious Diseases, 10*, 1856–1858.

Jay, M. T., Garrett, V., Mohle-Boetani, J. C., Barros, M., Farrar, J. A., Rios, R., et al. (2004). A multistate outbreak of *Escherichia coli* O157:H7 infection linked to consumption of beef tacos at a fast-food restaurant chain. (2004). *Clinical Infectious Diseases, 39*, 1–7.

Karmali, M. A., Steele, B. T., Petric, M., & Lim, C. (1983). Sporadic cases of haemolytic-uraemic syndrome associated with faecal cytotoxin producing *Escherichia coli* in stools. *Lancet, 1*(8325), 619–620.

Kassenborg, H. D., Hedberg, C. W., Hoekstra, M., Evans, M. C., Chin, A. E., Marcus, R., et al. for the Emerging Infectious Program FoodNet Working Group. (2004). Farm visits and undercooked hamburgers as major risk factors for sporadic *Escherichia coli* O157:H7 infection: Data from a case-control study in 5 FoodNet Sites. *Clinical Infectious Diseases, 38*(Suppl. 3), S271–278.

Koyange, L., Ollivier, G., Muyembe, J. J., Kebela, B., Gouali, M., & Germani, Y. (2004). Enterohemorrhagic *Escherichia coli* O157, Kinshasa. *Emerging Infectious Diseases, 10,* 968–969.

LeJeune, J. T., & Kauffman, M. D. (2005). Effect of sand and sawdust bedding materials on the fecal prevalence of *Escherichia coli* O157:H7 in dairy cows. *Applied and Environmental Microbiology, 71,* 326–330.

López, E. L., Prado-Jiménez, V., O'Ryan-Gallardo, M., & Contrini, M. M. (2000). Shigella and shiga toxin-producing *Escherichia coli* causing bloody diarrhea in Latin America. *Infectious Disease Clinics of North America, 14,* 41–65.

Low, J. C., McKendrick, I. J., McKechnie, C., Fenlon, D., Naylor, S. W., Currie, C., et al. (2005). Rectal carriage of *Escherichia coli* O157:H7 in slaughtered cattle. *Applied and Environmental Microbiology, 71,* 93–97.

Mead, P. S., & Griffin, P. M. (1998). *Escherichia coli* O157:H7. *Lancet, 352,* 1207–1212.

Michel, P., Wilson, J. B., Martin, S. W., Clarke, R. C., McEwen, S. A., & Gyles, C. L. (1999). Temporal and geographic distributions of reported cases of *Escherichia coli* O157:H7 associated with hemorrhagic colitis. *Journal of Clinical Microbiology, 23,* 869–872.

Mora, A., Blanco, J. E., Blanco, M., Alonso, M. P., Dhabi, G., Echeita, A., et al. (2005). Antimicrobial resistance of Shiga toxin (verotoxin)-producing *Escherichia coli* O157:H7 and non-O157 strains isolated from humans, cattle, sheep and food in Spain. *Research in Microbiology, 156,* 793–806.

Olsen, S. J., Miller, G., Breuer, T., Kennedy, M., Higgins, C., Walford, J., et al. (2002). A waterborne outbreak of *Escherichia coli* O157:H7 infections and hemolytic uremic syndrome: Implications for rural water systems. *Emerging Infectious Diseases, 8,* 370–375.

Osterholm, M. T. (2004). Foodborne disease: The more things change, the more they stay the same. *Clinical Infectious Diseases, 39,* 8–10.

Paunio, M., Peabody, R., Keskimaki, M., Kokki, M., Ruutu, P., Oinonen, S., et al. (1999). Swimming-associated outbreak of *Escherichia coli* O157:H7. *Epidemiology and Infection, 122,* 1–5.

Public Health Agency of Canada. (2005). An outbreak of *Escherichia coli* O157:H7 associated with a children's water spray park and identified by two rounds of pulsed-field gel electrophoresis testing. *Canada Communicable Disease Report, 31*(12), 133–140.

Rangel, J. M., Sparling, P. H., Crowe, C., Griffin, P. M., & Swerdlow, D. L. (2005). Epidemiology of *Escherichia coli* O157:H7 outbreaks, United States, 1982–2002. *Emerging Infectious Diseases, 11,* 603–609.

Ratiner, Y. A., Salmenlinna, S., Eklund, M., Keskimäki, M., & Siitonen, A. (2003). Serology and genetics of the flagellar antigen of *Escherichia coli* O157:H7a, 7c. *Journal of Clinical Microbiology, 41,* 1033–1040.

Reiss, G., Kunz, P., Koin, D., & Keeffe, E. B. (2006). *Escherichia coli* O157:H7 in nursing homes: Review of literature and report of recent outbreak. *Journal of the American Geriatrics Society, 54,* 680–684.

Safdar, N., Said, A., Gangnon, R. E., & Maki, D. G. (2002). Risk of hemolytic uremic syndrome after antibiotic treatment of *Escherichia coli* O157:H7 enteritis a meta-analysis. *Journal of the American Medical Association, 288,* 996–1001.

Schubert, C. (2001). Busting the gut busters. Virulent *E. coli* are revealing some weaknesses. *Science News, 160,* 74–76.

Slutsker, L., Ries, A. A., Greene, K. D., Wells, J. G., Hutwagner, L., & Griffin, P.M. *Escherichia coli* O157:H7 Study Group. (1997). *Escherichia coli* O157:H7 diarrhea in the United States: Clinical and epidemiologic features. *Annals of Internal Medicine, 126,* 505–513.

Steiner, T. S., Thielman, N. M., & Guerrant, R. L. (2006). Enteric *Escherichia coli* infections. In R. L. Guerrant, D. H. Walker, & P. F. Weller (Eds.), *Tropical infectious diseases* (2nd ed., pp. 201–219). Philadelphia: Churchill Livingstone Elsevier.

Tarr, P. I., Gordon, C. A., & Chandler, W. L. (2005). Shiga-toxin *Escherichia coli* and haemolytic uraemic syndrome. *Lancet, 365,* 1073–1086.

Tilden, J., Young, W., McNamara, A. M., Custer, C., Boesl, B., Lambert-Fair, M. A., et al. (1996). A new route of transmission for *Escherichia coli*: Infection from dry fermented salami. *American Journal of Public Health, 86,* 1142–1145.

Wang, G., & Doyle, M. P. (1998). Survival of enterohemorrhagic *Escherichia coli* O157:H7 in water. *Journal of Food Protection, 61,* 662–667.

Watanabe, Y., Ozasa, K., Mermin, J. H., Griffin, P. M., Masuda, K., Imashuku, S., et al. (1999). Factory outbreak of *Escherichia coli* O157:H7, *Heliobacter pylori*, and hepatitis C: Epidemiology, environmental survival, efficacy of disinfection and control measures. *Infection Control and Hospital Epidemiology, 22,* 306–315.

Weber, D. J., & Rutala, W. A. (2001). The emerging nosocomial pathogens *Cryptosporidium*, *Escherichia coli* O157:H7, *Heliobacter pylori*, and hepatitis C: Epidemiology, environmental survival, efficacy of disinfection, and control measures. *Infection control and Hospital Epidemiology, 22,* 306–315.

Weir, E., & Hay, K. (2006). *E. coli*—Sporadic case or an outbreak? *Canadian Medical Association Journal, 174,* 1711.

Wong, C. S., Jelacic, S., Habeeb, R. L., Watkins, S. L., & Tarr, P. I. (2000). The risk of the hemolytic-uremic syndrome after antibiotic treatment of *Escherichia coli* O157:H7 infections. *New England Journal of Medicine, 342,* 1930–1935.

Yoshitomi, K. J., Jinneman, K. C., & Weagant, S.D. (2006). Detection of Shiga toxin genes *stx*1, *stx*2, and the +93 *uid* A mutation of *E. coli* O157:H7/H- using SYBR® Green I in a real-time multiplex PCR. *Molecular and Cellular Probes, 20,* 31–41.

CHAPTER TEN

Emerging Fungal Infections

David S. Perlin

A 14-year-old boy with T-cell acute lymphoblastic leukemia was placed on chemoprophylaxis with trimethoprim–sulfamethoxazole and itraconazole to prevent systemic bacterial and fungal infections, respectively. During chemotherapy, he developed bilateral upper lobe pneumonia and was treated with antibacterial meropenem. The patient did not respond after 48 hours and was then treated with the polyene antifungal agent amphotericin B (AmB). A computed tomography (CT) scan showed lesions suspect for fungal infection. The patient therapy was switched to voriconazole, a broad-spectrum triazole antifungal. The lesions resolved within 10 days, suggesting an infection with *Aspergillus* spp. The patient was placed on voriconazole prophylaxis. After 6 months, he again developed pneumonia and was treated with AmB. Culture and histology findings of bronchoalveolar lavage fluid disclosed no microbial pathogens. Persistent fever led to resection of the infected lobe and discontinuation of chemotherapy. Microscopy of pulmonary tissue showed necrosis and broad hyphae suspect for Zygomycetes. He suffered from convulsions, spondylodiscitis, and a thromboembolic mass in his left cardiac ventricle. Cultures of the thrombus grew *Rhizopus microsporus*. Despite therapy with posaconazole, the boy died of progressive cardiac obstruction (van Well, van Groeningen, Debets-Ossenkopp, van Furth, & Zwaan, 2005).

This case report illustrates an emerging trend for patients at high risk for invasive fungal infections. Aggressive therapy with a new generation of highly active antifungal agents like voriconazole is counter selecting for rare fungi (e.g., Zygomycetes). Voriconazole has become the drug of choice for treating mould infections, especially those due to *Aspergillus* spp. Yet it has limited activity against Zygomycetes. Thus, selective pressure during therapy can result in rare infections, such as zygomycosis, that are largely refractory to conventional therapy (Imhof, Balajee, Fredricks, Englund, & Marr, 2004; Marty, Cosimi, & Baden, 2004; Oren, 2005; Pagano, Gleissner, & Fianchi, 2005).

Opportunistic fungal infections are widespread in immunosuppressed individuals, and the growing numbers of such life-threatening invasive fungal infections are often a consequence of advanced medical intervention for various cancers, acute leukemia, burns, gastrointestinal disease, and premature birth. Over the past four decades, fungal infections caused by *Candida* spp. have steadily increased and represent a significant cause of morbidity and mortality for severely ill patients (Henderson & Hirvela, 1996; Rapp, 2004; Wenzel, 1995). Fungal infections are the fourth leading cause of bloodstream infections in U.S. hospitals (Pfaller et al., 2000; Wisplinghoff et al., 2004). *Candida albicans* accounts for 45–60% of all such infections (Pfaller et al., 1999). Among human immunodeficiency virus-infected patients, meningoencephalitis due to *Cryptococcus neoformans* ranks among the most common acquired immunodeficiency syndrome (AIDS)-defining infections. Most fungi causing human disease have a low inherent virulence and are contained through the action of host defense systems. Yet, suppression of these systems by chemical or disease-related immune modulation allows fungi to flourish, potentially leading to topical mucosal and/or invasive fungal disease. Increasingly, non-*C. albicans* spp., non-*Aspergillus fumigatus* spp., other yeasts and moulds, and drug-resistant variants of common fungi are important causes of disease for high-risk patients (Marr, Carter, Boeckh, Martin, & Corey, 2002; Marr, Carter, Crippa, Wald, & Corey, 2002; see Table 10.1). This shift in invasive fungal infections is occurring as a consequence of changes in immunosuppressive and antineoplastic therapies and the use of broadly active antifungal agents for prophylaxis and empiric therapy (Wingard, 2005).

The treatment options for invasive fungal infections are limited. Unlike antibiotics for bacteria, there are relatively few chemical classes and targets represented by existing antifungal drugs. These classes include the polyene macrolides, flucytosine, the azoles, and echinocandins. Until recently, the pore-forming polyene AmB was the gold standard for therapy of invasive fungal disease. But AmB causes toxicity resulting in severe side effects, including renal insufficiency (Gallis, Drew, & Pickard, 1990). Newer lipid formulations reduce toxicity but do not eliminate it (Hann & Prentice, 2001). The triazole antifungal drugs comprise a large and important class of compounds that interfere with the cytochrome P450-dependent enzyme, lanosterol 14-demethylase, which is necessary for the biosynthesis of ergosterol, a fungal-specific membrane sterol. The first

Table 10.1. Fungal Mycoses and Common Pathogens

Disease	Candidiasis	Aspergillosis	Cryptococcosis	Scedosporium	Zygomycosis	Hyalohyphomycosis	Penicillosis	Histoplasmosis	Coccidioidomycosis	Blastomycosis	Paracoccidioidomycosis
Causative organisms	*Candida albicans* *C. glabrata* *C. parapsilosis* *C. krusei* *C. tropicalis* *C. lusitaniae* *C. guillmondei*	*Aspergillus fumigatus* *A. niger* *A. terreus* *A. lentilus* *A. nidulans*	*Cryptococcus neoformans*	*Pseudallescheria boydii* *Scedosporium prolificans*	*Rhizopus,* *Mucor* *Rhizomucor* *Absidia*	*Penicillium* *Paecilomyces* *Beauveria* *Fusarium* *Scopulariopsis*	*Penicillium marneffei*	*Histoplasma capsulatum* *Histoplasma dubosii*	*Coccidioides immitis*	*Blastomyces dermatitidis*	*Paracoccidioides brasiliensis*

generation triazole drug, fluconazole, is widely used, but it has a limited antifungal spectrum, and resistance can be a problem (Marr, 2004). The second generation triazole drugs (e.g., voriconazole and posaconazole) show better broad-spectrum reactivity and an ability to overcome azole resistance (Boucher, Groll, Chiou, & Walsh, 2004; Gupta & Tomas, 2003; Torres, Hachem, Chemaly, Kontoyiannis, & Raad, 2005). The echinocandin drugs (e.g., caspofungin and micafungin) are the newest approved class to treat serious mycoses due to yeasts and moulds (Denning, 2003). They inhibit glucan synthase, thereby preventing synthesis of (1,3)-β-D-glucan, an essential component of the fungal cell wall (Wiederhold & Lewis, 2003). These drugs are effective against most yeasts and moulds, although increasingly rare moulds are emerging that are insensitive to these therapies.

Infections due to moulds are particularly difficult to manage, with invasive aspergillosis (IA) being the most common filamentous fungal infection observed in immunocompromised patients and a leading cause of fungal mortality (Steinbach, Stevens, Denning, & Moss, 2003). *A. fumigatus* is the most dominant species causing invasive mould disease, although other *Aspergillus* spp. such as *A. flavus*, *A. niger*, *A. terreus*, and *A. versicolor* can be important. The incidence of IA was recently evaluated among 4,621 hematopoietic stem cell transplants (HSCT) and 4,110 solid organ transplants (SOT) at 19 sites in the United States over a 22-month period from March 2001 to December 2002. *A. fumigatus* represented 56% and 75% of all *Aspergillus* spp. isolates from the HSCT and SOT patients, respectively (Morgan et al., 2005). Risk factors for IA among transplant patients include host variables (age, underlying disease), transplant variables (stem cell source), and late complications (acute and chronic graft-versus-host disease [GVHD], corticosteroids, neutropenia, cytomegalovirus, and respiratory virus infection; Marr, Carter, Boeckh, et al., 2002).

Aspergillus is a dimorphic fungus that causes a variety of human diseases of varying severity depending on the host immune status. Three distinctive patterns of aspergillus-related lung disease are recognized, including IA, involving several organ systems; pulmonary aspergilloma; and allergic bronchopulmonary aspergillosis (ABPA; Hope, Walsh, & Denning, 2005a; Stevens et al., 2000). Aspergillosis is usually localized in the lungs and secondarily spreads to the brain. Dissemination occurs more frequently in severely immunocompromised patients receiving high-dose corticosteroids. Allergic bronchopulmonary aspergillosis is a hypersensitivity reaction that occurs in immunocompetent patients with asthma.

Invasive aspergillosis is difficult to diagnose, and a positive diagnosis is often confirmed postmortem (Stevens, 2002). The diagnosis of IA is most often made based on clinical and radiographic findings, which are nonspecific, since *Aspergillus* is rarely cultured from blood. Respiratory findings are varied but are often nonspecific, and a high index of suspicion is necessary in high-risk patients (Al-Alawi, Ryan, Flint, & Muller, 2005; Hope et al., 2005b). Signs include appearance of a crescent on CT scans, duration of neutropenia, and underlying disease (Kim et al., 2001). Surrogate markers of disease aid diagnosis and include cell wall antigens galactomannan and $(1,3)$-β-D-glucan, as well as detection of ribosomal nucleic acid (Verweij, 2005). Therapies are initiated empirically, often without ever establishing the diagnosis (Stevens et al., 2000). Invasive aspergillosis case definition is either considered proven, probable, or possible, as defined according to the joint guidelines of the European Organization for Research and Treatment of Cancer and the National Institutes of Health Mycoses Study Group. Current antifungal therapy for IA involves voriconazole, caspofungin, or amphotericin. *A. terreus* appears less susceptible to AmB than other *Aspergillus* spp., which necessitates the use of alternative antifungal agents (Steinbach et al., 2004). Similarly, *A. lentulus*, a close relative of *A. fumigatus,* shows decreased susceptibility to a broad range of antifungal agents, including polyene, azole, and echinocandin drugs (Balajee, Gribskov, Hanley, Nickle, & Marr, 2005).

Hyaline (colorless) septated filamentous fungi, such as the *Fusarium* spp., *Acremonium* spp., *Paecilomyces* spp., and *Trichoderma* spp., are increasingly being reported to cause invasive mycoses in severely ill patients (Walsh & Groll, 1999). Hyalohyphomycosis is a broad category of disease that now includes more than 30 different genera. Infections with *Fusarium* spp. and Zygomycetes increased during the late 1990s, especially in patients who received multiple transplants (Lionakis & Kontoyiannis, 2004; Marr, Carter, Crippa, et al., 2002; Nucci, 2003; Nucci et al., 2004). Dematiaceous septated filamentous fungi such as *Pseudallescheria boydii, Bipolaris* spp., and *Cladophialophora bantiana* cause pneumonia, sinusitis, and central nervous system (CNS) infection, and they are largely unresponsive to most therapies (Walsh & Groll, 1999). An increasing number of different members of the class of Zygomycetes are causing lethal infections. Finally, mycoses due to endemic organisms such *Penicillium marneffei, Coccidioides immitis,* and *Histoplasma capsulatum* often surge as a consequence of environmental exposures among immunosuppressed patients in endemic regions.

Fusarium infections are the second most frequent cause of invasive fungal disease among neutropenic cancer patients and are a major cause of disease in HSCT recipients (Lionakis & Kontoyiannis, 2004; Nucci et al., 2004). The largest number of cases of invasive *Fusarium* is in North America, and the most frequent cause of infection is *F. solani,* although species such as *F. oxysporum, F. verticillioides,* and others are known. Routes of infection include inhalation, aspiration, trauma, and contamination of intravascular devices. *Fusarium* spp. cause a wide range of superficial and systemic infections. Invasive *Fusarium* infections in neutropenic patients resemble acute IA with an added presence of cutaneous lesions (Lionakis & Kontoyiannis, 2004). Diagnosis is difficult and requires culture of the organism from blood or infected tissue with direct microscopic examination. Serological testing is not yet available, and molecular testing is just evolving (Kulik, Fordonski, Pszczolkowska, Plodzein, & Lapinski, 2004). Fusarium infections are often refractory to conventional antifungal therapy. Treatment requires therapy with AmB or posaconazole, along with aggressive surgical debridement of necrotic tissue. Prophylaxis with azole drugs is important for high-risk patients (Nucci, 2003).

Scedosporium comprises a group of filamentous fungi found in soil, sewage, and polluted water. The two major human pathogens within this genus are *Scedosporium apiospermum*, which is the asexual state of *Pseudallescheria boydii*, and *Scedosporium prolificans* (Tadros, Workowski, Siegel, Hunter, & Schwartz, 1998). Both resemble *Aspergillus* species, with branched septated hyphae. Infection can result from trauma and inhalation of contaminated water. These organisms cause systemic infection in immunocompromised hosts manifested as sinopulmonary, CNS, osteoarticular, ocular, endovascular, and lymphocutaneous disease. Dissemination of disease has a high associated mortality (>75%). *S. apiospermum* is the most frequent cause of cutaneous and fungal mycetoma in high-risk patients living in temperate regions. Patients at high risk include those receiving corticosteroids and immunosuppressive therapy for organ transplantation or those with underlying leukemia, lymphoma, systemic lupus, or Crohn's disease. Infections of the paranasal sinuses may lead to CNS disease with a poor prognosis. Scedosporium species are known to be refractory to AmB but do respond to triazole therapy with voriconazole (Panackal & Marr, 2004). Surgical resection or debridement of infected tissue is often the preferred treatment option.

The clinical importance of zygomycosis (mucormycosis) has significantly increased in recent years, with disease occurring posttransplantation in the presence of GVHD. There are three orders of the class Zygomycetes that cause human disease: the Mucorales, Mortierellales, and the Entomophthorales. The majority of human illness is caused by the Mucorales. While disease is most commonly linked to *Rhizopus* spp., other organisms are also associated with human infection, including *Mucor, Rhizomucor, Absidia, Apophysomyces, Saksenaea, Cunninghamella, Cokeromyces*, and *Syncephalastrum* spp. (Eucker, Sezer, Graf, & Possinger, 2001).

The most common route of transmission for Zygomycetes is inhalation of spores from the environment. Patients at highest risk for infections caused by Mucorales fungi include those with profound immunosuppression or diabetes, intravenous drug abusers, premature infants, those receiving deferoxamine, and recipients of bone marrow transplants. Mucormycosis commonly presents as rhinocerebral or pulmonary disease; gastrointestinal disease may also occur. Zygomycetes are the second most frequent cause of brain abscesses (Pagano, Caira, Falcucci, & Fianchi, 2005). Common features of pulmonary disease include fever, dyspnea, hemoptysis, and cavitation upon radiologic examination (Brown, 2005). The Mucorales are associated with angioinvasive disease, often leading to thrombosis, infarction of involved tissues, and tissue destruction. Host risk factors include diabetes mellitus, neutropenia, sustained immunosuppressive therapy, chronic steroid use, iron chelation therapy, broadspectrum antibiotic use, trauma, surgical wounds, needlesticks, or burns (Greenberg, Scott, Vaughn, & Ribes, 2004; Ribes, Vanover-Sams, & Baker, 2000; Safar et al., 2005). Most infections are acquired by inhalation, ingestion, or trauma. Rhinocerebral and pulmonary diseases are the most common manifestations, although cutaneous, gastrointestinal, and allergic diseases are also seen (Ribes et al., 2000). The incidence of Zygomycosis is reported to be as high as 8% in autopsied patients with leukemia and 2% in allogeneic bone marrow transplant patients (Greenberg et al., 2004). Diagnosis of mucormycosis is difficult and is based on culture methods or microscopy of clinical specimens, although new molecular tests are emerging (Greenberg et al., 2004). Mortality rates can be as high as 80% in infected transplant recipients. Therapy with lipid AmB and posaconazole must be started early and requires combinations of antifungal drugs, aggressive surgical debridement of necrotic tissue, and reversal of the underlying risk factors (Boucher et al., 2004; Brown, 2005; Safar et al., 2005).

Each year, a large number of individuals develop acute pulmonary infections from endemic fungi resulting in histoplasmosis, blastomycosis, or coccidioidomycosis. The pathogens can be cultured from patient sputum, exudates, or cerebrospinal fluid and are identified by histological evaluation, molecular probing, or sera immunochemistry. Most infections are self-limited, although treatment is necessary for patients with severe pneumonitis as well as various forms of chronic pulmonary and disseminated infections.

Coccidioidomycosis is caused by the dimorphic fungi in the genus *Coccidioides*, which persist as mycelia in the soil of desert areas of the southwestern United States, Northern Mexico, and scattered areas of Central and South America. *C. immitis* and *C. posadasii* are the predominant organisms that cause endemic and epidemic coccidioidomycosis (Viriyakosol, Fierer, Brown, & Kirkland, 2005). Natural infection occurs by inhalation of airborne arthroconidia, resulting in their conversion into a parasitic spherule-endospore phase. Such infections are typically mild but can be life threatening in some individuals. Exposure in some hosts results in immunity, which is associated with T-helper 1 (T_H1)-associated immune responses (Cox & Magee, 2004). *C. immitis* is classified as a select agent (bioterrorism agent) because of its relative ease of aerosol distribution and infection (Deresinski, 2003; Dixon, 2001). Recurrent outbreaks have driven the need for a human vaccine (Cole et al., 2004; Cox & Magee, 2004). Coccidioidomycosis can be detected serologically by determination of circulating antigen-specific immunoglobulin M antibodies. Most infections are self-limiting, although antifungal therapy with polyene or azole drugs may be required in more complicated cases (Goldman, Johnson, & Sarosi, 1999).

Pulmonary manifestations are the hallmark of histoplasmosis due to infections by the soil-dwelling dimorphic fungus *Histoplasma capsulatum*. The organism is endemic in North America but is also found in Central and South America. Clinical syndromes range from asymptomatic infection to diffuse alveolar disease causing respiratory difficulty and even death (Wheat, Conces, Allen, Blue-Hnidy, & Loyd, 2004). Inhalation of *H. capsulatum* spores is the usual mode of infection, with environmental exposure being the primary risk factor. Soil-rototilling at an Indiana elementary school in 2001 caused one of the largest outbreaks of histoplasmosis, with 523 students infected and 355 individuals who developed acute pulmonary histoplasmosis (Chamany et al., 2004). Serologic testing is important in the diagnosis of histoplasmosis. Detection of *H. capsulatum* antigen in bronchoalveolar lavage fluid is also helpful in patients with acute pulmonary histoplasmosis (Wheat et al., 2004). Histoplasmosis is mild and self-limited in most healthy individuals. Antifungal therapy is indicated for acute diffuse pulmonary infection, chronic pulmonary histoplasmosis, and progressive disseminated disease (Wheat et al., 2004).

Blastomycosis is an endemic mycosis in the central United States caused by a dimorphic fungus, *Blastomyces dermatitidis*. The organism produces epidemics of infection following a point source of infection or a sporadic endemic infection. Blastomycosis may result in subclinical illness, but it may present as progressive disease with either pulmonary or extrapulmonary disease (Bradsher, Chapman, & Pappas, 2003). Blastomycosis is difficult to recognize and is frequently misdiagnosed (Lemos, Baliga, & Guo, 2002), but new molecular diagnostic tools are emerging (Bialek, Gonzalez, Begerow, & Zelck, 2005). AmB and azole therapy are effective for both severe histoplasmosis and blastomycosis. Vaccines directed against *H. capsulatum* and *B. dermatitidis* are in development (Deepe, Wuthrich, & Klein, 2005).

Paracoccidioides brasiliensis is a dimorphic and thermoregulated fungus that is the causative agent of paracoccidioidomycosis (PCM), an endemic disease widespread in Latin America carrying a high mortality rate (Felipe et al., 2005; Simoes, Marques, & Bagagli, 2004). PCM is the most prevalent systemic mycosis in many countries in Latin America. Its distribution is limited to subtropical regions of Central and South America, where it is endemic. An estimated 10 million people are infected by this fungus, and up to 2% of them may develop the disseminated forms of the disease (de Almeida, 2005). After being inhaled, *P. brasiliensis* typically results in mild or subclinical disease in otherwise healthy individuals. Immunosuppression can result in reactivation and chronic infection of the lungs or other organs, especially mucous and cutaneous tissue, lymph nodes, adrenals, and the CNS. Brain CT or magnetic resonance imaging are useful for diagnosis but are not specific. Long-term antifungal therapy, usually involving itraconazole, is an effective treatment.

Penicillium marneffei is a major cause of infection in patients infected with human immunodeficiency virus in Southeast Asia, India, and China. In endemic regions, *P. marneffei* infection is regarded as an AIDS-defining illness, and the severity of the disease depends on the immunological status of the infected individual. Early diagnosis by serologic and molecular probing is important for diagnosing infection. Soil exposure, especially during the rainy season, has been suggested to be a critical risk factor (Vanittanakom, Cooper, Fisher, & Sirisanthana, 2006). *P. marneffei* is a dimorphic fungus that exists as a mould in the environment but forms elliptical yeast cells in tissue. Infection results from inhalation of airborne spores. The lungs are the primary site of infection, although disseminated infection is most apparent. Patients often present with papular skin lesions. Therapeutic management with AmB or voriconazole is effective. Use of azole drugs and control of any underlying immunosuppression are effective means of prophylaxis.

The increased use of antifungal agents in recent years has resulted in the development of resistance to these drugs (Marr, 2004). In particular, the widespread application of fluconazole and related triazole antifungals in AIDS and cancer patients promotes selection of resistant subpopulations by either inducing resistant subspecies of normally susceptible organisms like *C. albicans* or shifting colonization to more intrinsically resistant species such as *C. krusei* or *C. glabrata* (Hajjeh et al., 2004). A prominent association has evolved between prior exposure to azole-based antifungal drugs and development of resistance. This association is of concern due to the widespread use of triazole drugs for prophylaxis or preemptive therapy in high-risk patients. Clinical resistance to the newly approved echinocandins is only just emerging (Park et al., 2005).

REFERENCES

Al-Alawi, A., Ryan, C. F., Flint, J. D., & Muller, N. L. (2005). Aspergillus-related lung disease. *Canadian Respiratory Journal, 12,* 377–387.

Balajee, S. A., Gribskov, J. L., Hanley, E., Nickle, D., & Marr, K. A. (2005). *Aspergillus lentulus* sp. nov., a new sibling species of *A. fumigatus. Eukaryotic Cell, 4,* 625–632.

Bialek, R., Gonzalez, G. M., Begerow, D., & Zelck, U. E. (2005). Coccidioidomycosis and blastomycosis: Advances in molecular diagnosis. *FEMS Immunology and Medical Microbiology, 45,* 355–360.

Boucher, H. W., Groll, A. H., Chiou, C. C., & Walsh, T. J. (2004). Newer systemic antifungal agents: Pharmacokinetics, safety and efficacy. *Drugs, 64,* 1997–2020.

Bradsher, R. W., Chapman, S. W., & Pappas, P. G. (2003). Blastomycosis. *Infectious Disease Clinics of North America, 17,* 21–40.

Brown, J. (2005). Zygomycosis: An emerging fungal infection. *American Journal of Health-System Pharmacy, 62,* 2593–2596.

Chamany, S., Mirza, S. A., Fleming, J. W., Howell, J. F., Lenhart, S. W., Mortimer, V. D., et al. (2004). A large histoplasmosis outbreak among high school students in Indiana, 2001. *Pediatric Infectious Disease Journal, 23,* 909–914.

Cole, G. T., Xue, J. M., Okeke, C. N., Tarcha, E. J., Basrur, V., Schaller, R. A., et al. (2004). A vaccine against coccidioidomycosis is justified and attainable. *Medical Mycology, 42,* 189–216.

Cox, R. A., & Magee D. M. (2004). Coccidioidomycosis: Host response and vaccine development. *Clinical Microbiology Reviews, 17,* 804–839.

de Almeida, S. M. (2005). Central nervous system paracoccidioidomycosis: An overview. *Brazilian Journal of Infectious Diseases, 9,* 126–133.

Deepe, G. S., Jr., Wuthrich, M., & Klein, B. S. (2005). Progress in vaccination for histoplasmosis and blastomycosis: Coping with cellular immunity. *Medical Mycology, 43,* 381–389.

Denning, D. W. (2003). Echinocandin antifungal drugs. *Lancet, 362,* 1142–1151.

Deresinski, S. (2003). *Coccidioides immitis* as a potential bioweapon. *Seminars in Respiratory Infections, 18,* 216–219.

Dixon, D. M. (2001). *Coccidioides immitis* as a Select Agent of bioterrorism. *Journal of Applied Microbiology, 91,* 602–605.

Eucker, J., Sezer, O., Graf, B., & Possinger, K. (2001). Mucormycoses. *Mycoses, 44,* 253–260.

Felipe, M. S., Torres, F. A., Maranhao, A. Q., Silva-Pereira, I., Pocas-Fonseca, M. J., Campos, E. G., et al. (2005). Functional genome of the human pathogenic fungus *Paracoccidioides brasiliensis. FEMS Immunology and Medical Microbiology, 45,* 369–381.

Gallis, H. A., Drew, R. H., & Pickard, W. W. (1990). Amphotericin B: 30 years of clinical experience. *Reviews of Infectious Diseases, 12,* 308–329.

Goldman, M., Johnson, P. C., & Sarosi, G. A. (1999). Fungal pneumonias. The endemic mycoses. *Clinics in Chest Medicine, 20,* 507–519.

Greenberg, R. N., Scott, L. J., Vaughn, H. H., & Ribes, J. A. (2004). Zygomycosis (mucormycosis): Emerging clinical importance and new treatments. *Current Opinion in Infectious Diseases, 17, 517–525.*

Gupta, A. K., & Tomas, E. (2003). New antifungal agents. *Dermatology Clinics, 21, 565–576.*

Hajjeh, R. A., Sofair, A. N., Harrison, L. H., Lyon, G. M., Arthington-Skaggs, B. A., Mirza, S. A., et al. (2004). Incidence of bloodstream infections due to *Candida* species and in vitro susceptibilities of isolates collected from 1998 to 2000 in a population-based active surveillance program. *Journal of Clinical Microbiology, 42, 1519–1527.*

Hann, I. M., & Prentice, H. G. (2001). Lipid-based amphotericin B: A review of the last 10 years of use. *International Journal of Antimicrobial Agents, 17, 161–169.*

Henderson, V. J., & Hirvela, E. R. (1996). Emerging and reemerging microbial threats. Nosocomial fungal infections. *Archives of Surgery, 131, 330–337.*

Hope, W. W., Walsh, T. J., & Denning, D. W. (2005a). The invasive and saprophytic syndromes due to *Aspergillus* spp. *Medical Mycology, 43*(Suppl. 1), S207–238.

Hope, W. W., Walsh, T. J., & Denning, D. W. (2005b). Laboratory diagnosis of invasive aspergillosis. *Lancet Infectious Diseases, 5, 609–622.*

Imhof, A., Balajee, S. A., Fredricks, D. N., Englund, J. A., & Marr, K. A. (2004). Breakthrough fungal infections in stem cell transplant recipients receiving voriconazole. *Clinical Infectious Diseases, 39, 743–746.*

Kim, M. J., Lee, K. S., Kim, J., Jung, K. J., Lee, H. G., & Kim, T. S. (2001). Crescent sign in invasive pulmonary aspergillosis: Frequency and related CT and clinical factors. *Journal of Computer Assisted Tomography, 25, 305–310.*

Kulik, T., Fordonski, G., Pszczolkowska, A., Plodzein, K., & Lapinski, M. (2004). Development of PCR assay based on ITS2 rDNA polymorphism for the detection and differentiation of Fusarium sporotrichioides. *FEMS Microbiology Letters, 239*(1), 181–186.

Lemos, L. B., Baliga, M., & Guo, M. (2002). Blastomycosis: The great pretender can also be an opportunist. Initial clinical diagnosis and underlying diseases in 123 patients. *Annals of Diagnostic Pathology, 6, 194–203.*

Lionakis, M. S., & Kontoyiannis D. P. (2004). *Fusarium* infections in critically ill patients. *Seminars in Respiratory Critical Care Medicine, 25, 159–169.*

Marr, K. A. (2004). Invasive *Candida* infections: The changing epidemiology. *Oncology, 18*(Suppl. 13), 9–14.

Marr, K. A., Carter, R. A., Boeckh, M., Martin, P., & Corey, L. (2002). Invasive aspergillosis in allogeneic stem cell transplant recipients: Changes in epidemiology and risk factors. *Blood, 100, 4358–4366.*

Marr, K. A., Carter, R. A., Crippa, F., Wald, A., & Corey, L. (2002). Epidemiology and outcome of mold infections in hematopoietic stem cell transplant recipients. *Clinical Infectious Diseases, 34, 909–917.*

Marty, F. M., Cosimi, L. A., & Baden, L. R. (2004). Breakthrough zygomycosis after voriconazole treatment in recipients of hematopoietic stem-cell transplants. *New England Journal of Medicine, 350, 950–952.*

Morgan, J., Wannemuehler, K. A., Marr, K. A., Hadley, S., Kontoyiannis, D. P., & Walsh, T. J. (2005). Incidence of invasive aspergillosis following hematopoietic stem cell and solid organ transplantation: Interim results of a prospective multicenter surveillance program. *Medical Mycology, 43*(Suppl. 1), S49–58.

Nucci, M. (2003). Emerging moulds: *Fusarium, Scedosporium* and Zygomycetes in transplant recipients. *Current Opinion in Infectious Diseases, 16,* 607–612.

Nucci, M., Marr, K. A., Queiroz-Telles, F., Martins, C. A., Trabasso, P., Costa, S., et al. (2004). *Fusarium* infection in hematopoietic stem cell transplant recipients. *Clinical Infectious Diseases, 38,* 1237–1242.

Oren, I. (2005). Breakthrough zygomycosis during empirical voriconazole therapy in febrile patients with neutropenia. *Clinical Infectious Diseases, 40,* 770–771.

Pagano, L., Caira, M., Falcucci, P., & Fianchi, L. (2005). Fungal CNS infections in patients with hematologic malignancy. *Expert Review of Anti-Infective Therapy, 3,* 775–785.

Pagano, L., Gleissner, B., & Fianchi, L. (2005). Breakthrough zygomycosis and voriconazole. *Journal of Infectious Diseases, 192,* 1496–1497.

Panackal, A. A., & Marr, K. A. (2004). *Scedosporium/Pseudallescheria* infections. *Seminars in Respiratory Critical Care Medicine, 25,* 171–181.

Park, S., Kelly, R., Kahn, J. N., Robles, J., Hsu, M. J., Register, E., et al. (2005). Specific substitutions in the echinocandin target Fks1p account for reduced susceptibility of rare laboratory and clinical *Candida* sp. isolates. *Antimicrobial Agents and Chemotherapy, 49,* 3264–3273.

Pfaller, M. A., Jones, R. N., Doern, G. V., Sader, H. S., Messer, S. A., Houston, A., et al. (2000). Bloodstream infections due to *Candida* species: SENTRY antimicrobial surveillance program in North America and Latin America, 1997–1998. *Antimicrobial Agents and Chemotherapy, 44,* 747–751.

Pfaller, M. A., Messer, S. A., Hollis, R. J., Jones, R. N., Doern, G. V., Brandt, M. E., et al. (1999). Trends in species distribution and susceptibility to fluconazole among blood stream isolates of Candida species in the United States. *Diagnostic Microbiology and Infectious Disease, 33,* 217–222.

Rapp, R. P. (2004). Changing strategies for the management of invasive fungal infections. *Pharmacotherapy, 24*(2, Pt. 2), 4S–28; quiz 29S–32.

Ribes, J. A., Vanover-Sams, C. L., Baker, D. J. (2000). Zygomycetes in human disease. *Clinical Microbiology Reviews, 13,* 236–301.

Safar, A., Marsan, J., Marglani, O., Al-Sebeihi, K., Al-Harbi, J., & Valvoda, M. (2005). Early identification of rhinocerebral mucormycosis. *Journal of Otolaryngology, 34,* 166–171.

Simoes, L. B., Marques, S. A., & Bagagli, E. (2004). Distribution of paracoccidioidomycosis: Determination of ecologic correlates through spatial analyses. *Medical Mycology, 42,* 517–523.

Steinbach, W. J., Benjamin, D. K., Jr., Kontoyiannis, D. P, Perfect, J. R., Lutsar, I., Marr, K. A., et al. (2004). Infections due to *Aspergillus terreus*: A multicenter retrospective analysis of 83 cases. *Clinical Infectious Diseases, 39,* 192–198.

Steinbach, W. J., Stevens, D. A., Denning, D. W., & Moss, R. B. (2003). Advances against aspergillosis. *Clinical Infectious Diseases, 37*(Suppl. 3), S155–156.

Stevens, D. A. (2002). Diagnosis of fungal infections: Current status. *Journal of Antimicrobial Chemotherapy, 49*(Suppl. 1), 11–19.

Stevens, D. A., Kan, V. L., Judson, M. A., Morrison, V. A., Dummer, S., Denning, D. W., et al. (2000). Practice guidelines for diseases caused by *Aspergillus*. Infectious Diseases Society of America. *Clinical Infectious Diseases, 30*, 696–709.

Tadros, T. S., Workowski, K. A., Siegel, R. J., Hunter, S., & Schwartz, D. A. (1998). Pathology of hyalohyphomycosis caused by *Scedosporium apiospermum* (*Pseudallescheria boydii*): An emerging mycosis. *Human Pathology, 29*, 1266–1272.

Torres, H. A., Hachem, R. Y., Chemaly, R. F., Kontoyiannis, D. P., & Raad, I. I. (2005). Posaconazole: A broad-spectrum triazole antifungal. *Lancet Infectious Diseases, 5*, 775–785.

Vanittanakom, N., Cooper, C. R., Jr., Fisher, M. C., & Sirisanthana, T. (2006). *Penicillium marneffei* infection and recent advances in the epidemiology and molecular biology aspects. *Clinical Microbiology Reviews, 19*, 95–110.

van Well, G. T., van Groeningen, I., Debets-Ossenkopp, Y. J., van Furth, A. M., & Zwaan, C. M. (2005). Zygomycete infection following voriconazole prophylaxis. *Lancet Infectious Diseases, 5*, 594.

Verweij, P. E. (2005). Advances in diagnostic testing. *Medical Mycology, 43*(Suppl. 1), S121–124.

Viriyakosol, S., Fierer, J., Brown, G. D., & Kirkland, T. N. (2005). Innate immunity to the pathogenic fungus *Coccidioides posadasii* is dependent on Toll-like receptor 2 and Dectin-1. *Infectious Immunity, 73*, 1553–1560.

Walsh, T. J., & Groll, A. H. (1999). Emerging fungal pathogens: Evolving challenges to immunocompromised patients for the twenty-first century. *Transplant Infectious Disease, 1*, 247–261.

Wenzel, R. P. (1995). Nosocomial candidemia: Risk factors and attributable mortality. *Clinical Infectious Disease, 20*, 1531–1534.

Wheat, L. J., Conces, D., Allen, S. D., Blue-Hnidy, D., & Loyd, J. (2004). Pulmonary histoplasmosis syndromes: Recognition, diagnosis, and management. *Seminars in Respiratory Critical Care Medicine, 25*, 129–144.

Wiederhold, N. P., & Lewis, R. E. (2003). The echinocandin antifungals: An overview of the pharmacology, spectrum and clinical efficacy. *Expert Opinion on Investigational Drugs, 12*, 1313–1333.

Wingard, J. R. (2005). The changing face of invasive fungal infections in hematopoietic cell transplant recipients. *Current Opinion in Oncology, 17*, 89–92.

Wisplinghoff, H., Bischoff, T., Tallent, S. M., Seifert, H., Wenzel, R. P., & Edmond, M. B. (2004). Nosocomial bloodstream infections in US hospitals: Analysis of 24,179 cases from a prospective nationwide surveillance study. *Clinical Infectious Diseases, 39*, 309–317.

CHAPTER ELEVEN

Hantavirus Pulmonary Syndrome

James E. Cheek and Amy V. Groom

In 1993, a young, previously healthy, athletic American Indian man died shortly after collapsing at the funeral of his fiancée in New Mexico. The two deaths signaled the beginning of an intense search for a mysterious killer of young, healthy adults living in sparsely populated rural areas of the American West. Both young people had died of acute/adult respiratory distress syndrome (ARDS), a condition resulting from multiple etiologies including trauma, severe infections, and some environmental toxins. Particularly worrisome to clinicians was the rapid course of the illness; both victims had succumbed within 24 hours. Because plague was known to be endemic in the region, pneumonic plague was the first diagnosis to be ruled out. At that point, clinicians and public health authorities began systematically to work through a long list of known infectious agents and environmental toxins such as phosgene gas, a toxin produced in World War I and still routinely used in the area to control prairie dogs. Phosgene, however, turned out to be nothing more than a tantalizing hypothesis as no evidence could be found that the two victims had been exposed.

The initial response of public health authorities in the region was to search for additional cases of the illness while simultaneously gathering information to develop working hypotheses on the etiology. Within a week of the first two cases, four additional cases of severe respiratory illness in young, previously healthy adults were identified. These cases occurred within the previous 6 months and were spread over an area of 40,000 square miles and 12 medical facilities. Epidemiologists immediately began to develop a case–control study to help identify the etiology of this mysterious disease, but the etiology remained elusive. Although pathologic changes found in tissues of victims were consistent with some viral infections, a specific causative agent was not readily identified.

A breakthrough finally came 2 weeks into the investigation when scientists at the Viral Special Pathogens Branch at the Centers for Disease Control and Prevention (CDC) observed a consistently positive test result while testing patients' serum samples against a panel of known viral hemorrhagic fever agents. Surprisingly, the samples tested positive for two strains of hantavirus, an agent found in Eurasia, but convalescent titers from one of the few surviving patients confirmed the diagnosis as a hantavirus. The causative hantavirus, eventually named Sin Nombre virus (SNV), was isolated in culture from small mammal carriers in the region. Ultimately, 17 people were affected in the outbreak and 14 died.

Named for the Hantaan River in South Korea where the prototype virus (Hantaan) was first isolated in 1976 (Lee, Lee, & Johnson, 1978), the genus *Hantavirus* contains at least 30 viruses that are found worldwide (Peters, Mills, Spiropoulou, Zaki, & Rollin, 2006). Members of the Bunyaviridae family, hantaviruses are icosahedral, lipid-enveloped, tri-segmented negative-sense RNA viruses. Transmission within rodent populations occurs horizontally via scratching and biting, resulting in a lifelong asymptomatic infection (Mills, 2005; Root, Black, Calisher, Wilson, & Beaty, 2004). Vertical transmission of hantavirus from parent to offspring has not been demonstrated in rodents or in humans (Howard et al., 1999; Mills et al., 1997). Hantaviruses are not associated with illness in their rodent hosts, although infectious virus may be shed through an infected rodent's saliva, urine, and feces. Virus transmission to humans occurs when aerosols of rodent excreta are inhaled. It may also be spread through the bite of an infected rodent, contamination of broken skin with infected rodent saliva or excreta, and possibly the ingestion of contaminated food or water (CDC, 2002; Khan & Ksiazek, 2000). Transmission to humans can result in a range of illnesses, depending on the particular hantavirus, including hemorrhagic fever with renal syndrome, nephropathia epidemica, and hantavirus pulmonary syndrome (HPS; Peters, et al., 2006). Although human-to-human transmission of an HPS-causing hantavirus has been documented in Argentina (Martinez et al., 2005), a review of HPS cases found no evidence to suggest that this has occurred in the United States (Wells et al., 1997) or in neighboring Chile (Castillo et al., 2004). Hantaviruses associated with HFRS have been isolated in rodent species worldwide, though most commonly in Asia and Europe. Hantaviruses associated with HPS, however, have been found only in the Americas, with more than 1,900 cases identified throughout North, Central, and South America as of December 31, 2004 (Pan-American Health Organization, 2006).

Prior to 1993, hantaviruses found in indigenous rodent populations in the United States, such as the Prospect Hill virus carried by meadow voles (*Microtus pennsylvanicus*), were not linked to human disease (Yanagihara, 1990). In 1993, however, environmental conditions in the southwestern United States set the stage for the recognition of HPS and the causative hantavirus, SNV (Nichol et al., 1993). Since then, other hantaviruses that cause HPS have been identified in the United States, each associated with a primary rodent carrier species: Black Creek Canal virus (Glass et al., 1998; Khan, Gaviria et al., 1996), Bayou virus (Morzunov et al., 1995), Monongahela virus (Rhodes et al., 2000), and New York virus (Hjelle et al., 1995).

Distinct from one another, all of these HPS-causing viruses are part of the same clade (a group that shares a common ancestor) and are found among members of the Muridae subfamily Sigmodontinae. Sigmodontine rodents are found exclusively in the New World, which may explain why HPS is unique to the Americas (Yates et al., 2002). In the United States, SNV is responsible for the majority of HPS cases. The rodent host for SNV is the deer mouse (*Peromyscus maniculatus*) and is found extensively throughout Canada and the United States (Peters et. al., 2006). A largely rural species, *P. maniculatus* can invade suburban and urban dwellings (Kuenzi, Douglass, White, Bond, & Mills, 2001).

Environmental determinants of risk for hantavirus infection primarily reflect factors associated with an abundance of small mammal carriers of the virus. Clearly, risk of acquiring SNV rises with greater numbers of *P. maniculatus* in the environment. Increases in rodent populations appear to occur cyclically and are one of many factors that contribute to heightened risk of hantavirus infection in humans. Ecologists recently developed a hypothesis called the "trophic cascade" to describe this cycling (Yates et al., 2002). Indeed, the initial case—control study of HPS in the southwestern United States found an elevated risk for households with more mice present (Zeitz et al., 1995). Factors affecting rodent population density may be biotic, in the form of predation and competition, or abiotic, such as weather.

Predictive models of changing patterns of risk over large geographic areas can be developed for abiotic factors. Much of the variation in vegetation in the U.S. Southwest, for example, is thought to reflect the influence of the El Niño Southern Oscillation (ENSO) phenomenon, which has an effect on rodent populations (Glass et al., 2000). ENSO, a recurring, cyclical oceanic/atmospheric disruption in the tropical Pacific, affects weather patterns around world. In the southwestern United States, this disruption causes an increase in precipitation, resulting in more vegetation. The abundant shelter and food provided by this vegetation improve rodent habitat, creating ideal conditions for a rodent population increase

(Engelthaler et al., 1999). The relationship between this phenomenon and human risk, however, is a more complex one. Predicting human risk spatially and temporally may not be a simple linear correlation, with more rain equaling more mice, and therefore more human risk (Mills, Yates, Ksiazek, Peters, & Childs, 1999). Concomitant with fluctuations in population density, seroprevalence in rodent populations can vary dramatically over time and geographical location. Long-term studies have shown that the highest seroprevalence among mice often occurs the second or third year after an El Niño year when rodent populations mature before going into decline (Boone et al., 2002; Yates et al., 2002).

To date, most predictive studies of HPS seek to define the mathematical relationship among remotely sensed satellite variables and human risk. Such studies are relatively large scale, using changes in landscape features visible by high altitude satellites such as the National Aeronautics and Space Administration's Landsat or the National Oceanic and Atmospheric Administration's Advanced Very High Resolution Recorder (AVHRR). One study linked rainfall and temperature to HPS cases (Engelthaler et al., 1999). Glass and colleagues (2000) developed a model using Landsat data to predict high-risk areas for HPS transmission in the Southwest up to 1 year before an outbreak may occur. A subsequent study showed that changes in small mammal populations with the highest prevalence of SNV infection could be identified using the same model (Glass et al., 2002). Such modeling has proven useful in hantavirus prevention activities.

The majority (96%) of HPS cases in the United States are caused by SNV and are inextricably linked to the ecology of its rodent host, *P. maniculatus* (CDC, 2006). *P. maniculatus* has a wider range of habitats compared to other U.S. hantavirus hosts. They also tend to favor peridomestic settings and have a higher population density than these other species and, as a result, are more likely to come into contact with humans (Kuenzi et al., 2001). Although most (95%) of HPS cases have occurred west of the Mississippi River, cases have been identified in the eastern United States including New England and, most recently, West Virginia (CDC, 2004).

As of May 2006, 438 confirmed HPS cases in 30 states had been identified (CDC, 2006). The state with the highest incidence of cases is New Mexico, site of the original 1993 outbreak (Douglass, Calisher, & Bradley, 2005). About 63% of all reported cases occurred in men. The mean age for HPS cases is 38 years (range 10–83 years), with more cases occurring among adults than children (CDC, 2006). Recent studies of HPS in Panama, however, found 9% of children aged 4 to 10 years were seropositive for hantavirus (Choclo or Calabazo virus), suggesting that some hantaviruses may infect children (Armien et al., 2004). A case series of patients in New Mexico, aged 10 to 15 years who were infected with SNV, described clinical features almost identical to adult HPS patients, including a 37% fatality rate, making it unlikely that pediatric HPS cases in the United States would be missed (Ramos, Overturf, Crowley, Rosenberg, & Hjelle, 2001). Although the majority of HPS cases in the United States have occurred in Whites, HPS has disproportionately affected American Indians, who account for about 19% of HPS cases. The case fatality rate across all groups is 36% (CDC, 2006).

HPS cases occur year-round with seasonal peaks in the spring and summer in the southwestern United States. As mentioned earlier, this observation is likely attributable to environmental factors that favor increases in rodent populations, combined with seasonal activities that increase human–rodent contact. Specific activities identified with increased risk of HPS include peridomestic cleaning and agricultural activities (Zeitz et al., 1995). In particular, cleaning or entering seldom-used, rodent-infested structures has been found to put people at increased risk of hantavirus infection (CDC, 2002). Occupational and recreational exposures have also been reported among HPS case patients, although less frequently. Persons living in manufactured homes such as mobile homes may be particularly vulnerable to exposure.

HPS cases are defined by the CDC (2006) as those that meet the following clinical criteria: (a) a febrile illness (temperature greater that 101° F) characterized by bilateral, diffuse interstitial edema that may radiographically resemble ARDS with respiratory compromise requiring supplemental oxygen developing within 72 hours of hospitalization, occurring in a previously healthy person; or (b) an unexplained respiratory illness resulting in death with an autopsy examination demonstrating non-cardiogenic pulmonary edema without an identifiable cause. In order to be confirmed, cases must also have confirmed serologic evidence (detection of hantavirus-specific immunoglobulin [Ig] M or rising titers of IgG), positive reverse transcriptase polymerase chain reaction (RT-PCR) results for hantavirus RNA, or positive immunohistochemical results for hantavirus antigen in tissues (CDC, 2006). The clinical course of HPS is characterized by three phases—prodromal, cardiopulmonary, and convalescent—thought to reflect the effects of immune-mediated tissue injury. The incubation period appears to be between 9 to 33 days, with a median of 14–17 days (Khan et al., 2001; Young et al., 2000). The ensuing prodromal stage lasts for 3 to 4 days and is characterized by a nonspecific influenza-like illness consisting of fever, chills, malaise, and often severe myalgias affecting the large muscle groups (e.g., legs, shoulders, thighs, and lower back; Peters, Simpson, & Levy, 1999). Other frequent symptoms include nausea, vomiting, diarrhea, headache, malaise, and, in later stages, cough. Less frequently, patients have abdominal pain, shortness of breath, dizziness, and arthralgias. Rarely do patients complain of sore throat or show signs of rhinorrhea or otitis (Moolenaar et al., 1995). Patients often are sent home only to return within 24–28 hours, sometimes in florid respiratory failure. Thrombocytopenia (platelet count less than 150,000) is usually present at this stage and is an important clue to suspecting HPS (Peters et al., 1999).

After the prodrome, a shock stage (cardiopulmonary phase) begins that lasts for several days until recovery or death ensue. It is characterized by ever-increasing respiratory and cardiovascular system compromise, the latter resulting from a direct myocardial depressant effect. Patients exhibit severe shortness of breath with development of tachypnea and tachycardia. In addition, as fluid leaves the vascular space there is hemoconcentration, seen as an elevated hematocrit, and a marked decline in O_2 saturation. Of the first 100 HPS patients, 84% required intubation with mechanical ventilation for a median of 4 days (Khan, Khabbaz, et al., 1996). Chest radiographs reveal diffuse interstitial pulmonary infiltrates that may progress to bibasilar infiltrates (Peterson, Bastian, & Tatton, 1996). The final stage (called diuretic or convalescent) is signaled by a return of the cardiac index to normal. A relatively rapid resolution of symptoms occurs over 1 to 2 days in the final stage, with most patients taken off mechanical ventilation. Residual pulmonary deficits and cognitive impairment consistent with anoxic brain injury have been described (Hopkins, Larson-Lohr, Weaver, & Bigler, 1998). Renal impairment may be a component of infection with Sin Nombre and related viruses, and renal failure has been described (Dara, Albright, & Peters, 2005).

Milder cases of HPS associated with SNV have been reported in the United States. Although prodromal symptoms, thrombocytopenia, and hemoconcentration appear as they do in classic HPS cases, these infections typically do not include severe pulmonary involvement (Kitsutani et al., 1999). In contrast to hantaviruses in the United States, hantaviruses in Central and South America are more frequently associated with flushing of the head and neck, hemorrhagic manifestations, and mild renal impairment causing proteinuria, hematuria, and casts, as well as classic HPS. In addition, disease may be much milder than HPS, based on evidence of frequent infection as shown by high seropositivity rates in some Central and South American rural populations (Armien et al., 2004; Ferrer et al., 1998).

Diagnosis of HPS in the prodromal stage may be difficult due to the nonspecific symptoms and may be confused with influenza, pneumonia, and unexplained ARDS. Early distinguishing features of HPS patients are the presence of myalgias and the usual absence of sore throat, rhinorrhea, otitis, sinusitis, nasal congestion, or lobar infiltrates on chest x-ray (CDC, 1999; Moolenaar et al., 1995). Nausea, vomiting and abdominal pain may be severe. Thrombocytopenia is the only consistent (and often the earliest) laboratory sign, with the rapidly falling platelet count useful in distinguishing HPS from other infectious diseases such as bacterial sepsis, plague, tularemia, and borreliosis (Peters et al., 1999). Diagnosis is by serologic testing such as Western blot assay or a recombinant immunoblot assay (Peters et al., 1999). Diagnosis may also be made from viral identification using RT-PCR on clots, biopsies, or postmortem tissues (Zaki et al., 1996).

Treatment of HPS is primarily supportive, with antiviral agents playing a minimal role. A clinical trial of intravenous ribavirin proved inconclusive, although results suggested no benefit (Mertz et al., 2004). Supportive care of persons with HPS is based on early detection and treatment of shock and hypoxia (CDC, 1999). Intensive care unit management is most successful with early use of careful hemodynamic monitoring, preferably with pulmonary artery catheterization, judicious intravascular volume resuscitation, mechanical ventilation, and early use of inotropic agents such as dobutamine and amrinone (CDC, 1999). Volume replacement requires careful administration of fluids to avoid exacerbating pulmonary edema. The nursing management of critically ill patients with HPS has been described by Goodman and Griego (1998). In some patients with elevated lactate levels (greater than 4 mmol/L) and other signs correlated with death, salvage therapy using extracorporeal membrane oxygenation has been successful (Crowley et al., 1998).

No vaccine is currently available for SNV. Prevention guidelines developed by the CDC (2002) in cooperation with state health departments and others focus on reducing contact between humans and rodents and limiting human contact with rodent excreta by addressing three key areas: preventing rodents from entering the home, preventing rodents from living around the home, and taking appropriate precautions when cleaning out rodent-infested structures. These guidelines stress the importance of limiting rodent access to food, water, and shelter both inside and outside the home and sealing off buildings. A community-based study demonstrated that with relatively inexpensive rodent proofing, rural homes could reduce the number of wild mice entering the dwelling (Hopkins et al., 2002). The CDC guidelines also suggest methods to trap rodents and clean out rodent-infested areas safely. Simply removing mice without simultaneously rodent proofing a dwelling, however, may lead to an increase in infected mice entering the home (Douglass, Kuenzi, Williams, Douglass, & Mills, 2003). See Appendix C.

EMERGING INFECTION?

The question may be asked that since hantaviruses have been known about for years in Eurasia, is HPS really an emerging infection? Clearly, it is a newly recognized disease, and SNV and other American hantaviruses are newly recognized pathogens, just as *Bartonella, Legionella, Ehrlichia, Anaplasma* (see chapters 3, 15, and 16, respectively), and others are. But is HPS a new disease? Probably not, based on genetic mutation; rather, it is a virus that has coevolved with its rodent host over many years (Nichol et al., 1993; Yates et al., 2002). Furthermore, serological evidence from as early as 1959 (Frampton, Lanser, & Nichols, 1995) indicates that HPS has been causing disease in humans for many years. This idea is further supported by the oral history of Pueblo people of the Southwest who describe an association between abundant vegetation and mice and increased human mortality. Indeed, some have even speculated that HPS may have played a role in the dramatic disappearance of pre-Pueblo cultures throughout the Southwest in ancient times (Chastel, 1998). Most likely, HPS has always been a rare disease, appearing in sparsely populated rural areas. Because a chance clustering of two cases in patients seen by the same physicians occurred in 1993, the disease was investigated rather than being ascribed to a nonspecific viral pneumonia. Without such clustering, cases would have been widely separated geographically and temporally, with little likelihood of detection.

THE FUTURE

The key to preventing hantavirus infection is to continue unraveling the complex relationship among the ecology of rodent hosts, the environment, and human risk. To this end, ongoing longitudinal rodent studies on factors affecting infection among carrier species are an important area of research (Mills et al., 1999). Information gathered from satellite images may help in developing predictive models to determine the level of human risk and ultimately assist in prevention efforts (Glass et al., 2000; Glass et al., 2002).

Finally, supporting surveillance and enhancing our understanding of the pathology and treatment of HPS is critical and may yield information applicable to other viral respiratory diseases, such as avian influenza. Recently published descriptions of lethal cases of pandemic influenza from 1918 (Taubenberger & Morens, 2006) share striking similarities with florid HPS, suggesting that there may be similar immune mechanisms involved in the two diseases. In addition, there are several other similarities between the two diseases including (a) jumps from nonhuman species, (b) severe disease affecting predominantly healthy young adults, and (c) clinical courses characterized by rapid development of ARDS and subsequent death. Further research into HPS could prove useful well beyond the somewhat limited number of human cases, especially given current concerns regarding the possibility of an impending influenza pandemic similar to that of 1918 associated with avian influenza.

REFERENCES

Armien, B., Pascale, J. M., Bayard, V., Munoz, C., Mosca, I., Guerrero, G., et al. (2004). High seroprevalence of hantavirus infection on the Azuero Peninsula of Panama. *American Journal of Tropical Medicine and Hygiene, 70*, 682–687.

Boone, J. D., McGwire, K. C., Otteson, E. W., Debaca, R. S., Kuhn, E. A., & St. Jeor, S. C. (2002). Infection dynamics of Sin Nombre virus after a widespread decline in host populations. *American Journal of Tropical Medicine and Hygiene, 67*, 310–318.

Castillo, C., Villagra, E., Sanhueza, L., Ferres, M., Mardones, J., & Mertz, G. J. (2004). Prevalence of antibodies to hantavirus among family and health care worker contacts of persons with hantavirus cardiopulmonary syndrome: Lack of evidence for nosocomial transmission of Andes virus to health care workers in Chile. *American Journal of Tropical Medicine and Hygiene, 70*, 302–304.

Centers for Disease Control and Prevention. (1999). *Hantavirus pulmonary syndrome clinical update.* Atlanta, GA: Author.

Centers for Disease Control and Prevention. (2002). Hantavirus pulmonary syndrome—United States: Updated recommendations for risk reduction. *Morbidity and Mortality Weekly Report, 51*, 1–12.

Centers for Disease Control and Prevention. (2004). Two cases of hantavirus pulmonary syndrome—Randolph County, West Virginia, July 2004. *Morbidity and Mortality Weekly Report, 53*, 1086–1089.

Centers for Disease Control and Prevention. (2006). *Hantavirus.* Retrieved January 3, 2007, from http://www.cdc.gov/ncidod/diseases/hanta/hps/noframes/caseinfo.htm

Chastel, C. (1998). Were hantaviruses eventually responsible for the lost Anasazi culture? *Acta Virologica, 42*, 353.

Crowley, M. R., Katz, R. W., Kessler, R., Simpson, S. Q., Levy, H., Hallin, G. W., et al. (1998). Successful treatment of adults with severe hantavirus pulmonary syndrome with extracorporeal membrane oxygenation. *Critical Care Medicine, 26*, 409–415.

Dara, S. I., Albright, R. C., & Peters, S. G. (2005). Acute Sin Nombre hantavirus infection complicated by renal failure requiring hemodialysis. *Mayo Clinic Proceedings, 80*, 703–704.

Douglass, R. J., Calisher, C. H., & Bradley, K. C. (2005). State-by-state incidences of hantavirus pulmonary syndrome in the United States, 1993–2004. *Vectorborne and Zoonotic Diseases, 5*, 189–192.

Douglass, R. J., Kuenzi, A. J., Williams, C. Y., Douglass, S. J., & Mills, J. N. (2003). Removing deer mice from buildings and the risk for human exposure to Sin Nombre virus. *Emerging Infectious Diseases, 9*, 390–392.

Engelthaler, D. M., Mosley, D. G., Cheek J. E., Levy, C. E., Komatsu, K. K., Ettestad, P., et al. (1999). Climatic and environmental patterns associated with hantavirus pulmonary syndrome, Four Corners region, United States. *Emerging Infectious Diseases, 5,* 87–94.

Ferrer, J. F., Jonsson, C. B., Esteban, E., Galligan, D., Basombrio, M. A., Peralta-Ramos, M., et al. (1998). High prevalence of hantavirus infection in Indian communities of the Paraguayan and Argentinean Gran Chaco. *American Journal of Tropical Medical and Hygiene, 59,* 438–444.

Frampton, J. W., Lanser, S., & Nichols, C. R. (1995). Sin Nombre virus infection in 1959. *Lancet, 346,* 781–782.

Glass, G. E., Cheek, J. E., Patz, J. A., Shields, T. M., Doyle, T. J., Thoroughman, D. A., et al. (2000). Using remotely sensed data to identify areas at risk for hantavirus pulmonary syndrome. *Emerging Infectious Diseases, 6,* 238–247.

Glass, G. E., Livingstone, W., Mills, J. N., Hlady, W. G., Fine, J. B., Biggler, W., et al. (1998). Black Creek Canal virus infection in *Sigmodon hispidus* in southern Florida. *American Journal of Tropical Medicine and Hygiene, 59,* 699–703.

Glass, G. E., Yates, T. L., Fine, J. B., Shields, T. M., Kendall, J. B., Hope, A. G., et al. (2002). Satellite imagery characterizes local animal reservoir populations of Sin Nombre virus in the southwestern United States. *Proceedings of the National Academy of Science, 99,* 16817–16822.

Goodman, D., & Griego, L. (1998). Hantavirus pulmonary syndrome: Implications for critical care nurses. *Critical Care Nurse, 18*(1), 23–30.

Hjelle, B. J., Krolikowski. J., Torrez-Martinez, N., Chavez-Giles, F., Vanner, C., & Laposata, E. (1995). Phylogenetically distinct hantavirus implicated in a case of hantavirus pulmonary syndrome in the northeastern United States. *Journal of Medical Virology, 46,* 21–27.

Hopkins, A. S., Whitetail-Eagle, J., Corneli, A. L., Person, B., Ettestad, P. J., Dimenna, M., et al. (2002). Experimental evaluation of rodent exclusion methods to reduce hantavirus transmission to residents in a Native American community in New Mexico. *Vector Borne and Zoonotic Diseases, 2,* 61–68.

Hopkins, R. O., Larson-Lohr, V., Weaver, L. K., & Bigler, E. D. (1998). Neuropsychological impairments following hantavirus pulmonary syndrome. *Journal of International Neuropsychology and Sociology, 4,* 190–196.

Howard, M. J., Doyle, T. J., Loster, F. T., Zaki, S. R., Khan, A. S., Petersen, E. A., et al. (1999). Hantavirus pulmonary syndrome in pregnancy. *Clinical Infectious Diseases, 29,* 1538–1544.

Khan, A. S., Gaviria, M., Rollin, P. E., Hlady, W. G., Ksiazek, T. G., Armstrong, L. R., et al. (1996). Hantavirus pulmonary syndrome in Florida: Association with the newly identified Black Creek Canal virus. *American Journal of Medicine, 100,* 46–48.

Khan, A. S., Khabbaz, R. F., Armstrong, L. R., Holman, R. C., Bauer, S. P., Graber, J., et al. (1996). Hantavirus pulmonary syndrome: The first 100 U.S. cases. *Journal of Infectious Diseases, 173,* 1297–1303.

Khan, A. S., & Ksiazek, T. G. (2000). Diseases caused by hantaviruses. In G. T. Strickland (Ed.), *Hunter's tropical medicine and emerging infectious diseases* (8th ed., pp. 228–293). Philadelphia: W. B. Saunders.

Khan, A. S., Graves, T. K., Fritz, C. L., Young, J. C., Metzger, K. B., Humphreys, J. G., et al. (2001). The incubation period of hantavirus pulmonary syndrome. *American Journal of Tropical Medicine and Hygiene, 62,* 714–717.

Kitsutani, P. T., Denton, R. W., Fritz, C. L., Murray, R. A., Todd, R. L., Pape, W. J., et al. (1999). Acute Sin Nombre hantavirus infection without pulmonary syndrome, United States. *Emerging Infectious Diseases, 5,* 701–705.

Kuenzi, A. J., Douglass, R. J., White, D., Jr., Bond, C. W., & Mills, J. N. (2001). Antibody to Sin Nombre virus in rodents associated with peridomestic habitats in west central Montana. *American Journal of Tropical Medicine and Hygiene, 64,* 137–146.

Lee, H. W., Lee, P. W., & Johnson, K. M. (1978). Isolation of the etiologic agent of Korean hemorrhagic fever. *Journal of Infectious Diseases, 137,* 298–308.

Martinez, V. P., Bellomo, C., San Juan, J., Pinna, D., Forlenza, R., Elder, M., et al. (2005). Person-to-person transmission of Andes Virus. *Emerging Infectious Diseases, 11,* 1848–1853.

Mertz, G. J., Miedzinski, L., Goade, D., Pavia, A. T., Hjelle, B. J., Hansbarger, C. O., et al. (2004). Placebo-controlled, double-blind trial of intravenous ribavirin for the treatment of hantavirus cardiopulmonary syndrome in North America. *Clinical Infectious Diseases, 39,* 1307–1313.

Mills, J. N. (2005). Regulation of rodent-borne viruses in the natural host: Implications for human disease. *Archives of Virology, 19*(Suppl.), 45–57.

Mills, J., Ksiazek, T., Ellis, B., Rollin, P., Nichol, S., Yates, T., et al. (1997). Patterns of association with host and habitat: Antibody reactivity with Sin Nombre virus in small mammals in the major biotic communities of the southwestern United States. *American Journal of Tropical Medicine and Hygiene, 56,* 273–284.

Mills, J. N., Yates, T. L., Ksiazek, T. G., Peters, C. J., & Childs, J. E. (1999). Long-term studies of hantavirus reservoir populations in the southwestern United States: Rationale, potential, and methods. *Emerging Infectious Diseases, 5,* 95–101.

Moolenaar, R. L., Dalton, C., Lipman, H. B., Umland, E. T., Gallaher, M., Duchin, J. S., et al. (1995). Clinical features that differentiate hantavirus pulmonary syndrome from three other acute respiratory illnesses. *Clinical Infectious Diseases, 21,* 643–649.

Morzunov, S. P., Feldmann, H., Spiropoulou, C. F., Semenova, V. A., Rollin, P. E., Ksiazek, T. G., et al. (1995). A newly recognized virus associated with a fatal case of hantavirus pulmonary syndrome in Louisiana. *Journal of Virology, 69,* 1980–1983.

Nichol, S. T., Spiropoulou, C. F., Morzunov, S., Rollin, P. E., Ksiazek, T. G., Feldmann, H., et al. (1993). Genetic identification of a hantavirus associated with an outbreak of acute respiratory illness. *Science, 262,* 914–917.

Pan American Health Organization. (2006). *Number of cases and deaths from hantavirus pulmonary syndrome (HPS) (Region of the Americas, 1993–2004).* Retrieved January 1, 2006, from http://www.paho.org/english/ad/dpc/cd/hantavirus-1993-2004.htm

Peters C. J., Mills, J. N., Spiropoulou, C., Zaki, S. R., & Rollin, P. E. (2006). Hantaviruses. In R. L. Guerrant, D. H. Walker, & P. F. Weller (Eds.), *Tropical infectious diseases: Principles, pathogens, & practice* (2nd ed., pp. 762–780). Philadelphia: Churchill Livingstone Elsevier.

Peters, C. J., Simpson, G. L., & Levy, H. (1999). Spectrum of hantavirus infection: Hemorrhagic fever with renal syndrome and hantavirus pulmonary syndrome. *Annual Review of Medicine, 50*, 531–545.

Peterson, M. C., Bastian, B. V., & Tatton, J. A. (1996). Radiologic findings of the hantavirus pulmonary syndrome. *Western Journal of Medicine, 164*, 76–77.

Ramos, M. M., Overturf, G. D., Crowley, M. R., Rosenberg, R. B., & Hjelle, B. (2001). Infection with Sin Nombre hantavirus: Clinical presentation and outcome in children and adolescents. *Pediatrics, 108*, 27–33.

Rhodes, L. V., III, Huang, C., Sanchez, A. J., Nichol, S. T., Zaki, S. R., Ksiazek, T. G., et al. (2000). Hantavirus pulmonary syndrome associated with Monongahela virus. Pennsylvania. *Emerging Infectious Diseases, 6*, 616–621.

Root, J. J., Black, W. C., Calisher, C. H., Wilson, K. R., & Beaty, B. J. (2004). Genetic relatedness of deer mice (*Peromyscus maniculatus*) infected with Sin Nombre virus. *Vector-borne and Zoonotic Diseases, 4*, 149–157.

Taubenberger, J. K., & Morens, D. M. (2006). 1918 influenza: The mother of all pandemics. *Emerging Infectious Diseases, 12*, 15–22.

Wells, R. M., Young, J., Williams, R. J., Armstrong, L. R., Busico, K., Khan, A. S., et al. (1997). Hantavirus transmission in the United States. *Emerging Infectious Diseases, 3*, 361–365.

Yanagihara, R. (1990). Hantavirus infection in the United States: Epizootiology and epidemiology. *Review of Infectious Diseases, 12*, 449–457.

Yates, T. L., Mills, J. N., Parmenter, C. A., Ksiazek, T. G., Parmenter, R. R., Vande Castle, J. R., et al. (2002). The ecology and evolutionary history of an emergent disease: Hantavirus pulmonary syndrome. *BioScience, 52*, 989–998.

Young, J. C., Hansen, G. R., Graves, T. K., Deasy, M. P., Humphreys, J. G., Fritz, C. L., et al. (2000). The incubation period of hantavirus pulmonary syndrome. *American Journal of Tropical Medicine and Hygiene, 62*, 714–717.

Zaki, S. R., Khan, A. S., Goodman, R. A., Armstrong, L. R., Greer, P. W., Coffield, L. M., et al. (1996). Retrospective diagnosis of hantavirus pulmonary syndrome, 1978–1993: Implications for emerging infectious diseases. *Archives of Pathology and Laboratory Medicine, 120*, 134–139.

Zeitz, P. S., Butler, J. C., Cheek, J. E., Samuel, M. C., Childs, J. E., Shands, L. A., et al. (1995). A case-control study of hantavirus pulmonary syndrome during an outbreak in the southwestern United States. *Journal of Infectious Diseases, 171*, 864–870.

CHAPTER TWELVE

Hepatitis C

Victoria Davey

JW, a healthy 36-year-old biology professor at a small midwestern college, visited his physician for an annual physical. He reported that for the past 6 months he had felt more tired than usual at the end of his work day and found little energy to devote to weekend activities. He attributed these changes to the onset of middle age, to the complacency of his mid-career status, and, most troubling to him, being less apt to exercise regularly. JW's medical history was brief and unhelpful: an appendectomy at 15 years of age, a concussion sustained during a pickup football game in graduate school, and a hospitalization for an atypical pneumonia at age 30. He drank an occasional glass of wine or beer; he was married to a college professor and had two elementary school-aged daughters.

The physician performed a physical examination and obtained laboratory studies, including a complete blood count, blood chemistries, and liver function tests. The physical examination was normal except for mild tenderness in the epigastric region. There was no spleen tip felt; the liver was 2 cm by percussion. Results of the laboratory tests were normal except for an elevated serum alanine aminotransferase (ALT) of 345 units/L (laboratory normal 6–41 units/L) and aspartate aminotransferase of 139 units/L (laboratory normal 9–34 units/L). Concerned, the physician called JW to discuss a plan for evaluation of the abnormal liver function tests and to review JW's medical and social history again. Specifically, he asked JW for history of blood product transfusion, transplantation, use of recreational or "street" drugs, and whether he had received injections where there was a possibility that nonsterile equipment was used. He asked for a sexual history including number of partners, history of payment for sex, and risky sexual practices. Most of the additional history shed little light on the abnormal liver function tests except for the fact that in 1990, while JW was an undergraduate and considering a health care career, he had been employed as a phlebotomist at a large inner city hospital. JW recalled the trauma of receiving an accidental deep needlestick while discarding phlebotomy equipment into an overly full sharps container and the several months of anxious serial testing for human immunodeficiency virus (HIV) that followed but ended, happily, with negative results. The incident had long been put out of JW's mind.

With this history, JW's physician included serology for antibodies to hepatitis C by enzyme-linked immunosorbent assay (ELISA or EIA), HIV ELISA, and hepatitis B surface antigen in the laboratory evaluation. The HIV and hepatitis B studies were negative, but the hepatitis C EIA was positive and was confirmed by recombinant immunoblot assay (RIBA) and a positive qualitative test for hepatitis C RNA. The physician informed JW that he suspected chronic hepatitis C, most likely as a result of the long-forgotten needlestick, and would need to plan for further evaluation, possible treatment, and some lifestyle considerations, including avoidance of alcohol.

JW's story is typical of many hepatitis C patients. His exposure occurred many years in the past, and he lacked major symptoms of liver disease. He complained of some fatigue, but it was not disturbing enough to cause him to seek special medical attention. The positive hepatitis C serology was discovered, as it often is, when an individual seeks medical care for an unrelated event. JW's physician initiated a number of interventions for the newly diagnosed patient: educational sessions and provision of written materials for JW and his wife to help them understand the illness, the possibilities of transmission, and options for treatment. He was scheduled for an appointment with a hepatologist for further evaluation of the hepatitis C infection.

After the causative agents of two transmissible types of hepatitis, A and B, were identified in the 1960s and 1970s, it was evident that at least one other agent, initially called "non-A, non-B," was responsible for hepatic disease in a large number of transfusion recipients and injection drug users (Thomas & Seeff, 2005). This third agent, hepatitis C virus (HCV), is a single-stranded RNA virus of the Flaviviridae family that includes several viruses important in causing human disease: dengue (see chapter 7), West Nile fever (see chapter 23), Japanese encephalitis, yellow fever, and St. Louis encephalitis (Robertson et al., 1998). HCV was isolated and sequenced in 1989, and an assay for detection in serum was approved in 1992 (Alter et al., 1989; Choo et al., 1989; McHutchison & Bacon, 2005). HCV is genetically diverse, existing as at least 6 major genotypes, each with more than 50 subtypes designated as 1a, 1b, etc. While some HCV genotypes have worldwide distribution, there are distinct differences in prevalence as well as regional distribution (Shepard, Finelli, & Alter, 2005; Simmonds et al., 2005). This genetic variability is one reason HCV may avoid detection and destruction by the human immune system and also helps explain its varied natural history, treatment responsiveness, and the difficulties faced in developing an effective HCV vaccine (De Francesco & Migliaccio, 2005; Houghton & Abrignani, 2005).

The overall prevalence of positive hepatitis C serology, denoting past exposure to hepatitis C, is 1.8% of the U.S. population, or an estimated 3.9 million people. Approximately 2.7 million people in the United States have chronic hepatitis C infection, and up to 170 million people world-wide are infected. Males in the 30–49-year-old age group have the highest prevalence (Alter et al., 1999; Centers for Disease Control and Prevention [CDC], 2004b; McHutchison & Bacon, 2005). Hepatitis C is endemic globally with prevalence estimates varying by country from a low of 0.6% (Germany) to 22% (Egypt). High prevalence rates are found in countries of Africa and southwestern Asia, although data are far from complete (Shepard et al., 2005). In the United States, prevalence studies also demonstrate a wide range. A national sero-study of users of the Department of Veterans Affairs (VA) health care system estimated a prevalence of 5.4% (reflecting, predominantly, traditional risk factors of past blood transfusion and injection drug use in the VA patient population; Dominitz et al., 2005). A study in Baltimore, Maryland, found an HCV prevalence of 15% and 18% among patients attending a clinic for sexually transmitted diseases and an urban emergency room, respectively (Thomas, 2000). The Third National Health and Nutrition Examination survey among noninstitutionalized U.S. civilians detected high HCV prevalence rates in African American and Mexican American men; however, when data were adjusted for transmission risk factors and socioeconomic variables, racial/ethnic and gender differences were not seen (Alter et al., 1999), although high prevalences are known to exist in specific age groups, for example, among African American men currently 40 to 59 years old, who have a prevalence of 6.1% (National Institutes of Health [NIH], 2002). Other subpopulations are a major cause for concern—incarcerated and homeless persons and injection drug users are known to have prevalence rates of 70 to 90% (CDC, 2003; NIH, 2002; Samuel, Bulterys, Jenison, & Doherty, 2005).

It is estimated that 30,000 new infections occur each year in the United States, although there has been a decline in the incidence of infection since 1989, when the virus was identified and serologic tests developed, leading in July 1992 to a safer blood supply and better understanding of risk behaviors (CDC, 2004a; McHutchison & Bacon, 2005). However, 8,000 to 10,000 people die annually of the consequences of the disease in the United States (CDC, 2004a), and hepatitis C is the leading cause of chronic liver diseases such as cirrhosis, end-stage liver disease, and liver cancer. It is the major reason for liver transplantation in the United States (NIH, 2002). Moreover, the number of chronic infections recognized is expected to increase as Americans with past risk factors for hepatitis C, including blood transfusion before donor screening, past occupational exposures, or injection drug use are found to be infected. Direct notification programs for those who received transfusions from donors who later tested positive for hepatitis C have been conducted (Buffington, Rowel, Hinman, Sharp, & Choi, 2001).

The major route of transmission is by direct percutaneous exposure to the blood of an infected person. This transmission may occur via transfusion of contaminated blood and blood products, exposure to contaminated medical equipment (through recreational or street drug use or through unsafe therapeutic injections), or transplantation of organs from an infected donor. With screening of blood products and blood donors, the incidence of posttransfusion HCV infection is now estimated to be less than 1 per 100,000 units of transfused blood in the United States (Shepard et al., 2005; Sulkowski, Mast, Seeff, & Thomas, 2000). The overwhelming majority of new cases of HCV in the United States and elsewhere currently occur in injection drug users or those who are exposed to contaminated medical equipment (Shepard et al., 2005). Because of common risk factors, one third or more of HIV-infected persons may also be coinfected with HCV (Backus, Boothroyd, & Deyton, 2005; Sulkowski et al., 2000).

HCV transmission from patients to health care workers via accidental needlestick, or exposure to blood via mucous membranes and conjunctiva, has been reported, although fortunately it appears increasingly rare with the use of standard (universal) precautions and safer needle devices. The risk after needlestick exposure to an HCV-infected patient has been reported to range from 1.8% to 8%, with the greatest risk from a deep puncture with a blood-contaminated hollow-bore needle (Boal, Hales, & Ross, 2005; Fry, 2005; Thomas, 2000; Yazdanpanah et al., 2005). Transmission from health care providers to patients has also been described infrequently, including one case of six patients who were infected by a surgeon (Esteban et al., 1996). Hepatitis C-infected health care workers are generally considered to be at low risk for transmission to patients. Recommendations for practice restrictions should be individualized to a health care worker's specific job duties (CDC, 1998; Thomson & Finch, 2005).

Nosocomial transmission has been described. A contaminated colonoscope was implicated in the transmission of HCV from one patient to others (Bronowicki et al., 1997). Patients have been infected through use of contaminated multidose vials used during anesthesia (Gremion & Cerny, 2005), through unsafe therapeutic injection practices (Faustini et al., 2005), and during hemodialysis (Savey et al., 2005). Inadvertent transmission during preventive health campaigns has also been described, such as in injection therapy for schistosomiasis in Egypt (Habib et al., 2001). Tattooing, acupuncture, human bites, sharing of body jewelry, and medical folk practices such as scarification rituals have been associated with HCV transmission, although these practices are considered to be isolated, lower-level risks for transmission (Daniel & Sheha, 2005; McHutchison & Bacon, 2005; Samuel et al, 2005; Thomas, 2000; Thomson & Finch, 2005).

HCV can be transmitted sexually; HCV RNA has been detected in saliva and semen, although the efficiency of sexual transmission is much less than that of direct percutaneous blood exposure. High HCV prevalence is found in commercial sex workers and those with multiple sex partners, especially 50 partners and more (CDC, 1998; Shepard et al., 2005; Thomas, 2000). Unprotected sexual intercourse between long-term steady partners demonstrated HCV seroprevalence rates of 4.4% in the partner, with risk of infection increasing with the length of the relationship (Tong et al., 1995). Perinatal transmission rates from an HCV-infected mother to her infant are reported to be from 0% to 8.4% in various studies (Shepard et al., 2005; Tajiri et al., 2001; Thomas, 2000). There is an increased risk of transmitting HCV perinatally in those women with high HCV viral load, viremia at delivery, and/or HIV coinfection. In particular, women with HIV and hepatitis C coinfection are recommended to consider cesarean delivery and avoid breast-feeding (Shepard et al., 2005; Tajiri et al., 2001; Thomson & Finch, 2005).

After infection, HCV virus can be measured in blood (by HCV RNA) in 2 to 3 weeks, and 90% of infected persons have measurable HCV antibodies within 3 months. In contrast to other types of viral hepatitis, only about 20% of infected persons develop symptoms of hepatitis C within the first month or two after infection (NIH, 2002; Thomas & Seeff, 2005). Some persons with acute hepatitis C or asymptomatic infection clear the infection, but 65% to 85% of those who are infected develop chronic, lifelong infection (defined as presence of HCV RNA in serum for 6 months or more) that results in a spectrum of disease from mild illness to cirrhosis and end-stage liver disease. Individuals may remain asymptomatic for decades, not realizing that they are infected. During this time, they may transmit HCV to others (NIH, 2002; Thomas & Seeff, 2005). Eventually, infected persons may recognize nonspecific symptoms such as malaise, fatigue, anorexia, right-sided abdominal pain, and weight loss. Chronic hepatitis C is characterized not only by persistent presence of HCV in the blood, but also by fluctuations in levels of serum ALT. Studies have demonstrated variability in hepatitis C disease progression—women, young age at infection, White race, and normal immune function are associated with clearing of HCV after infection, while men, older age at infection, African American race, and those who are immunosuppressed are more likely to develop persistent disease (NIH, 2002; Thomas & Seeff, 2005; Wiese et al., 2005). Chronic hepatitis C infection may have extrahepatic effects, also. Mixed cryoglobulinemia is the most studied; but reports of Sjögren syndrome, diabetes, and thyroid disease appear in the literature as well (Ali & Zein, 2005).

The liver damage caused by HCV appears to be not a direct effect of the viral infection but from the inflammatory response to it—immune system cells that attack hepatocytes displaying HCV markers (Gremion & Cerny, 2005). In persons with chronic HCV infection, approximately 20% will develop cirrhosis over the 20–30-year period after initial infection, but disease progression may be accelerated in males, in persons with coinfection with hepatitis B or HIV, persons with heavy alcohol intake, and persons with nonalcoholic liver disease (McHutchison & Bacon, 2005). Manifestations of progression to cirrhosis include portal hypertension with ascites, edema, esophageal varices, bleeding, jaundice, prothrombin time prolongation, hypoalbuminemia, and hepatic encephalopathy (Everson, 2005). Hepatocellular carcinoma may develop in those with HCV-related cirrhosis; the annual rate of development is estimated at 1–4% annually (Thomas & Seeff, 2005). Since most persons currently living with hepatitis C were infected between 1960 and 1990, and given the long quiescent period before severe manifestations of chronic hepatitis C are apparent, the societal burden of hepatitis C is projected to dramatically increase between 2005 and 2020. Hospitalizations, cases of cirrhosis, cases of hepatocellular carcinoma, the need for liver transplantation for hepatitis C-related liver failure, and hepatitis C-related deaths will increase manyfold (Everson, 2005; McHutchison & Bacon, 2005).

The long indolent period of hepatitis C infection, coupled with the presence of infectious HCV in the blood, allows this disease to go unrecognized and to be transmitted by its apparently healthy host. Health care providers must recognize persons at risk and recommend testing for them. Risk factors for hepatitis C overlap with those of other bloodborne virus infections like HIV and hepatitis B. Persons with longstanding HIV or hepatitis B may not have been tested for hepatitis C since the serologic test for HCV was developed after that for hepatitis B or HIV, and the high rates of prevalence of HCV have only recently been recognized. Table 12.1 lists persons at risk for HCV infection.

Early diagnosis allows for implementation of practices to reduce transmission and to provide early treatment to limit disease progression before significant liver damage occurs. Serologic tests for presence of antibody to hepatitis C are reliable and accurate. These tests include EIA for use in screening and RIBA, the latter usually employed as a confirmatory

Table 12.1. Persons Who Should Consider Testing for Hepatitis C

- Persons who ever injected illegal drugs, including those who injected once or a few times many years ago and do not consider themselves drug users
- Persons who received clotting factor concentrates produced before 1987
- Persons who were ever on chronic (long-term) hemodialysis
- Persons with persistently abnormal alanine aminotransferase levels
- Persons who were notified that they received blood from a donor who later tested positive for HCV infection
- Persons who received a transfusion of blood or blood components before July 1992
- Persons who received an organ transplant before July 1992
- Health care, emergency medical, and public safety workers who have had needlesticks, sharps, or mucosal exposures to HCV-positive blood
- Children born to HCV-positive mothers

Source: Centers for Disease Control and Prevention, 1998.

test. Diagnostic tests that directly detect HCV RNA include both quantitative and qualitative polymerase chain reaction and branched DNA signal amplification assay (Desombere, Van Vlierberghe, Couvent, Clinckspoor, & Leroux-Roels, 2005). HCV RNA measurement provides a useful technique to follow the response to therapy or to diagnose HCV in an immunocompromised patient who does not mount a measurable antibody response, thus leading to false-negative serologic tests (Desombere et al., 2005; NIH, 2002).

Drug therapies for hepatitis C have improved steadily over the past two decades. Therapy is given with the aim of clearing detectable levels of virus from serum and, ultimately, to prevent long-term liver damage. Currently, optimal therapy is considered to be the combination of an immunomodulatory drug, pegylated interferon alfa, and an antiviral drug, ribavirin, given for 24 to 48 weeks (depending on mid-treatment course response and HCV genotype). Treatment should be considered for all persons with hepatitis C but is especially recommended for those whose disease is most likely to progress to cirrhosis. This includes those with persistent abnormal ALT levels, circulating HCV RNA, and moderate to severe hepatitis and fibrosis on biopsy (Hoofnagle & Seeff, 2006; McHutchison & Bacon, 2005; NIH, 2002). The combination of pegylated interferon alfa and ribavirin will cure about 50% of persons with hepatitis C. However, success rates vary greatly by HCV genotype, and the list of contraindications to the drugs is long, the treatment is very expensive, and side effects can be daunting (Hoofnagle & Seeff, 2006; McHutchison & Baker, 2005). Relapses are common, and better therapies are needed for patients who need retreatment or are in special categories, like those who develop acute hepatitis C or recurrent hepatitis C after receiving a liver transplantation. Inexpensive and effective simple drug regimens are needed to treat the many millions of people worldwide infected with hepatitis C. New antiviral drugs and immunomodulatory agents are in Phase I and II clinical trials and are expected to increase the available pool of drugs and therapeutic options (DeFrancesco & Migliaccio, 2005).

Many people currently living with hepatitis C acquired it through infected blood products. The discovery of the virus, the development of sensitive tests to detect it, and efficient and thorough means to eliminate it in plasma-derived products (such as blood-clotting factors and immunoglobulin) mean that blood products are no longer a major transmission consideration in those countries where these blood-product screening measures are used. But there is ongoing transmission via injection drug use in the developed world and via exposure to contaminated blood products or medical equipment in the developing world. A safe and effective preventive hepatitis C vaccine has been sought for more than a decade. Because of characteristics of hepatitis C, including its genetic variability and a lack of understanding of the human immune response to HCV infection, development of a preventive vaccine has been elusive, although prospects are improving with some recent discoveries (Houghton & Abrignani, 2005). Therapeutic vaccines that would stimulate the immune system of an already infected person to respond to the virus are also the subject of research efforts (Houghton & Abrignani, 2005).

While therapies and improved vaccines are being developed, there is a great need for all health care providers to be aware of the current and coming burden of hepatitis C, to teach patients about hepatitis management and transmission prevention, to enable at-risk persons to reduce their risk of HCV infection by providing treatment for substance use, and to teach the avoidance of exposure to potentially infected blood or body fluids (see Table 12.2).

SUMMARY

Chronic HCV infection frequently results in serious liver disease. An estimated 2.7 million Americans and 170 million persons around the world are thought to have chronic hepatitis C. The disease frequently develops over decades and causes few symptoms so that people are often not aware that they are infected until they have manifestations of serious liver disease. HCV is transmitted by contact with blood or tissue of an infected person through transfusion of blood or blood products, organ or tissue transplantation, sharing of needles or medical equipment between persons without adequate sterilization, and, less frequently, high-risk sexual

Table 12.2. Primary and Secondary Prevention of Hepatitis C Infection

---

Primary prevention—the best ways to prevent hepatitis C infection are as follows:

- Exclude HCV-positive donors, or persons at high risk for HCV, from donating blood, plasma, tissue, organs, or semen.
- Inactivate viruses in clotting factor concentrates and other plasma-derived products.
- Counsel clients to discontinue use of illegal drugs.
- If drugs are used, counsel clients never to share or reuse needles, syringes, water, or any part of "works," including straws used intranasally.
- Counsel clients not to share razors, toothbrushes, body jewelry, or manicure equipment items that might be contaminated with blood.
- Counsel patients that the best way to avoid sexually transmitted diseases including HIV, hepatitis B, and, to an extent, hepatitis C is to not have sex or to have sex with one monogamous partner.
- Counsel patients to use male or female condoms correctly, every time they engage in sex.

Secondary prevention—for persons who have hepatitis C, the best ways to protect the liver from further damage are as follows:

- Follow the recommendations of your health care provider.
- Avoid alcohol.
- Do not use illegal drugs.
- Do not take medicines, including over-the-counter, herbal, or alternative medicines, without the recommendation of your health care provider.
- Maintain a healthy body weight.
- Get vaccinated for hepatitis A and B.
- Get tested for human immunodeficiency virus, and consider treatment if positive.

Source: Centers for Disease Control and Prevention, 1998; Thomas & Seeff, 2005.

practices and an infected mother to her child. Nosocomial transmission infrequently occurs. Many risk factors for hepatitis C overlap those of other bloodborne diseases, like HIV and hepatitis B. Coinfection with other bloodborne viruses may accelerate the rate of hepatitis C progression. Since 1992, blood and blood products in the United States are considered safe from HCV, although transmission through contaminated blood products and medical equipment continues to be a problem in the developing world. Transmission by sharing needles or illegal drug equipment continues to be a major route of HCV transmission everywhere. Health care providers of every discipline need to know the risk factors for hepatitis C and to consider hepatitis C risk in every patient. The best way to reduce transmission and prevent progression of HCV infection is to know what the risks are, to test for it, to educate persons at risk about prevention and lifestyle alteration, to treat those eligible, and to facilitate research in all facets of the disease.

REFERENCES

Ali, A., & Zein, N. N. (2005). Hepatitis C infection: A systemic disease with extrahepatic manifestations. *Cleveland Clinic Journal of Medicine, 72,* 1005–1008.

Alter, H. J., Purcell, R. H., Shih, J. W., Melpolder, J. C., Houghton, M., Choo, Q.-L., et al. (1989). Detection of antibody to hepatitis C in prospectively followed transfusion recipients with acute and chronic non-A, non-B hepatitis. *New England Journal of Medicine, 321,* 1494–1500.

Alter, M. J., Kruszon-Moran, D., Nainan, O. V., McQuillan, G. M., Fengxiang, G., Moyer, L. A, et al. (1999). The prevalence of hepatitis C infection in the United States, 1988 through 1994. *New England Journal of Medicine, 341,* 556–562.

Backus, L. I., Boothroyd, D., & Deyton, L. R. (2005). HIV, hepatitis C and HIV/hepatitis C virus co-infection in vulnerable populations. *AIDS, 19*(Suppl. 3), S13–19.

Boal, W. L., Hales, T., & Ross, C. S. (2005). Blood-borne pathogens among firefighters and emergency technicians. *Prehospital Emergency Care, 9*(2), 236–247.

Bronowicki, J. P., Venard, V., Botté, C., Monhoven, N., Gastin, I., Choné, L., et al. (1997). Patient-to-patient transmission of hepatitis C virus during colonoscopy. *New England Journal of Medicine, 337,* 237–240.

Buffington, J., Rowel, R., Hinman, J. M., Sharp, K., & Choi, S. (2001). Lack of awareness of hepatitis C risk among persons who received blood transfusions before 1990. *American Journal of Public Health, 91,* 47–48.

Centers for Disease Control and Prevention. (1998). Recommendations for prevention and control of hepatitis C virus (HCV) infection and HCV-related chronic disease. *Morbidity and Mortality Weekly Report, 47*(RR-19), 1–39.

Centers for Disease Control and Prevention. (2003). Prevention and control of infections with hepatitis in correctional settings. *Morbidity and Mortality Weekly Report, 52*(RR-01), 1–33.

Centers for Disease Control and Prevention. (2004a). *Disease burden from viral hepatitis A, B, and C in the United States.* Retrieved February 26, 2006, from http://www.cdc.gov/ncidod/diseases/hepatitis/resource/PDFs/disease_burden2004.pdf

Centers for Disease Control and Prevention. (2004b). *Hepatitis Surveillance Report No. 59.* Atlanta, GA: U.S. Department of Health and Human Services. Retrieved February 26, 2005, from http://www.cdc.gov/ncidod/diseases/hepatitis/resource/PDFs/hep_surveillance_59.pdf

Choo, Q.-L., Kuo, G., Weiner, A. J., Overby, L. R., Bradley, D. W., & Houghton, M. (1989). Isolation of a CDNA clone derived from a blood-borne non-A, non-B viral hepatitis genome. *Science, 244,* 359–362.

Daniel, A. R., & Sheha, T. (2005). Transmission of hepatitis C through swapping body jewelry. *Pediatrics, 116,* 1264–1265.

De Francesco, R., & Migliaccio, G. (2005). Challenges and successes in developing new therapies for hepatitis C. *Nature, 436,* 953–960.

Desombere I., Van Vlierberghe H., Couvent S., Clinckspoor, F., Leroux-Roels, G. (2005). Comparison of qualitative (COBAS AMPLICOR HCV 2.0 versus VERSANT HCV RNA) and quantitative (COBAS AMPLICOR HCV monitor 2.0 versus VERSANT HCV RNA 3.0) assays for hepatitis C virus (HCV) RNA detection and quantification: impact on diagnosis and treatment of HCV infections. *Journal of Clinical Microbiology, 43*, 2590–2597.

Dominitz, J. A., Boyko, E. J., Koepsell, T. D., Heagerty, P. J., Maynard, C., Sporleder J. L., et al. (2005). Elevated prevalence of hepatitis C injection in users of United States veterans medical centers. *Hepatology, 41*(1), 88–96.

Esteban, J. I., Gomez, J., Martell, M., Cabot, B., Quer, J., Camps, J., et al. (1996). Transmission of hepatitis C virus by a cardiac surgeon. *New England Journal of Medicine, 334*, 550–560.

Everson, G. T. (2005). Management of cirrhosis due to chronic hepatitis C. *Journal of Hepatology, 42*, S45–74.

Faustini, A., Capobianchi, M. R., Martinelli, M., Abbate, I., Cappiello, G., & Perucci, C. A. (2005). A cluster of hepatitis C virus infections associated with ozone-enriched transfusion of autologous blood in Rome, Italy. *Infection Control and Hospital Epidemiology, 26*, 763–7.

Fry, D. E. (2005). Occupational blood-borne diseases in surgery. *American Journal of Surgery, 190*, 249–254.

Gremion, C., & Cerny, A. (2005). Hepatitis C virus and the immune system: A concise review. *Reviews in Medical Virology, 15*(4), 235–268.

Habib, M., Mohamed, M. K., Abdel-Aziz, F., Magder, L. S., Abdet-Hamid, M., Gamil, F., et al. (2001). Hepatitis C virus infection in a community in the Nile delta: Risk factors for seropositivity. *Hepatology, 33*, 248–233.

Hoofnagle J. H., & Seeff, L. B. (2006). Peginterferon and ribaviran for chronic hepatitis C. *New England Journal of Medicine, 355*, 2444–2451

Houghton, M., & Abrignani, S. (2005). Prospects for a vaccine against hepatitis C. *Nature, 436*, 961–966.

McHutchison, J. G., & Bacon, B. R. (2005). Chronic hepatitis C: An age wave of disease burden. *American Journal of Managed Care, 11*, S286–295.

National Institutes of Health. (2002). *Management of hepatitis C: 2002. National Institutes of Health Consensus Conference Statement, June 10–12, 2002.* Retrieved February 21, 2006, from http://consensus.nih.gov/2002/2002HepatitisC2002116html.htm

Robertson, B., Myers, G., Howard, C., Brettin, T., Bukh, J., Gaschen, B., et al. (1998). Classification, nomenclature, and database development for hepatitis C virus (HCV) and related viruses: Proposals for standardization. *Archives of Virology, 143*, 2493–2503.

Samuel, M. C., Bulterys, M., Jenison, S., & Doherty, P. (2005). Tattoos, incarceration and hepatitis B and C among street-recruited injection drug users in New Mexico, USA: Update. *Epidemiology and Infection, 133*, 1146–1148.

Savey, A., Simon, F., Izopet, J., Lepoutre, A., Fabry, J., & Desenclos, J. C. (2005). A large nosocomial outbreak of hepatitis C virus infections at a hemodialysis center. *Infection Control and Hospital Epidemiology, 26*, 752–760.

Shepard, C. W., Finelli, L., & Alter, M. J. (2005). Global epidemiology of hepatitis C virus infection. *Lancet Infectious Diseases, 5,* 558–567.

Simmonds, P., Bukh, J., Combet, C., Deleage, G., Enomoto, G., & Feinstone, S., et al. (2005). Consensus proposals for a unified system of nomenclature of hepatitis C virus genotypes. *Hepatology, 42,* 962–973.

Sulkowski, M. S., Mast, E. E., Seeff, L. B., & Thomas, D. L. (2000). Hepatitis C virus infection as an opportunistic disease in persons infected with human immunodeficiency virus. *Clinical Infectious Diseases, 30,* S77–84.

Tajiri, H., Miyoshi, Y., Funada, S., Etani, Y., Abe, J., Onodera, T., et al. (2001). Prospective study of mother-to-infant transmission of hepatitis C virus. *Pediatric Infectious Diseases Journal, 20,* 10–14.

Thomas, D. L. (2000). Hepatitis C epidemiology. *Current Topics in Microbiology and Immunology, 242,* 25–41.

Thomas, D. L., & Seeff, L. B. (2005). Natural history of hepatitis C. *Clinics in Liver Disease, 9,* 383–398.

Thomson, B. J., & Finch, R. G. (2005). Hepatitis C virus infection. *Clinical Microbiology and Infectious Diseases, 11,* 86–94.

Tong, M. J., Lai, P. P. C., Hwang, S.-J., Lee, S.-Y., Co, R. L., Chien, R. N., et al. (1995). Evaluation of sexual transmission in patients with hepatitis C infection. *Clinical and Diagnostic Virology, 3,* 39–47.

Wiese, M., Grungrieff, K., Guthoff, W., Lafrenz, M., Oesen, U., Porst, H., et al. (2005). Outcome in a hepatitis C (genotype 1b) single source outbreak in Germany—A 25-year multicenter study. *Journal of Hepatology, 43,* 550–552.

Yazdanpanah Y., De Carli, G., Migueres, B., Lot, F., Campins, M., Colombo, C., et al. (2005). Risk factors for hepatitis C virus transmission to health care workers after occupational exposure: a European case control study. *Clinical Infectious Diseases, 41,* 1423–1430.

CHAPTER THIRTEEN

HIV/AIDS

Inge B. Corless

An emerging disease has all the drama of a good mystery—in some cases, an unknown assailant, one or more victims, and various clues as to the mode and method of assault. Human immunodeficiency virus/acquired immunodeficiency syndrome (HIV/AIDS) was and, to some extent, remains a mystery and cause of continuing debate. But it is a "cold case" no longer as we know the cause and increasingly the intricacies of attack. The jury is still out, however, as to the cure and or a biological mode of prevention. In this chapter the evidence and debate on the cause of AIDS and how it arose in humans and subsequently became a pandemic will be reviewed, along with an examination of the current epidemiology, pathogenicity, approaches to therapy, vaccine development efforts, and the political and economic ramifications of HIV/AIDS.

In the United States, the condition that came to be known as HIV/AIDS was first recognized by physicians who noted uncommon presentations of disease such as *Pneumocystis carinii* pneumonia (PCP, now *Pneumocystis jiroveci*) and Kaposi sarcoma in young homosexual men and by a clerk at the Centers for Disease Control (CDC) who observed frequent requests for pentamidine, a drug used to treat PCP, a formerly rare condition (CDC, 1981a, 1981b; Friedman-Kien, 1981; Gottlieb et al., 1981; Masur et al., 1981; Shilts, 1987). These observations marked the beginning of awareness of the HIV/AIDS epidemic in the United States.

Clinicians and scientists hypothesized early on that the disease, which induced severe immunosuppression, followed a transmission pattern similar to that of hepatitis B, a belief verified by the identification of transfusion-related infection in 1982 (CDC, 1982). The cause of the immunosuppression was first identified by the Pasteur Institute's

Luc Montagnier (Barré-Sinoussi et al., 1983) as lymphadenopathy virus, thereafter by Gallo (Popovic, Sarngadharan, Read, & Gallo, 1984; Sarngadharan, Popovic, Bruch, Schupbach, & Gallo, 1984) as human T-cell lymphotropic virus type III, and by Levy (Levy et al., 1984) as AIDS-associated retrovirus (ARV). A special committee designated to determine one name for the newly identified organism resolved the differing nomenclature. The organism was named "human immunodeficiency virus" and the resultant disease "acquired immunodeficiency syndrome" (Coffin et al., 1986). HIV is a retrovirus that has two types, HIV-1 and HIV-2. HIV-1 is composed of three groups: M for main; N for non-M, non-O; and O for outlier. There are subtype designations within the groups. In group M, there are subtype or clade designations A–K (Hahn, Shaw, De Cock, & Sharp, 2000; Robertson et al., 2000).

Although the virus had a name, HIV as the cause of AIDS was challenged by Duesberg (1988), who argued that HIV did not comply with all of Koch's postulates, the ground rules of whether an organism causes a disease. In particular, Duesberg (1989, 1991, 1994) argued that HIV could not be isolated from all individuals who are immunosuppressed, thereby violating one of Koch's postulates. Advances in technology and the resultant identification of the presence of HIV refute this claim. Scientists have examined the evidence regarding myths about HIV as the cause of AIDS and have overwhelmingly concluded that HIV is the cause of AIDS (Ascher, Sheppard, Winkelstein, & Vittinghoff, 1993; Delaney, 2000; Hillis, 2000; Joint United Nations Programme on HIV/AIDS, 2005; Kurth, 1990; National Institute of Allergy and Infectious Diseases, 2000a, 2000b).

Even though the cause of AIDS has been scientifically established, questions about how HIV became established in humans has been a source of controversy since humans are not the natural host. Apparently HIV became established in humans through cross-species transmission, and this makes AIDS a zoonosis. The simian lentivirus, simian immunodeficiency virus (SIV) of sooty mangabeys, was the source of HIV-2, and HIV-1 arose from the SIV from chimpanzees (SIVcpz), the *Pan troglodytes troglodytes* subspecies (Stebbing, Gazzard, & Douek, 2004). Zoonotic transmission to humans has been documented on multiple occasions, and SIV has been demonstrated to replicate in human peripheral mononuclear cells in vitro (Grimm, Beer, Hirsch, & Clouse, 2003).

The manner in which trans-species crossover of HIV occurred was the cause of vigorous debate. Hahn and colleagues (2000) outlined two competing hypotheses. The one Hahn and her colleagues favored is that exposure to animal blood in the course of hunting, butchering, and ingestion of raw bush meat accounted for the transmission of HIV from primate to human. The point of initial transmission must have occurred multiple times to result in epidemic spread and is accounted for through a combination of factors, including urbanization, disruption of family life through jobs at a distance from families leading to risky sexual behaviors, prostitution, cultural mores that promote men having numerous sexual partners, and the use of unsterilized needles for both medicinal and recreational drug injections. While these sociocultural factors contribute to the transmission of an infection that has already gotten a toehold, the factors in and of themselves are necessary but not sufficient for a pandemic.

The other hypothesis noted by Hahn and associates (2000) has been proposed by a number of individuals including Curtis (1992), Elswood and Stricker (1994), and Hooper (1999). This hypothesis is that SIVcpz was present in the kidney substrate used in the propagation of oral polio virus (OPV) for vaccination trials in the Belgian Congo in the 1950s. Elswood and Stricker focused on simian virus 40 contamination of early polio vaccine and viewed this as a means of transmitting a simian precursor of HIV to man. Hooper investigated the various clues, interviewed key informants who were present at the conduct of the oral polio vaccine trials in Africa or who had knowledge of them, examined the travels of various armies and other migrations, and consulted with world-renowned scientists. He listed 27 arguments for the OPV contamination thesis and 4 against the hypothesis. In his view, the argument against the OPV connection boils down to the lack of definitive evidence. Specifically against the hypothesis are that most of the animals used for the oral polio vaccine were from different species than the ones from which HIV originated and that the M group of HIV-1 is believed to have originated 10–50 years before the vaccine trials began (Hahn et al., 2000; Korber et al., 2000; Korber, Theiler, & Wolinsky, 1998). Additional data from four groups of researchers found no evidence of chimpanzee DNA in an analysis of multiple oral polio vaccine samples, and thus there appeared to be no support for the introduction of HIV to humans through OPV (Poinar, Kuch, & Paabo, 2001).

Geographical association is demonstrated by both HIV-1 and HIV-2. HIV-2 is particularly associated with areas in West Africa such as Senegal, Guinea-Bissau, Guinea Conakry, Cote d'Ivoire, Sierra Leone, and Liberia. HIV-1 group N infections have been found primarily in Cameroon. Groups M, N, and O have all been found in Gabon, Equatorial Guinea, Cameroon, and the Republic of the Congo (Congo-Brazzaville; Hahn et al., 2000). The clades of Group M have been found worldwide, with clade B predominant in North America and Europe; clades B and BF in Latin America; clades B and C in North Africa and the Middle East; clades A, C, D, F, G, H, J, K and CRF (a recombinant type) in sub-Saharan Africa; clades A, B, and AB in Eastern Europe and Central Asia; clades B, C, and BC in East Asia; and clades B and AE in South and Southeast

Asia (Simon, Ho, & Abdool Karim, 2006). This picture of regional clade dominance is likely to change with time and the travel of HIV-infected individuals.

In 2005, 4.1 million persons were newly infected with HIV and an estimated 2.8 million died from HIV/AIDS. At the end of 2005, an estimated 38.6 million (33.4 million–46.0 million) people were living with HIV infection; of these, 25 million were in sub-Saharan Africa (UNAIDS, 2006). Women are increasingly affected, now comprising about 42% of those living with HIV. Over 70% of HIV-infected women live in sub-Saharan Africa (Simon et al., 2006). Since the onset of the pandemic, an estimated 65 million persons have been infected with HIV/AIDS, with 25 million deaths worldwide from the disease (CDC, 2006; Simon et al., 2006).

In the United States, an estimated 1,039,000 to 1,185,000 persons are living with HIV/AIDS (Glynn & Rhodes, 2005), possibly 24–27% of whom are not aware of their infection. Through 2004, the total estimated number of diagnosed AIDS cases in the United States was 944,305. Most (73%) were male, although this percentage is lower than previously. Most (66%) infected persons were from ethnic minority groups, an increase from prior years. The overall rate per 100,000 population in the United States is 136.5 for HIV infection and 176.2 for AIDS.

The states and territories with highest rates for AIDS in adults and adolescents are the District of Columbia (2,091.2), New York (458.7), the Virgin Islands (346.9), Puerto Rico (339.4), Florida (301.7), and Maryland (304.6). The overall rate per 100,000 for children under 13 years diagnosed with HIV is 7.4, whereas the rate of AIDS is 2.7. The states and territories with the highest rates of AIDS per 100,000 for children under 13 years of age are the District of Columbia (45.5), the Virgin Islands (13.1), and Florida (8.6). Not all states collect name-based HIV data, so comparisons are more difficult. Nonetheless, the rates of HIV for children in those states and territories reporting are significantly higher including New York (29.1) and New Jersey (16.1) but not the Virgin Islands (9.5) (CDC, 2005).

Transmission of HIV occurs by sexual contact; blood, including transfusions; contaminated injection equipment and needles; and an infected mother to her child during the perinatal period, including breast-feeding (Lashley, 2006). The hallmark of HIV infection is immunosuppression, leading to decreased $CD4^+$ cells and derangements of the immune system. Opportunistic illnesses, infections, and neoplasms result. Many of these infections were not seen or were seen only rarely in humans, especially in developed countries, before the AIDS pandemic. Since their initial recognition, some of these illnesses and conditions have been increasingly noticed, sometimes in the immunocompetent person. These include infections with such organisms and diseases as *Cryptosporid-ium* (see chapter 5), microsporidia (see chapter 3), West Nile virus (see chapter 23), multidrug-resistant tuberculosis (see chapter 20), Kaposi sarcoma (see chapter 24), cervical intraepithelial neoplasia (see chapter 24), *Rhodococcus equi, Penicillium marneffei* (see chapter 10), hepatitis C (see chapter 12), *Bartonella* (see chapter 3), unusual forms of *Candida* (see chapter 10), atypical mycobacteria, *Cyclospora* (see chapter 6), and others. Many of these are discussed in tables in Appendices A and B. In persons with HIV infection, these infections may:

- be more likely to be disseminated,
- have an atypical presentation,
- be more severe,
- have atypical locations,
- progress rapidly, and
- be difficult to treat (Lashley, 2000).

Emerging infectious diseases often appear disproportionately in those with HIV infection. The surveillance definition and clinical categories of AIDS may be found at the CDC Web site (http://www.cdc.gov). However, since the emergence of highly active antiretroviral treatment (HAART), "the median time to the first AIDS event after starting HAART decreased over time" (May et al., 2006, p. 455).

Although drug therapy with HAART, as well as prophylaxis for in-fections, has reduced HIV-related morbidity and mortality, debate about when to initiate treatment has been answered for the moment with the decisions to initiate treatment for those with 200–350 × 10^9 CD4 cells/L and for those with defined opportunistic infections (Bartlett & Gallant, 2005; Hammer et al., 2006). In resource-limited countries, the protocol is to initiate treatment for those with CD4 counts of 200 and below and for those with defined opportunistic infections. As new information emerges, treatment guidelines are amended to reflect the latest data (Department of Health and Human Services, 2005).

The standard of care for initiation of therapy currently is based on CD4$^+$ count. Drug treatment also takes into account such factors as level of plasma HIV RNA and the potential for poor medication adherence, among other factors. The need for strict adherence to sometimes complex drug regimens remains a key challenge to successful antiretroviral treat-ment of HIV-infected persons, although this concern is being alleviated to some degree with the emergence of regimens of one combination drug pill per day. Nonetheless, because persons living with HIV disease may take numerous drugs simultaneously, however formulated, the potential for side effects is significant.

Various government agencies have issued and updated guidelines for treatment. These guidelines are available on-line from the HIV/AIDS Treatment Information Service (http://hivatis.org) and include current and past recommendations for adult/adolescent, pediatric, and perinatal treatment. Once antiretroviral treatment has been initiated, treatment goals are aimed at durable suppression of viral load, restoration and/or preservation of immunologic function, improvement in the quality of life, and reduction of HIV-related morbidity and mortality.

Three classes of antiretroviral drugs are available for use in the treatment of HIV infection—reverse transcriptase inhibitors (RTIs), consisting of nucleoside RTIs (NRTIs) and nonnucleoside RTIs (NNRTIs); protease inhibitors (PIs); and entry inhibitors. These drugs act by different mechanisms to inhibit viral replication. Currently, there are a number of NRTIs, NNRTIs, PIs, and several entry inhibitor drugs including emtricitabine (T-20), maraviroc, vicriviroc, and eight others in various stages of investigation. A greater interest in the development of CCR5 antagonists (entry inhibitors) is apparent from the number of such drugs in process. Integrase inhibitors are also in development.

Currently more than 10 antiretroviral agents/combinations have been approved by the Food and Drug Administration for once per day use (Coffey, 2006). Atripla, a new once per day ARV, was introduced more widely at the XVI International AIDS meeting in Toronto. It must be noted that few efficacy studies have been completed on once daily regimens. Given that these medications are taken only once per day, adherence becomes all the more important.

An approach to once per day therapy is a beginning period with initial induction therapy and then switching to monotherapy (Sherer, 2006). This approach, however, is of concern to some clinicians. Although some side effects might be prevented and drug costs reduced, the concern is that resistance might develop more rapidly under these circumstances.

Many other drugs are in various stages of development and clinical testing. Because of the high costs of these drugs, individuals in the United States needing assistance may gain access to HIV-related medications through the AIDS Drug Assistance Program (ADAP) and national pharmaceutical industry patient assistance/expanded access programs (AIDS Treatment Data Network, 2006).

As exciting as the developments in antiretroviral drug therapy have been, the lack of access to medications worldwide—often because of high cost, the complexity of the regimens, the need to treat side effects, and the scarcity of practitioners with the necessary expertise and equipment—all combine to make the current therapies inaccessible to much of the world's people. Development of generic drugs in Brazil and India has made antiretroviral therapy available at reduced costs. Indeed, Brazil has decided to provide antiretroviral therapy to all of its infected citizens. In other countries, such as South Africa, determining who is to have access to insufficient supplies places health care providers in an untenable position reminiscent of the early days of hemodialysis and kidney transplantation.

Even when antiretroviral medications are available, concerns about viral resistance remain. It is suggested that resistance testing be performed on individuals with newly diagnosed acute or recent infection with HIV. Gallant (2005) indicates there is increasing support for resistance testing being conducted for chronically infected, treatment-naive patients as well.

If all persons currently infected were given access to antiretroviral medications, the problem of HIV/AIDS would not be resolved. Unless the rate of new infections is curtailed, the costs of drug provision will far outstrip the capacity to provide such drugs. The two major approaches to prevention are behavioral and pharmacological (namely, the development of a vaccine). Even if behavioral changes succeeded with consensual sexual behaviors, nonconsensual behaviors such as rape would still need to be addressed. Gang rape as an instrument of war and politics creates the conditions for rapid spread of infection. Further, the status of women in many societies, the paucity of occupational options for women, and dependency on men for economic benefits and protection combine to make women vulnerable for HIV transmission (Cohen & Durham, 1993). Such conditions make the development of a vaccine all the more urgent. Unfortunately, such development is still not on the horizon. However, even a vaccine that is 50% effective will reduce the incidence of new infections provided that the vaccinated do not engage in a greater number of risky behaviors.

Development of a vaccine must address the mutability of the human immunodeficiency virus as well as the variety of its presentation in different clades. Eliciting an antibody response indicative of resistance rather than exposure is another challenge. Last, whether to deploy a less than maximally effective vaccine is a major subject of debate. Is it better to protect some people rather than none at all? Will the imperfect protection of today's vaccines preclude later inoculation with a more advanced product? Will vaccination convey the potentially mistaken perception of protection and lead to engagement in risky behaviors? If a perfect vaccine is not available, when is a "good" vaccine good enough? The answers to these questions are not the answers to a mystery but to profound scientific, ethical, and philosophical issues. And the answers are not without political consequences. The tentative answer appears to be in favor of the good vaccine.

The infection of large portions of the adult population (30–40% in some African countries) will also have profound political, economic, and demographic consequences. The deaths of parents of young children often leave AIDS orphans without food and shelter, let alone the money for school fees. Unless these children are educated, their ability to participate in the economic sector will be impaired, potentially leading to political destabilization. The ramifications of this pandemic are profound on every level.

While there are numerous scientific mysteries still to be solved, the social and political issues may be the most elusive to solution. Although the means of transmission are well known, individuals still engage in risky behaviors. Even if everyone requiring therapy were to receive it, infected individuals who do not know their status would account for further increases in infected persons. Finally, the ARV rollout is hindered by a lack of human resources and, in particular, nurses. Task shifting may increase the recognized responsibilities of nurses in resource-limited settings.

This lack of human resources is one of several challenges that need to be addressed according to Kim and Farmer (2006). The other challenges include making available first-, second-, and third-line drugs at prices accessible to resource-limited countries; the rebuilding of the public health infrastructure; provision of services such as food, transportation to clinics, child care, and housing to those in extreme poverty; a commitment to expanding access to second-line drugs for drug-resistant AIDS and malaria; and the development of a vaccine and new classes of therapeutics (Kim & Farmer, 2006). Finally, male circumcision has been shown to decrease transmission from females to males. The translational aspect of this finding is a source of vivid debate. Given that implementation of male circumcision will not be universally acceptable, the need for female microbicides becomes all the more urgent. The Gates Foundation has made development of a female microbicide a priority for its funding.

A good mystery ends with the detective having brought the pieces of the puzzle into alignment, resulting in a neat solution. In this case, while the assailant and modes of attack have been identified, how to prevent further attacks, if not a mystery, is still a subject of much debate.

REFERENCES

AIDS Treatment Data Network. (2006). AIDS drug assistance programs. Retrieved August 20, 2006, from http://www.atdn.org/access/states/index.html

Ascher, M., Sheppard, H., Winkelstein, W., & Vittinghoff, E. (1993). Does drug use cause AIDS? Nature, 362, 103–104.

Barré-Sinoussi. F., Chermann, J., Rey, F., Nugeyre, M. T., Chamaret, S., Gruest, J., et al. (1983). Isolation of a T-lymphotropic retrovirus from a patient at risk for acquired immune deficiency syndrome (AIDS). Science, 220, 868–871.

Bartlett, J. G., & Gallant, J. E. (2005). 2005–2006 medical management of HIV infection. Baltimore, MD: Johns Hopkins University Centennial.

Centers for Disease Control. (1981a). Kaposi's sarcoma and pneumocystis pneumonia among homosexual men—New York City and California. *Morbidity and Mortality Weekly Report, 30*, 305–308.

Centers for Disease Control. (1981b). *Pneumocystis* pneumonia—Los Angeles. *Morbidity and Mortality Weekly Report, 30*, 250–252.

Centers for Disease Control. (1982). Possible transfusion-associated acquired immune deficiency syndrome (AIDS)—California. *Morbidity and Mortality Weekly Report, 31*, 652–654.

Centers for Disease Control and Prevention. (2005). *HIV/AIDS Surveillance Report, 17*, 1–54. Retrieved December 24, 2006, from http://www.cdc.gov/HIV/topics/surveillance/resources/reports/2005report/pdf2005Surveillance Report.pdf

Centers for Disease Control and Prevention. (2006). The global HIV/AIDS pandemic. *Morbidity and Mortality Weekly Report, 55*, 841–844.

Coffey, S. (2006). *Options for once-daily dosing of antiretrovirals. AETC National Resource Center.* Retrieved August 21, 2006, from http://www.aids-ed.org/aidsetc?page=et-03-00-01

Coffin, J., Haase, A., Levy, J. A., Montagnier, L., Oroszlan, S., Teich, N., et al. (1986). What to call the AIDS virus? *Nature, 321*, 10.

Cohen, F. L., & Durham, D. (Eds.). (1993). *Women, children and HIV/AIDS.* New York: Springer.

Curtis, T. (1992, March 19). The origin of AIDS. *Rolling Stone, 54*–63.

Delaney, M. (2000). *HIV/AIDS and the distortion of science.* Retrieved December 15, 2006, from http://www.aegis.org/topics/mdelaney.html

Department of Health and Human Services. (2005). *Guidelines for the use of antiretroviral agents in HIV-1-infected adults and adolescents.* Retrieved December 15, 2006, from http://AIDSinfo.nih.gov

Duesberg, P. (1988). HIV is not the cause of AIDS. *Science, 241*, 524, 517.

Duesberg, P. (1989). Human immunodeficiency virus and acquired immunodeficiency syndrome: Correlation but not causation. *Proceedings of the National Academy of Science, USA, 86*, 755–764.

Duesberg, P. (1991). AIDS epidemiology: Inconsistencies with human immunodeficiency virus and with infectious disease. *Proceedings of the National Academy of Science, USA, 88*, 1575–1579.

Duesberg, P. (1994). Infectious AIDS—Stretching the germ theory beyond its limits. *International Archives of Allergy and Immunology, 103*(2), 118–127.

Elswood, B., & Stricker, R. (1994). Polio vaccines and the origin of AIDS. *Medical Hypotheses, 42*, 347–354.

Friedman-Kien, A. (1981). Disseminated Kaposi's sarcoma syndrome in young homosexual men. *Journal of the American Academy of Dermatology, 5*, 468–471.

Gallant, J. E. (2005). Antiretroviral drug resistance and resistance testing. *Topics in HIV Medicine, 13*, 138–142.

Glynn, M., & Rhodes, P. (2005). Estimated HIV prevalence in the United States at the end of 2003. National HIV Prevention Conference; June, Atlanta. Abstract 595.

Gottlieb, M., Schroff, R., Schanker, H., Weisman, J. D., Fan, P. T., Wolf, R. A., et al. (1981). *Pneumocystis carinii* pneumonia and mucosal candidiasis in previously healthy homosexual men: Evidence of a new acquired cellular immunodeficiency. *New England Journal of Medicine, 305,* 1425–1431.

Grimm, T. A., Beer, B. E., Hirsch, V. M., & Clouse, K. A. (2003). Simian immunodeficiency viruses from multiple lineages infect human macrophages: Implications for cross-species transmission. *Journal of the Acquired Immune Deficiency Syndrome, 32,* 362–369.

Hahn, B., Shaw, G., De Cock, K., & Sharp, P. (2000). AIDS as a zoonosis: Scientific and public health implications. *Science, 287,* 607–614.

Hammer, S. M., Saag, M. S., Schechter, M., Montaner, J. S. G., Schooley, R. T., Jacobsen, D. M., et al. (2006). Treatment for adult HIV infection: 2006 recommendations of the International AIDS Society—USA Panel. *Journal of the American Medical Association, 296,* 827–843.

Hillis, D. (2000). Origins of HIV. *Science, 288,* 1757, 1759.

Hooper, E. (1999). *The river: A journey to the source of HIV and AIDS.* New York: Little Brown.

Joint United Nations Programme on HIV/AIDS. (2005). *AIDS epidemic update: 2005.* Retrieved from http://www.unaids.org/epi/2005/doc/report_pdf.asp

Kim, J. Y., & Farmer, P. (2006). AIDS in 2006—Moving toward one world, one hope? *The New England Journal of Medicine, 355,* 645–647.

Korber, B., Muldoon, M., Theiler, J., Gao, F., Gupta, R., Lapedes, A., et al. (2000). Timing the ancestor of the HIV-1 pandemic strains. *Science, 288,* 1789–1796.

Korber, B., Theiler, J., & Wolinsky, S. (1998). Limitations of a molecular clock applied to considerations of the origins of HIV-1. *Science, 280,* 1868–1871.

Kurth, R. (1990). Does HIV cause AIDS? An updated response to Duesberg's theories. *Intervirology, 31,* 301–314.

Lashley, F. R. (2000). The clinical spectrum of HIV infection and its treatment. In J. D. Durham & F. R. Lashley (Eds.), *The person with HIV/AIDS: Nursing perspectives* (3rd ed., pp. 167–270). New York: Springer.

Lashley, F. R. (2006). Transmission and epimioloy of HIV/AIDS: A global view. *Nursing Clinics of North America, 41,* 339–354.

Levy, J., Hoffman, A., Kramer, S., Landis, J., Shimabukuro, J. M., & Oshiro, L. S. (1984). Isolation of lymphocytopathic retroviruses from San Francisco patients with AIDS. *Science, 225,* 840–842.

Masur, H., Michelis, M. A., Greene, J. B., Onorato, I., Stouwe, R. A., Hoizman, R. S., et al. (1981). An outbreak of community-acquired *Pneumocystis carinii* pneumonia: Initial manifestation of cellular immune dysfunction. *New England Journal of Medicine, 305,* 1431–1438.

May, M. T., Sterne, J. A., Costaqliola, D., Sabin, C. A., Phillips, A. N., Justice, A. C., et al., & The Antiretroviral Therapy (ART) Cohort Collaboration. (2006). HIV treatment response and prognosis in Europe and North America in the first decade of highly antiretroviral therapy: A collaborative analysis. *Lancet, 368,* 451–458.

National Institute of Allergy and Infectious Diseases. (2000a). *The evidence that HIV causes AIDS. Fact Sheet.* Retrieved December 15, 2006, from http://www.niaid.nih.gov/factsheets/evidhiv.htm

National Institute of Allergy and Infectious Diseases. (2000b). *The relationship between the human immunodeficiency virus and the acquired immunodeficiency syndrome.* Retrieved December 15, 2006, from http://www.niaid. nih.gov/publications/hivaids/all.htm

Poinar, H., Kuch, M., & Paabo, S. (2001). Molecular analyses of oral polio vaccine samples. *Science, 292,* 743–744.

Popovic, M., Sarngadharan, M., Read, E., & Gallo, R. (1984). Detection, isolation, and continuous production of cytopathic retroviruses (HTLV-III) from patients with AIDS and pre-AIDS. *Science, 224,* 497–500.

Robertson, D. L., Anderson, J. P., Bradac, J. A., Carr, K., Foley, B., Funkhouser, R. K., et al. (2000). HIV-1 nomenclature proposal. *Science, 288,* 55–57.

Sarngadharan, M., Popovic, M., Bruch, L., Schupbach, J., & Gallo, R. C. (1984). Antibodies reactive with human T-lymphotropic retroviruses (HTLV-III) in the serum of patients with AIDS. *Science, 224,* 506–508.

Scherer, R. (2006). Unresolved management issues in HIV. *A newsletter update from the 16th International AIDS Conference—Issue #2, 5*(4), 2–4.

Shilts, R. (1987). *And the band played on.* New York: Penguin Books.

Simon, V., Ho, D. D., & Abdool Karim, Q. (2006). HIV/AIDS epidemiology, pathogenesis, prevention, and treatment. *The Lancet, 368*(9534), 489–504.

Stebbing, J., Gazzard, B., & Douek, D. C. (2004). Where does HIV live? *New England Journal of Medicine, 350,* 1872–1880.

UNAIDS. (2006). *2006 report on the global AIDS epidemic* (chap. 6–7). Geneva, Switzerland: Joint United Nations Programme on HIV/AIDS.

CHAPTER FOURTEEN

Avian Influenza A (H5N1)

James Mark Simmerman and Timothy M. Uyeki

Kumawari is a 30-year-old woman who lives in a poor urban neighborhood in Jakarta, Indonesia. Her small concrete block house with a tin roof is similar to those of her 38 extended family members who live nearby. Narrow dirt paths and open sewers separate the houses. Until recently, the small community shared the responsibility for about 20 ducks and 60 chickens. One day, two of the community's hens suddenly became sick. Crouching low, with feathers ruffled and unsteady, the hens died within 24 hours of first becoming ill. During each of the next 10 days, more chickens became sick and died rapidly, many displaying severely discolored, swollen combs and wattles. Fearing that all of her hens would soon die and that her family would not benefit from the nutrition these chickens provide, Kumawari and her 10-year-old daughter, Muriara, caught two hens and prepared them for their family to eat. Once the chickens were boiled and fried, several other family members and neighbors consumed the birds.

Four days later, Kumawari woke with a severe headache, fever, nausea, and vomiting. By that afternoon, Muriara was also vomiting and febrile and had developed diarrhea, but no other family members were ill. Chills and muscle aches set in a few hours later and, not having the financial resources to afford medical care, both women remained at home. Extended family members provided nursing care until the fourth day when they could no longer avoid a visit to the hospital. Both received intravenous fluids to treat their dehydration, and that night they both abruptly developed a severe, dry cough and dyspnea. Chest x-rays taken the next morning showed patchy bilateral infiltrates, and intravenous broad-spectrum antibiotics were begun. As is the practice in many poor hospitals, family members provided much of the nursing care in the hospital.

Over the next 3 days, Kumawari became severely ill and required intubation and mechanical ventilation. A blood test showed leukopenia and thrombocytopenia. She developed pulmonary edema, and her chest x-ray showed a virtual "whiteout" in all lung fields. On the fourth day of hospitalization, Kumawari died despite aggressive medical care.

Muriara's illness progressed more slowly, and she was intubated the day her mother died. As Muriara began to recover slowly several days later, reports began to surface that several members of her extended family and other persons from the community were also ill. The district hospital outpatient clinic began to see increasing numbers of patients with influenza-like symptoms. While some patients became rapidly ill and were hospitalized, others seemed to have a milder form of illness. Five days after their initial contact with Kumawari and her daughter, two nurses called in sick with vomiting and fever.

An investigation by central disease control authorities began, and the next day, the national public health laboratory reported that a respiratory specimen taken from Kumawari had tested positive for influenza type A, but negative for hemagglutinin (HA) subtypes 1 and 3. The specimen was forwarded to a regional World Health Organization (WHO) reference laboratory and, 2 days later, the diagnosis of avian influenza A (H5N1) virus infection was made. By this time, more than 50 patients, mostly children and young adults, had become ill and 22 had been hospitalized at several hospitals in the area. Local supplies of personal protective equipment (PPE) were rapidly depleted as reports of the first nurse to succumb from the infection reached the news media. International public health authorities mobilized available PPE and antiviral drugs as hundreds of additional persons reported to hospitals. At the same time, infectious disease hospitals in Kuala Lumpur, Malaysia, and Bangkok, Thailand, announced they had also admitted multiple patients with suspiciously similar clinical presentations and histories and were awaiting test results. As countries began to impose travel restrictions, the world braced for the public health crisis looming in the difficult months ahead.

Wild waterfowl, gulls, and shorebirds are the natural reservoirs for influenza type A viruses. Influenza A viruses representing all 16 subtypes of HA and 9 subtypes of neuraminidase (NA) have been isolated from waterfowl (Stallknecht, Shane, Zwank, Senne, & Kearney, 1990; Suarez & Schultz-Cherry, 2000). Until the emergence of highly pathogenic H5N1, influenza A viruses in waterfowl were considered to be in evolutionary stasis, causing mainly asymptomatic infections (Hulse-Post et al., 2005; Suarez, 2000; Webster, Bean, Gorman, Chambers, & Kawaoka, 1992; Webster, Sharp, & Claas, 1995). In contrast, many influenza A virus subtypes have been documented to cause symptomatic infection in perching birds, marine mammals, horses, pigs, cats, and dogs (Crawford et al., 2005; Kaye & Pringle, 2005; Liu et al., 2003; Swayne & Suarez, 2000). Until 1997, however, only subtypes H1, H2, and H3 had been associated with clinically significant disease in humans.

In 1997 in Hong Kong, 18 human cases of avian influenza A (H5N1) infection and 6 deaths occurred concurrently with outbreaks in domestic poultry (Mounts et al., 1999; Shortridge et al., 1998). Until this event, avian influenza A viruses had not been associated with severe disease in humans. The fear of the potential of the H5N1 virus to cause a human pandemic prompted the culling of millions of poultry in Hong Kong and the implementation of extensive measures to prevent further spread (Sims et al., 2003).

Due to their low fidelity polymerase and segmented genome, influenza A viruses are characterized by extreme genetic variability (Lin, Gregory, Bennett, & Hay, 2004; Wu & Yan, 2005). In addition, cross-species transmission events appear to accelerate the rates of mutations (Guan et al., 2003; Li et al., 2004; Webster, 1997). Across much of Asia, it is common practice to both raise and market multiple bird species and pigs in close proximity to humans, creating an ideal environment for the development of new influenza A virus reassortants that are potentially capable of causing disease in humans (Choi, Seo, Kim, Webby, & Webster, 2005; Kung et al., 2003; Peiris et al., 2001; Webster, 2004). In addition, international agribusinesses that maintain production facilities in many Asian countries and produce billions of poultry in crowded conditions may also favor the development and distribution of new avian influenza A virus strains (Kwon et al., 2005; Thomas et al., 2005). Finally, the interaction of wild migratory waterfowl with domestic ducks and chickens appears to have contributed to the geographic spread of the H5N1 virus (Hubalek, 2004; Krauss et al., 2004; Ligon, 2005; Liu et al., 2005). In fewer than 10 years since the virus was identified in Hong Kong, it has become endemic in much of East Asia and was identified in Europe and Africa in 2006 (Lee et al., 2005; WHO, 2006a).

The precursor to the H5N1 virus identified in Hong Kong in 1997 was first detected in geese in the Guangdong province of China in 1996. Despite extensive control measures, new H5N1 reassortants emerged and caused outbreaks among birds in Hong Kong in 2000 and 2001 and probably killed two out of three infected humans in 2002 (Guan et al., 2002; Peiris et al., 2004; Sturm-Ramirez et al., 2004). In 2001, H5N1 viruses were isolated from live wet poultry markets in Vietnam (Nguyen et al., 2005). In 2003, highly pathogenic avian influenza H5N1 viruses began to cause massive mortality in large-scale commercial poultry farms in Thailand, Cambodia, China, Indonesia, Japan, Laos, South Korea, and Vietnam (Centers for Disease Control and Prevention [CDC], 2004; Tiensin et al., 2005). As of February 2004, 23 human H5N1 cases and 18 deaths (78% case fatality rate) had been reported in Vietnam and Thailand ("Avian Influenza A," 2004). A fatal Chinese H5N1 case from November 2003 was reported in June 2006 (Zhu et al., 2006).

By December 2006, 10 countries including Cambodia, China, Indonesia, Egypt, Turkey, Azerbaijan, and Iraq had reported human fatalities, and WHO had recorded 261 confirmed human cases with 157 (60%) deaths (WHO, 2006b). H5N1 is now endemic among poultry in East and Southeast Asia. Infection and culling has resulted in the deaths of more than 200 million poultry in 30 countries, major economic losses to large agribusinesses, and negative impacts on rural household income (Food & Agriculture Organization, 2006; Maltsoglu & Rapsomanikis, 2005).

Influenza viruses belong to the family Orthomyxoviridae and have three antigenic types: influenza A, B, and C. Only influenza types A and B viruses are known to cause human disease, and only type A viruses have been documented to cause human pandemics. Influenza virions are enveloped particles of spherical or slightly elongated dimensions measuring from 80 to 120 nm in diameter. The genome consists of single-stranded, negative-sense RNA in eight gene segments that code for 10 proteins (Wright & Webster, 2001).

The major surface glycoproteins, HA and NA, play primary roles in transmission and pathogenesis of human influenza viruses. Specific antibody against HA is protective, but minor antigenic changes occur frequently and new strains can infect and cause disease in persons who have antibody against other related but antigenically distinct strains. Antibody to NA may help modify disease severity. Sixteen different HA (differing by at least 30% in their nucleotide homology) and nine different NA subtypes have been identified. Of these, only viruses with combinations of HA 1, 2, and 3 and NA 1 and 2 were known to cause severe disease in humans until the occurrence of H5N1 infection in humans in 1997. Briefly, NA promotes the release of virus from infected cells, inhibits the aggregation of new virions, and facilitates their spread to other respiratory tract cells (Colman, 1994). HA mediates receptor binding and membrane fusion of influenza virus and is the primary target for infectivity-neutralizing antibodies (Skehel & Wiley, 2000). While the determinants of viral tropism and receptor specificity are polygenic, HA is believed to be the key molecule in pathogenesis (Gamblin et al., 2004).

The receptor specificity of HA is directly relevant to the ability of H5N1 viruses to cross the species barrier (Suzuki et al., 2000). Human influenza viruses bind preferentially to cells with sialic acid receptors containing $\alpha,2,6$-galactose linkages while avian viruses bind preferentially those containing $\alpha,2,3$-galactose linkages (Stephenson, Wood, Nicholson, & Zambon, 2003). However, there is evidence that even a single amino acid substitution in the HA gene can alter the receptor specificity of avian H5N1 viruses, providing them with an ability to bind to receptors optimal for human influenza viruses (Gambaryan et al., 2005). The implications of such a mutation are significant. The H1N1 virus that caused a massive pandemic in 1918 was also of avian origin and had acquired a preference for the S-α,2,6-galactose receptors (Glaser et al., 2005; Taubenberger et al., 2005; Tumpey et al., 2005). Close monitoring of the genetic evolution and receptor-binding preference of H5N1 viruses is a public health priority.

The presence of multiple basic amino acids at the HA cleavage site is also characteristic of highly pathogenic avian strains (Claas et al., 1998; Subbarao et al., 1998). While the current H5N1 viruses have been found to possess this predictor for increased pathogenicity, it is interesting to note that the 1918 pandemic H1N1 virus did not (Tumpey et al., 2005).

Since its identification in humans in 1997, the H5N1 virus has undergone rapid evolution demonstrated by development of multiple genotypes (Guan et al., 2002), antigenic changes (Horimoto et al., 2004; WHO, 2005b), increased pathogenicity and extrapulmonary disease (de Jong et al., 2005; Govorkova et al., 2005; Liu et al., 2005; Maines et al., 2005), an extended host range (Kuiken et al., 2004; Thanawongnuwech et al., 2005), increasing numbers of human clusters (Olsen, Ungchusak, et al., 2005; Kandun, et al., 2006), and development of resistance to antiviral medications that inhibit the M2 ion channel (adamantanes; Bright et al., 2005; Guan & Chen, 2005). In addition, one case report has documented the development of resistance to the NA inhibitor oseltamivir (Le et al., 2005). The latter developments are of great public health importance as antiviral medications are key public health tools to combat a future pandemic (Ferguson et al., 2005; Hayden, 2001; Longini et al., 2005).

While these developments are worrying, other research suggests that avian influenza viruses are not easily transmissible to humans and that extensive molecular changes may be required for a human pandemic virus to emerge. Receptors specific for attachment by most avian influenza A viruses were found to be distributed primarily in the human lower respiratory tract, and H5N1 virus was shown to predominantly attach to type II pneumocytes, alveolar macrophages, and nonciliated cuboidal epithelial cells in terminal bronchioles of the lower respiratory tract. These findings suggest that the inability of current H5N1 viruses to attach to upper respiratory tract tissues may limit human-to-human virus transmissibility (Shinya et al., 2006; Van Riel et al., 2006).

Another study employing a comparative ferret model and plasmid-based reverse genetic methods to generate H5N1 reassortant viruses also demonstrated the complexity of the genetic basis for transmissibility of influenza viruses. Neither human influenza H3N2 surface proteins nor human influenza virus internal proteins were sufficient for a 1997 H5N1 virus to develop pandemic characteristics, even after serial passages in ferrets (Maines et al., 2006).

The epidemiology of human infection with H5N1 virus is incompletely understood, but each new case affords an important opportunity to advance what is known about this pathogen. Human influenza is principally transmitted through droplet spread, while fomite and aerosol transmission each have a role in certain situations. Although the routes of transmission for H5N1 have not been definitively established, most patients have had direct exposure to infected birds, including butchering, consuming incompletely cooked or raw poultry products, and handling fighting cocks or other poultry being commonly reported (Beigel et al., 2005). A case–control study in Thailand found that the most significant H5N1 risk factor was having direct contact with dead poultry; poultry deaths in or near the house or performing activities with close poultry exposure were also associated with H5N1 disease during 2004 (Areechokchai, Jiraphongsa, Laosiritaworn, Hanshaoworakul, & O'Reilly, 2006).

Such exposures suggest that pharyngeal or gastrointestinal inoculation of the virus may be an important method of transmission. Even so, contact with sick poultry has not been identified in all cases. Importantly, while chickens infected with H5N1 rapidly develop symptoms that can signal a risk for potential human exposure, domestic ducks can remain apparently healthy while continuing to excrete virus (Chen et al., 2004; Sturm-Ramirez et al., 2005). This has ominous implications for widespread human exposures in Asia where duck husbandry is very common. Because the human population has no effective immunity to H5N1 influenza, confirmation of efficient and sustained human-to-human transmission will likely signal the start of the next global influenza pandemic. While transmission directly from infected poultry explains most cases to date, small clusters of human cases are increasingly reported, suggesting the possibility of limited person-to-person transmissions (Kandun et al., 2006; Olsen, Ungchusak, et al., 2005).

Of particular concern was a cluster of seven deaths in a single family that occurred in May 2006 in North Sumatra Province, Indonesia. The epidemiological evidence suggested that human-to-human transmission may have occurred during close and prolonged contact with the index case during the late stages of her illness. In addition, for the first time, epidemiological and virological data suggested the possibility of a third generation of transmission from the index patient, to a child, and then to another adult. Analysis of the viruses isolated from these patients showed that all were entirely avian in origin without evidence of genetic reassortment (WHO, 2006d).

Documenting human-to-human transmission is complicated by many factors, including the high frequency of potential confounding exposures to ill poultry or surfaces contaminated with feces, delays in the initiation of epidemiologic investigations, and limited availability of clinical specimens of adequate quality. To date, no evidence of sustained, efficient person-to-person transmission of H5N1 virus has been identified, but the potential for the development of efficient human-to-human transmission highlights the need for rapid epidemiological investigation of H5N1 cases and their contacts. The World Health Organization has issued guidance on the prompt identification of clusters and the immediate implementation of control measures to contain or slow a developing pandemic, and many countries have begun training their public health workers to conduct such a response (WHO, 2006e).

The possibility of mild or asymptomatic H5N1 virus infection is supported by epidemiological studies conducted during the 1997 outbreak. One health care worker had no symptoms and one colleague had mild respiratory illness, but both seroconverted for H5N1 antibody (Buxton Bridges et al., 2000). Another study among poultry workers estimated that 10% had been infected (Bridges et al., 2002). A 2004 community survey in northern Vietnam suggested that mild H5N1 infections may be more common than currently appreciated, but this study did not include laboratory confirmation (Thorson, Petzold, Nguyen, & Ekdahl, 2006). A serosurvey of case contacts and persons with presumably intense exposures in rural Cambodia in 2005 did not support the widespread occurrence of mild or asymptomatic disease (Vong et al., 2005). A small number of clinically mild H5N1 cases were reported in Turkey but the extent and role of mild H5N1 cases in the epidemiology of H5N1 remains unknown.

Therefore, case finding for H5N1 has focused primarily on hospitalized cases of severe acute respiratory infection. Early identification of an expanded spectrum of illness with H5N1 infection is of public health importance as it may represent a key change toward a virus with increased pandemic potential.

Most clinical descriptions of H5N1 are from patients hospitalized with severe pneumonia. While most cases in 2004 were identified in children or young adults, patients from across the age spectrum were identified in 2005. In June 2006, WHO published a review of the epidemiology of 205 laboratory-confirmed human H5N1 cases (WHO, 2006d). From December 1, 2003 to April 30, 2006, the median age of H5N1 cases was 20 years (range 3 months–75 years), and the male to female ratio was 0.9. The median duration from illness onset to hospitalization was 4 days (range 0–18 days), and the median duration from illness onset to death was 9 days (range 2–31 days). Overall observed mortality was 56%. The highest mortality was 73% in cases aged 10–19 years, and the lowest case fatality was 18% in cases aged >50 years.

The incubation period for H5N1 ranges from 2–8 days with a median of 4 days (Beigel et al., 2005; Tran et al., 2004). This incubation period appears to be longer than that for human influenza viruses, in which the incubation period is 1–4 days with a median of 2 days (Cate, 1987). Nearly all patients present with high fever and systemic influenza-like symptoms such as nausea, headache, and myalgia. Upper respiratory symptoms are usually but not always present. A few case reports have documented atypical syndromes, including patients whose primary symptoms are gastrointestinal (Apisarnthanarak et al., 2004) or neurological (de Jong et al., 2005a). Diarrhea is common and may precede the onset of respiratory symptoms by several days (Apisarnthanarak et al., 2004). Clinically significant lymphopenia and mild to moderate thrombocytopenia are common laboratory findings (Tran et al., 2004). Lower respiratory tract symptoms are usually found on admission to the hospital, with dyspnea developing in a median of 5 days from onset of illness in one group of patients in Thailand (Chotpitayasunondh et al., 2005). A variety of radiographic abnormalities usually follow closely after the onset of dyspnea including diffuse, multifocal, or patchy infiltrates; interstitial infiltrates; or lobular consolidation. Pleural effusions are uncommon (Bay et al., 2002). In many patients, the clinical course worsens over several days with the onset of acute respiratory distress syndrome and the characteristic diffuse "groundglass" infiltrates on chest x-ray. Death is commonly preceded by multiorgan failure (Beigel et al., 2005; Chan, 2002; Chotpitayasunondh et al., 2005). One observational study showed an association between high H5N1 viral load and elevated cytokine levels in fatal cases. This suggests that early antiviral treatment may be needed to suppress H5N1 viral replication to prevent the inflammatory response that appears to contribute sustantially to the pathogenesis of H5N1 disease (de Jong et al. 2006).

Laboratory diagnosis is complicated by the difficulty in obtaining properly collected and well-maintained clinical specimens. Often, H5N1 infection has not been suspected until late in the course of illness or even after death (Ungchusak et al., 2005). Isolation of H5N1 virus from respiratory specimens using embryonated hen's eggs or tissue cell culture under enhanced Biosafety Level 3 (BSL-3) conditions is the gold standard. Reverse transcriptase polymerase chain reaction (RT-PCR) testing of respiratory specimens is most frequently used to diagnose H5N1 infection due to its high sensitivity and speed. Throat and lower respiratory tract specimens appear to have higher yield for detecting H5N1 virus than nasal specimens. Stool specimens have tested positive for viral RNA and yielded virus isolates (Beigel et al., 2005; de Jong et al., 2005a).

Serologic testing for evidence of H5N1 antibody is technically complex and requires the need to use live H5N1 virus under BSL-3 laboratory conditions. When properly timed acute and convalescent serum samples have been collected, the microneutralization assay with confirmatory Western blot assay is highly sensitive and specific (Rowe et al., 1999). The traditional hemagglutination-inhibition test (HI) does not require live virus and effectively detects increases in human influenza antibody in serum. However, HI is insensitive for the detection of human antibody responses to avian influenza H5 hemagglutinin, even in the presence of high titers of neutralizing antibody after confirmed infection. A modified HI test using horse red blood cells has been developed (Stephenson et al., 2003) and is being field tested in several countries. Rapid antigen influenza diagnostic tests are much less sensitive than PCR methods and are not currently recommended for the purpose of detecting H5N1 (Chotpitayasunondh et al., 2005; Woolcock & Cardona, 2005).

In most cases, religious beliefs and social customs have prevented postmortem analyses. Early reports have found severe pulmonary injury with histopathological changes of diffuse alveolar damage and hyaline membrane formation similar to pneumonia due to human influenza virus infection (Guarner et al., 2000; To et al., 2001; Uiprasertkul et al., 2005). One autopsy report found evidence of H5N1 viral replication in the lungs and intestinal tract (Uiprasertkul et al., 2005).

Across East and Southeast Asia, billions of terrestrial and aquatic poultry are raised annually for personal consumption, sale, ornamental collection, and gaming purposes. In one recent survey in rural Thailand, 74% of households raised at least one type of poultry (Olsen, Laosiritaworm, Pattanasin, Prapasiri & Dowell, 2005). In addition, international trafficking in wild Asian birds is an ongoing environmental and potential human health problem (Karesh, Cook, Bennett, & Newcomb, 2005; Van Borm et al., 2005). These activities result in frequent, and potentially intense, human exposures as well the distribution of avian influenza viruses across international borders.

In both rural and poor urban settings, multiple avian species and swine are often raised in close proximity to each other, increasing the risk of cross-species transmissions and reassortment events (Ito et al., 1998; Webster & Hulse, 2004). In addition to the economic importance of these activities, such practices are often deeply rooted in social and religious customs. For example, the consumption of raw duck blood is considered a delicacy in Vietnam but constitutes a substantial risk of avian influenza infection (CDC, 2005).

While affluent Hong Kong has made substantial progress in controlling avian influenza through farm and market regulations (Kung et al., 2003), most Asian countries lack human and financial resources required to improve biosecurity significantly in traditional farming practices. The situation is particularly severe for millions of Asia's poorest citizens, for whom the loss of poultry to H5N1 infection or culling to control the disease can have dire nutritional consequences. The threat of large-scale poultry culling acts as a significant deterrent for villagers to report poultry outbreaks to veterinary authorities. Further, visibly ill chickens are often butchered and eaten by poverty-stricken families, a behavior that has been implicated in the increasing number of fatal human cases (Center for Infectious Disease Research and Policy, 2005).

A small number of antiviral medicines play an important role in the control of influenza infection and are a key component in the pandemic influenza plans of most countries (Groeneveld & van der Noordaa, 2005; Monto, 2003). In May 2006, WHO also published guidelines on the use of antiviral medicines in the clinical management of human H5N1 cases (WHO, 2006f).

The adamantane derivatives (amantadine and rimantadine) block the ion channel function of the M2 protein and have been used for treatment and prophylaxis of influenza A viruses for more than 30 years (Belshe, Smith, Hall, Betts, & Hay, 1988; Dolin et al., 1982). Prior to 2000, fewer than 2% of all influenza A/H3 viruses isolated worldwide demonstrated resistance to adamantanes (Ziegler et al., 1999). However, recent surveillance has revealed an alarming increase in the incidence of adamantine resistance, with 160 of 1304 (12.3%) global isolates being resistant in 2004. In China 109 of 149 (73.2%) of influenza H3 isolates in 2004 were found to be resistant (Bright et al., 2005). In 2005, 91% of influenza isolates in the United States were also resistant, leading the CDC to recommend that adamantanes not be used to treat influenza virus infection during the 2005/2006 season (CDC, 2006). In addition, H5N1 viruses isolated in the 1997 Hong Kong outbreak were uniformly susceptible to adamantanes, but most human and most avian A (H5N1) isolates tested since 2003 have been resistant (Bright et al., 2005; Ilyushina, Govorkova, & Webster, 2005). The disturbing increase in resistance to adamantanes suggests that these drugs will be of limited value in response to a future influenza pandemic.

Oseltamivir and zanamivir belong to a newer class of antiviral agents that inhibit the viral enzyme NA and have proven to reduce the length and severity of infection from human influenza A and B when early treatment is initiated, reduce viral shedding, and be effective prophylactics (Hayden et al., 1999, 2004). However, the effectiveness of NA inhibitors used for late treatment of severe H5N1 illness is unknown. The lack of proven effectiveness with late antiviral treatment could be due to induction of proinflammatory cytokines as a major factor in pathogenesis of H5N1 (Chan et al., 2005). The ideal dose and duration of treatment for H5N1 infection have not been established, but research in the mouse model suggests that higher doses and longer than standard treatment periods may be necessary (Yen, Monto, Webster, & Gorvokova, 2005)

Due to the widespread resistance of H5N1 to adamantanes, many countries have elected to establish national stockpiles of oseltamivir as one measure of pandemic preparedness (Ferguson et al., 2005; Longini et al., 2005; Ward, Small, Smith, Suter, & Dutkowski, 2005). Accordingly, the development of resistance to NA inhibitors is of major public health importance.

Naturally occurring oseltamivir-resistant influenza viruses have not been identified (McKimm-Breschkin et al., 2003). Resistant variants appear to develop infrequently during treatment, particularly in young children who receive inadequate weight-based unit doses (Kiso et al., 2004). Some evidence suggests that these resistant variants may have reduced biological fitness in terms of infectivity, pathogenicity, and replicative ability (Carr et al., 2002; Yen et al., 2005). Of particular concern is the isolation of an H5N1 virus with partial resistance to oseltamivir in a Vietnamese girl in 2005 who was treated for 11 days and survived (Le et al., 2005). A second study from Vietnam reported high-level resistance to oseltamivir in two of eight patients. One of these patients died despite the early initiation of antiviral therapy at currently recommended levels (de Jong et al., 2005b). These findings underscore the importance of global monitoring for drug resistance and the judicious use of antiviral medications (Mishin, Hayden, & Gubareva, 2005).

The unprecedented spread and virulence of avian influenza A (H5N1) in poultry and ongoing sporadic human infections raise concern that this influenza virus could cause the next human pandemic. An effective response requires political transparency and the close cooperation of animal and human health authorities at every level. In most countries, the capacity of the veterinary health system lags well behind that of human public health, and significant resources will be required to correct this deficit. In much of Asia, H5N1 is now endemic in poultry, and early hopes of eradication appear unlikely. Coordinated efforts should aim to reduce the amount of virus circulating in domestic poultry flocks and to decrease the risk of avian-to-human infection, thereby minimizing the potential for development of an H5N1 strain capable of efficient and sustained human-to-human transmission.

Although new H5N1 cases in humans continue to be identified, they remain relatively uncommon. Control of the infection in poultry through improved biosecurity in farming and marketing is a priority. In response to massive losses during outbreaks in 2003 and 2004, the commercial poultry sector has taken effective steps to reduce H5N1 infection. However, changing animal husbandry practices in millions of small backyard farms in rural and urban settings is a daunting challenge. Systematic poultry surveillance, accurate laboratory diagnosis, separation of domestic poultry from wild birds, rapid culling of infected flocks, strict movement restrictions, and restocking or adequate financial compensation to farmers are key components of an effective control program (Food and Agriculture Organization, 2004). Countries that choose to vaccinate poultry as one component of a broader control program must have reliable systems in place to assure vaccine quality and proper administration, to monitor efficacy, and to provide long-term funding to sustain the vaccination program.

Public education campaigns to discourage behaviors known to be associated with the risk of bird-to-human transmission are essential to prevent illness and deaths. Likewise, family members and health care workers must be educated and equipped with PPE as appropriate to reduce the risk of human-to-human transmission. Because early symptoms of H5N1 infection are nonspecific, surveillance for H5N1 infection has focused primarily on severe respiratory illness in hospitals. Improving laboratory diagnostic capacity to detect H5N1 virus is essential. Development of a rapid and accurate diagnostic H5N1 test that could be conducted in simple hospital laboratories would represent a major scientific advance. Serological surveys should be regularly undertaken to monitor for mild or asymptomatic illness that could suggest the virus has become better adapted to humans.

Each new human case merits investigation. Multiple, sequential clinical specimens should be collected and viruses promptly submitted to a WHO collaborating laboratory. Molecular analysis of the H5N1 genome is essential to monitor for changes in host affinity, genetic reassortment, antigenic drift, and antiviral resistance and to ensure virus strains used to develop pandemic influenza vaccines are current (WHO, 2005a). Reverse genetic methods have been used to develop nonvirulent H5N1 vaccine strains (Lipatov, Webby, Govorkova, Krauss, & Webster, 2005). Development of clade 1 and clade 2 H5N1 virus vaccine candidates continues in several countries, while an unadjuvanted clade 1 H5N1 virus vaccine was shown to be safe in adults but required high doses to promote immunogenicity (Treanor, Campbell, Zangwill, Rowe, & Wolff, 2006). Clinical research to better describe the natural history of illness, determine transmission risks, and develop more effective treatment protocols is a priority.

H5N1 avian influenza is a threat to animal and human health worldwide. It is possible that we are now witnessing events similar to those that led to the 1918 influenza pandemic that claimed at least 40 million lives (Taubenberger et al., 2005; Tumpey et al., 2005). A long-term, multisectoral approach and sustained funding are needed to control the disease in poultry and to prepare for a possible human influenza pandemic.

REFERENCES

Apisarnthanarak, A., Kitphati, R., Thongphubethik, K., Patoomanunt, P., Anthanont, P., Auwanit, W., et al. (2004). Atypical avian influenza (H5N1). *Emerging Infectious Diseases, 10,* 1321–1324.

Areechokchai, D., Jiraphongsa, C., Laosiritaworn, Y., Hanshaoworakul, W., & O'Reilly, M. (2006). Investigation of avian influenza (H5N1) outbreak in humans—Thailand, 2004. *Morbidly and Mortality Weekly Report,* 55(Suppl. 1), 3–6.

Avian influenza A (H5N1). (2004). *Weekly Epidemiological Record. 79,* 65–70.

Beigel, J. H., Farrar, J., Han, A. M., Hayden, F. G., Hyer, R., de Jong, M. D., et al. (2005). Avian influenza A (H5N1) infection in humans. *New England Journal of Medicine, 353,* 1374–1385.

Bay, A., Etlik. O., Oner, A. F., Unal, O., Arslan, H., Bora, A. et al. (2007). Radiological and clinical course of pneumonia in patients with avian influenza H5N1. *European Journal of Radiology, 61,* 245–250.

Belshe, R. B., Smith, M. H., Hall, C. B., Betts, R., & Hay, A. J. (1988). Genetic basis of resistance to rimantadine emerging during treatment of influenza virus infection. *Journal of Virology, 62,* 1508–1512.

Bridges, C. B., Lim, W., Hu-Primmer, J., Sims, L., Fukuda, K., Mak, K. H., et al. (2002). Risk of influenza A (H5N1) infection among poultry workers, Hong Kong, 1997–1998. *Journal of Infectious Diseases, 185,* 1005–1110.

Bright, R. A., Medina, M. J., Xu, X., Perez-Oronoz, G., Wallis, T. R., Davis, X. M., et al. (2005). Incidence of adamantane resistance among influenza A (H3N2) viruses isolated worldwide from 1994 to 2005: A cause for concern. *Lancet, 366,* 1175–1181.

Buxton Bridges, C., Katz, J. M., Seto, W. H., Chan, P. K., Tsang, D., Ho, W., et al. (2000). Risk of influenza A (H5N1) infection among health care workers exposed to patients with influenza A (H5N1), Hong Kong. *Journal of Infectious Diseases, 181,* 344–348.

Carr, J., Ives, J., Kelly, L., Lambkin, R., Oxford, J., Mendel, D., et al. (2002). Influenza virus carrying neuraminidase with reduced sensitivity to oseltamivir carboxylate has altered properties in vitro and is compromised for infectivity and replicative ability in vivo. *Antiviral Research, 54,* 79–88.

Cate, T. R. (1987). Clinical manifestations and consequences of influenza. *American Journal of Medicine, 82,* 15–19.

Centers for Disease Control and Prevention. (2004). Outbreaks of avian influenza A (H5N1) in Asia and interim recommendations for evaluation and reporting of suspected cases—United States, 2004. *Morbidity and Mortality Weekly Report, 53,* 97–100.

Centers for Disease Control and Prevention. (2005, October 28). *Recent avian influenza outbreaks in Asia and Europe.* Retrieved December 15, 2006, from the CDC Web site: http://www.cdc.gov/flu/avian/outbreaks/asia.htm

Centers for Disease Control and Prevention. (2006). High levels of adamantane resistance among influenza A (H3N2) viruses and interim guidelines for use of antiviral agents—United States, 2005–06 influenza season. *Morbidity and Mortality Weekly Report, 55,* 44–46.

Chan, M. C., Cheung, C. Y., Chui, W., Tsao, S. W., Nicholls, J. M., Chan, Y. O., et al. (2005). Proinflammatory cytokine responses induced by influenza A (H5N1) viruses in primary human alveolar and bronchial epithelial cells. *Respiratory Research, 6,* 135.

Chan, P. K. (2002). Outbreak of avian influenza A(H5N1) virus infection in Hong Kong in 1997. *Clinical Infectious Diseases, 34*(Suppl. 2), S58–64.

Chen, H., Deng, G., Li, Z., Tian, G., Li, Y., Jiao, P., et al. (2004). The evolution of H5N1 influenza viruses in ducks in southern China. *Proceedings of the National Academy of Sciences, USA, 101,* 10452–10457.

Choi, Y. K., Seo, S. H., Kim, J. A., Webby, R. J., & Webster, R. G. (2005). Avian influenza viruses in Korean live poultry markets and their pathogenic potential. *Virology, 332,* 529–537.

Chotpitayasunondh, T., Ungchusak, K., Hanshaoworakul, W., Chunsuthiwat, S., Sawanpanyalert, P., Kijphati, R., et al. (2005). Human disease from influenza A (H5N1), Thailand, 2004. *Emerging Infectious Diseases, 11,* 201–209.

Claas, E. C., Osterhaus, A. D., van Beek, R., De Jong, J. C., Rimmelzwaan, G. F., Senne, D. A., et al. (1998). Human influenza A H5N1 virus related to a highly pathogenic avian influenza virus. *Lancet, 351,* 472–477.

Colman, P. M. (1994). Influenza virus neuraminidase: Structure, antibodies, and inhibitors. *Protein Science, 3,* 1687–1696.

Crawford, P. C., Dubovi, E. J., Castleman, W. L., Stephenson, I., Gibbs, E. P., Chen, L., et al. (2005). Transmission of equine influenza virus to dogs. *Science, 311,* 1241–1242.

de Jong, M. D., Bach, V. C., Phan, T. Q., Vo, M. H., Tran, T. T., Nguyen, B. H., et al. (2005a). Fatal avian influenza A (H5N1) in a child presenting with diarrhea followed by coma. *New England Journal of Medicine, 352,* 686–691.

de Jong, M. D., Simmons, C. P., Thanh, T. T., Hien, V. M., Smith, G. J., Chau, T. N. et al. (2006). Fatal outcome of human influenza A (H5N1) is associated with high viral load and hypercytokinemia. *Nature Medicine, 12,* 1203–1207.

de Jong, M. D., Tran, T. T., Truong, H. K., Vo, M. H., Smith, G. H., Nguyen, V. C., et al. (2005b). Oseltamivir resistance during treatment of influenza A (H5N1) infection. *New England Journal of Medicine, 353,* 2667–2672.

Dolin, R., Reichman, R. C., Madore, H. P., Maynard, R., Linton, P. N., Webber-Jones, J., et al. (1982). A controlled trial of amantadine and rimantadine in the prophylaxis of influenza A infection. *New England Journal of Medicine, 307,* 580–584.

Ferguson, N. M., Cummings, D. A., Cauchemez, S., Fraser, C., Riley, S., Meeyai, A., et al. (2005). Strategies for containing an emerging influenza pandemic in Southeast Asia. *Nature, 437,* 209–214.

Food and Agriculture Organization. (2004). *FAO recommendations on the prevention, control and eradication of highly pathogenic avian influenza (HPAI) in Asia* (FAO Position Paper). Rome: Food and Agriculture Organization, A.P.A.H. Division, Editor.

Food and Agriculture Organization. (2006, August 9). Update on the avian influenza situation as of June 19, 2006. *FAOAidenews, 40.* Available from the FAO Web site, http://www.fao.org/ag/againfo/subjects/en/health/diseases-cards/avian_update.html

Gambaryan A, Tuzikov A, Pazynina G, Bovin N, Balish A, Klimov A. (2006). Evolution of the receptor binding phenotype of influenza A (H5) viruses. *Virology, 344(2),* 432–8.

Gamblin, S., Haire, L., Russell, R., Stevens, D., Xiao, B., Ha, Y., et al. (2004). The structure and receptor binding properties of the 1918 influenza hemagglutinin. *Science, 303*, 1838–1842.

Glaser, L., Stevens, J., Zamarin, D., Wilson, I. A., Garcia-Sastre, A., Tumpey, T. M., et al. (2005). A single amino acid substitution in 1918 influenza virus hemagglutinin changes receptor binding specificity. *Journal of Virology, 79*, 11533–11536.

Goto, H., & Kawaoka, Y. (1988). A novel mechanism for the acquisition of virulence by a human influenza A virus. *Proceedings of the National Academy of Sciences, USA, 95*, 10224–10228.

Govorkova, E. A., Rehg, J. E., Krauss, S., Yen, H. L., Guan, Y., Peiris, M., et al. (2005). Lethality to ferrets of H5N1 influenza viruses isolated from humans and poultry in 2004. *Journal of Virology, 79*, 2191–2198.

Groeneveld, K., & van der Noordaa, J. (2005). Use of antiviral agents and other measures in an influenza pandemic. *Netherlands Journal of Medicine, 63*, 339–343.

Guan, Y., & Chen, H. (2005). Resistance to anti-influenza agents. *Lancet, 366*, 1139–1140.

Guan, Y., Peiris, J. S., Lipatov, A. S., Ellis, T. M., Dyrting, K. C., Krauss, S., et al. (2002). Emergence of multiple genotypes of H5N1 avian influenza viruses in Hong Kong SAR. *Proceedings of the National Academy of Sciences, USA, 99*, 8950–8955.

Guan, Y., Peiris, J. S., Poon, L. L., Dyrting, K. C., Ellis, T. M., Sims, L., et al. (2003). Reassortants of H5N1 influenza viruses recently isolated from aquatic poultry in Hong Kong SAR. *Avian Diseases, 47*(3 Suppl.), 911–913.

Guarner, J., Shieh, W. J., Dawson, J., Subbarao, K., Shaw, M., Ferebb, T., et al. (2000). Immunohistochemical and in situ hybridization studies of influenza A virus infection in human lungs. *American Journal of Clinical Pathology, 114*, 227–233.

Hayden, F. G. (2001). Perspectives on antiviral use during pandemic influenza. *Philosophical Transactions of the Royal Society of London B. Series B, Biological Sciences, 356*, 1877–1884.

Hayden, F. G., Atmar, R. L, Schilling, M., Johnson, C., Poretz, D., Paar, D., et al. (1999). Use of the selective oral neuraminidase inhibitor oseltamivir to prevent influenza. *New England Journal of Medicine, 341*, 1336–1343.

Hayden, F. G., Belshe, R., Villanueva, C., Lanno, R., Hughes, C., Small, I., et al. (2004). Management of influenza in households: A prospective, randomized comparison of oseltamivir treatment with or without postexposure prophylaxis. *Journal of Infectious Diseases, 189*, 440–449.

Horimoto, T., Fukuda, N., Iwatsuki-Horimoto, K., Guan, Y., Lim, W., Peiris, M., et al. (2004). Antigenic differences between H5N1 human influenza viruses isolated in 1997 and 2003. *Journal of Veterinary Medical Science, 66*, 303–305.

Hubalek, Z. (2004). An annotated checklist of pathogenic microorganisms associated with migratory birds. *Journal of Wildlife Diseases, 40*, 639–659.

Hulse-Post, D. J., Sturm-Ramirez, K. M., Humberd, J., Seiler, P., Govorkova, E. A., Krauss, S., et al. (2005). Role of domestic ducks in the propagation and biological evolution of highly pathogenic H5N1 influenza viruses in Asia. *Proceedings of the National Academy of Sciences, USA, 102,* 10682–10687.

Ilyushina, N. A., Govorkova, E. A., & Webster, R. G. (2005). Detection of amantadine-resistant variants among avian influenza viruses isolated in North America and Asia. *Virology, 341,* 102–106.

International Office of Epizootics (2005, October 20). *Highly pathogenic avian influenza in Romania.* Retrieved October 20, 2005 from http://www.oie.int/eng/info/hebdo/a_current.htm#Sec10

Ito, T., Couceiro, J. N., Kelm, S., Baum, L. G., Krauss, S., Castrucci, M. R., et al. (1998). Molecular basis for the generation in pigs of influenza A viruses with pandemic potential. *Journal of Virology, 72,* 7367–7373.

Kandun, I. N., Wibisono, H., Sedyaningsih, E. R., Yusharmen, Hadisoedarsuno, W., Purba, W. et al. (2006). Three Indonesian clusters of H5N1 virus infection in 2005. *New England Journal of Medicine, 355,* 2186–2194.

Karesh, W. B., Cook, R. A., Bennett, E. L., & Newcomb, J. (2005). Wildlife trade and global disease emergence. *Emerging Infectious Diseases, 11,* 1000–1002.

Kaye, D., & Pringle, C. R. (2005). Avian influenza viruses and their implication for human health. *Clinical Infectious Diseases, 40,* 108–112.

Kiso, M., Mitamura, K., Sakai-Tagawa, Y., Shiraishi, K., Kawakami, C., Kimura, K., et al. (2004). Resistant influenza A viruses in children treated with oseltamivir: Descriptive study. *Lancet, 364,* 759–765.

Krauss, S., Walker, D., Pryor, S. P., Niles, L., Chenghong, L., Hinshaw, V. S., et al. (2004). Influenza A viruses of migrating wild aquatic birds in North America. *Vector-Borne and Zoonotic Diseases, 4,* 177–189.

Kuiken, T., Rimmelzwaan, G., van Riel, D., van Amerongen, G., Baars, M., Fouchier, R., et al. (2004). Avian H5N1 influenza in cats. *Science, 306,* 241.

Kung, N. Y., Guan, Y., Perkins, N. R., Bissett, L., Ellis, T., Sims, L., et al. (2003). The impact of a monthly rest day on avian influenza virus isolation rates in retail live poultry markets in Hong Kong. *Avian Diseases, 47*(3 Suppl.), 1037–1041.

Kwon, Y. K., Joh, S. J., Kim, M. C., Sung, H. W., Lee, Y. J., Choi, J. G., et al. (2005). Highly pathogenic avian influenza (H5N1) in the commercial domestic ducks of South Korea. *Avian Pathology, 34,* 367–370.

Le, Q. M., Kiso, M., Someya, K., Sakai, Y. T., Nguyen, T. H., Nguyen, K. H., et al. (2005). Avian flu: Isolation of drug-resistant H5N1 virus. *Nature, 437,* 1108.

Lee, C. W., Suarez, D. L., Tumpey, T. M., Sung, H. W., Kwon, Y. K., Lee, Y. J., et al. (2005). Characterization of highly pathogenic H5N1 avian influenza A viruses isolated from South Korea. *Journal of Virology, 79,* 3692–3702.

Li, K. S., Guan, Y., Wang, J., Smith, G. J., Xu, K. M., Duan, L., et al. (2004). Genesis of a highly pathogenic and potentially pandemic H5N1 influenza virus in eastern Asia. *Nature, 430,* 209–213.

Ligon, B. L. (2005). Avian influenza virus H5N1: A review of its history and information regarding its potential to cause the next pandemic. *Seminars in Pediatric Infectious Diseases, 16,* 326–35.

Lin, Y. P., Gregory, V., Bennett, M., & Hay, A. (2004). Recent changes among human influenza viruses. *Virus Research, 103,* 47–52.

Lipatov, A. S., Webby, R. J., Govorkova, E. A., Krauss, S., & Webster, R. G. (2005). Efficacy of H5 influenza vaccines produced by reverse genetics in a lethal mouse model. *Journal of Infectious Diseases, 191,* 1216–1220.

Liu, J., Xiao, H., Lei, F., Zhu, Q., Qin, K., Zhang, X. W., et al. (2005). Highly pathogenic H5N1 influenza virus infection in migratory birds. *Science, 309,* 1206.

Liu, M., Guan, Y., Peiris, M., He, S., Webby, R. J., Perez, D., et al. (2003). The quest of influenza A viruses for new hosts. *Avian Diseases, 47*(3 Suppl.), 849–856.

Longini, I. M., Jr., Nizam, A., Xu, S., Ungchusak, K., Hanshaoworakul, W., Cummings, D. A., et al. (2005). Containing pandemic influenza at the source. *Science, 309,* 1083–1087.

Maines, T. R., Chen, L. M., Mtsuoka, Y., Chen, H., Rowe, T., & Ortin, J., et al. (2006). Lack of transmission of H5N1 avian-human reassortant influenza viruses in a ferret model. *Proceedings of the National Academy of Sciences, USA, 103,* 12121–12126.

Maines, T. R., Lu, X. H., Erb, S. M., Edwards, L., Guarner, J., Greer, P. W., et al. (2005). Avian influenza (H5N1) viruses isolated from humans in Asia in 2004 exhibit increased virulence in mammals. *Journal of Virology, 79,* 11788–11800.

Maltsoglu, I., & Rapsomanikis, G. (2005, June). *FAO pro-poor livestock policy initiative. The contribution of livestock to household income in Vietnam: A household typology based analysis* (Working Paper No. 21). Rome: Food and Agricultural Organization of the United Nations.

McKimm-Breschkin, J., Trivedi, T., Hampson, A., Hay, A., Klimov, A., Tashiro, M., et al. (2003). Neuraminidase sequence analysis and susceptibilities of influenza virus clinical isolates to zanamivir and oseltamivir. *Antimicrobial Agents and Chemotherapy, 47,* 2264–2272.

Mishin, V. P., Hayden, F. G., & Gubareva, L. V. (2005). Susceptibilities of antiviral-resistant influenza viruses to novel neuraminidase inhibitors. *Antimicrobial Agents and Chemotherapy, 49,* 4515–4520.

Monto, A. S. (2003). The role of antivirals in the control of influenza. *Vaccine, 21,* 1796–1800.

Mounts, A. W., Kwong, H., Izurieta, H. S., Ho, Y., Au, T., Lee, M., et al. (1999). Case-control study of risk factors for avian influenza A (H5N1) disease, Hong Kong, 1997. *Journal of Infectious Diseases, 180,* 505–508.

Nguyen, D. C., Uyeki, T. M., Jadhao, S., Maines, T., Shaw, M., Matsuoka, Y., et al. (2005). Isolation and characterization of avian influenza viruses, including highly pathogenic H5N1, from poultry in live bird markets in Hanoi, Vietnam, in 2001. *Journal of Virology, 79,* 4201–4212.

Olsen, S., Laosiritaworn, Y., Pattanasin, S., Prapasiri, P., & Dowell, S. F. (2005). Poultry-handling practices during avian influenza outbreak, Thailand. *Emerging Infectious Diseases, 11,* 1601–1603.

Olsen, S., Ungchusak, K., Sovann, L., Uyeki, T. M., Dowell, S. F., Cox, N. J., et al. (2005). Family clustering of avian influenza A (H5N1). *Emerging Infectious Diseases, 11,* 1799–1801.

Oner, A. F., Bay, A., Arslan, S., Akdeniz, H., Sahin, H. A., Cesur, Y. et al. (2006). Avian influenza A (H5N1) infection in eastern Turkey in 2006. *New England Journal of Medicine, 355,* 2179–2185.

Peiris, J. S., Guan, Y., Markwell, D., Ghose, P., Webster, R. G., & Shortridge, K. F. (2001). Cocirculation of avian H9N2 and contemporary "human" H3N2 influenza A viruses in pigs in southeastern China: Potential for genetic reassortment? *Journal of Virology, 75,* 9679–9686.

Peiris, J. S., Yu, W. C., Leung, C. W., Cheung, C. Y., Ng, W. F., Nicholls, J. M., et al. (2004). Re-emergence of fatal human influenza A subtype H5N1 disease. *Lancet, 363,* 617–619.

Rowe, T., Abernathy, R. A., Hu-Primmer, J., Thompson, W. W., Lu, X., Lim, W., et al. (1999). Detection of antibody to avian influenza A (H5N1) virus in human serum by using a combination of serologic assays. *Journal of Clinical Microbiology, 37,* 937–943.

Shinya, K., Ebina, M., Yamada, S., Ono, M., Kasai, N., & Kawaoka, Y. (2006). Avian flu: Influenza virus receptors in the human airway. *Nature, 440,* 312–399.

Shortridge, K. F., Zhou, N. N., Guan, Y., Gao, P., Ito, T., Kawaoka, Y., et al. (1998). Characterization of avian H5N1 influenza viruses from poultry in Hong Kong. *Virology, 252,* 331–342.

Sims, L. D., Ellis, T. M., Liu, K. K., Dyrting, K., Wong, H., Peiris, M., et al. (2003). Avian influenza in Hong Kong 1997–2002. *Avian Diseases, 47*(3 Suppl.), 832–838.

Skehel, J. J., & Wiley, D. C. (2000). Receptor binding and membrane fusion in virus entry: The influenza hemagglutinin. *Annual Review of Biochemistry, 69,* 531–569.

Stallknecht, D. E., Shane, S. M., Zwank, P. J., Senne, D. A., & Kearney, M. T. (1990). Avian influenza viruses from migratory and resident ducks of coastal Louisiana. *Avian Diseases, 34,* 398–405.

Stephenson, I., Wood, J. M., Nicholson, K. G., & Zambon, M. C. (2003). Sialic acid receptor specificity on erythrocytes affects detection of antibody to avian influenza haemagglutinin. *Journal of Medical Virology, 70,* 391–398.

Sturm-Ramirez, K. M., Ellis, T., Bousfield, B., Bissett, L., Dyrting, K., Rehg, J. E., et al. (2004). Reemerging H5N1 influenza viruses in Hong Kong in 2002 are highly pathogenic to ducks. *Journal of Virology, 78,* 4892–4901.

Sturm-Ramirez, K. M., Hulse-Post, D. J., Govorkova, E. A., Humberd, J., Seiler, P., Puthavathana, P., et al. (2005). Are ducks contributing to the endemicity of highly pathogenic H5N1 influenza virus in Asia? *Journal of Virology, 79,* 11269–11279.

Suarez, D. L. (2000). Evolution of avian influenza viruses. *Veterinary Microbiology, 74,* 15–27.

Suarez, D. L., & Schultz-Cherry, S. (2000). Immunology of avian influenza virus: A review. *Developmental and Comparative Immunology, 24,* 269–283.

Subbarao, K., Klimov, A., Katz, J., Regnery, H., Lim, W., Hall, H., et al. (1998). Characterization of an avian influenza A (H5N1) virus isolated from a child with a fatal respiratory illness. *Science, 279,* 393–396.

Suzuki, Y., Ito, T., Suzuki, T., Holland, R. E., Jr., Chambers, T. M., Kiso, M., et al. (2000). Sialic acid species as a determinant of the host range of influenza A viruses. *Journal of Virology, 74,* 11825–11831.

Swayne, D. E., & Suarez, D. L. (2000). Highly pathogenic avian influenza. *Revue Scientifique et Technique, 19,* 463–482.

Taubenberger, J. K., Reid, A. H., Lourens, R. M., Wang, R., Jin, G., & Fanning, T. G. (2005). Characterization of the 1918 influenza virus polymerase genes. *Nature, 437,* 889–893.

Thanawongnuwech, R., Amonsin, A., Tantilertcharoen, R., Damrongwatana-pokin, S., Theamboonlers, A., Payungporn, S., et al. (2005). Probable tiger-to-tiger transmission of avian influenza H5N1. *Emerging Infectious Diseases, 11,* 699–701.

Thomas, M. E., Bouma, A., Ekker, H. M., Fonken, A. J., Stegeman, J. A., & Nielen, M. (2005). Risk factors for the introduction of high pathogenicity avian influenza virus into poultry farms during the epidemic in the Netherlands in 2003. *Preventive Veterinary Medicine, 69,* 1–11.

Thorson, A., Petzold, M., Nguyen, T. K., & Ekdahl, K. (2006). Is exposure to sick or dead poultry associated with flulike illness? A population-based study from a rural area in Vietnam with outbreaks of highly pathogenic avian influenza. *Archives of Internal Medicine, 166,* 119–123.

Tiensin, T., Chaitaweesub, P., Songserm, T., Chaisingh, A., Hoonsuwan, W., Buranathai, C., et al. (2005). Highly pathogenic avian influenza H5N1, Thailand, 2004. *Emerging Infectious Diseases, 11,* 1664–1672.

To, K. F., Chan, P. K., Chan, K. F., Lee, W. K., Lam, W. Y., & Wong, K. F. (2001). Pathology of fatal human infection associated with avian influenza A H5N1 virus. *Journal of Medical Virology, 63,* 242–246.

Tran, T. H., Nguyen, T. L., Nguyen, T. D., Luong, T. S., Pham, P. M., Nguyen, V. C., et al. (2004). Avian influenza A (H5N1) in 10 patients in Vietnam. *New England Journal of Medicine, 350,* 1179–1188.

Treanor, J. J., Campbell, J. D., Zangwill, K. M., Rowe, T., & Wolff, M. (2006). Safety and immunogenicity of an inactivated subvirion influenza A (H5N1) vaccine. *New England Journal of Medicine, 354,* 1343–1351.

Tumpey, T. M., Basler, C. F., Aguilar, P. V., Zeng, H., Solorzano, A., Swayne, D. E., et al. (2005). Characterization of the reconstructed 1918 Spanish influenza pandemic virus. *Science, 310,* 77–80.

Uiprasertkul, M., Puthavathana, P., Sanasiriwut, K., Pooruk, P., Srisook, K., Peiris, M., et al. (2005). Influenza A H5N1 replication sites in humans. *Emerging Infectious Diseases, 11,* 1036–1041.

Ungchusak, K., Auewarakul, P., Dowell, S. F., Kitphati, R., Auwanit, W., Putha-vathana, P., et al. (2005). Probable person-to-person transmission of avian influenza A (H5N1). *New England Journal of Medicine, 352,* 333–340.

Van Borm, S., Thomas, I., Hanguet, G., Lambrecht, B., Boschmans, M., Dupont, G., et al. (2005). Highly pathogenic H5N1 influenza virus in smuggled Thai eagles, Belgium. *Emerging Infectious Diseases, 11,* 702–705.

Van Riel, D., Munster, V. J., de Wit, E., Rimmelzwaan, G. F., Fouchier, R. A. M., Osterhaus, D. M. E., et al. (2006). H5N1 virus attachment to lower respiratory tract. *Science, 312*(5772), 399.

Vong, S., Coghlan, B., Mardy, S., Holl, D., Seng, H., Ly, S. et al. (2006). Low frequency of poultry-to-human H5N1 virus transmission, Southern Cambodia, 2005. *Emerging Infectious Diseases, 12*: 1542–1547.

Ward, P., Small, I., Smith, J., Suter, P., & Dutkowski, R. (2005). Oseltamivir (Tamiflu) and its potential for use in the event of an influenza pandemic. *Journal of Antimicrobial Chemotherapy, 55*(Suppl. 1), 15–21.

Webster, R. G. (1997). Influenza virus: Transmission between species and relevance to emergence of the next human pandemic. *Archives of Virology. Supplementum, 13,* 105–113.

Webster, R. G. (2004). Wet markets—A continuing source of severe acute respiratory syndrome and influenza? *Lancet, 363,* 234–236.

Webster, R. G., Bean, W. J., Gorman, O. T., Chambers, T. M., & Kawaoka, Y. (1992). Evolution and ecology of influenza A viruses. *Microbiological Reviews, 56,* 152–179.

Webster, R. G., & Hulse, D. J. (2004). Microbial adaptation and change: Avian influenza. *Review Scientifique et Technique, 23,* 453–465.

Webster, R. G., Sharp, G. B., & Claas, E. C. (1995). Interspecies transmission of influenza viruses. *American Journal of Respiratory and Critical Care Medicine, 152*(4 Pt. 2), S25–30.

Woolcock, P. R., & Cardona, C. J. (2005). Commercial immunoassay kits for the detection of influenza virus type A: Evaluation of their use with poultry. *Avian Diseases, 49,* 477–481.

World Health Organization. (2005a, December 20). *Epidemic and pandemic alert and response.* Retrieved January 1, 2006, from http://www.who.int/csr/disease/influenza/pandemic/en/index.html

World Health Organization. (2005b). Evolution of H5N1 avian influenza viruses in Asia. *Emerging Infectious Diseases, 11,* 1515–1521.

World Health Organization. (2006a, April 3). *Avian influenza situation in Egypt—Update 2.* Retrieved August 9, 2006, from http://www.who.int/csr/don/2006_04_03/en/

World Health Organization. (2006b, May 31). *Avian influenza situation in Indonesia—Update 16.* Retrieved January 1, 2006, from http://www.who.int/crs/don/2006_05_31/en/print.html

World Health Organization. (2006c, August 9). *Cumulative number of confirmed human cases of avian influenza A/(H5N1) reported to WHO.* Retrieved December 1, 2006, from http://www.who.int/csr/disease/avian_influenza/country/cases_table_2006_08_09/en/index.html

World Health Organization. (2006d). Epidemiology of WHO-confirmed human cases of avian influenza A (H5N1) infection. *Weekly Epidemiological Record, 81,* 249–257.

World Health Organization. (2006e). *WHO pandemic influenza protocol for rapid response and containment.* Retrieved August 15, 2006, from http://www.who.int/csr/disease/avian_influenza/guidelines/draftprotocol/en/index.html

World Health Organization. (2006f, May 2006). *WHO Rapid Advice Guidelines on pharmacological management of humans infected with avian influenza A (H5N1) virus.* Retrieved January 1, 2006, from http://www.who.int/medicines/publications/WHO_PSM_PAR_2006.6.pdf

Wright, P., & Webster, R. (2001). Orthomyxoviruses. In D. M. Knipe, P. M. Howley, D. E. Griffin, R. A. Lamb, M. A. Martin, B. Roizman et al. (Eds.), *Field's virology* (pp. 1533–1579). Philadelphia: Lippincott Williams & Wilkins.

Wu, G., & Yan, S. (2005). Mutation features of 215 polymerase proteins from different influenza A viruses. *Medical Science Monitor, 11*(10), BR367–372.

Yen, H. L., Herlocher, L. M., Hoffmann, E., Matrosovich, M. N., Monto, A. S., Webster, R. G., et al. (2005). Neuraminidase inhibitor-resistant influenza viruses may differ substantially in fitness and transmissibility. *Antimicrobial Agents and Chemotherapy, 49,* 4075–4084.

Yen, H. L., Monto, A. S., Webster, R. G., & Govorkova, E. A. (2005). Virulence may determine the necessary duration and dosage of oseltamivir treatment for highly pathogenic A/Vietnam/1203/04 influenza virus in mice. *Journal of Infectious Diseases, 192,* 665–672.

Ziegler, T., Hemphill, M. L., Ziegler, M. L., Perez-Oronoz, G., Klimov, A. I., Hampson, A. W., et al. (1999). Low incidence of rimantadine resistance in field isolates of influenza A viruses. *Journal of Infectious Diseases, 180,* 935–939.

Zhu, Q. Y., Qin, E. D., Wang, W., Yu, J., Liu, B. H., Hu, Y., et al. (2006). Fatal infection with influenza A (H5N1) virus in China. *New England Journal of Medicine, 354,* 2731–2732.

CHAPTER FIFTEEN

Legionellosis

Legionnaires Disease and Pontiac Fever

Christina R. Phares and Matthew R. Moore

In July 1976, during the annual American Legion convention in Philadelphia, an outbreak of a severe form of pneumonia occurred among attendees at the convention hotel. Between July 2 and August 3, 1976, 182 persons were infected, 147 (81%) required hospitalization, and 29 (16%) died (Fraser et al., 1977). Scientists at the Centers for Disease Control and Prevention (CDC) identified a previously unknown pathogen from autopsy lung specimens. The new pathogen was named *Legionella pneumophila*, and the clinical syndrome, Legionnaires disease (McDade et al., 1977). Subsequently, through stored serum samples, investigators determined retrospectively that *Legionella* had caused earlier outbreaks, including one at the same hotel in 1974, one at a psychiatric hospital in 1965, and one at a meat packing plant in 1957 (Osterholm et al., 1983; Terranova, Cohen, & Fraser, 1978; Thacker et al., 1978). Sporadic cases from 1947 were also found (McDade, Brenner, & Bozeman, 1979).

Legionella is a gram-negative, aerobic, unencapsulated bacillus. At least 49 species and 71 serogroups of *Legionella* have been identified. One species, *L. pneumophila*, causes over 90% of cases of Legionnaires disease in the United States and Europe (Fields, Benson, & Besser, 2002). Rarely, non-*pneumophila Legionella* species have been associated with Legionnaires disease in the United States, including *L. longbeachae*, *L. micdadei*, *L. dumoffii*, and *L. bozemanii* (Fields et al., 2002). In Australia, unlike the United States and Europe, many cases of Legionnaires disease are caused by *L. longbeachae*, although *L. pneumophila* still causes the majority of cases (Edelstein & Cianciotto, 2005; Yu et al., 2002). *Legionellae* are ubiquitous in freshwater environments, including lakes, rivers, thermally polluted ponds, and wet soil (Fliermans et al., 1981; Steele, 1996). Natural freshwater environments, however, have rarely been implicated as a source of human disease. Man-made water environments are the principal reservoirs of *Legionella* species that cause human disease because they allow for the growth, amplification, and dissemination of the bacteria. *Legionellae* require temperatures of 25–42° C and environments with appropriate nutritional requirements. These nutritional requirements are met within intracellular environments, and *Legionellae* survive as intracellular parasites of free living protozoa, especially amoebae (Breiman et al., 1990; Fields, Fields, et al., 1993; Fields, Sanden, & Barbaree, 1993; Fields, Shotts, Feeley, Gorman, & Martin, 1984). Other factors, such as water stagnation and the presence of biofilm and sediment, enhance the amplification of *Legionellae* in water systems, making man-made environments ideal conditions for the growth and amplification of *Legionellae*.

Two clinically and epidemiologically distinct syndromes are caused by *Legionella*: Legionnaires disease and Pontiac fever. Legionnaires disease is a form of pneumonia that can be severe and that may include systemic symptoms such as fever, diarrhea, abdominal pain, and delirium. Other symptoms can include a nonproductive cough, headache, and myalgia. *Legionella* species are thought to cause 2% to 14% of adult community-acquired pneumonia cases in the United States (Marston et al., 1997; Vergis, Akbas, & Yu, 2000). Persons with compromised immune systems and underlying medical conditions—such as the elderly, smokers, persons with chronic cardiovascular or pulmonary conditions, and users of immunosuppressive drugs—are most susceptible. Extrapulmonary infection can also occur in this population, although it is rare (Cunha, 2006). It is less common to diagnose Legionnaires disease in young, healthy persons. It is not surprising, therefore, that the attack rate for Legionnaires disease in outbreaks is low, less than 5%, and that mortality can be high, ranging from 5% to 30% (Benin, Benson, & Besser, 2002; Hoge & Breiman, 1991). The incubation period for Legionnaires disease is usually reported as 2–10 days, although cases have been documented 14 days or more after exposure (Den Boer et al., 2002; Fraser et al., 1977).

The first reported outbreak of Pontiac fever occurred in 1968 in Southfield, Michigan (Glick et al., 1978). In contrast to Legionnaires disease, Pontiac fever is a self-limited, nonfatal, nonpneumonic illness that presents with influenza-like symptoms such as malaise, fever, chills, headache, and myalgia. It has a shorter incubation period than Legionnaires disease, usually 24–48 hours. Unlike Legionnaires disease, it generally affects persons without underlying medical conditions and has a high attack rate (up to 95%). In patients with Pontiac fever, it is difficult to demonstrate actively replicating *Legionella*. Recent evidence suggests that the symptoms of Pontiac fever are caused by exposure to endotoxin released by dead *Legionella* (Castor et al., 2005; Fields et al., 2001). Outbreaks of legionellosis can manifest as both Legionnaires disease and Pontiac fever (Benin, Benson, Arnold et al., 2002).

Man-made water environments that produce aerosols also promote transmission via inhalation. Water droplets of 1–5 microliters can reach alveoli in the lung, where they are retained and have the ability to cause disease in susceptible persons (Mathieu et al., 2006). Man-made fresh-water environments that have been implicated in the dissemination of *Legionella* include cooling towers, evaporative condensers, whirlpools, and spas, as well as sources that use potable water from plumbing systems such as showers, cool-mist humidifiers, and supermarket ultrasonic misting machines (Den Boer et al., 2002; Garcia-Fulgueiras et al., 2003; Greig et al., 2004; Kura et al., 2006; Lepine et al., 1998; Mahoney et al., 1992; Nguyen et al., 2006). If *Legionellae* are present in these water systems, each type of system has the ability to disseminate water droplets containing bacteria to susceptible persons.

The largest outbreak of Legionnaires disease occurred in 2001 in Murcia, Spain. Aerosols contaminated with *L. pneumophila* serogroup 1 released from cooling towers resulted in an estimated 650 cases, including 449 confirmed cases, within a 1-month period (Garcia-Fulgueiras et al., 2003). Other large outbreaks of Legionnaires disease include one in Melbourne, Australia, associated with a cooling tower on an aquarium, resulting in 125 cases and 4 deaths (Greig et al., 2004); one in Bovenkar-spel, Netherlands, associated with a whirlpool spa on display at a flower show, resulting in 188 cases and 21 deaths (Den Boer et al., 2002); and another in Toronto, Canada, associated with a cooling tower on a long-term care facility, resulting in 127 cases and 20 deaths (Henry, Young, & Walker, 2005).

Investigations of common-source outbreaks associated with cooling towers have demonstrated that contaminated aerosols can travel long distances to transmit disease. Transmission is greatest within 0.4–0.8 km of the source (Addiss et al., 1989; Brown et al., 1999), although transmission can occur at much longer distances (Nguyen et al., 2006). Weather conditions may also enhance transmission (Fisman et al., 2005).

Hospitals and long-term care facilities pose unique challenges for the prevention of Legionnaires disease because they often have older, complex plumbing systems, numerous sources of aerosol transmission are often present, and highly susceptible persons are concentrated in one location. Numerous outbreaks of health care-acquired legionellosis have been reported. Although the majority have been associated with potable water, cooling towers are another confirmed source of transmission (Campins et al., 2000; Johnson et al., 1985; Garcia-Fulgeiras et al., 2003; Greig et al., 2004; Nguyen et al., 2006).

As advances in technology have improved medical care, persons with underlying medical conditions are more likely to be active in their communities and to travel for business and pleasure. Therefore, although *Legionellae* have been in the natural environment for centuries, it is only in the 20th century that technologic advances have provided the ideal setting for multiplication of the bacterium, effective dissemination, and contact with a sizable number of susceptible hosts (Breiman & Butler, 1998).

Four methods are currently available to diagnosis Legionnaires disease: culture of the organism from respiratory secretions or lung tissue, detection of *Legionella* urinary antigen by either enzyme immunoassay or radioimmunoassay, paired acute- and convalescent-phase serologic testing, and direct fluorescent antibody. Of the four, *Legionella* urinary antigen detection and culture are most commonly used (Cunha, 2006).

Culture of respiratory secretions is nearly 60% sensitive and 100% specific (Fields et al., 2002). *Legionellae* are fastidious and require special media and conditions for growth; techniques for culturing other respiratory pathogens will not detect *Legionella*. Therefore, the clinician and microbiologist must always consider *Legionella* in the differential diagnosis of pneumonia so that sputum samples can be appropriately evaluated. Also, unlike culture of respiratory secretions for other pathogens, colonization of the upper airway with *Legionella* does not occur, and specimen quality is not a limitation to recovery of the organism (Ingram & Plouffe, 1994). An advantage of culture as a diagnostic method for Legionnaires disease is that culture techniques will isolate all *Legionella* species. Also, molecular typing techniques can be used to determine whether two or more cases are related to each other. Furthermore, an isolate obtained from an environmental source can be compared with a clinical isolate to determine if the water environment is the source of the *Legionella* causing disease. Without directly comparing environmental and clinical isolates, it is difficult to implicate a source definitively in a case of Legionnaires disease.

Urine antigen testing has become the most common type of testing for Legionnaires disease in the United States (Benin, Benson, et al., 2002). Urinary antigen tests are simple to perform and give results much sooner than culture. Obtaining a urine sample is often easier than obtaining a sputum sample. Commercially available tests detect only *L. pneumophila* serogroup 1, with specificity approaching 100% (Fields et al., 2002). *L. pneumophila* serogroup 1 causes the majority of cases of Legionnaires disease in the United States and Europe; however, cases due to other species and serogroups may go undiagnosed if the evaluation is limited to urinary antigen tests. Also, without a clinical isolate, it is not possible to use molecular techniques to identify an environmental source of a case or outbreak.

Serologic testing is not useful for clinical decision making because of the need to obtain convalescent sera 3 to 6 weeks following the acute illness. Serology can be useful in epidemiologic studies where culture and urine antigen testing may not be feasible for some patients. Single serologic specimens are not useful under any circumstances (Plouffe et al., 1995).

Because *Legionella* is an intracellular pathogen, those antibiotics that achieve high intracellular concentration are most effective. The traditional use of erythromycin has largely been replaced by newer agents such as azithromycin and levofloxacin (Yu et al., 2004). These can achieve high pulmonary concentrations. None of the beta-lactams, monobactams, aminoglycosides, or phenicols are active against *Legionella* infection (Edelstein & Cianciotto, 2005).

Legionnaires disease is underdiagnosed and underreported in the United States. An estimated 8,000 to 18,000 hospitalized cases of Legionnaires disease occur yearly, yet fewer than 2,000 reports per year are received at the CDC (CDC, 2005b; Marston et al., 1997). Legionellosis is reportable in all states in the United States.

Travelers are exposed to many potential *Legionella* sources, including evaporative coolers (Garcia-Fulgueiras et al., 2003), potable water systems (Joseph et al., 1996), and whirlpool spas in hotels and aboard cruise ships (CDC, 2005a; Jernigan et al., 1996). The first outbreak of Legionnaires disease described in 1976 was travel related and is an example of how a concentration of susceptible hosts exposed to a single source can result in an outbreak. Because the incubation period is relatively long, onset of illness is often after travelers return home to different locations, making travel-associated outbreaks difficult to detect. In Europe, surveillance for Legionnaires disease has focused on detecting travel-associated clusters and outbreaks. In 1997, 29% of European cases were community acquired, 16% were nosocomial, and 22% were travel related (World Health Organization, 1998). Recently, the CDC and state health departments have increased efforts to improve surveillance for travel-associated legionellosis (Council of State and Territorial Epidemiologists, 2005).

Surveillance for Legionnaires disease in health care settings is especially important because health care facilities include concentrations of patients who are highly susceptible to *Legionella* infection. A case of Legionnaires disease is considered to be a definite nosocomial case if it is laboratory confirmed and occurs in a patient who has been hospitalized continuously for 10 days or more before the onset of symptoms. A case is considered a possible case of nosocomial Legionnaires disease if the infection is laboratory confirmed and occurs 2–9 days after hospital admission. From 1980 through 1998, 35% of cases reported to the CDC were designated as possibly or definitely nosocomial, and 28% of those were associated with an outbreak (Benin, Benson, et al., 2002).

Efforts to prevent the transmission of *Legionellae* from the environment to susceptible hosts have focused on either altering aquatic environments so they no longer support the growth of *Legionellae* or on reducing the exposure of susceptible hosts to potentially contaminated aerosols. Several published guidelines are available to reduce transmission of *Legionellae* to susceptible persons and minimize the risk of community- and travel-acquired legionellosis. The American Society of Heating, Refrigerating and Air-Conditioning Engineers (ASHRAE) has published guidelines to diminish the risk of legionellosis associated with building water systems (ASHRAE Standard Project Committee, 2000). Also, specific guidelines for reducing the transmission of *Legionella* in public spas and hot tubs are available (CDC, 1997).

Guidelines to reduce the transmission of *Legionellae* in health care environments are available from several organizations (Allegheny County Health Department, 1997; CDC, 1997, 2000, 2004; State of Maryland Department of Health and Mental Hygiene, 2000; Texas Department of State Health Services, 1999). An area of controversy among these guidelines is the extent to which routine environmental sampling is recommended for potable water systems in health care facilities. In Allegheny County, Pennsylvania, routine environmental sampling is recommended for all hospitals, with the frequency of sampling dependent on hospital size (Allegheny County Health Department, 1997). The Maryland Department of Health and Mental Hygiene recommends routine environmental sampling of water systems within acute care hospitals. However, the frequency of sampling should be driven by institution-specific risk assessments (State of Maryland Department of Health and Mental Hygiene, 2000). Finally, the Texas Department of State Health Services recommends that all acute care hospitals conduct a risk assessment to determine whether and how often environmental sampling should be performed (Texas Department of State Health Services, 1999). Recommendations from the CDC acknowledge that routine sampling may be used as part of an overall Legionnaires disease prevention strategy in transplant settings (CDC, 2000). However, because of the lack of evidence that routine sampling independently leads to reduced risk of Legionnaires disease in health care settings, the CDC does not have a recommendation for or against this strategy in nontransplant settings (CDC, 2004).

Although there are multiple guidelines to diminish the risk of transmission from specific sources and settings, community-wide prevention strategies are lacking. Some evidence suggests that improved disinfection of municipal water supplies is feasible. In the United States, chlorine is the chemical most commonly used for residual disinfection of municipal drinking water. Monochloramine is also frequently used and has the advantage of reacting less with organic material in water; therefore, it persists in effective concentrations in longer distribution systems. The risk of health care-associated Legionnaires disease appears to be lower in hospitals served by municipalities that use monochloramine as opposed to chlorine (Heffelfinger et al., 2000; Kool, Carpenter, & Fields, 1999). In addition, *Legionella* colonization of water distribution systems declines significantly when municipal water systems convert their primary residual disinfectant from chlorine to monochloramine (Flannery et al., 2006; Moore et al., 2006). While municipal water systems are unlikely to convert to monochloramine solely for the prevention of Legionnaires disease, this benefit is an important public health consideration. Finally, introduction of monochloramine directly into health care facility water systems could provide another option for prevention of health care-associated Legionnaires disease.

CONCLUSION

Twentieth century advances in technology have contributed to the emergence of *Legionella* as a human pathogen. Surveillance, use of appropriate diagnostic tests, and reporting of all cases are critical public health steps that can identify outbreaks and, through the implementation of disinfection procedures, prevent additional cases.

REFERENCES

Addiss, D. G., Davis, J. P., LaVenture, M., Ward, P. J., Hutchinson, M. A., & McKinney, R. M. (1989). Community-acquired Legionnaires' disease associated with a cooling tower: Evidence for longer-distance transport of *Legionella pneumophila. American Journal of Epidemiology, 130, 557–568.*

Allegheny County Health Department. (1997). *Approaches to the prevention and control of Legionella infection in Allegheny County health care facilities* (2nd ed.). Pittsburgh, PA: Author.

ASHRAE Standard Project Committee 12-2000 (2000). *Minimizing the risk of Legionellosis associated with building water systems.* Atlanta, GA: American Society of Heating, Refrigerating and Air-Conditioning Engineers.

Benin, A. L., Benson, R. F., Arnold, K. E., Fiore, A. E., Cook, P. G., Williams, L. K., et al. (2002). An outbreak of travel-associated Legionnaires disease and Pontiac fever: The need for enhanced surveillance of travel-associated legionellosis in the United States. *Journal of Infectious Diseases, 185, 237–243.*

Benin, A. L., Benson, R. F., & Besser, R. E. (2002). Trends in Legionnaires disease, 1980–1998: Declining mortality and new patterns of diagnosis. *Clinical Infectious Diseases, 35*, 1039–1046.

Breiman, R. F., & Butler, J. C. (1998). Legionnaires' disease: Clinical, epidemiological, and public health perspectives. *Seminars in Respiratory Infections, 13*, 84–89.

Breiman, R. F., Fields, B. S., Sanden, G. N., Volmer, L., Meier, A., & Spika, J. S. (1990). Association of shower use with Legionnaires' disease. Possible role of amoebae. *Journal of the American Medical Association, 263*, 2924–2926.

Brown, C. M., Nuorti, P. J., Breiman, R. F., Hatchcock, A. L., Fields, B. S., Lipman, H. B., et al. (1999). A community outbreak of Legionnaires' disease linked to hospital cooling towers: An epidemiological method to calculate dose of exposure. *International Journal of Epidemiology, 28*, 353–359.

Campins, M., Ferrer, A., Callis, L., Pelaz, C., Cortes, P. J., Pinart, N., et al. (2000). Nosocomial Legionnaire's disease in a children's hospital. *Pediatric Infectious Disease Journal, 19*, 228–234.

Castor, M. L., Wagstrom, E. A., Danila, R. N., Smith, K. E., Naimi, T. S., Besser, J. M., et al. (2005). An outbreak of Pontiac fever with respiratory distress among workers performing high-pressure cleaning at a sugar-beet processing plant. *Journal of Infectious Diseases, 191*, 1530–1537.

Centers for Disease Control and Prevention. (1997). *Final recommendations to minimize transmission of Legionnaires' disease from whirlpool spas on cruise ships*. Atlanta, GA: U.S. Department of Health and Human Services.

Centers for Disease Control and Prevention. (2000). Guidelines for preventing opportunistic infections among hematopoietic stem cell transplant recipients: Recommendations of CDC, the Infectious Disease Society of America, and the American Society of Blood and Marrow Transplantation. *Morbidity and Mortality Weekly Report, 49*(RR-10), 36–38.

Centers for Disease Control and Prevention. (2004). Guidelines for preventing healthcare-associated pneumonia, 2003. *Morbidity and Mortality Weekly Report, 53*(RR-3), 1–36.

Centers for Disease Control and Prevention. (2005a). Cruise-ship–associated Legionnaires disease, November 2003–May 2004. *Morbidity and Mortality Weekly Report, 54*, 1153–1155.

Centers for Disease Control and Prevention. (2005b). Summary of notifiable diseases—United States, 2003. *Morbidity and Mortality Weekly Report, 52*, 16.

Council of State and Territorial Epidemiologists. (2005). *Strengthening surveillance for travel-associated legionellosis and revised case definition for Legionnaires' disease*. Position paper presented at the Annual Conference of the Council of State and Territorial Epidemiologists, Albuquerque, NM.

Cunha, B. A. (2006). The atypical pneumonias: Clinical diagnosis and importance. *Clinical Microbiology and Infections, 12*, 12–24.

Den Boer, J. W., Yzerman, E. P., Schellekens, J., Lettinga, K. D., Boshuizen, H. C., Van Steenbergen, J. E., et al. (2002). A large outbreak of Legionnaires' disease at a flower show, the Netherlands, 1999. *Emerging Infectious Diseases, 8,* 37–43.

Edelstein, P. H., & Cianciotto, N. P. (2005). *Legionella.* In G. L. Mandell, J. E. Bennett, & R. Dolin (Eds.), *Mandell, Douglas, and Bennett's principles and practice of infectious diseases* (6th ed., pp. 2711–2724). Philadelphia: Churchill Livingstone Elsevier.

Fields, B., Sanden, G. N., & Barbaree, J. M. (1993). *Legionella* and protozoa: Interaction of a pathogen and its natural host. In J. M. Barbaree, R. Breiman, & A. Dufour (Eds.), *Legionella: Current status and emerging perspectives* (pp. 129–136). Washington, DC: American Society for Microbiology.

Fields, B. S., Benson, R. F., & Besser, R. E. (2002). *Legionella* and Legionnaires' disease: 25 years of investigation. *Clinical Microbiology Reviews, 15,* 506–526.

Fields, B. S., Fields, S. R., Loy, J. N., White, E. H., Steffens, W. L., Shotts, E. B., et al. (1993). Attachment and entry of *Legionella pneumophila* in *Hartmannella vermiformis. Journal of Infectious Diseases, 167,* 1146–1150.

Fields, B. S., Haupt, T., Davis, J. P., Arduino, M. J., Miller, P. H., & Butler, J. C. (2001). Pontiac fever due to *Legionella micdadei* from a whirlpool spa: Possible role of bacterial endotoxin. *Journal of Infectious Diseases, 184,* 1289–1292.

Fields, B. S., Shotts, E. B., Jr., Feeley, J. C., Gorman, G. W., & Martin, W. T. (1984). Proliferation of *Legionella pneumophila* as an intracellular parasite of the ciliated protozoan *Tetrahymena pyriformis. Applied and Environmental Microbiology, 47,* 467–471.

Fisman, D. N., Lim, S., Wellenius, G. A., Johnson, C., Britz, P., Gaskins, M., et al. (2005). It's not the heat, it's the humidity: Wet weather increases legionellosis risk in the greater Philadelphia metropolitan area. *Journal of Infectious Diseases, 192,* 2066–2073.

Flannery, B., Gelling, L. B., Vugia, D. J., Weintraub, J. M., Salerno, J. J., Conroy, M. J., et al. (2006). Reducing *Legionella* colonization of water systems with monochloramine. *Emerging Infectious Diseases, 12,* 588–596.

Fliermans, C. B., Cherry, W. B., Orrison, L. H., Smith, S. J., Tison, D. L., & Pope, D. H. (1981). Ecological distribution of *Legionella pneumophila. Applied and Environmental Microbiology, 41,* 9–16.

Fraser, D. W., Tsai, T. R., Orenstein, W., Parkin, W. E., Beecham, H. J., Sharrar, R. G., et al. (1977). Legionnaires' disease: Description of an epidemic of pneumonia. *New England Journal of Medicine, 297,* 1189–1197.

Garcia-Fulgueiras, A., Navarro, C., Fenoll, D., Garcia, J., Gonzalez-Diego, D., Jimenez-Bunaules, T., et al. (2003). Legionnaires' disease outbreak in Murcia, Spain. *Emerging Infectious Diseases, 9,* 915–921.

Glick, T. H., Gregg, M. B., Berman, B., Mallison, G., Rhodes, W. W., Jr., & Kassanoff, I. (1978). Pontiac fever: An epidemic of unknown etiology in a health department. *American Journal of Epidemiology, 107,* 149–160.

Greig, J. E., Carnie, J. A., Tallis, G. F., Ryan, N. J., Tan, A. G., Gordon, I. R., et al. (2004). An outbreak of Legionnaires' disease at the Melbourne Aquarium,

April 2000: Investigation and case-control studies. *Medical Journal of Australia, 180,* 566–572.

Heffelfinger, J., Fridkin, S. K., Kool, J., Fraser, V., Hageman, J., Kupronis, B, et. al. (2000). *Association between monochloramine use by municipal water treatment plants and nosocomial Legionnaires' disease.* Paper presented at the Fourth Decennial Conference, Centers for Disease Control and Prevention, Atlanta, GA.

Henry, B., Young, J. G., & Walker, D. (2005). *Report of the expert panel on the Legionnaires' disease outbreak in the city of Toronto—September/October 2005.* Toronto, Canada: Ministry of Health and Long-Term Care.

Hoge, C. W., & Breiman, R. F. (1991). Advances in the epidemiology and control of *Legionella* infections. *Epidemiologic Reviews, 13,* 329–340.

Ingram, J. G., & Plouffe, J. F. (1994). Danger of sputum purulence screens in culture of *Legionella* species. *Journal of Clinical Microbiology, 32,* 209–210.

Jernigan, D. B., Hofmann, J., Cetron, M. S., Genese, C. A., Nuorti, J. P., Fields, B. S., et al. (1996). Outbreak of Legionnaires' disease among cruise ship passengers exposed to a contaminated whirlpool spa. *Lancet, 347,* 494–499.

Johnson, J. T., Yu, V. L., Best, M. G., Vickers, R. M., Goetz, A., Wagner, R., et al. (1985). Nosocomial legionellosis in surgical patients with head-and-neck cancer: Implications for epidemiological reservoir and mode of transmission. *Lancet, 2*(8450), 298–300.

Joseph, C., Morgan, D., Birtles, R., Pelaz, C., Martin-Bourgon, C., Black, M., et al. (1996). An international investigation of an outbreak of Legionnaires disease among UK and French tourists. *European Journal of Epidemiology, 12,* 215–219.

Kool, J. L., Carpenter, J. C., & Fields, B. S. (1999). Effect of monochloramine disinfection of municipal drinking water on risk of nosocomial Legionnaires' disease. *Lancet, 353,* 272–277.

Kura, F., Amemura-Maekawa, J., Yagita, K., Endo, T., Ikeno, M., Tsuji, H., et al. (2006). Outbreak of Legionnaires' disease on a cruise ship linked to spa-bath filter stones contaminated with *Legionella pneumophila* serogroup 5. *Epidemiology & Infection, 134,* 385–391.

Lepine, L. A., Jernigan, D. B., Butler, J. C., Pruckler, J. M., Benson, R. F., Kim, G., et al. (1998). A recurrent outbreak of nosocomial Legionnaires' disease detected by urinary antigen testing: Evidence for long-term colonization of a hospital plumbing system. *Infection Control and Hospital Epidemiology, 19,* 905–910.

Mahoney, F. J., Hoge, C. W., Farley, T. A., Barbaree, J. M., Breiman, R. F., Benson, R. F., et al. (1992). Communitywide outbreak of Legionnaires' disease associated with a grocery store mist machine. *Journal of Infectious Diseases, 165,* 736–739.

Mandell, G. L., Douglas, R. G., Bennett, J. E., & Dolin, R. (2005). Mandell, Douglas, and Bennett's principles and practice of infectious diseases, 6th ed. New York: Elsevier/Churchill Livingstone, 2005 (pp. 2711–2724).

Marston, B. J., Plouffe, J. F., File, T. M., Jr., Hackman, B. A., Salstrom, S. J., Lipman, H. B., et al. (1997). Incidence of community-acquired pneumonia requiring hospitalization. Results of a population-based active surveillance Study in Ohio. The Community-Based Pneumonia Incidence Study Group. *Archives of Internal Medicine, 157,* 1709–1718.

Mathieu, L., Robine, E., Deloge-Abarkan, M., Ritoux, S., Pauly, D., Hartemann, P., et al. (2006). *Legionella* bacteria in aerosols: Sampling and analytical approaches used during the Legionnaires disease outbreak in Pas-de-Calais. *Journal of Infectious Disease, 193,* 1333–1335.

McDade, J. E., Brenner, D. J., & Bozeman, F. M. (1979). Legionnaires' disease bacterium isolated in 1947. *Annals of Internal Medicine, 90,* 659–661.

McDade, J. E., Shepard, C. C., Fraser, D. W., Tsai, T. R., Redus, M. A., & Dowdle, W. R. (1977). Legionnaires' disease: Isolation of a bacterium and demonstration of its role in other respiratory disease. *New England Journal of Medicine, 297,* 1197–1203.

Moore, M. R., Pryor, M., Fields, B., Lucas, C., Phelan, M., & Besser, R. E. (2006). Introduction of monochloramine into a municipal water system: Impact on colonization of buildings by *Legionella* spp. *Applied and Environmental Microbiology, 72,* 378–783.

Nguyen, T. M., Ilef, D., Jarraud, S., Rouil, L., Campese, C., Che, D., et al. (2006). A community-wide outbreak of Legionnaires disease linked to industrial cooling towers—How far can contaminated aerosols spread? *Journal of Infectious Diseases, 193,* 102–111.

Osterholm, M. T., Chin, T. D., Osborne, D. O., Dull, H. B., Dean, A. G., Fraser, D. W., et al. (1983). A 1957 outbreak of Legionnaires' disease associated with a meat packing plant. *American Journal of Epidemiology, 117,* 60–67.

Plouffe, J. F., File, T. M., Jr., Breiman, R. F., Hackman, B. A., Salstrom, S. J., Marston, B. I., et al. (1995). Reevaluation of the definition of Legionnaires' disease: Use of the urinary antigen assay. Community-Based Pneumonia Incidence Study Group. *Clinical Infectious Diseases, 20,* 1286–1291.

State of Maryland Department of Health and Mental Hygiene. (2000). *Report of the Maryland Scientific Working Group to Study Legionella in Water Systems in Healthcare Institutions* (pp. 1–27). Baltimore, MD: Author.

Steele, T. W. (1996). The ecology of *Legionella longbeachae* in Australia. *Medical Journal of Australia, 164,* 703–704.

Terranova, W., Cohen, M. L., & Fraser, D. W. (1978). 1974 outbreak of Legionnaires' disease diagnosed in 1977. Clinical and epidemiological features. *Lancet, 2,* 122–124.

Texas Department of State Health Services. (1999). *Report of the Texas Legionnaires' Disease Task Force.* Austin, TX: Author.

Thacker, S. B., Bennett, J. V., Tsai, F., Fraser, D. W., McDade, J. E., Shepard, C. C., et al. (1978). An outbreak in 1965 of severe respiratory illness caused by the Legionnaires' disease bacterium. *Journal of Infectious Diseases, 138,* 512–519.

Vergis, E. N., Akbas, E., & Yu, V. L. (2000). *Legionella* as a cause of severe pneumonia. *Seminars in Respiratory and Critical Care Medicine, 21,* 295–304.

World Health Organization. (1998). Legionnaires' disease in Europe, 1997. *Weekly Epidemiological Record, 73,* 257–261.

Yu, V. L., Greenberg, R. N., Zadeikis, N., Stout, J. E., Khashab, M. M., Olson, W. H., et al. (2004). Levofloxacin efficacy in the treatment of community-acquired legionellosis. *Chest, 125,* 2135–2139.

Yu, V. L., Plouffe, J. F., Pastoris, M. C., Stout, J. E., Schousboe, M., Widmer, A., et al. (2002). Distribution of *Legionella* species and serogroups isolated by culture in patients with sporadic community-acquired legionellosis: An international collaborative survey. *Journal of Infectious Diseases, 186,* 127–128.

CHAPTER SIXTEEN

Lyme Disease, Ehrlichiosis, Anaplasmosis, and Babesiosis

Felissa R. Lashley

Since the mid-1970s, more than 20 tickborne infectious diseases have been newly identified in humans. Among these emerging diseases, several are clinically important in the United States:

- Lyme disease, usually caused by *Borrelia burgdorferi*, a spirochete, was first recognized in North America in the 1970s.
- Ehrlichiosis, which is caused in humans by *Ehrlichia chaffeensis*, came to attention in 1986.
- Anaplasmosis, caused by *Anaplasma phagocytophilum*, was formerly classified as an ehrlichiosis, as described later in this chapter.
- Babesiosis, a parasitic infection, usually caused by *Babesia microti*, has been increasingly recognized in recent years.

All of these diseases have usual animal reservoirs. Societal and environmental changes—such as building suburban and country residential dwellings that increasingly encroach on wooded areas near where deer, large mammals, and certain types of wild rodents usually live—facilitate spread. Humans can then come into contact with these microbes through routine maintenance such as gardening and yard work and via pets that may carry ticks into yards and homes. More leisure time to pursue outdoor activities such as hiking, fishing, and camping in meadows and wooded areas also affords opportunities for exposure. Changes in weather and climate such as global warming and increased rainfall can increase reservoir and vector populations. Vectorborne diseases are discussed in general in chapter 3. Preventive measures are shown in Appendix C, Table C.4. Lyme disease, ehrlichiosis, anaplasmosis, and babesiosis are considered here.

LYME DISEASE

Lyme disease is the most frequent tickborne disease in North America, and more than 200,000 cases have been reported to the Centers for Disease Control and Prevention (CDC) since 1982, with approximately 20,000 new cases each year (Aguero-Rosenfeld, Wang, Schwartz, & Wormser, 2005; Ogden et al., 2006). The recognition of Lyme disease began with a phone call to the state health department in November 1975 from a mother in Old Lyme, Connecticut, who reported a cluster of 12 cases of a disease that had been diagnosed as juvenile rheumatoid arthritis. Four of these people lived on the same street (Steere, Malawista, Snydman, & Andiman, 1976; Steere et al., 1977). This report was quickly followed by that of another mother in the same community, who told investigators at the Yale Rheumatology Clinic and the state health department about arthritis occurring in herself, her husband, two of their children, and several neighbors (Steere et al., 1977).

Researchers began investigating cases of clustering arthritis in Lyme, Old Lyme, and East Haddam, Connecticut, believing that they were not typical juvenile or another type of rheumatoid arthritis. In all, 51 persons, 39 children, and 12 adults comprised the sample investigated at that time, with information that some cases began in 1972. The investigators believed that an arbovirus might be responsible, and tests were performed for the Ross River, chikungunya, and O' nyong-nyong viruses. The tests were negative. Thus, investigators referred to this arthritis as a new or previously unrecognized clinical entity and called it Lyme arthritis (Steere et al., 1976, 1977). As investigations moved forward, an arthropod vector was suspected (Steere et al., 1977). The typical skin lesion known as erythema migrans, a bull's-eye rash, was described in earlier literature in Europe and in a 1970 report in the United States from Connecticut (Parola & Raoult, 2001; Scrimenti, 1970), suggesting earlier times of emergence without recognition of a new agent.

In the United States, Lyme disease is caused by the gram-negative bacterial spirochete complex *B. burgdorferi* sensu lato, but in Europe, *Borrelia afzelii* and *Borrelia garinii* can also cause infection (Steere, 2005). *B. burgdorferi* has been described as one of the most complex bacteria known (Stricker, Lautin, & Burrascano, 2006). The organism is transmitted to humans by the deer or black-legged tick, specifically *Ixodes scapularis* (also called *Ixodes dammini*), *Ixodes pacificus* in the West, and others (Steere, 2005). The life cycle of the tick occurs over a 2-year period and involves the evolution from eggs to the feeding of the larva, particularly on the white-footed mouse and other small rodents such as chipmunks, where *B. burgdorferi* may be acquired. The life cycle progresses through a nymphal stage the next spring, with feeding again on mice, to adult stages when the adult ticks feed on and attach to white-tailed deer or other large mammals where they mate and may fall off (Strickland, 2000). In the Pacific northwest, the life cycle involves woodrats and lizards. Ticks of the *Ixodes* genus can hide in ground litter and leaf litter and find hosts from the tips of grass and shrubs. They prefer shade with high humidity.

Humans are incidental hosts (Strickland, 2000). The size of the nymphs that may attach to humans is about that of a poppy seed and thus can be difficult to detect. While humans may encounter the ticks during recreational activities such as hiking, fishing, and camping in meadows and wooded areas, or when doing activities such as clearing brush, ticks can also be encountered in the backyards of suburban dwellings, as humans have expanded their housing into formerly wooded areas where deer may live. Furthermore, household pets such as cats may carry ticks into yards and homes. Therefore, preventing tick bites is an important aspect of preventing tickborne diseases (see Appendix C, Table C.4). There is a potential for *Borrelia* to be transmitted by blood transfusion but this occurrence has not yet been documented in humans (Alter, Stramer & Dodd, 2007).

It is yet unclear what human factors are associated with an increased predisposition to acquiring Lyme disease from a tick. One factor does appear to be the length of time the tick is attached to the body. Persons to whom the tick is attached for less than 24 hours appear to have a smaller risk of acquiring Lyme disease (Steere, 2005). The Lone Star ticks usually found in the Southeast have been increasing in number in New England. They are more aggressive and are known to be able to transmit such diseases as ehrlichiosis, Rocky Mountain spotted fever, and tularemia but are not yet known to transmit Lyme disease ("Lone Star tick," 2006). Rather recently, it has been realized that these ticks may be coinfected with the agents of babesiosis, anaplasmosis, and ehrlichiosis, transmitting multiple infective agents together. These diseases are discussed later in this chapter.

Lyme disease became a nationally notifiable disease in January 1991. Although cases have been reported from 49 of the 50 states and the District of Columbia, more than 90% are reported from 8 northeastern and mid-Atlantic states (New York, Connecticut, Pennsylvania, New Jersey, Maryland, Rhode Island, Massachusetts, and Delaware) and two north-central states (Wisconsin and Minnesota; Aguero-Rosenfeld et al., 2005; Phillips,

Burrascano, Horowitz, Savely, & Stricker, 2006). Cases have also been reported from Europe, Asia, Australia, and other locales (Steere, 2005).

Lyme disease can cause acute and chronic manifestations that may be localized and/or disseminated and multisystem, with both early and late signs and symptoms (Steere, 2005). Signs and symptoms often differ among cases seen in the United States and in Europe, perhaps due to the difference in causative organism strains. In the United States, in about three quarters of patients, Lyme disease begins 7 to 14 days (range 3 to 30) after a tick bite, most commonly with the appearance of the previously described skin lesion known as erythema migrans that appears at the site of the tick bite (Wormser, 2006). Often, the person may not be aware of being bitten. This is called Stage 1, localized infection. The macule/papule expands over days or weeks to form a large round lesion that measures at least 5 cm to 15 cm (and can be up to 50 cm) with partial central clearing and a red outer border that can be hot to the touch (Bratton & Corey, 2005; Steere, 2005). There may also be flu-like symptoms, which some believe is evidence of dissemination (Aguero-Rosenfeld et al., 2005).

Stage 2 is early disseminated infection and occurs several days to weeks after the initial lesion. Manifestations may include multiple skin lesions as described above that may even coalesce, malaise, fatigue, headache, fever, chills, lymphadenopathy, sore throat, conjunctivitis, cough, migratory muscle pains, and, in some men, testicular swelling. Meningeal irritation with headache and neck pain and stiffness and encephalopathy with mentation difficulty may occur. Even if untreated, these symptoms may remit for a period of time, and patients may have intermittent and changing symptoms. About 5% develop cardiac involvement such as atrioventricular block.

Stage 3 is a late stage of persistent infection that can be seen months to years after infection, especially in untreated or inadequately treated persons. One of the most frequent symptoms is arthritis. The arthritis is generally asymmetric and oligoarticular, and the knee is nearly always a site. Arthritis may become chronic in 10% to 20% of persons. Certain *HLA* alleles, especially *DRB1*0401* and *DRB*0101*, are associated with chronic Lyme arthritis, possibly resulting from an autoimmune response (Radolf, 2005; Steere, 2005). Such *HLA* associations are seen with other forms of arthritis (Lashley, 2005). About 5% of untreated patients may develop chronic neurological symptoms, especially spinal radicular pain and paresthesias. In Europe, ataxia, cognitive impairment, 7th and 8th cranial nerve neuropathy, and bladder dysfunction may be seen (Steere, 2005). Chronic inflammatory eye disease such as keratitis may be seen, and in Europe, acrodermatitis chronica atrophicans can occur years after infection or, if present early, can last for many years (Steere, 2005). Even when Lyme disease is appropriately treated, a percentage of persons continue to have symptoms such as musculoskeletal pain, neurocognitive impairment, fatigue, and/or arthritis (Klempner et al., 2005; Radolf, 2005). This condition is known as posttreatment chronic Lyme disease (PTCLD). Some believe that PTCLD results from deep persistent infection, while others believe that it is not due to either infection or inflammation. Some believe that the original diagnosis in these instances was in error (Radolf, 2005; Strickland, 2000). In any case, those affected have impaired health-related quality of life (Klempner et al., 2005).

Diagnosis may be by direct detection methods such as culture or molecular methods, and the best results appear to be from skin biopsies or synovial fluid. Antibody detection through serology has a low sensitivity in Stage 1 but is improved in Stages 2 and 3 (Wilske, 2005). There are varying opinions on whether diagnostic testing is needed and the best approach for such testing. Usually, the history of the tick bite and characteristic signs (especially the characteristic skin lesion) and symptoms suffice for diagnosis (Wormser, 2006).

Detailed treatment protocols have been developed and disseminated for different situations (Steere, 2005; Wormser et al., 2006). It is important to treat Lyme disease early and completely. In a 10- to 20-year follow-up study, patients with Lyme disease who developed facial palsy and were not initially treated with antibiotics had more residual deficits, even though these were mild (Kalish et al., 2001). Practice guidelines recommend doxycycline, 100 mg twice daily, or amoxicillin, 500 mg three times daily, for 14 to 21 days for early localized or disseminated Lyme disease, and other therapy may be used in cases of severe manifestations such as neurologic or cardiac complications (Wormser, 2006). Doxycycline has the advantage of also being effective against human granulocytic anaplasmosis (HGA) and human monocytic ehrlichiosis (HME), which is useful since persons may be coinfected. Wormser (2006) recommends single-dose doxycycline prophylaxis in persons bitten by a tick that was attached for at least 36 hours in endemic areas. Treatment is generally recommended for pregnant women with Lyme disease (Walsh, Mayer, & Baxi, 2007). A vaccine against Lyme disease was marketed but was withdrawn in 2002. Persons with Lyme disease may be coinfected with ehrlichiosis, anaplasmosis, or babesiosis, and coinfection should be considered when planning treatment (Wormser, 2006).

EHRLICHIOSIS AND ANAPLASMOSIS

In 1986, human ehrlichial infections in North America were first identified in Ft. Chaffee, Arkansas (McQuiston, Paddock, Holman, & Childs, 1999). The agent was subsequently named E. chaffeensis and was found to cause HME. In 1992 and 1993, an outbreak of ehrlichiosis in the Midwest was recognized but was realized to be due to an agent distinct from *E. chaffeensis*. The agent was closely related to *Ehrlichia phagocytophila* and *Ehrlichia equi*. becoming known as the human granulocytic ehrlichiosis (HGE) agent. The causative agent in this outbreak resulted in HGE, now known as human granulocytic anaplasmosis (HGA). Many changes in taxonomy and nomenclature have occurred in recent years. The agent causing HGA is now designated as *Anaplasma phagocytophilum* (Dumler, 2005; Parola, Davoust, & Raoult, 2005; Wormser et al., 2006).

A. *phagocytophilum*, *E. chaffeensis*, and *Neorickettsia* (formerly *Ehrlichia*) *sennetsu* are small α-proteobacteria that are obligate intracellular pathogens (Dunning-Hotopp et al., 2006). Those known to be human rather than animal pathogens are relatively few at this time. These are (a) *E. chaffeensis* causing HME; (b) *A. phagocytophilum* causing HGA; (c) *Ehrlichia ewingii*, a known pathogen of dogs recently recognized as a human pathogen, which was first reported from Missouri in 1999, is known to cause human ewingii ehrlichiosis, and is similar to HME and HGA in many ways; (d) *N. sennetsu*, which has been known to cause an illness similar to mononucleosis in Japan and Malaysia and was first reported upon in 1985; and (e) *Ehrlichia canis*, mainly affecting dogs but with reported human asymptomatic infection (Buller et al., 1999; Dumler, 2005; Dunning-Hotopp et al., 2006; Parola et al., 2005). The tick vector for *E. chaffeensis* is the Lone Star tick (*Amblyomma americanum*), and the white-tailed deer is the principal wildlife reservoir, although it has been suggested that wild canids such as coyotes and domestic dogs may hold a future potential for cross-species transmission. The Lone Star tick is also the vector for the more recently identified *E. ewingii* (CDC, 2006; Parola et al., 2005). For *A. phagocytophilum*, the *I. scapularis* and *I. pacificus* ticks appear to be insect vectors while white-tailed deer, mice, and other small mammals are important reservoirs (Parola et al., 2005). Distribution of HGA is now worldwide, while HME has been documented only in the United States, especially in south-central and southeastern states such as Missouri, Oklahoma, Tennessee, Arkansas, and Maryland (Dumler, 2005; Parola et al., 2005).

Signs and symptoms follow a tick bite. In HME, onset ranges from 1 to 4 weeks, and with HGA the incubation period is typically 7 to 10 days. The clinical and laboratory findings of both HME and HGA are similar, especially at onset. Symptoms at onset for both include fever, headache, chills, myalgia, and malaise (CDC, 2006). In HME, vomiting occurs in a little more than one third, as does a petechial, macular, or maculopapular rash, which is seen more frequently in children than adults. A cough occurs in about 25%. Central nervous system findings such as meningitis and encephalitis, other gastrointestinal symptoms, pharyngitis, and conjunctivitis may be seen. Laboratory findings may include leukopenia, thrombocytopenia, and elevated transaminase levels. About half require hospitalization, and the typical case fatality rate is about 3.1%. The clinical course for HGA is very similar to HME with the exception that rash is rarely present, and a nonproductive cough, arthralgia, nausea, and anorexia are seen. In regard to laboratory findings, leukopenia and thrombocytopenia are often seen. The case fatality rate is about 1%, although about half of patients may require hospitalization. Both HME and HGA tend to occur in adults around 50 years of age, although cases can occur at any age (Amsden, Warmack, & Gubbins, 2005; Dumler, 2005; Parola et al., 2005; Schutze, 2006). Most patients recover completely within 2 months.

Both HME and HGA can have a range of severity from asymptomatic or mild illness through life-threatening illness and death. A complete description of management can be found in documents from the CDC (2006) and the Infectious Diseases Society of America (Wormser et al., 2006). For both HME and HGA, diagnosis is through serologic methods such as indirect immunofluorescence assays (IFA) and polymerase chain reaction (PCR) assays for detection of specific recombinant RNA gene targets and DNA. Early treatment with doxycycline is important in avoiding severe illness, although sometimes complications develop despite treatment (Buckingham, 2005; Parola et al., 2005; Schutze, 2006). However, chronic illness similar to that following Lyme disease is not recognized. Persons with ehrlichiosis or anaplasmosis may be coinfected with Lyme disease and/or babesiosis.

BABESIOSIS

Babesiosis is a zoonotic disease caused by protozoal parasites of the genus *Babesia*. These organisms are sometimes known as piroplasms because of their pear-like shape (Conrad et al., 2006; Levine, 1971). There are more than 100 species known. Among those affecting humans, *B. microti* is the major species found in the United States, especially in the eastern portion, while a newly recognized strain of *Babesia* called WA-1 was found on the West Coast in 1991 and MO-1 was identified in Missouri in 1992 (Gelfand & Vannier, 2005; Mylonakis, 2001). In Europe, *Babesia bovis* and *Babesia divergens* are the species recognized to cause human disease (Amsden et al., 2005; Leiby, 2006). It has been suggested that this *B. microti* should be reclassified as a member of the *Theileria* genus (Uilenberg, 2006). In 1956, the first human case was recognized in a splenectomized man in Yugoslavia, followed by a 1966 report from California and a 1969 report from Nantucket, Massachusetts (Gelfand & Vannier, 2005; Skrabolo & Deanovic, 1957). Babesiosis may be an ancient disease. It has been suggested that the plague of the pharaoh's cattle known as murrain, referred to in Exodus 9:3, was actually babesiosis (Gelfand & Vannier, 2005). The most common geographic locations in the United States for babesiosis are the northeast, especially on the offshore islands of Connecticut, Rhode Island, Massachusetts, and New York, and the upper Midwest, especially Wisconsin (Amsden et al., 2005).

Babesiosis is transmitted from its usual animal reservoir to humans via a tick vector. In the eastern United States, the usual tick vector is *I. scapularis*, also called *I. dammini*, while in Europe, *Ixodes ricinus*, the hard-bodied cattle tick, is the common vector. Human babesiosis has been described in the United States outside the range of the usual vector, and thus either the range may be expanding or a similar *Ixodes* tick may also be a vector. In the United States, common hosts are the white-footed mouse (a major reservoir), the white-tailed deer, and other large and small mammals that include field mice, rats, and chipmunks and occasionally bats, certain birds, and lizards. Babesiosis may also be acquired via blood transfusion, and the number occurring in this way has sharply increased, mainly due to *B. microti* (Leiby, 2006). Most cases occur between June and August (Amsden et al., 2005). Some neonatal cases of babesiosis have been found to be congenital (Fox et al., 2006).

The incubation period for tickborne *Babesia* infection ranges from 1 week to several weeks and is shorter for those cases from blood transfusion (Buckingham, 2005; Leiby, 2006). In Europe, most of the symptomatic cases have been in asplenic or immunocompromised persons; however, this is not the case in the United States. *Babesia* invade the erythrocytes, launching a complicated cycle. Thus, laboratory findings commonly include hemolytic anemia signs. Signs and symptoms include fever, chills, sweating, malaise, fatigue, weakness, headache, and myalgia and may appear malaria-like. Also seen may be arthralgia, nausea, vomiting, anorexia, abdominal pain, sore throat, conjunctival redness, depression, emotional lability, dark urine, and mild hepatosplenomegaly. Anemia, thrombocytopenia, and evidence of hemolysis may be seen. Infection can also be asymptomatic (Amsden et al., 2005; Buckingham, 2005; Gelfand & Vannier, 2005). Severe illness can occur in about 5% and can be fatal. Severity is more common in those over 50 years of age. Children generally have milder disease (Buckingham, 2005). Complications can include myocardial infarction, pulmonary edema, adult respiratory distress syndrome, disseminated intravascular coagulation, renal failure, and death (Amsden et al., 2005). Diagnosis is by examination of blood smears, serology, and PCR analysis. Standard therapy has been a combination of clindamycin and quinine but frequently results in adverse reactions. A combination of atovaquone plus azithromycin appears as effective with fewer adverse effects (Amsden et al., 2005; Vial & Gorenflot, 2006; Wormser et al., 2006). Sometimes exchange transfusion is done, especially for those with parasitemia at or above 10% or severe system compromise (Wormser et al., 2006). For tickborne cases, preventive measures to avoid tick bites is recommended, as shown in Appendix C, Table C.4. Coinfection with Lyme disease is relatively common, so the practitioner should test for concurrent infection, especially if a rash is present.

SUMMARY

These tickborne diseases provide examples of how changes in human activities result in increased opportunities for exposure to emerging infectious disease agents. In a short 25 years, Lyme disease has progressed from a virtually unknown problem to a clinically significant endemic disease in parts of the northeastern United States. Preventive measures for tick bites are considered in Appendix C, Table C.4.

REFERENCES

Aguero-Rosenfeld, M. E., Wang, G., Schwartz, I., & Wormser, G. P. (2005). Diagnosis of Lyme borreliosis. *Clinical Microbiology Reviews, 18,* 484–509.

Alter, H. J., Stramer, S. L., & Dodd, R. Y. (2007). Emerging infectious diseases that threaten the blood supply. *Seminars in Hematology, 44,* 32–41.

Amsden, J. R., Warmack, S., & Gubbins, P. O. (2005). Tick-borne bacterial, rickettsial, spirochetal, and protozoal infectious diseases in the United States: A comprehensive review. *Pharmacotherapy, 25,* 191–210.

Bratton, R. L., & Corey, R. (2005). Tick-borne disease. *American Family Physician, 71,* 2323–2330.

Buckingham, S. C. (2005). Tick-borne infections in children. *Pediatric Drugs, 7,* 163–176.

Buller, R. S., Arens, M., Hmiel, S. P., Paddock, C. D., Sumner, J. W., Rikhisa, Y., et al. (1999). *Ehrlichia ewingii,* a newly recognized agent of human ehrlichiosis. *New England Journal of Medicine, 341,* 148–155.

Centers for Disease Control and Prevention. (2006). Diagnosis and management of tickborne rickettsial diseases: Rocky Mountain spotted fever, ehrlichioses, and anaplasmosis—United States. *Morbidity and Mortality Weekly Report, 55*(RR-4), 1–29.

Conrad, P. A., Kjemstrup, A. M., Carreno, R. A., Thomford, J., Wainwright, K., Eberhard, M. et al. (2006). Description of *Babesia duncanin* sp. (Apicomplexa: Babesiidae) from humans and its differentiation from other prioplasms. *International Journal of Parasitology, 36,* 779–789.

Dumler, J. S. (2005). *Anaplasma* and *Ehrlichia* infection. *Annals of the New York Academy of Sciences, 1063*, 361–373.

Dunning-Hotopp, J. C., Lin, M., Madupu, R., Crabtree, J., Angiuoli, S. V., Eisen, J., et al. (2006). Comparative genomics of emerging human ehrlichiosis agents. *PLoS Genetics, 2*(2), 208–223.

Fox, L. M., Wingerter, S., Ahmed, A., Arnold, A., Chou, J., Rhein, L., et al. (2006). Neonatal babesiosis: Case report and review of the literature. *Pediatric Infectious Disease Journal, 25*, 169–173.

Gelfand, J. A., & Vannier, E. (2005). *Babesia* species. In G. L. Mandell, J. E. Bennett, & R. Dolin (Eds.), *Mandell, Douglas, and Bennett's principles and practice of infectious diseases* (6th ed., pp. 3209–3215). New York: Elsevier Churchill Livingstone.

Kalish, R. A., Kaplan, R. F., Taylor, E., Jones-Woodward, L., Workman, K., & Steere, A. C. (2001). Evaluation of study patients with Lyme disease, 10–20 year follow-up. *Journal of Infectious Diseases, 183*, 453–460.

Klempner, M. S., Wormser, G. H., Wade, K., Trevino, R. P., Tang, J., Kaslow, R. A., et al. (2005). A case-control study to examine HLA haplotype associations in patients with posttreatment chronic Lyme Disease. *Journal of Infectious Diseases, 192*, 1010–1013.

Lashley, F. R. (2005). *Clinical genetics in nursing practice* (3rd ed.). New York: Springer.

Leiby, D. A. (2006). Babesiosis and blood transfusion: Flying under the radar. *Vox Sanguinis, 90*, 157–165.

Levine, N. D. (1971). Taxonomy of piroplasms. *Transactions of the American Microscopy Society, 90*, 2–33.

Lone Star tick—USA: New England. (2006, July 24). *ProMED Digest, 328*, unpaginated.

McQuiston, J. H., Paddock, C. D., Holman, R. C., & Childs, J. E. (1999). The human ehrlichioses in the United States. *Emerging Infectious Diseases, 5*, 635–642.

Mylonakis, E. (2001). When to suspect and how to monitor babesiosis. *American Family Physician, 63*, 1969–1976.

Ogden, N. H., Maarouf, A., Barker, I. K., Bigras-Poulin, M., Lindsay, L. R., Morshed, M. G., et al. (2006). Climate change and the potential for range expansion of the Lyme disease vector *Ixodes scapularis* in Canada. *Journal of Medical Entomology, 43*, 403–414.

Parola, P., Davoust, B., & Raoult, D. (2005). Tick-and flea-borne rickettsial emerging zoonoses. *Veterinary Research, 36*, 469–492.

Parola, P., & Raoult, D. (2001). Ticks and tickborne bacterial diseases in humans: An emerging infectious threat. *Clinical Infectious Diseases, 32*, 897–928.

Phillips, S. E., Burrascano, J. J., Horowitz, R., Savely, V. R., & Stricker, R. B. (2006). Lyme disease testing. *Lancet Infectious Disease, 6*, 122.

Radolf, J. (2005). Posttreatment chronic Lyme disease—What it is not. *Journal of Infectious Diseases, 192*, 948–949.

Schutze, G. E. (2006). Ehrlichiosis. *Pediatric Infectious Disease Journal, 25*, 71–72.

Scrimenti, R. J. (1970). Erythema chronicum migrans. *Archives of Dermatology*, *102*, 104–105.

Skrabolo, Z., & Deanovic, Z. (1957). Piroplasmosis in man. *Documenta de Medicina Geographica et Tropica*, *9*, 11–16.

Steere, A. C. (2005). *Borrelia burgdorferi* (Lyme disease, Lyme borreliosis). In G. L. Mandell, J. E. Bennett, & R. Dolin (Eds.), *Mandell, Douglas, and Bennett's principles and practice of infectious diseases* (6th ed., pp. 2798–2809). New York: Elsevier Churchill Livingstone.

Steere, A. C., Malawista, S. E., Snydman, D. R., & Andiman, W. A. (1976). A cluster of arthritis in children and adults in Lyme, Connecticut. *Arthritis and Rheumatism*, *19*, 824.

Steere, A. C., Malawista, S. E., Snydman, D. R., Shope, R. E., Andiman, W. A., Ross, M. R., et al. (1977). Lyme arthritis: An epidemic of oligoarticular arthritis in children and adults in three Connecticut communities. *Arthritis and Rheumatism*, *20*, 7–16.

Stricker, R. B., Lautin, A., & Burrascano, J. J. (2006). Lyme disease: The quest for magic bullets. *Chemotherapy*, *52*, 53–59.

Strickland, G. T. (Ed.). (2000). *Hunter's tropical medicine and emerging infectious diseases*. Philadelphia: W. B. Saunders.

Uilenberg, G. (2006). *Babesia*—a historical overview. *Veterinary Parasitology*, *138*, 3–10.

Vial, H. J., & Gorenflot, A. (2006). Chemotherapy against babesiosis. *Veterinary Parasitology*, *138*, 147–160.

Walsh, C. A., Mayer, E. W., & Baxi, L. V. (2007). Lyme disease in pregnancy: Case report and review of the literature. *Obstetric and Gynecologic Survey*, *62*, 41–50.

Wilske, B. (2005). Epidemiology and diagnosis of Lyme borreliosis. *Annals of Medicine*, *37*, 568–579.

Wormser, G. P. (2006). Early Lyme disease. *New England Journal of Medicine*, *354*, 2794–2801.

Wormser, G. P., Dattwyler, R. J., Shapiro, E. D., Halperin, J. J., Steere, A. C., Klepner, M. S., et al. (2006). The clinical assessment, treatment, and prevention of Lyme disease, human granulocytic anaplasmosis, and babesiosis: Clinical practice guidelines by the Infectious Diseases Society of America. *Clinical Infectious Diseases*, *43*, 1089–1134.

CHAPTER SEVENTEEN

Malaria

Barbara A. Goldrick

The first case of malaria secondary to inpatient nursing practices in the United States was reported by Jain et al. (2005). Patient 1 was a 14-year-old female from Maryland with a history of cerebral palsy who was admitted to a Maryland tertiary hospital for placement of a feeding tube. Patient 2 was a 9-year-old boy who was being treated for *Plasmodium falciparum* malaria, presumably acquired on a recent trip to Gambia. Patients 1 and 2 shared a semiprivate room in a pediatric unit for approximately 24 hours before Patient 1 was discharged. A week after discharge and 17 days after sharing the semiprivate room with Patient 2, Patient 1 was admitted to another hospital for a fever work up. She was discharged after 3 days with a diagnosis of a viral illness. However, persistent fever and pancytopenia developed and resulted in her readmission to the first tertiary care hospital 23 days after sharing the room with Patient 2. Patient 1's leukocyte count was 1,890 cells/mm^3, hematocrit was 35.2%, platelets were 47,000/mm^3, and total bilirubin was 1.5 mg/dL. Six days after admission, Patient 1 had a peripheral blood smear that was positive for *P. falciparum* with a 12% parasitemia. She had no history of recent travel or transfusion. She was treated successfully with three blood transfusions and intravenous quinidine and doxycycline; she was discharged 14 days after her second admission. An epidemiologic investigation indicated that reuse of saline flush syringes by nurses in the Maryland tertiary care hospital pediatric unit was the most likely source of nosocomial transmission of *P. falciparum*, which was confirmed by molecular genotyping (Jain et al., 2005). This case illustrates the need for stringent infection control practices when providing health care.

Of all infectious diseases, rarely have those other than malaria had such a devastating effect upon the social and economic development of countries over time. Malaria is among the top 10 fatal diseases in the world and therefore is a major public health problem, posing the greatest risk to children and pregnant women. It also places travelers to endemic areas at risk and increases imported cases to nonendemic areas (World Health Organization [WHO], 2005a). Worldwide annual estimates of malaria cases vary between 350 and 500 million, with 1.5 to 2.7 million deaths, 90% of which occur in poor nations such as those in Africa's tropical Sahara, where 75% of the malaria deaths occur among children. In addition to Africa, two thirds of the remaining malaria cases occur in only three countries: Brazil, India, and Sri Lanka (WHO, 2005a).

The causative agent of malaria is a one-cell protozoan, *Plasmodium*, which invades body cells, becoming an intracellular parasite. The four species that affect humans, *P. falciparum, P. vivax, P. malariae,* and *P. ovale,* vary in their virulence depending upon the age of the host and other factors. Of the four species of *Plasmodium* that cause human infection, *P. falciparum* is associated with the highest degree of morbidity and mortality and requires rapid diagnosis and treatment with appropriate antimalarial compounds and supportive care. In addition, *P. falciparum* poses the biggest challenge in terms of development of resistance to chloroquine and other antimalarial drugs (Centers for Disease Control and Prevention [CDC], 2005d; Franco-Paredes & Santos-Preciado, 2006).

Transmission occurs through the bite of an infected female *Anopheles* mosquito, in which the parasite can complete the "invertebrate host" half of its life cycle. Once inside a human host, the parasite undergoes division and maturation, primarily within liver and red blood cells, where it can evade the immune system. Mosquitoes, in turn, also can become infected by biting an infected human or animal (CDC, 2005b). Although rare, transmission of malaria can also occur through blood transfusions, organ transplantation, sharing needles, or maternal transmission to a fetus ("congenital malaria"; CDC, 2005d). The incubation period in most cases varies from 7 to 30 days. The shorter periods are observed most frequently with *P. falciparum* and the longer ones with *P. malariae* (CDC, 2005d).

Signs and symptoms of malaria are often nonspecific and can vary with different species of the parasite; however, fever is usually present. Other symptoms may include headache, chills, increased sweating, back pain, myalgia, diarrhea, nausea, vomiting, and cough. *P. falciparum* infection is characterized by a high level of parasitemia, renal failure, severe hemolysis and anemia, pulmonary edema, and a variety of serious neurologic abnormalities. These complications lead to a high incidence of mortality among those infected with the parasite (CDC, 2005c). In countries where cases of malaria are infrequent, these symptoms may be misdiagnosed as influenza. Conversely, in countries where malaria is endemic, patients often will treat themselves without seeking diagnostic confirmation of malaria (CDC, 2005c).

Diagnosis of malaria includes detection of the parasite in a stained peripheral blood smear by basic light microscopy, which can differentiate between species and determine the parasitic load. This method is still used, especially in resource-poor settings (Moody, 2002). Molecular techniques have been developed and are used where possible (Collins & Jeffrey, 2005).

As noted above, severe malaria can result in neurologic abnormalities, acute respiratory distress syndrome, acute kidney failure, cardiovascular collapse, and shock (CDC, 2005c). Without treatment, infection with the *Plasmodium* parasite can rapidly become life threatening, especially in children. Prompt diagnosis requires that malaria be included in the differential diagnosis of illness in a febrile person, especially those with a history of travel to an endemic malaria area. Therefore, a travel history among febrile patients who are international visitors, immigrants, refugees, migrant laborers, and international travelers is important.

Malaria is endemic in 105 countries, including Mexico, Central and South America, the Dominican Republic, Haiti, Africa, Asia (including the Indian subcontinent, Southeast Asia, and the Middle East), Eastern Europe, and the South Pacific (CDC, 2005e). However, emergence and reemergence of malaria is occurring in other regions of the world, especially in newly independent countries. Environmental change and increases in the numbers of displaced persons and refugees have contributed to the spread of malaria. International travelers, military personnel, and migrant workers from endemic areas import malaria to nonendemic areas, resulting in local spread.

In 2004, 1,324 malaria cases among persons in the United States and its territories were reported to the CDC. These represented an increase of 3.6% from the 1,278 cases reported in 2003. Of the 2004 cases of malaria, 775 were among U.S. civilians, 32 cases were among military personnel, and 282 cases among foreign civilians. The additional 235 cases had no civilian status recorded. All but four reported cases were imported. The majority of imported cases (68%) were acquired in Africa; an additional 15% each were acquired in Asia and the Americas, respectively. Within the Americas, the majority of imported malaria cases (70%) were acquired in Central America and the Carribbean, followed by South America (20%) and Mexico (18%). The CDC reports that in recent years cases among U.S. civilians have increased, while cases among foreign-born civilians have decreased. These trends are likely due to increased travel among U.S.

citizens to endemic malaria regions and decreased immigration from these areas since 2001 (CDC, 2006).

The 32 cases of imported malaria among U.S. military personnel in 2004 were reported by state health departments; therefore, these data may not include all reported malaria cases identified during malaria surveillance activities conducted by the Department of Defense. Twenty-six (81%) of military personnel provided information about malaria chemoprophylaxis: six (23.1%) were not using any chemoprophylaxis, and two (7.7%) had adhered to an incorrect regimen. In addition, less than a quarter (21%) of civilians who acquired malaria abroad reported that they had followed a chemoprophylaxis regimen recommended by the CDC for the area to which they had traveled (CDC, 2006). One case of induced malaria, caused by blood transfusion, was reported in 2003 in a 69-year-old male from Texas who had upper gastrointestinal bleeding and was transfused with two units of packed red blood cells. An epidemiologic investigation, which included donor traceback of the patient's transfusions, determined that one donor was an 18-year-old Ghanaian man who had immigrated to Houston in 2002. Although blood smear examination and polymerase chain reaction performed on the specimen from the Ghanaian donor were negative for the presence of malaria parasites or parasite DNA, his mother reported that he had been treated for malaria in Ghana 2 years earlier. Serology using indirect immunofluorescence antibody testing indicated elevated titers of antibodies to several *Plasmodium* species, signifying previous malaria infection (CDC, 2005f).

Outbreaks involving locally acquired mosquito-transmitted malaria have been reported in the United States, with the most recent outbreak occurring in Palm Beach County, Florida, when an outbreak of eight cases of *P. vivax* malaria occurred between July and September 2003. Although endemic malaria has been eradicated from Florida since the early 1950s, because of its climate, proximity of human and mosquito populations, and the frequent travel of its residents and visitors from endemic malaria areas, Florida is vulnerable to sporadic, small outbreaks of locally acquired mosquito-borne transmission of malaria. This latest outbreak demonstrated the potential for reemergence of malaria in the United States despite intensive surveillance and vector-control strategies (CDC, 2003).

Treatment of malaria should not be initiated until the diagnosis is confirmed by laboratory studies. However, when there is strong clinical suspicion of malaria in the presence of severe disease and obtaining prompt laboratory confirmation is impractical, presumptive treatment should be started immediately. Treatment should be guided by three main factors: the infecting *Plasmodium* species, the clinical status of the patient, and the drug susceptibility of the infecting parasites as determined by the geographic area where the infection was acquired (CDC, 2005h).

The drug of choice for treatment of malaria is chloroquine phosphate; however, malaria is chloroquine resistant in most endemic countries (CDC, 2005h). Quinine sulfate is used in combination with other drugs for treatment of chloroquine-resistant malaria. In severe cases, parenteral quinidine gluconate may be indicated. Therefore, the location of the patient's exposure to malaria is important in treatment decisions. For treatment options in the United States, see CDC's *Malaria Treatment Guidelines* at http://www.cdc.gov/malaria/pdf/treatmenttable.pdf.

In 2005, the CDC reported a case of late relapse *P. ovale* malaria in a 23-year-old Nigerian man living in Philadelphia, Pennsylvania. The patient had been treated several times for malaria in Nigeria, with his most recent treatment 6 years before onset of his illness in the United States. The patient was seen in an emergency room after 10 days of nocturnal fevers, chills, and night sweats, occurring every 48–72 hours. He had a history of identical symptoms that had been treated empirically for malaria while he lived in Nigeria, but he reported no prior unexplained episodes of fever during the 4 years since immigrating to the United States. The patient reported that he had no recent travel to any area where malaria is endemic and had not traveled outside of the Philadelphia area since immigrating. The patient was discharged with a 7-day treatment regimen of quinine and doxycycline. His symptoms resolved within 48 hours. A subsequent screen for glucose-6-phosphate dehydrogenase deficiency was negative (a requirement for primaquine), and a 14-day course of primaquine (30 mg daily) was administered. At a 4-month follow-up, the patient reported no further symptoms. This report illustrates the importance of taking a detailed travel and immigration history when evaluating unexplained fever and considering malaria in the differential diagnosis (CDC, 2005a).

Malaria infection in pregnant women is associated with high risks of morbidity and mortality for both the mother and fetus. Malaria infection during pregnancy can lead to miscarriage, premature delivery, low birth weight, congenital infection, and/or perinatal death. Pregnant women are three times more likely to develop severe malaria disease than nonpregnant women acquiring infections from the same area due to a reduced immune response. In addition, malaria parasites sequester and replicate in the placenta (CDC, 2005i). Pregnant women are particularly susceptible to *P. falciparum* malaria (Duffy & Fried, 2005).

Prompt treatment with chloroquine (as with nonpregnant adult patients) is recommended for uncomplicated malaria in pregnant women that is caused by *P. malariae*, *P. vivax*, *P. ovale*, or chloroquine-sensitive *P. falciparum* infection. However, for pregnant women diagnosed with uncomplicated malaria caused by chloroquine-resistant *P. falciparum* infection, prompt treatment with quinine sulfate and clindamycin is recommended (CDC, 2005i). Several antimalarial combination therapies containing artemisinin and its derivatives, artemether and artesunate, have been developed and have been used in a total of 53 countries since 2001. These countries have adopted one of the WHO-recommended artemisinin-based combination therapies, with several countries providing them as a first-line course of treatment and a few countries using them as a second-line course of treatment (WHO, 2005a). Barnes et al. (2005) reported that an artemisinin-based combination treatment policy in South Africa, along with vector control measures, reduced malaria-related outpatient cases and admissions by 99% and malaria-related deaths by 97% in that region. Artemisinin, an extract of sweet wormwood commonly used in Chinese herbal medicine, is recommended only for treatment and not for prophylaxis; however, it is not licensed for use in the United States. Additional information on the treatment of malaria in pregnant women in the United States can be found in the CDC *Malaria Treatment Guidelines*.

The inappropriate use of antimalarial drugs during the past century has contributed to the current situation of antimalarial drug resistance. Antimalarial drugs were distributed on a large scale in endemic areas as monotherapies and were generally poorly managed. When used alone, antimalarial drugs rapidly lose their effectiveness as the malaria parasites develop resistance. However, combining drugs with different targets in the malaria parasite cycle delays resistance (WHO, 2005a).

In June 2005, the Bill and Melinda Gates Foundation, which had already donated $150 million toward the development of a malaria vaccine, provided additional grants totaling $437 million, approximately 20% of which was earmarked specifically for global malaria research. Also in June 2005, President Bush pledged more than $1.2 billion over 5 years to be launched in 2006 to fight malaria in Africa by providing funds for treated mosquito netting, indoor spraying, and the distribution of new, effective drug regimens, such as artemisinin-based combination treatments in target countries. This initiative, aimed to inspire other G8 countries and private foundations to contribute to the campaign, could cut malaria deaths in half within 5 years in Africa (Magill & Panosian, 2005).

Magill and Panosian (2005) point out that while tens of millions of dollars are intended to bring much-needed artemisinin-based combination treatments to people in malaria-plagued Africa, the U.S. government still has no plans to ensure that potentially lifesaving, Food and Drug Administration (FDA)-approved treatments, such as intravenous artesunate, intravenous quinine, or oral artemisinins, are available in the United States.

Travelers or U.S. military personnel recently returning from Africa who are diagnosed with *P. falciparum*, with signs and symptoms that warrant immediate parenteral treatment, will have neither intravenous quinine nor oral, rectal, or intravenous artemisinins, which have been approved by the FDA, available to them in the United States. In many U.S. hospitals, intravenous quinidine gluconate, the single parenteral antimalarial agent that is available in this country, is not available since most cardiologists in North America have stopped using intravenous quinidine as an antiarrhythmic agent. However, Eli Lilly, the manufacturer of quinidine gluconate, continues to maintain supplies despite the lack of a commercial market for the drug and will ship the drug quickly to a U.S. health care facility if a patient needs intravenous antimalarial treatment.

Antimalarial drugs do not prevent initial infection from a mosquito bite, but they do prevent the development of the malaria parasite cycle in the blood, thereby preventing disease. Correct doses of antimalarial drugs for prophylaxis must be taken on schedule, and doses should not be missed. Conversely, overdosage can be fatal. It is important to note that chemoprophylaxis with common schizonticides (those that affect blood-stage parasites) does not prevent infection with *P. vivax* and *P. ovale* and can mask symptoms of initial infection (Schwartz, Parise, Kozarsky, & Cetron, 2003). Therefore, the addition of 2 weeks of premaquine phosphate therapy is recommended for deployed military personnel and travelers to endemic malaria areas (Malaria Foundation International, 2005). Common chemoprophylaxis antimalarial drugs and dosages for travelers can be found at the CDC Web site at http://www.cdc.gov/travel/malariadrugs2.htm (CDC, 2005g). Although several malaria vaccines are currently in development, none are available at this time, and it will likely be at least a decade before any are available (Greenwood, Bojang, Whitty, & Targett, 2005). Additional information about the WHO malaria prevention and control initiatives can be found at the following Web sites: Malaria Foundation International Global Malaria Initiatives at http:/www.malaria.org and Roll Back Malaria at http://rbm.who.int (WHO, 2005b).

All health care providers should include malaria in the differential diagnosis in febrile patients with a history of travel to endemic malaria areas. They should also consider malaria as a possible diagnosis among patients who are experiencing fevers with alternating sweats and chills who have no obvious cause or travel history. As noted above, prompt diagnosis of malaria is essential in a febrile person, especially those with a history of travel to a *P. falciparum* endemic area. Therefore, obtaining a travel history from febrile patients who are international visitors, immigrants, refugees, migrant laborers, and international travelers is an important early intervention.

REFERENCES

Barnes, K. I., Durrheim, D. N., Little, F., Jackson, A. Mehta, U., Allen, E., et al. (2005). Effect of artemether-lumefantrine policy and improved vector control on malaria burden in KwaZulu—Natal, South Africa [Electronic version]. *PLOS Medicine, 2*(11), e330. Retrieved December 15, 2006, from http://medicine.plosjournals.org/archive/1549-1676/2/11/pdf/10.1371_journal.pmed.0020330-S.pdf

Centers for Disease Control and Prevention. (2003). Local transmission of *Plasmodium vivax* malaria—Palm Beach County, Florida, 2003. *Morbidity and Mortality Weekly Report, 52,* 908–911.

Centers for Disease Control and Prevention. (2005a). Late relapse of *Plasmodium ovale* malaria—Philadelphia, Pennsylvania, November 2004. *Morbidity and Mortality Weekly Report, 54,* 1231–1233.

Centers for Disease Control and Prevention. (2005b). *Malaria biology.* Retrieved December 15, 2006, from http://www.cdc.gov/malaria/biology/life_cycle.htm

Centers for Disease Control and Prevention. (2005c). *Malaria disease.* Retrieved December 15, 2006, from http://www.cdc.gov/malaria/disease.htm

Centers for Disease Control and Prevention. (2005d). *Malaria epidemiology.* Retrieved December 15, 2006, from http://www.cdc.gov/malaria/distribution_epi/epidemiology.htm

Centers for Disease Control and Prevention. (2005e). *Malaria geographic distribution.* Retrieved December 15, 2006, from http://www.cdc.gov/malaria/distribution_epi/distribution.htm

Centers for Disease Control and Prevention. (2005f). Malaria surveillance—United States, 2003. *Morbidity and Mortality Weekly Report, 54*(SS-02), 25–39.

Centers for Disease Control and Prevention. (2005g). *Malaria travel drugs.* Retrieved December 15, 2006, from http://www.cdc.gov/travel/malariadrugs2.htm

Centers for Disease Control and Prevention. (2005h). *Malaria treatment, Part 2.* Retrieved December 15, 2006, from http://www.cdc.gov/malaria/diagnosis_treatment/clinicians2.htm

Centers for Disease Control and Prevention. (2005i). *Malaria treatment, Part 3.* Retrieved December 15, 2006, from http://www.cdc.gov/malaria/diagnosis_treatment/clinicians3.htm

Centers for Disease Control and Prevention (2006). Malaria Surveillance—United States, 2004. *Morbidity and Mortality Weekly Report, 55*(SS04); 23–37.

Collins W. E., & Jeffrey, G. M. (2005). *Plasmodium ovale*: Parasite and disease. *Clinical Microbiology Reviews, 18,* 570–581.

Duffy, P. E., & Fried, M. (2005). Malaria in the pregnant woman. *Current Topics in Microbiology and Immunology, 295,* 169–200.

Franco-Paredes, C., & Santos-Preciado, J. I. (2006). Problem pathogens: Prevention of malaria in travellers. *Lancet Infectious Diseases, 6,* 139–149.

Greenwood, B., Bojang, K., Whitty, C., & Targett, G. (2005). Malaria. *Lancet, 365,* 1487–1498.

Jain, S. K., Persaud, D., Perl, T. M., Pass, M. A., Murphy, K. M., Pisciotta, M., et al. (2005). Nosocomial malaria and saline flush. *Emerging Infectious Diseases, 11,* 1097–1099.

Magill, A., & Panosian, C. (2005). Making antimalarial agents available in the United States. *New England Journal of Medicine, 353,* 335–337.

Malaria Foundation International. (2005). *Global malaria initiatives.* Retrieved December 15, 2006, from http:/www.malaria.org

Moody, A. (2002). Rapid diagnostic tests for malaria parasites. *Clinical Microbiology Reviews, 15,* 66–78.

Schwartz, E., Parise, M., Kozarsky, P., & Cetron, M. (2003). Delayed onset of malaria—Implications for chemoprophylaxis in travelers. *New England Journal of Medicine, 349,* 1510–1516.

World Health Organization. (2005a). *Malaria.* Retrieved December 15, 2006, from http://w3.whosea.org/EN/Section10/Section21/Section334.htm

World Health Organization. (2005b). *Roll back malaria. ACT: The way forward for treating malaria.* Retrieved, December 15, 2006, from http://www.rbm. who.int/cmc_upload/0/000/015/364/RBMInfosheet_9.htm

CHAPTER EIGHTEEN

Metapneumovirus

Bernadette G. van den Hoogen, Albert D. M. E.
Osterhaus, and Ron A. M. Fouchier

In 2001, a previously unknown virus was isolated in the Netherlands from 28 hospitalized children who suffered from severe respiratory tract infections (RTIs) that were epidemiologically unrelated. Twenty-seven of the patients were below the age of 5 years, and 13 of these were infants between 1 and 12 months old. The clinical symptoms of these children were largely similar to the RTI caused by respiratory syncytial virus (RSV), ranging from severe cough to bronchiolitis and pneumonia, often accompanied by high fever, myalgia, and vomiting. Some of these patients were hospitalized and needed mechanical ventilation (van den Hoogen et al., 2001).

Acute RTIs are a major cause of morbidity and mortality in adults and children worldwide, and costs attributable to acute RTI in both general practices and hospitals are an important burden on national health care budgets (Monto, 2002). In past decades, a plethora of etiological agents of RTI have been identified, but a significant proportion still cannot be attributed to known pathogens. Electron microscopy and genetic analyses upon RNA arbitrarily primed polymerase chain reaction (PCR) revealed that this newly isolated virus belonged to the *Pneumovirinae* subfamily of the *Paramyxoviridae* family (van den Hoogen et al., 2001; van den Hoogen, Bestebroer, Osterhaus, & Fouchier, 2002). The subfamily *Pneumovirinae* contains two genera, with RSV and avian pneumovirus (APV) as the type species of the *Pneumovirus* and the *Metapneumovirus* genus, respectively. Based on genome organization and sequence similarities to APV, the newly discovered virus was named human metapneumovirus (hMPV).

Avian pneumovirus (APV), previously known as turkey rhinotracheitis virus, was first described in 1976 as the causative agent of respiratory tract disease in turkeys (Cook, 2000). Seroprevalence studies have demonstrated that hMPV has circulated for at least 50 years in the human population (van den Hoogen et al., 2001). It is thus likely that hMPV emerged in humans a long time ago after a zoonosis caused by APV and has since been endemic in humans. This scenario may be similar to that for influenza A viruses in humans, which also emerged from an avian source, but for influenza A viruses such zoonoses occur more frequently.

EPIDEMIOLOGY

Worldwide surveys for the incidence rates of hMPV have demonstrated that the virus circulates on every continent, primarily among the pediatric population. In the pediatric population, hMPV accounts for approximately 5–25% of the reported RTIs, depending on factors such as season, collection and detection methods used, inclusion criteria for the cohorts, and whether other respiratory viruses were included in the surveys. Researchers at Vanderbilt University Medical Center have evaluated the role of hMPV in RTIs among otherwise healthy hospitalized children under the age of 5 years prospectively over more than 20 years. In this cohort, 12% of lower RTIs were attributable to hMPV infection. In addition, hMPV was detected in 5% of the children suffering from upper RTIs (Williams et al., 2004). The combined results of all studies conducted among children indicate that the peak age for hMPV infection in otherwise healthy children, leading to severe disease requiring hospitalization, is 4 to 6 months. In contrast, the peak age for RSV infection-induced severe disease is between 0 and 2 months (van den Hoogen et al., 2003; Williams et al., 2004; Williams et al., 2006).

In surveys among hospitalized patients of all ages, hMPV has been detected frequently in patients older than 5 years of age. Many of these patients were immunocompromised individuals or patients with underlying disease such as chronic obstructive pulmonary disease, asthma, and cancer (van den Hoogen, Osterhaus, & Fouchier, 2004). Although hospitalized adults suffering from severe RTI due to hMPV infection often have underlying disease or impaired immunity, healthy adults are also at risk for severe disease resulting in hospitalization. Kaye, Skidmore, Osman, Weinbren, & Warren (2006) reported the presence of hMPV in 5.4% of adults hospitalized for severe RTI. In the general community, both young adults and the elderly suffer from hMPV infection that leads to medically attended illnesses, with incidence rates ranging from 1% to 9%. However, frail elderly people with hMPV infections appear to seek medical attention more frequently (Falsey, Criddle, & Walsh, 2006; Kaye et al., 2006).

Most studies have demonstrated that hMPV infections occur mainly during the winter season in temperate regions and in late spring and summer seasons in the subtropics, similar to RSV and influenza virus infections (Chano, Rousseau, Laferriere, Couillard, & Charest, 2005; Robinson, Lee, Bastien, & Li, 2005). In most epidemiological studies, RSV is the most common cause of bronchiolitis in the first half of the winter RSV epidemics, while in the second half hMPV and RSV may occur with similar frequencies. When hMPV epidemics start after the RSV season, hMPV is often the primary cause of bronchiolitis among pediatric patients (Williams et al., 2004). Human metapneumovirus has been detected around the year, including in the summer months, in contrast to RSV and influenza virus, which cause more restricted epidemics (van den Hoogen, Osterhaus, et al., 2004; Williams et al., 2004; Williams et al., 2006). Although hMPV causes yearly epidemics of RTI, the incidence rates vary from year to year or between locations. For example, in a 25-year surveillance, incidence rates varied from 0% to 31%. Human metapneumovirus is the second most detected pathogen after RSV in pediatric wards and has been detected as frequently as RSV in immunocompromised individuals; thus, it is no surprise that nosocomial hMPV infections have been reported. In a study by Williams, Martino, et al. (2006), nosocomial transmissions were reported for 45% of the infections. These findings should influence the protocols for prevention of nosocomial infections followed in many health care facilities for children with RTI, such as patient isolation and cohorting criteria. The timely diagnosis of hMPV is important to prevent nosocomial infections.

GENETIC AND ANTIGENIC VARIATION

When hMPV was first described as the causative agent of RTI in children, at least two genetic lineages were identified (van den Hoogen et al., 2001). These lineages have now been reported to circulate around the globe. Later, genetic analyses of the F and G membrane proteins of numerous hMPV isolates identified two main genetic lineages (A and B), each consisting of two sublineages (A1, A2, B1, B2). Whereas the F protein revealed approximately 95% amino acid sequence identity between viruses from the two lineages, the G protein shared only 30% identity (van den Hoogen, Herfst, et al., 2004). Virus neutralization assays using virus lineage-specific ferret antisera demonstrated a 12-fold to a greater than 100-fold difference in virus neutralization titers between viruses from the two main lineages. Classical virology studies have used a definition of a homologous-to-heterologous virus neutralization titer of more than 16 as a definition of serotypes. On the basis of this definition, the large antigenic differences, and the high sequence divergence between the two main lineages, two serotypes of hMPV were defined (van den Hoogen, Herfst, et al., 2004). It should be noted that in studies with sera collected from experimentally infected hamsters and nonhuman primates, large differences in virus neutralizing antibody titers were not observed, but antibody titers against the homologous virus were somewhat higher than against the heterologous viruses (Skiadopoulos et al., 2004). In these animal models, reinfection with both homologous and heterologous viruses did not occur when challenged within 6 weeks after primary infection. This contrasts to the findings in a study in cynomolgus macaques that were challenged 3–8 months after infection and which were not protected from either homologous or heterologous infection in their upper respiratory tract (van den Hoogen et al., in press).

It is important to note that, in humans, heterologous reinfections within 1 month after primary infection have been reported in an otherwise healthy infant (Ebihara, Endo, Ishiguro, et al., 2004) and that seroprevalence studies and virus incidence studies have indicated that reinfections in humans occur frequently (Ebihara, Endo, Kikuta, et al., 2004; Leung, Esper, Weibel, & Kahn, 2005; van den Hoogen et al., 2001). Reinfections during childhood are no surprise since it is well established that children mount a poor antibody response upon primary respiratory virus infection (Crowe & Williams, 2003). Since hMPV infections have been described in the adult population despite probable infections earlier in life, it is likely that infections can occur throughout life due to incomplete protective immune responses or acquisition of new genotypes. At this moment it is uncertain whether, and if so at what age, young infants develop neutralizing antibodies against the F, G, or other viral proteins and what the longevity is of those antibody responses.

CLINICAL FEATURES

A wide spectrum of clinical symptoms associated with hMPV infection has been reported in patients of all ages, ranging from mild to severe RTI requiring hospitalization (van den Hoogen et al., 2001; Williams et al., 2004; Williams et al., 2006). Clinical symptoms of hMPV-infected children include fever, nonproductive cough, rhinorrhea, wheezing, and dyspnea. Resulting diagnoses may range from rhinopharyngitis to bronchiolitis and/or pneumonia and asthma-associated illnesses. In addition, diarrhea, vomiting, rash, febrile seizures, feeding difficulties, conjunctivitis, and, in a high percentage of the patients, otitis media have been reported (Williams et al., 2006). The wide spectrum of hMPV-induced illnesses reported thus far are similar to those caused by RSV and influenza virus infections. Although hMPV-related disease ranges from mild to severe in young infants, virus infections in immunocompromised individuals or patients with underlying disease such as asthma can be extremely severe; deaths related to hMPV infection in those patients have been reported (Noyola et al., 2005; van den Hoogen, Osterhaus, et al., 2004). hMPV has also been detected as the sole pathogen in postmortem samples from the brain and lung of patients with fatal encephalitis (Schildgen et al., 2005). This result, in addition to the development of febrile seizures and convulsions reported in hMPV-infected children, suggests that a clinical study of central nervous system complications is warranted (Kashiwa, Shimozono, & Takao, 2004; Suzuki et al., 2005).

Human metapneumovirus infections among healthy adults and the elderly have not been studied in detail. The virus has been associated with flu-like illnesses and colds in healthy adults (Sasaki et al., 2005; van den Hoogen, Osterhaus, et al., 2004). Falsey et al. (2006) observed a higher rate of flu-like illnesses among young adults, although older adults experienced more dyspnea and wheezing, and those with cardiopulmonary conditions were ill for nearly twice as long as younger adults.

The role of viral RTIs in acute and chronic asthma has been a subject of much debate and research. Several studies have indicated an association between hMPV infection and asthma. Williams, Tollefson, et al. (2005) demonstrated a significant association between hMPV infection and wheezing among children younger than 3 years, especially during the midwinter months. In children 3 years of age and older, no significant association was detected and rhinovirus was detected most often (Williams, Tollefson, et al., 2005). These researchers also showed that hMPV is associated with acute asthma exacerbation in adults (Williams, Crowe, et al., 2005). Other studies have found asthma to be more frequently associated with rhinoviruses than with hMPV (Jartti et al., 2004; Rawlinson et al., 2003). Studies aiming at the identification of an association between hMPV and asthma are problematic because asthma is a difficult clinical diagnosis in children younger than 2 years of age, the population most at risk for hMPV infection. Although hMPV is frequently detected in patients with asthma exacerbations, and one of the profound clinical signs of hMPV infection is wheezing, it is not yet clear whether or not the virus is associated with the induction of or predisposition for asthma.

DIAGNOSIS

Although hMPV has circulated in humans for more than 50 years and probably much longer, the virus escaped attention because it replicates poorly in the cell cultures that are routinely used for respiratory virus diagnosis. Moreover, the virus is dependent on trypsin in cell-cultures and is highly sensitive to freeze thawing. Human metapneumovirus was initially isolated and propagated in tertiary monkey kidney cells, but several laboratories have shown LLC-MK2 and Vero cell lines to be permissive as well (Deffrasnes, Cote, & Boivin, 2005; MacPhail et al., 2004). However, hMPV replicates slowly, and even upon blind passage in these cell lines cytopathic effects are difficult to observe, and immunostaining may be necessary.

The antigenic and genetic variability of hMPV has implications for the development of serological tests and reverse transcriptase (RT)-PCR assays. Serological tests based on a single hMPV prototype may be less sensitive for the detection of virus isolates with different antigenic properties. Immunofluorescence staining of clinical specimens is a method commonly used in clinical virology laboratories for rapid diagnosis (Irmen & Kelleher, 2000). Such antigen detection assays have now been described for the detection of hMPV, based on monoclonal antibodies against the fusion and matrix protein of hMPV (Ebihara, Endo, Ma, Ishiguro, & Kikuta, 2005; Landry, Ferguson, Cohen, Peret, & Erdman, 2005; Percivalle, Sarasini, Visai, Revello, & Gerna, 2005). For RT-PCR assays, it has been shown to be important to design primers based on regions that are conserved between viruses of the different genetic lineages (Agapov et al., 2006; Maertzdorf et al., 2004).

PREVENTION AND TREATMENT

There is no specific treatment for metapneumovirus infection. Supportive care may include supplemental oxygen, and in vitro activity has been found for ribavirin but is not currently recommended for treatment (Principi, Bosis, & Esposito, 2005). The clinical impact of hMPV in the pediatric and elderly population warrants the development of vaccines. Recently, reverse genetics techniques have been designed to produce hMPV from plasmid DNA (Biacchesi, Skiadopoulos, Tran, et al., 2004; Herfst et al., 2004). These techniques are now used to develop live attenuated vaccines by deleting nonessential genes, and such viruses have been found to induce protective antibodies in animals (Biacchesi, Skiadopoulos, Yang, et al., 2004; Buchholz et al., 2005). Chimeric viruses consisting of a parainfluenza virus backbone in which the fusion protein of hMPV was inserted were also found to represent interesting vaccine candidates. Such viruses induced antibodies against both the vector and hMPV, resulting in protective immunity in animal models (Skiadopoulos et al., 2006; Tang et al., 2005).

REFERENCES

Agapov, E., Sumino, K. C., Gaudreault-Keener, M., Storch, G. A., & Holtzman, M. J. (2006). Genetic variability of human metapneumovirus infection: Evidence of a shift in viral genotype without a change in illness. *Journal of Infectious Diseases, 193,* 396–403.

Biacchesi, S., Skiadopoulos, M. H., Tran, K. C., Murphy, B. R., Collins, P. L., & Buchholz, U. J. (2004). Recovery of human metapneumovirus from cDNA: Optimization of growth in vitro and expression of additional genes. *Virology, 321,* 247–259.

Biacchesi, S., Skiadopoulos, M. H., Yang, L., Lamirande, E. W., Tran, K. C., Murphy, B. R., et al. (2004). Recombinant human metapneumovirus lacking the small hydrophobic SH and/or attachment G glycoprotein: Deletion of G yields a promising vaccine candidate. *Journal of Virology, 78,* 12877–12887.

Buchholz, U. J., Biacchesi, S., Pham, Q. N., Tran, K. C., Yang, L., Luongo, C. L., et al. (2005). Deletion of M2 gene open reading frames 1 and 2 of human metapneumovirus: Effects on RNA synthesis, attenuation, and immunogenicity. *Journal of Virology, 79,* 6588–6597.

Chano, F., Rousseau, C., Laferriere, C., Couillard, M., & Charest, H. (2005). Epidemiological survey of human metapneumovirus infection in a large pediatric tertiary care center. *Journal of Clinical Microbiology, 43,* 5520–5525.

Cook, J. K. (2000). Avian rhinotracheitis. *Scientific and Technical Review of the International Office International des Épizooties, 19,* 602–613.

Crowe, J. E. J., & Williams, J. V. (2003). Immunology of viral respiratory tract infection in infancy. *Paediatric Respiratory Reviews, 4,* 112–119.

Deffrasnes, C., Cote, S., & Boivin, G. (2005). Analysis of replication kinetics of the human metapneumovirus in different cell lines by real-time PCR. *Journal of Clinical Microbiology, 43,* 488–490.

Ebihara, T., Endo, R., Ishiguro, N., Nakayama, T., Sawada, H., & Kikuta, H. (2004). Early reinfection with human metapneumovirus in an infant. *Journal of Clinical Microbiology, 42,* 5944–5946.

Ebihara, T., Endo, R., Kikuta, H., Ishiguro, N., Ishiko, H., Hara, M., et al. (2004). Human metapneumovirus infection in Japanese children. *Journal of Clinical Microbiology, 42,* 126–132.

Ebihara, T., Endo, R., Ma, X., Ishiguro, N., & Kikuta, H. (2005). Detection of human metapneumovirus antigens in nasopharyngeal secretions by an immunofluorescent-antibody test. *Journal of Clinical Microbiology, 43,* 1138–1141.

Falsey, A. R., Criddle, M. C., & Walsh, E. E. (2006). Detection of respiratory syncytial virus and human metapneumovirus by reverse transcription polymerase chain reaction in adults with and without respiratory illness. *Journal of Clinical Virology, 35,* 46–50.

Gerna, G., Campanini, G., Rovida, F., Sarasini, A., Lilleri, D., Paolucci, S., et al. (2005). Changing circulation rate of human metapneumovirus strains and types among hospitalized pediatric patients during three consecutive winter-spring seasons. *Archives of Virology, 150,* 2365–2375.

Herfst, S., de Graaf, M., Schickli, J. H., Tang, R. S., Kaur, J., Yang, C. F., et al. (2004). Recovery of human metapneumovirus genetic lineages A and B from cloned cDNA. *Journal of Virology, 78,* 8264–8270.

Irmen, K. E., & Kelleher, J. J. (2000). Use of monoclonal antibodies for rapid diagnosis of respiratory viruses in a community hospital. *Clinical and Diagnostic Laboratory Immunology, 7,* 396–403.

Jartti, T., Lehtinen, P., Vuorinen, T., Osterback, R., van den Hoogen, B. G., Osterhaus, A. D., et al. (2004). Respiratory picornaviruses and respiratory syncytial virus as causative agents of acute expiratory wheezing in children. *Emerging Infectious Diseases, 10,* 1095–1101.

Kashiwa, H., Shimozono, H., & Takao, S. (2004). Clinical pictures of children with human metapneumovirus infection: Comparison with respiratory syncytial virus infection. *Japanese Journal of Infectious Diseases, 57,* 80–82.

Kaye, M., Skidmore, S., Osman, H., Weinbren, M., & Warren, R. (2006). Surveillance of respiratory virus infections in adult hospital admissions using rapid methods. *Epidemiology and Infection, 134,* 792–798.

Landry, M. L., Ferguson, D., Cohen, S., Peret, T. C., & Erdman, D. D. (2005). Detection of human metapneumovirus in clinical samples by immunofluorescence staining of shell vial centrifugation cultures prepared from three different cell lines. *Journal of Clinical Microbiology, 43,* 1950–1952.

Leung, J., Esper, F., Weibel, C., & Kahn, J. S. (2005). Seroepidemiology of human metapneumovirus (hMPV) on the basis of a novel enzyme-linked immunosorbent assay utilizing hMPV fusion protein expressed in recombinant vesicular stomatitis virus. *Journal of Clinical Microbiology, 43,* 1213–1219.

Ludewick, H. P., Abed, Y., van Niekerk, N., Boivin, G., Klugman, K. P., & Madhi, S. A. (2005). Human metapneumovirus genetic variability, South Africa. *Emerging Infectious Diseases, 11,* 1074–1078.

MacPhail, M., Schickli, J. H., Tang, R. S., Kaur, J., Robinson, C., Fouchier, R. A., et al. (2004). Identification of small-animal and primate models for evaluation of vaccine candidates for human metapneumovirus (hMPV) and implications for hMPV vaccine design. *Journal of General Virology, 85*(Pt. 6), 1655–1663.

Maertzdorf, J., Wang, C. K., Brown, J. B., Quinto, J. D., Chu, M., de Graaf, M., et al. (2004). Real-time reverse transcriptase PCR assay for detection of human metapneumoviruses from all known genetic lineages. *Journal of Clinical Microbiology, 42,* 981–986.

Monto, A. S. (2002). Epidemiology of viral respiratory infections. *American Journal of Medicine, 112*(Suppl. 6A), 4S–12S.

Noyola, D. E., Alpuche-Solis, A. G., Herrera-Diaz, A., Soria-Guerra, R. E., Sanchez-Alvarado, J., & Lopez-Revilla, R. (2005). Human metapneumovirus infections in Mexico: Epidemiological and clinical characteristics. *Journal of Medical Microbiology, 54*(Pt. 10), 969–974.

Percivalle, E., Sarasini, A., Visai, L., Revello, M. G., & Gerna, G. (2005). Rapid detection of human metapneumovirus strains in nasopharyngeal aspirates and shell vial cultures by monoclonal antibodies. *Journal of Clinical Microbiology, 43,* 3443–3446.

Principi, N., Bosis, S., & Esposito, S. (2005). Human metapneumovirus in paediatric patients. *Clinical Microbiology and Infection, 12,* 301–308.

Rawlinson, W. D., Waliuzzaman, Z., Carter, I. W., Belessis, Y. C., Gilbert, K. M., & Morton, J. R. (2003). Asthma exacerbations in children associated with rhinovirus but not human metapneumovirus infection. *Journal of Infectious Diseases, 187,* 1314–1318.

Robinson, J. L., Lee, B. E., Bastien, N., & Li, Y. (2005). Seasonality and clinical features of human metapneumovirus in children in North Alberta. *Journal of Medical Virology, 76,* 98–105.

Sasaki, A., Suzuki, H., Saito, R., Sato, M., Sato, I., Sano, Y., et al. (2005). Prevalence of human metapneumovirus and influenza virus infections among Japanese children during two successive winters. *Pediatric Infectious Disease Journal, 24,* 905–908.

Schildgen, O., Glatzel, T., Geikowski, T., Scheibner, B., Matz, B., Bindl, L., et al. (2005). Human metapneumovirus RNA in encephalitis patient. *Emerging Infectious Diseases, 11,* 467–470.

Skiadopoulos, M. H., Biacchesi, S., Buchholz, U. J., Amaro-Carambot, E., Surman, S. R., Collins, P. L., et al. (2006). Individual contributions of the human metapneumovirus F, G, and SH surface glycoproteins to the induction of neutralizing antibodies and protective immunity. *Virology, 345,* 492–501.

Skiadopoulos, M. H., Biacchesi, S., Buchholz, U. J., Riggs, J. M., Surman, S. R., Amaro-Carambot, E., et al. (2004). The two major human metapneumovirus genetic lineages are highly related antigenically, and the fusion (F) protein is a major contributor to this antigenic relatedness. *Journal of Virology, 78,* 6927–6937.

Suzuki, A., Watanabe, O., Okamoto, M., Endo, H., Yano, H., Suetake, M., et al. (2005). Detection of human metapneumovirus from children with acute otitis media. *Pediatric Infectious Disease Journal, 24,* 655–657.

Tang, R. S., Mahmood, K., MacPhail, M., Guzzetta, J. M., Haller, A. A., Liu, H., et al. (2005). A host-range restricted parainfluenza virus type 3 (PIV3) expressing the human metapneumovirus (hMPV) fusion protein elicits protective immunity in African green monkeys. *Vaccine, 23,* 1657–1667.

van den Hoogen, B. G., Bestebroer, T. M., Osterhaus, A. D., & Fouchier, R. A. (2002). Analysis of the genomic sequence of a human metapneumovirus. *Virology, 295,* 119–132.

van den Hoogen, B. G., de Jong, J. C., Groen, J., Kuiken, T., de Groot, R., Fouchier, R. A., et al. (2001). A newly discovered human pneumovirus isolated from young children with respiratory tract disease. *Nature Medicine, 7,* 719–724.

van den Hoogen, B. G., Herfst, S., Sprong, L., Cane, P. A., Forleo-Neto, E., de Swart, R. L., et al. (2004). Antigenic and genetic variability of human metapneumoviruses. *Emerging Infectious Diseases, 10,* 658–666.

van den Hoogen, B. G., Osterhaus, A. D., & Fouchier, R. A. (2004). Clinical impact and diagnosis of human metapneumovirus infection. *Pediatric Infectious Disease Journal, 23*(1 Suppl.), S25–S32.

van den Hoogen, B. G., van Doornum, G. J., Fockens, J. C., Cornelissen, J. J., Beyer, W. E., Groot, R. R., et al. (2003). Prevalence and clinical symptoms of human metapneumovirus infection in hospitalized patients. *Journal of Infectious Diseases, 188*, 1571–1577.

van den Hoogen, B. G., Herfst, S., de Graaf, M., Sprong, L., van Lavieren, R., van Amerongen, G., et al. (2007). Experimental infection of macaques with human metapneumovirus induces transient protective immunity. *Journal of General Virology.* (in press)

Williams, J. V., Crowe, J. E., Jr., Enriquez, R., Minton, P., Peebles, R. S., Jr., Hamilton, R. G., et al. (2005). Human metapneumovirus infection plays an etiologic role in acute asthma exacerbations requiring hospitalization in adults. *Journal of Infectious Diseases, 192*, 1149–1153.

Williams, J. V., Harris, P. A., Tollefson, S. J., Halburnt-Rush, L. L., Pingsterhaus, J. M., Edwards, K. M., et al. (2004). Human metapneumovirus and lower respiratory tract disease in otherwise healthy infants and children. *New England Journal of Medicine, 350*, 443–450.

Williams, J. V., Martino, R., Rabella, N., Otegui, M., Parody, R., Heck, J. M., et al. (2005). A prospective study comparing human metapneumovirus with other respiratory viruses in adults with hematologic malignancies and respiratory tract infections. *Journal of Infectious Diseases, 192*, 1061–1065.

Williams, J. V., Tollefson, S. J., Heymann, P. W., Carper, H. T., Patrie, J., & Crowe, J. E. (2005). Human metapneumovirus infection in children hospitalized for wheezing. *Journal of Allergy and Clinical Immunology, 115*, 1311–1312.

Williams, J. V., Wang, C. K., Yang, C. F., Tollefson, S. J., House, F. S., Heck, J. M., et al. (2006). The role of human metapneumovirus in upper respiratory tract infections in children: A 20-year experience. *Journal of Infectious Diseases, 193*, 387–395.

CHAPTER NINETEEN

Monkeypox and Other Emerging *Orthopoxvirus* Infections

Kurt D. Reed

On May 24, 2003, the Wisconsin Division of Public Health (WDPH) was notified of a 3-year-old girl hospitalized in central Wisconsin with fever and cellulitis of the finger after a bite from a prairie dog on May 13. The family had purchased two prairie dogs several days earlier at a swap meet where a wide variety of animals can be purchased or traded as pets. The prairie dog became ill on May 13 with skin lesions, ocular discharge, and lymphadenopathy; it died on May 20 and an enlarged lymph node was submitted for bacterial culture. On May 24, a gram-negative bacillus was isolated, raising the possibility of tularemia or plague. This concern was communicated to public health officials. However, the organism was subsequently identified as an *Acinetobacter spp.* and considered to be a contaminant. On June 2, the WDPH learned of a similar illness in a meat inspector who lived in southeastern Wisconsin. He also worked as a distributor of exotic animals, was bitten and scratched by a prairie dog on May 18, and experienced a febrile illness associated with a nodular skin lesion at the scratch site that began on May 23. He was hospitalized, and tularemia and plague were considered in the clinical differential diagnosis.

By June 3 investigators from the WDPH determined that this individual had sold the prairie dogs to the index patient's family at the swap meet, creating an epidemiologic link between two cases from different regions of Wisconsin. On June 2, the WDPH was notified that Marshfield Laboratories (Marshfield, Wisconsin) had ultrastructural evidence of a poxvirus

287

from a vesiculopustular skin lesion from the mother of the index case. The mother had also received bites and scratches from the ill prairie dog and experienced an influenza-like illness and vesiculopustular eruption at the sites of trauma. On June 4, particles consistent with orthopoxvirus were visualized by negative-stain electron microscopy (EM) of cell-culture supernatants from the mother and the prairie dog. On June 6, polymerase chain reaction (PCR) by the Centers for Disease Control and Prevention (CDC) Poxvirus Section revealed monkeypox-virus (MPV)-specific DNA signatures from biopsies from multiple patients from southeastern Wisconsin. Additionally, DNA sequencing confirmed identity with the hemagglutinin gene (HA) sequences derived from a western Africa clade of MPV. By June 9, 11 patients from central and southeastern Wisconsin were identified with confirmed or suspected MPV. All of the patients had direct contact with prairie dogs sold by the distributor (Reed et al., 2004).

Subsequent trace-back and trace-forward investigations by the WDPH, the CDC, and other state and federal agencies revealed that the distributor had purchased 39 prairie dogs from a supplier in northeastern Illinois. On May 3, the distributor had transported an ill Gambian giant rat that had recently been imported from Ghana along with 15 prairie dogs and 94 other animals. Ultimately, it was determined that several of the rodents imported from western Africa were ill with MPV and the outbreak had extended well beyond Wisconsin. In the final analysis, 72 cases (37 laboratory confirmed) were reported from Wisconsin, Illinois, Indiana, Missouri, and Kansas. The peak of the onset of illness occurred between May 29 and June 9, 2003, and no further cases were reported after June 22 (CDC, 2003). Significant effort was directed toward determining whether or not MPV had spread to wild rodent populations in North America. To date there is no evidence that a sylvan cycle of monkeypox transmission has occurred.

MPV is an uncommon viral zoonosis caused by a member of the genus *Orthopoxvirus*. The disease is important to public health because the virus has a close genetic relationship to variola virus and is capable of causing a clinical syndrome that closely resembles smallpox. The genus *Orthopoxvirus* includes four species that are known to infect humans: variola virus, MPV, vaccinia virus (used for smallpox vaccination), and cowpox virus. Other orthopoxviruses, such as ectromelia (mousepox), have been implicated in human infections, but the evidence is less compelling (Reynolds et al., 2006).

MPV was named based on its association with nine outbreaks of vesicular exanthems among captive primates in laboratories and zoos during the 1950s and 1960s. The first cases of human disease were not reported until 1970 in Zaire (now the Democratic Republic of Congo [DRC]). Prior cases of human MPV undoubtedly occurred in central

Africa but were confused with smallpox or varicella zoster (chickenpox). Since its initial recognition, MPV has been documented to occur both sporadically and during outbreaks of rash illness among humans throughout central and western Africa. It is considered by some to be the most important orthopoxvirus now that smallpox is eradicated (Nalca, Rimoin, Bavari, & Whitehouse, 2005).

Renewed interest in human MPV was generated by the unexpected emergence of the disease in the midwestern United States associated with the importation of infected rodents from western Africa as described above (Reed et al., 2004). Additionally, MPV is considered a potential agent of biological terrorism (see chapter 27). This chapter reviews the 2003 outbreak of MPV in North America as well as current knowledge of the epidemiologic, clinical, and laboratory features of MPV infections. Although the emphasis is on MPV, relevant information related to other orthopoxvirus infections of medical concern, such as variola, vaccinia, and cowpox viruses, are also included in the discussion.

Variola virus has a host range that is restricted to humans in natural settings. Infection is easily transmitted by large-droplet aerosols and close contact with infectious persons or sloughed scab material. Vaccinia virus is of uncertain origin but is of great importance to medicine because it is cross-protective as a vaccine against other orthopoxvirus infections. Disease related to vaccinia virus is usually limited to adverse reactions to vaccinia vaccination for smallpox. Rare cases of disseminated disease in infants or immunocompromised hosts occur when they come in contact with a recently vaccinated individual.

MPV and cowpox are zoonotic pathogens, that is, both viruses are maintained in nature by mammalian reservoirs with humans being regarded as incidental hosts. Compared to MPV, cowpox virus infections are relatively rare and can be acquired from infected cows but more commonly from exposure to other infected animals such as rats, domestic cats, or captive elephants in zoos or circuses. Most cowpox lesions are confined to the hands and resemble vesicles occurring after smallpox vaccination. Systemic infections have been reported and can be quite severe (Damon & Esposito, 2003).

At the genetic level, orthopoxviruses have large, complex, double-stranded DNA virus genomes that code for over 200 potential protein products. Two genetic clades of MPV are recognized: a Congo basin-derived clade associated with 2–10% mortality in unvaccinated individuals and a west African clade associated with milder illness and very low mortality (Chen et al., 2005).

Human MPV has probably occurred in central and western Africa for hundreds, if not thousands, of years but was overshadowed by smallpox until variola virus was eradicated in central Africa in the late 1960s.

Although it is clear that MPV is maintained in animal reservoirs, there is surprisingly little detailed information on the enzootic cycle MPV maintains in nature. Humans and monkeys are considered incidental hosts, and the reservoirs that amplify the virus in natural settings are probably the numerous rodent or squirrels species that inhabit the sub-Saharan rain forests. This notion is supported by laboratory studies that indicate that MPV has a broad host range and can infect numerous species of small mammals (Breman, 2000).

One concern is that MPV could emerge from central Africa and replace smallpox as a more global health problem. Detailed studies of the epidemiology of MPV suggest that this is unlikely to occur. World Health Organization (WHO) surveillance studies performed between 1981 and 1986 in the DRC revealed that the majority (>70%) of cases were associated with an animal source of infection and the remainder were due to secondary transmission. Most cases occurred in children, and the mean age was 4.4 years. Although the rate of secondary transmission was several times higher than that observed during the 1970s, in no instance did the chain of transmission go beyond four generations, suggesting that MPV has low potential for epidemic spread. More recently, extended interhuman transmission of MPV has been observed in a hospital in the DRC where up to six sequential transmission cycles were hypothesized to have occurred (Learned et al., 2005). This pattern of more sustained transmission suggests that MPV might have the capacity to undergo genetic changes that could result in it becoming better adapted as a human pathogen. Transmission can be from person-to-person via oropharyngeal exudates, direct contact with infected animals via inoculation, or ingestion (Reynolds et al., 2006; Sale, Melski, & Stratman, 2006).

The reported cases of human MPV declined after formal WHO surveillance ended in 1986. From 1986 to 1992 only 13 cases were reported in the medical literature, and none were reported from 1993 to 1995. This trend suddenly reversed in 1996–1997 when more than 500 cases of suspected MPV were reported in the Kasai-Oriental province of the DRC. This outbreak was associated with a low fatality rate (1–5%) and high person-to-person transmission (78%) compared to previous outbreaks. Since many of these suspected cases were not laboratory confirmed, some authors have speculated that the majority of cases were actually due to varicella rather than MPV (Hutin et al., 2001). From 1998 to 2002 over 1,200 cases of MPV were reported to the DRC Ministry of Health. Of those cases that were laboratory confirmed, patient age ranged from 10 months to 38 years with a mean of 16.5 years (Kebela, 2004). Active and passive surveillance for MPV continues on the African continent but is hampered by political unrest and lack of adequate public health resources.

Most of the patients in the U.S. outbreak discussed above had mild, self-limited disease in comparison to the more severe illness reported among African patients. The milder illness can be explained in part by the fact that many of the adults who were infected had previously received smallpox vaccination. Additionally, the strain of MPV associated with the U.S. outbreak was of western African origin and is known to be less virulent than Congo basin-derived strains. Of 69 patients for whom data are available, 18 were hospitalized. No deaths were reported. Two pediatric patients had serious clinical illness; one child had severe encephalitis requiring treatment in an intensive care unit for 14 days, and the other had diffuse pox lesions and painful cervical and tonsillar lymphadenopathy and oropharyngeal lesions (Anderson, Frenkel, Homann, & Guffey, 2003; Huhn et al., 2005).

Observational studies of human MPV occurring in central and western Africa during the 1980s showed an incubation period of 10–14 days and a period of infectivity during the first week of rash. MPV enters the body through skin abrasions, the mucosa of the upper respiratory tract, or ingestion. During primary viremia, the virus migrates to regional lymph nodes and then disseminates throughout the body with the appearance of a rash. A prodrome of fever and malaise typically occurs 1 to 2 days prior to rash onset and is associated with lymphadenopathy in around 90% of cases. The distribution of lymphadenopathy is variable and can include submandibular, cervical, axillary, and inguinal areas or a combination of these sites. Because smallpox is rarely associated with significant lymphadenopathy, this clinical feature is a key distinguishing feature between the two diseases.

The rash of MPV begins as papular lesions of 1–5 mm in diameter that progress through vesicular, pustular, and crusted stages over a period of 14–21 days. The crusts eventually slough off, leaving depressed scars. Case descriptions from Africa emphasize a centrifugal pattern of spread that becomes generalized over time. However, centripetal rash similar to that described for chickenpox has been described in a few cases (Nalca et al., 2005). Several unique clinical manifestations were noted among patients infected during the 2003 outbreak of MPV in the United States. These included focal hemorrhagic necrosis, particularly at the sites of bites or scratches, and erythematous flares that are probably more apparent on light skin (Reed et al., 2004). The list of differential diagnoses for the rash lesions of MPV is long and includes smallpox, chickenpox, orf, milker's nodule, erythema multiforme, drug eruptions, rickettsialpox, and eczema herpeticum.

Extracutaneous manifestations of MPV infection include cough, pharyngitis, chest tightness, diarrhea, myalgias, back pain, and nausea. Complications can include secondary skin and soft tissue infections

(20%), pneumonitis (12%), ocular involvement (5%), and, rarely, encephalitis (<1%; Nalca et al., 2005). Prior smallpox vaccination modulates the clinical course of human MPV in a number of aspects. In general, vaccinated patients experience a milder illness and have lower morbidity and mortality. The rash tends to be more pleomorphic in vaccinated individuals and more closely resembles chickenpox. Clinical manifestations may be influenced by mode of transmission, strain virulence, and host characteristics such as nutritional status and prior smallpox vaccination (Sale et al., 2006).

Human MPV is a reportable disease, and state and local public health departments should be notified immediately of any suspected cases. Although the history and clinical characteristics can be helpful in differentiating between MPV and other causes of vesiculopustular eruptions, every attempt should be made to confirm cases by laboratory testing. The CDC recommends the following laboratory criteria for diagnosing human MPV cases: (a) isolation of MPV in culture, (b) demonstration of MPV DNA by PCR testing in a clinical sample, (c) electron microscopic evidence of an orthopoxvirus in the absence of exposure to another orthopoxvirus, and (d) immunohistochemical evidence of an orthopoxvirus in tissue in the absence of exposure to another orthopoxvirus. Most diagnostic laboratories in the United States have limited experience with isolating orthopoxviruses from clinical specimens and should refer specimens from suspected cases to the appropriate state health laboratory or to the CDC. In the United States, possession, transfer, and handling of positive MPV cultures is regulated under the Select Agent Rule (42 CFR).

MPV grows well in established cell culture lines, such as rhesus monkey kidney cells and Vero cells. Cytopathic effect usually occurs within 1 to 4 days and is characterized by plaques of elongated and rounded cells with prominent cytoplasmic bridging and formation of syncytium. Another approach to virus isolation is the use of embryonated eggs, but this is not available to most clinical laboratories. Clinical samples that are appropriate for virus isolation include biopsies and touch preparations of skin lesions, lymph nodes, oropharyngeal swabs, and whole blood during the prodromal stage. MPV-infected clinical samples can be handled safely in the laboratory by personnel who have received smallpox vaccination within the past 10 years and who use strict Biosafety Level 2 containment (Damon & Esposito, 2003).

A number of molecular diagnostic tests are available to aid in the definitive diagnosis of MPV infections. DNA-based tests, such as PCR with restriction endonuclease digestion or sequencing of the HA, can confirm the identity of an orthopoxvirus to the species level and can be accomplished in just a few hours. This method is based on the use of primers EACP1 and EACP2 (for Old World orthopoxviruses) or NACP1 and NACP2 (for New World orthopoxviruses) to produce amplicons for further analysis (Damon & Esposito, 2003). Additional PCR protocols are available.

Electron microscopy is an important frontline method for the laboratory diagnosis of poxvirus infections because it is a simple technique that can rapidly exclude varicella (a herpesvirus) from the differential diagnosis (Curry, Appleton, & Dowsett, 2006; Hazelton & Gelderblom, 2003). Transmission EM of tissue biopsies reveals virions with dumbbell-shaped inner cores highly characteristic of poxviruses. However, this technique does not distinguish between orthopoxviruses and the other genera of poxviruses. When vesicle fluid or tissue culture supernatants are examined by negative-stain EM with phosphotungstic acid or other heavy metal, orthopoxviruses have a distinctive brick-shaped appearance with regularly spaced threadlike ridges on the exposed surfaces. In contrast, parapoxviruses appear ovoid with spiraling crisscross surface projections. Negative stain EM of cell culture supernatants provided the first clues that the 2003 U.S. outbreak was due to an orthopoxvirus (Reed et al., 2004).

The histopathology of MPV mirrors the clinical progression of the skin lesions. Early lesions show ballooning degeneration of basal keratinocytes and spongiosis of a mildly acanthotic epidermis. This progresses to full-thickness necrosis of a markedly acanthotic epidermis containing few viable keratinocytes. The histologic differential diagnosis includes herpes simplex, varicella, and other poxviruses (Bayer-Garner, I.B. 2005). Electron microscopy will reliably distinguish between herpesvirus and poxvirus infections. Identification of MPV and other orthopoxvirus infections by immunoserologic methods has been difficult because of the close antigenic relationship shared among this group of viruses. Neutralization tests with hyperimmune sera, hemagglutination inhibition assays, and enzyme-linked immunosorbent assay are available to detect orthopox-specific antibodies in patient sera, but the efficacy of these assays ranges from 50% to 95%. Currently, there is no serologic test that is sensitive and specific for identifying MPV infections that is widely available in most clinical diagnostic laboratories (Damon & Esposito, 2003). However, serological testing has proven useful in epidemiologic studies. A retrospective study of individuals potentially exposed to MPV in the 2003 U.S. outbreak revealed three cases of asymptomatic infection that occurred in persons who had been vaccinated against smallpox decades earlier (Hammarlund et al., 2005).

Vaccination with vaccinia virus is around 85% protective and is indicated for persons investigating animal or human MPV cases, health care workers caring for infected patients, and laboratory workers who handle specimens that may contain MPV. Vaccination within 4 days after initial close contact with a confirmed MPV case is recommended by the CDC and should be considered up to 14 days after exposure. Vaccinia immune globulin may be considered as a prophylactic for exposed persons with impaired T-cell function who would not be candidates for vaccination (Di Giulio & Eckburg, 2004).

Treatment of severe illness with vaccinia immune globulin should be considered, but no data are currently available documenting efficacy in treating human MPV. Additionally, there are no currently licensed antiviral drugs for treating MPV. Cidofovir is a broad-spectrum antiviral drug with known activity against cytomegalovirus and many other DNA viruses, including MPV. Although clinical experience with the use of cidofovir in human MPV infections is limited, antiviral treatment with that agent was more effective than postexposure smallpox vaccination in a cynomolgus monkey (*Macaca fascicularis*) model (Stittelaar et al., 2006).

Transmission of MPV within hospitals has been described, but the overall risk appears low. The CDC recommends a combination of standard, contact, and droplet precautions for infection control purposes. Airborne precautions should be implemented whenever possible. All laboratory specimens should be handled in a biological safety cabinet (Fleischauer et al., 2005). The 2003 U.S. outbreak was a sobering reminder of the impact emerging infectious diseases can have on public health. That emergence of MPV in North America was linked directly to the importation of rodents from west Africa and subsequent comingling of these animals with native fauna. Based on that information, it is clear that the primary prevention strategy for MPV in the New World is to limit importation of infected animal reservoirs. On June 11, 2003, the CDC and the Food and Drug Administration issued a joint order prohibiting the importation of all African rodents into the United States. The order also banned within the United States any sale, distribution, transport, or release into the environment of prairie dogs and six specific genera of African rodents. The joint order was enacted as part of the public health response to the first cases of human MPV in North America. On November 4, 2003, the joint order was replaced by an interim final rule that maintained the importation ban. Animals can still be imported for scientific, exhibition, or educational purposes with a valid permit issued by the CDC.

REFERENCES

Anderson, M. G., Frenkel, L. D., Homann, S., & Guffey, J. (2003). A case of severe monkeypox disease in an American child: Emerging infections and changing professional values. *Pediatric Infectious Disease Journal, 22,* 1093–1096.

Bayer-Garner, I. B. (2005). Monkeypox virus: Histologic, immunohistochemical and electron-microscopic findings. *Journal of Cutaneous Pathology, 32,* 28–34.

Breman, J. G. (2000). Monkeypox: An emerging infection for humans? In M. W. Scheld, W. A. Craig, & J. M. Hughes (Eds.), *Emerging infections 4* (45–67). Washington DC: ASM Press.

Centers for Disease Control and Prevention. (2003). Update: Multistate outbreak of monkeypox—Illinois, Indiana, Kansas, Missouri, Ohio, and Wisconsin. *Morbidity and Mortality Weekly Report, 52,* 642–646.

Chen, N., Li, G., Liszewski, M. K., Atkinson, J. P., Jahrling, P. B., Feng, Z., et al. (2005). Virulence differences between monkeypox virus isolates from west Africa and the Congo basin. *Virology, 340,* 46–63.

Curry, A., Appleton, H., & Dowsett, B. (2006). Application of transmission electron microscopy to the clinical study of viral and bacterial infections: Present and future. *Micronesica, 37,* 91–106.

Damon, I. K., & Esposito, J. J. (2003). Poxviruses that infect humans. In P. R. Murray, E. J. Barron, J. H. Jorgensen, M. A. Pfaller, & R. H. Yolken (Eds.), *Manual of clinical microbiology* (8th ed.). Washington, DC: ASM Press.

Di Giulio, D. B., & Eckburg, P. B. (2004). Human monkeypox: An emerging zoonosis. *Lancet Infectious Diseases, 4,* 15–25.

Fleischauer, A. T., Kile, J. C., Davidson, M., Fischer, M., Karem, K. L., Teclaw, R., et al. (2005). Evaluation of human-to-human transmission of monkeypox from infected patients to health care workers. *Clinical Infectious Diseases, 40,* 689–694.

Hammarlund, E., Lewis, M. W., Carter, S. V., Amanna, I., Hansen, S. G., Strelow, L. I., et al. (2005). Multiple diagnostic techniques identify previously vaccinated individuals with protective immunity against monkeypox. *Nature Medicine, 11,* 1005–1011.

Hazelton, P. R., & Gelderblom, H. R. (2003). Electron microscopy for rapid diagnosis of infectious agents in emergent situations. *Emerging Infectious Diseases, 9,* 294–303.

Huhn, G. D., Bauer, A. M., Yorita, K., Graham, M. B., Sejvar, J., Likos, A., et al. (2005). Clinical characteristics of human monkeypox, and risk factors for severe disease. *Clinical Infectious Diseases, 41,* 1742–1751.

Hutin, Y. J., Williams, R. J., Malfait, P., Pebody, R., Loparev, V. N., Ropp, S. L., et al. (2001). Outbreak of human monkeypox, Democratic Republic of Congo, 1996 to 1997. *Emerging Infectious Diseases, 7,* 434–438.

Kebela, B. (2004). Le profil épidémiologique de monkeypox en RDC, 1998–2002. [The epidemiologic profile of monkeypox in RDC, 1998 to 2002]. *Bulletin Épidémiologique de la République Démocratique du Congo, 29,* 2.

Learned, L. A., Reynolds, M. G., Wassa, D. W., Li, Y., Olson, V. A., Karem, K., et al. (2005). Extended interhuman transmission of monkeypox in a hospital community in the Republic of the Congo, 2003. *American Journal of Tropical Medicine and Hygiene, 73,* 428–434.

Nalca, A., Rimoin, A. W., Bavari, S., & Whitehouse, C. A. (2005). Reemergence of monkeypox: Prevalence, diagnostics, and countermeasures. *Clinical Infectious Diseases, 41,* 1765–1771.

Reed, K. D., Melski, J. W., Graham, M. B., Regnery, R. L., Sotir, M. J., Wegner, M. V., et al. (2004). The detection of monkeypox in humans in the Western Hemisphere. *New England Journal of Medicine, 350,* 342–350.

Reynolds, M., G., Yorita, K. L., Kuehnert, M. J., Davidson, W. B., Huhn, G. D., Holman, R., et al. (2006). Clinical manifestations of human monkeypox influenced by route of infection. *Journal of Infectious Diseases, 194,* 773–780.

Sale, T. A., Melski, J. W., & Stratman, E. J. (2006). Monkeypox: An epidemiologic and clinical comparison of African and US disease. *Journal of the American Academy of Dermatology, 55,* 478–481.

Stittelaar, K. J., Neyts, J., Naesens, L., van Amerongen, G., van Lavieren, R. F., Holy, A., et al. (2006). Antiviral treatment is more effective than smallpox vaccination upon lethal monkeypox virus infection. *Nature, 439,* 745–748.

CHAPTER TWENTY

Multidrug-Resistant Tuberculosis

Neil W. Schluger

M. T., a 45-year-old man, presented to the chest clinic complaining of fever, cough, and a 15-pound weight loss. The patient, a recent immigrant from the former Soviet Union, had a history of tuberculosis that had been treated several years ago. He was unsure of his treatment while in the Soviet Union, but he states that the medications were changed frequently. After being released, he took his medications sporadically, as he could not afford all the drugs that were prescribed for him. Since entering the United States, he has had no medical care. On examination the patient was a thin male. He had rhonchi over the upper left lung field. A chest radiograph showed a cavitary infiltrate in the left upper lobe, and a sputum sample contained numerous acid-fast bacilli. He was started on a regimen of six antituberculous medications, including isoniazid, rifampin, pyrazinamide, ethambutol, streptomycin, and levofloxacin, all of which were administered by directly observed therapy (DOT). A sputum culture was positive for *Mycobacterium tuberculosis* 2 weeks after beginning therapy. Two months after beginning treatment, the mycobacteriology laboratory reported that the patient's isolate was resistant to rifampin and isoniazid. These drugs were discontinued, and the patient was treated with the remaining drugs. Streptomycin injections were discontinued after 9 months, and the patient received ethambutol, pyrazinamide, and levofloxacin for a total of 18 months. He regained all the weight he had lost, and sputum cultures were negative for the last 15 months of his therapy. He continues to do well.

This case illustrates many of the important principles involved in understanding the epidemiology, pathogenesis, diagnosis, and treatment of multidrug-resistant tuberculosis (MDR-TB). In this chapter all of these areas will be reviewed in detail.

Both tuberculous infection and TB are caused by the tubercle bacilli *Mycobacterium* spp. that include *M. tuberculosis, M. africanum, M. bovis,* and *M. microti. M. tuberculosis* is the most common and most important in the United States. *M. tuberculosis* is a nonmotile, non-spore-forming, rod-shaped bacillus that has no capsule and does not produce toxin. It is known as acid fast because of staining characteristics. It can survive for long periods under adverse conditions. Like other microbes, it can mutate and affect characteristics such as drug sensitivity, which is the focus of this chapter. *M. tuberculosis* can cause pulmonary or extrapulmonary TB. Common symptoms of pulmonary TB include cough (usually productive), fatigue or malaise, anorexia, weight loss, low-grade fever, sweating and/or chills at night, and dull, aching chest pain or tightness (Brodie, & Schluger, 2005). Extrapulmonary TB may include systemic symptoms and those related to the affected organ system.

Tuberculosis remains the leading cause of death due to infection in the world today among persons older than 5 years of age. The global burden of disease due to *M. tuberculosis* is staggering. The World Health Organization (WHO) estimates that roughly one third of the world's population, or some 2 billion people, are infected with *M. tuberculosis* (Dye, Watt, Bleed, Hosseini, & Raviglione, 2005). Of these, between 8 and 12 million people will actually develop active disease each year (new or incident cases). At any given time there are approximately 16 million total prevalent cases in the world, and 2–3 million people die each year of TB around the world. The vast majority (95%) of both cases and deaths due to TB occur in resource-poor countries, with most cases found in sub-Saharan Africa, South and Southeast Asia, and parts of South America. In some of these regions, the annual case rate exceeds 300 cases per 100,000 population annually. By contrast, in the United States, the case rate for TB in 2005 was a historic low of 4.8 cases per 100,000 population (Centers for Disease Control and Prevention [CDC], 2006). Current public health activities in the United States are aimed both at keeping the overall incidence of TB at low levels and preventing the reemergence of MDR-TB (Taylor, Nolan, & Blumberg, 2005).

Drug-resistant TB was first noted to develop soon after the introduction of streptomycin as the first useful antibiotic with activity against *M. tuberculosis.* When used as a single agent, as was the case in the early clinical trials of the drug, initial exhilaration over treatment success was soon tempered with the realization that most patients taking the single agent soon failed therapy or relapsed with organisms resistant to streptomycin (Dean et al., 2002). This problem was alleviated by the coadministration of isoniazid and streptomycin together, although soon after the introduction of isoniazid in the early 1950s resistance to this drug was noted as well.

The truly modern era of chemotherapy for TB began in the 1970s with the introduction of rifampin, which allowed the shortening of chemotherapy regimens to 9 and eventually 6 months (Leibert & Rom, 2004). This simplified treatment programs greatly, although resistance to rifampin was noted in a few regions around the world, notably in a report in the mid-1980s from the Philippines. However, as culture and drug susceptibility testing for M. *tuberculosis* is not routinely performed in many parts of the world because of the substantial expense involved, true and systematic estimates of the prevalence of MDR-TB (now generally defined as cases of TB that are resistant to at least both isoniazid and rifampin) is not known.

Renewed attention to and concern about MDR-TB arose again in the early 1990s when a sharp rise in drug-resistant TB cases was noted in New York City (Frieden et al., 1993). This rise accompanied an overall increase in TB cases that was caused by a dismantling of the city's public health infrastructure; a deterioration in the living conditions among the indigent, with increased use of homeless shelters and a larger percentage of incarcerated persons; and the AIDS epidemic, which facilitated rapid transmission of TB cases among extremely vulnerable populations. In addition, inadequate infection control procedures in hospitals and prisons, as well as poor prescribing practices of physicians caring for TB cases, contributed greatly to the emergence of MDR-TB as a significant threat to the public health in New York City. In 1992, New York City reported a total of 450 cases of MDR-TB out of an overall caseload of 3,811 persons with TB. In other words, 11.8% of all cases of TB in New York City in that year were due to MDR-TB. Remarkably, in 1999, the MDR-TB case burden in New York City had fallen to only 30 out of a total of 1,460, or only 2% of the total, and this low level of MDR-TB has been maintained to the present (Munsiff et al., 2006). The reasons behind this dramatic turnaround have been extensively described and will be discussed later in this chapter.

Globally, little was known about the prevalence of drug-resistant TB until the WHO conducted the first global survey in 1994 and reported the results a few years later (Pablos-Mendez et al., 1998). The results of this survey sparked great concern in the global public health community. Thirty-five countries, representing every region of the world, were surveyed. No region was found to be without MDR-TB cases, and in some regions the incidence of MDR-TB was astoundingly high. Countries as diverse as the Dominican Republic, India, Latvia, Estonia, Russia, and Côte d'Ivoire had rates of MDR-TB that ranged from 7% to 22% of total cases. As these countries have extremely high overall rates of TB (in the state of Delhi, India, the TB case rate may be as high as 450 cases/100,000 population), the absolute numbers of MDR-TB patients in these nations are quite high. In prisons in parts of the former Soviet Union, the TB case rate may be as high as 4,000/100,000 population, and some reports indicate that MDR-TB cases constitute at least 20% of this total (CDC, 1999; Kimerling et al., 1999; Viljanen et al., 1998).

An update of the WHO's report of the global burden of MDR-TB completed in 1999 indicated that in several regions of the world the problem is getting worse, not better (WHO, 2000). In Denmark and Germany, although the absolute numbers are small, MDR cases have increased by 50%. In Estonia, MDR-TB cases now account for 18% of the total TB burden. Other regions or countries where MDR-TB cases have continued to rise include China (Henan and Zhejiang), India (Tamil Nadu), Iran, Mozambique, Russia (Tomsk), Israel, Italy, and Mexico (Baja California, Oaxaca, and Sinaloa). Because of the ease and frequency with which persons travel around the globe in the current age, it is reasonable to expect that MDR-TB cases will continue to appear in every region of the world for the next many years (Ormerod, 2005; Schluger, 2000). The most recent analysis by the WHO indicates that just three countries, China, India, and the Russian Federation, account for nearly two-thirds of MDR-TB cases in the world, and 4.3% of all TB cases worldwide are MDR (Zignol et al., 2006). Strains of highly resistant M. *tuberculosis*, termed XDR (extensively drug-resistant), have been isolated, mostly from patients with HIV infection in South Africa (Gandhi et al., 2006). They are resistant to nearly all drugs available to treat TB, and are associated with extraordinarily high rates of mortality.

Compounding the gravity of the above situation is the fact that no new class of drugs has been developed since the introduction of rifamycins in the late 1960s and early 1970s. This situation is not likely to improve in the near future. From the perspective of pharmaceutical manufacturers, TB drug development is economically unattractive, as most of the cases occur in countries with little money available to buy new agents (Pecoul, Chirac, Trouiller, & Pinel, 1999). This acts as a powerful disincentive for the development of new antibiotics for TB. In the last few years, however, there have been great efforts to develop new classes of drugs for the treatment of TB, spurred in large part by the efforts of the Global Alliance for TB Drug Development. Although at present there still has not been a new class of TB drugs introduced, several new compounds are in clinical trials, and there is hope that in the next 5 years there will be approval of at least one new class of drugs useful for treating MDR-TB. Of drugs already available, the quinolone class of antibiotics holds significant promise in treating MDR-TB (Nuermberger et al., 2005; Onyebujoh et al., 2005; Rosenthal et al., 2005).

Resistance to antimycobacterial drugs occurs naturally in any population of mycobacteria, although at different frequencies for different drugs. Resistance to isoniazid is found in approximately 1 in 10^6 organisms, which is the same frequency at which resistance to ethambutol occurs. On the other hand, resistance to rifampin is quite a bit less common, occurring spontaneously at a rate of about 1 in 10^8 organisms. These naturally occurring rates of resistance provide the basis for understanding the need for multidrug therapy of TB. If only a single drug were used (say, isoniazid), eventually the 1 in 10^6 organisms with naturally occurring resistance would be selected for and would lead to a treatment failure or relapse due to isoniazid-resistant TB. On the other hand, if two drugs were used initially (say, isoniazid and rifampin), naturally occurring resistance to both would be present in only 1 in 10^{14} organisms, and the likelihood of selecting for one of these would be very, very low. Not only does the natural occurrence of drug resistance explain the need for multidrug chemotherapy at the outset of treatment, but it also underlies the most important rule for treating cases of suspected drug resistance, namely, never add a single drug to a failing regimen.

In recent years, there has been substantial progress in the molecular understanding of the basis of antibiotic resistance in mycobacteria (Riska, Jacobs, & Alland, 2000). Resistance to isoniazid occurs as a result of mutations in genes that encode enzymes that normally convert isoniazid (INH) to its active form (catalase), or genes that produce proteins that normally bind INH to form a complex that prevents cell wall synthesis (inhA). Rifampin normally works by binding to the β subunit of RNA polymerase, thus interfering with RNA synthesis. Mutations in the *rpoB* gene prevent the rifampin from binding, and RNA synthesis continues uninterrupted. Streptomycin interferes with ribosomal protein synthesis, and mutations in the ribosomal protein gene *rrs* prevent this from occurring. The fluoroquinolones work by inhibiting a group of enzymes called DNA gyrases. Although the elucidation of the molecular basis of mycobacterial drug resistance may target drug development and may lead to rapid molecular-based diagnostic techniques, at present the clinical application of this information is somewhat limited (Drobniewski, Watterson, Wilson, & Harris, 2000; McNerney, Kiepiela, Bishop, Nye, & Stoker, 2000; Piatek et al., 2000).

In practice, a patient develops MDR-TB in one of two ways. The patient is either infected initially with a drug-resistant strain of *M. tuberculosis* (so-called primary drug resistance), or he or she is initially infected with a drug-susceptible strain and only later does this strain become resistant (so-called secondary drug resistance). A high prevalence of primary drug-resistant cases may indicate failure of an infection control program or treatment program (or both) so that vulnerable patients are exposed to infectious cases on an ongoing basis. On the other hand, a high prevalence of secondary drug resistance indicates a serious problem with either the prescribing practices of treating physicians (the wrong drugs are being used in an improper fashion) or in patient adherence to the medical regimen (patients may be taking their medicine sporadically and erratically). Unfortunately, neither of the circumstances leading to the development of secondary drug resistance is rare. Difficulties in compliance with TB treatment have been well chronicled (Cohen, 1997), and a study from a leading referral center found that in the typical case of MDR-TB, treating physicians had made an average of nearly four management errors per patient (Mahmoudi & Iseman, 1993).

There is nothing in the clinical presentation of the patient that leads one to suspect MDR-TB. Signs, symptoms, and radiographic findings are all indistinguishable from drug-susceptible TB. Rather, the major clinical clue to the presence of drug resistance is in the patient's history (Telzak et al., 1999). Drug resistance should be suspected in any patient with active TB who has a history of previously treated TB. In such cases, every effort must be made to obtain all the details of the patient's prior treatment. This includes not only all previous culture and drug susceptibility reports, but also records of the previous drug treatment regimen and the record of the patient's adherence to it. If a patient has relapsed after excellent adherence to a proper regimen, then in fact the development of drug resistance is extremely uncommon, and empiric therapy for drug resistance is not generally indicated. If on the other hand a patient develops relapse or treatment failure in the setting of poor adherence to the prescribed regimen, or the regimen turns out not to have been adequate based on the known drug susceptibility pattern, MDR-TB should be suspected.

When MDR-TB is suspected on clinical grounds, every effort should be made to obtain a relevant clinical specimen for culture and drug susceptibility testing. However, there will be a significant delay in treatment if drugs are held until drug susceptibility results are obtained, so empiric therapy must be instituted. When beginning treatment for MDR-TB on clinical grounds, there is one rule that must always be obeyed: *Never add a single agent to a failing (or failed) regimen*. One must assume that the patient is resistant to all previous drugs used, so the regimen to be used should contain at least two, and preferably at least three, drugs that the patient has not received before.

The selection of drugs used in the treatment of MDR-TB depends obviously on the pattern of drug resistance present. Although it is clear that the outcome of treatment for MDR-TB is not as good as it is for drug-susceptible TB (which is essentially always curable), recent studies demonstrate that aggressive therapy is associated with a very high likelihood of cure, especially in human immunodeficiency virus-negative persons (Burgos et al., 2005; Escudero, Pena, Alvarez-Sala, Vazquez, & Ortega, 2006; Quy et al., 2006).

Specific treatment regimens for MDR-TB are beyond the scope of this chapter, and as a general rule treatment of drug-resistant TB should be attempted only by persons with expertise in the field. In addition, treatment for MDR-TB can best be accomplished only in the setting of a program of DOT, so adherence to the therapeutic regimen can be assured. The use of tailored individual regimens for patients with drug-resistant isolates has come to be known as DOT-Plus, and this is an effective approach, although perhaps a costly one for many resource-limited settings (Farmer, 2001; Mukherjee et al., 2004).

The key drug in the treatment of TB is rifampin. If a patient has TB that is resistant to isoniazid and streptomycin, a regimen of rifampin, pyrazinamide, and ethambutol can be used for 6–9 months, and excellent results can generally be expected. In the relatively unusual setting of rifampin-monoresistant TB (seen primarily, for poorly understood reasons, in persons with acquired immunodeficiency syndrome [AIDS]; Sandman, Schluger, Davidow, & Bonk, 1999), a 9-month regimen of isoniazid, streptomycin, and pyrazinamide has been reported (in the pre-AIDS era) to be associated with a relapse rate of 5–6% (British Medical Research Council, 1977). On the other hand, if neither rifampin nor isoniazid can be used, treatment regimens will always need to be prolonged to 18–24 months (Iseman, 1993). In the case of isoniazid- and rifampin-resistant TB, the combination of an aminoglycoside such as streptomycin with a fluoroquinolone forms the cornerstone of the regimen. If these drugs can be used, particularly in combination with pyrazinamide, a good outcome can be expected. Patients in this circumstance will typically be treated with the aminoglycoside for the first 6–9 months of therapy, and the remaining drugs will be continued for a total of 18–24 months, depending on the extent of disease and response to treatment. If, on the other hand, the patient is resistant to isoniazid, rifampin, and all of the aminoglycosides (or the related drug capreomycin), the potential for a medical cure becomes less, and consideration for early surgical intervention to resect lung tissue at the site of disease should be given. Obviously, this can only be done if the disease is localized (Lallo, Naidoo, & Ambaram, 2006).

There have been several case reports of patients with drug-resistant TB being treated with regimens that include the antibiotic linezolid. Although there has been good response to this drug in terms of microbiologic criteria, its widespread use is severely limited by potential for severe toxicity, including bone marrow depression and peripheral neuropathy, and by its cost (Fortun et al., 2005; von der Lippe, Sandven, & Brubakk, 2006).

CONCLUSION

MDR-TB represents one of the most worrisome infectious diseases to emerge in the last several years because of the magnitude of the problem, the potential for significant morbidity and mortality, and the lack of new drugs at present or on the horizon with which to treat these infections

(Farmer et al., 1998). At present, careful prescribing and assurances of adherence to therapy are the best tools clinicians have to prevent the emergence and spread of MDR-TB.

REFERENCES

British Medical Research Council. (1977). Controlled trial of 6-month and 9-month regimens of daily and intermittent streptomycin plus isoniazid plus pyrazinamide for pulmonary tuberculosis in Hong Kong. The results up to 30 months. *American Review of Respiratory Disease, 115,* 727–735.

Brodie, D., & Schluger, N. W. (2005). The diagnosis of tuberculosis. *Clinics in Chest Medicine, 26,* 247–271.

Burgos, M., Gonzalez, L. C., Paz, E. A., Gourinis, E., Kawamura, L. M., Schecter, G., et al. (2005). Treatment of multidrug-resistant tuberculosis in San Francisco: An outpatient-based approach. *Clinical Infectious Diseases, 40,* 968–975.

Centers for Disease Control and Prevention. (1999). Primary multidrug-resistant tuberculosis—Ivanovo Oblast, Russia. *Morbidity and Mortality Weekly Report, 48,* 661–664.

Centers for Disease Control and Prevention. (2006). Trends in tuberculosis—United States, 2005. *Morbidity and Mortality Weekly Report, 55,* 305–308.

Cohen, F. L. (1997). Adherence to therapy in tuberculosis. *Annual Review of Nursing Research, 15,* 153–184.

Dean, G. L., Edwards, S. G., Ives, N. J., Matthews, G., Fox, E. F., Navaratne, L., et al. (2002). Treatment of tuberculosis in HIV-infected persons in the era of highly active antiretroviral therapy. *AIDS, 16*(1), 75–83.

Drobniewski, F. A., Watterson, S. A., Wilson, S. M., & Harris, G. S. (2000). A clinical, microbiological and economic analysis of a national service for the rapid molecular diagnosis of tuberculosis and rifampicin resistance in *Mycobacterium tuberculosis. Journal of Medical Microbiology, 49,* 271–278.

Dye, C., Watt, C. J., Bleed, D. M., Hosseini, S. M., & Raviglione, M. C. (2005). Evolution of tuberculosis control and prospects for reducing tuberculosis incidence, prevalence, and deaths globally. *Journal of the American Medical Association, 293,* 2767–2775.

Escudero, E., Peña, J. M., Alvarez-Sala, R., Vazquez, J. J., & Ortega A. (2006). Multidrug-resistant tuberculosis without HIV infection: Success with individualized therapy. *International Journal of Tuberculosis and Lung Disease, 10,* 409–414.

Farmer, P., Bayona, J., Becerra, M., Furin, J., Henry, C., Hiatt, H., et al. (1998). The dilemma of MDR-TB in the global era. *International Journal of Tuberculosis and Lung Disease, 2,* 869–876.

Fortun, J., Martin-Davila, P., Navas, E., Perez-Elias, M. J., Cobo, J., Tato, M., et al. (2005). Linezolid for the treatment of multidrug-resistant tuberculosis. *Journal of Antimicrobial Chemotherapy, 56,* 180–185.

Frieden, T. R., Sterling, T., Pablos-Mendez, A., Kilburn, J. O., Cauthen, G. M., & Dooley, S. W. (1993). The emergence of drug-resistant tuberculosis in New York City. *New England Journal of Medicine, 328,* 521–526.

Gandhi, N. R., Moll, A., Sturm, A. W., Pawinski, R., Govender, T., Lalloo, U. et al. (2006). Extensively drug-resistant tuberculosis as a cause of death in patients co-infected with tuberculosis and HIV in a rural area of South Africa. *Lancet, 368,* 1575-1580.

Iseman, M. D. (1993). Treatment of multidrug-resistant tuberculosis. *New England Journal of Medicine, 329,* 784–791.

Kimerling, M. E., Kluge, H., Vezhnina, N., Iacovazzi, T., Demeulenaere, T., Portaels, F., et al. (1999). Inadequacy of the current WHO re-treatment regimen in a central Siberian prison: Treatment failure and MDR-TB. *International Journal of Tuberculosis and Lung Disease, 3,* 451–453.

Lalloo, U. G., Naidoo, R., & Ambaram, A. (2006). Recent advances in the medical and surgical treatment of multi-drug resistant tuberculosis. *Current Opinion in Pulmonary Medicine, 12*(3), 179–185.

Leibert, E., & Rom, W. N. (2004). Principles of tuberculosis management. In W. N. Rom & S. M. Garay (Eds.), *Tuberculosis* (pp. 713–729). Philadelphia: Lippincott Williams & Wilkins.

Mahmoudi, A., & Iseman, M. D. (1993). Pitfalls in the care of patients with tuberculosis. Common errors and their association with the acquisition of drug resistance. *Journal of the American Medical Association, 270,* 65–68.

McNerney, R., Kiepiela, P., Bishop, K. S., Nye, P. M., & Stoker, N. G. (2000). Rapid screening of *Mycobacterium tuberculosis* for susceptibility to rifampicin and streptomycin. *International Journal of Tuberculosis and Lung Disease, 4,* 69–75.

Mukherjee, J. S., Rich, M. L,. Socci, A. R., Joseph, J. K., Viru, F. A,. Shin, S. S., et al. (2004). Programmes and principles in treatment of multidrug-resistant tuberculosis. *Lancet, 363,* 474–81.

Munsiff, S. S., Li, J., Cook, S., Piatek, A., Laraque, F., Ebrahimzadeh, A., et al. (2006). Trends in drug-resistant *Mycobacterium tuberculosis* in New York City, 1991–2003. *Clinical Infectious Diseases, 42,* 1702–1710.

Nuermberger, E., Tyagi, S., Williams, K. N., Rosenthal, I., Bishai, W. R., & Grosset, J. H. (2005). Rifapentine, moxifloxacin, or DNA vaccine improves treatment of latent tuberculosis in a mouse model. *American Journal of Respiratory and Critical Care Medicine, 172,* 1452–1456.

Onyebujoh, P., Zumla, A., Ribeiro, I., Rustomjee, R., Mwaba, P., Gomes, M., et al. (2005). Treatment of tuberculosis: Present status and future prospects. *Bulletin of the World Health Organization, 83,* 857–865.

Ormerod, L. P. (2005). Multidrug-resistant tuberculosis (MDR-TB): Epidemiology, prevention and treatment. *British Medical Bulletin, 73/74,* 17–24.

Pablos-Méndez, A., Raviglione, M. C., Laszlo, A., Binkin, N., Rieder, H. L., Bustreo, F., et al. (1998). Global surveillance for antituberculosis-drug resistance, 1994–1997. World Health Organization—International Union Against Tuberculosis and Lung Disease Working Group on Anti-Tuberculosis Drug Resistance Surveillance. *New England Journal of Medicine, 338,* 1641–1649.

Pecoul, B., Chirac, P., Trouiller, P., & Pinel, J. (1999). Access to essential drugs in poor countries: A lost battle? *Journal of the American Medical Association, 281,* 361–367.

Piatek, A. S., Telenti, A., Murray, M. R., El-Hajj, H., Jacobs, W. R., Jr., et al. (2000). Genotypic analysis of *Mycobacterium tuberculosis* in two distinct populations using molecular beacons: Implications for rapid susceptibility testing. *Antimicrobial Agents and Chemotherapy, 44,* 103–110.

Quy, H. T., Cobelens, F. G., Lan, N. T., Buu, T. N., Lambregts, C. S., Borgdorff, M. W. (2006). Treatment outcomes by drug resistance and HIV status among tuberculosis patients in Ho Chi Minh City, Vietnam. *The International Journal of Tuberculosis and Lung Disease, 10,* 45–51.

Riska, P. F., Jacobs, W. R., Jr., & Alland, D. (2000). Molecular determinants of drug resistance in tuberculosis. *International Journal of Tuberculosis and Lung Disease, 4*(2 Suppl. 1), S4–10.

Rosenthal I. M., Williams K., Tyagi S., Vernon A. A., Peloquin C. A., Bishai W. R., Grosset J. H., Nuermberger E. L. (2005). Weekly moxifloxacin and rifapentine is more active than the Denver regimen in murine tuberculosis. *American Journal of Respiratory and Critical Care Medicine, 172,* 1457–1462.

Sandman, L., Schluger, N. W., Davidow, A. L., & Bonk, S. (1999). Risk factors for rifampin-monoresistant tuberculosis: A case-control study. *American Journal of Respiratory and Critical Care Medicine, 159,* 468–472.

Schluger, N. W. (2000). The impact of drug resistance on the global tuberculosis epidemic. *International Journal of Tuberculosis and Lung Disease, 4*(2 Suppl. 1), S71–75.

Taylor, Z., Nolan, C. M., & Blumberg, H. M. (2005). Controlling tuberculosis in the United States. Recommendations from the American Thoracic Society, CDC, and the Infectious Diseases Society of America. *Morbidity and Mortality Weekly Report, 54*(RR-12), 1–81.

Telzak, E. E., Chirgwin, K. D., Nelson, E. T., Matts, J. P., Sepkowitz, K. A., Benson, C., et al. (1999). Predictors for multidrug-resistant tuberculosis among HIV-infected patients and response to specific drug regimens. Terry Beirn Community Programs for Clinical Research on AIDS (CPCRA) and the AIDS Clinical Trials Group (ACTG), National Institutes for Health. *International Journal of Tuberculosis and Lung Disease, 3,* 337–343.

Viljanen, M. K., Vyshnevskiy, B. I., Otten, T. F., Vyshnevskaya, E., Marjamaki, M., Soini, H., et al. (1998). Survey of drug-resistant tuberculosis in northwestern Russia from 1984 through 1994. *European Journal of Clinical Microbiology and Infectious Diseases, 17,* 177–183.

von der Lippe, B., Sandven, P., & Brubakk, O. (2006). Efficacy and safety of linezolid in multidrug resistant tuberculosis (MDR-TB)—A report of ten cases. *Journal of Infection, 52,* 92–96.

World Health Organization. (2000). *Global tuberculosis report 2000.* Geneva, Switzerland: World Health Organization.

Zignol, M., Hosseini, M. S., Wright, A., Weezenbeek, C. L., Nunn, P., Watt, C. J., et al. (2006). Global incidence of multidrug-resistant tuberculosis. *Journal of Infectious Diseases, 194,* 479–485.

CHAPTER TWENTY-ONE

Prion Diseases

Creutzfeldt–Jakob Disease and Other Transmissible Spongiform Encephalopathies

Felissa R. Lashley

Stephen, a 19-year-old Englishman, became the first officially acknowledged victim of what was then known popularly as "mad cow disease" or, more technically, bovine spongiform encephalopathy (BSE). Like most people, Stephen ate beef, and he had visited his aunt's farm every year for 8 years, coming into contact with cows as well as drinking unpasteurized milk. However, no cases of mad cow disease had been reported in his aunt's herd. The first hints of illness came in 1994 when Stephen's college grades were worse than expected. He became depressed and dizzy, and his parents watched him deteriorate into a living nightmare of madness and hallucinations. As his condition grew worse, he lost coordination and balance until he could no longer walk, swallow, talk, or move, until finally dying in May of 1995 (Rampton & Stauber, 1997).

In March of 1996, the British government announced that 10 young Britons, whose average age was 27 years, were dead or dying of what looked like Creutzfeldt–Jakob disease (CJD), a fatal neurodegenerative disorder that usually affects older persons. Thus, the condition was named new variant CJD, now usually called variant CJD (vCJD). A link was made between eating beef from cows with BSE and developing vCJD. Altered prions were believed to be the agent responsible (Brown, Will, Bradley, Asher, & Detwiler, 2001).

PRIONS

Prions are usually defined as normally occurring proteins that are widely expressed in the body and are components of the neuronal cell membrane (Mead, 2006). Prusiner (2001) defined prions as infectious proteins. The normal prion protein is known as PrP^C (C for cellular). Abnormally folded forms of the prion are pathogenic. When this particle is converted into an abnormal form or isoform, it is known as PrP^{SC} (SC for scrapie) or PrP^{Res} (Res for resistant). In its abnormal conformational form, it is resistant to proteinase K, an enzyme, and PrP accumulates in neurons, eventually causing cell damage or death (Ludlam & Turner, 2006). The recognition of prions, which are believed to be devoid of nucleic acids, caused considerable discussion and controversy in the scientific community but resulted ultimately in a Nobel prize in 1997 for Stanley B. Prusiner. He coined the term *prion*, which he originally referred to as the scrapie agent, discovered a new biological principle of infection, and published detailed work about the properties of prions beginning in 1977 (Prusiner, 1982). When the abnormal form of the prion comes into contact with the normal form, the previously normal form changes shape and becomes abnormal. How this change occurs is not yet known. Prion diseases then result from the accumulation of PrP^{SC}. Prions are considered to be the etiologic agents of a group of fatal neurodegenerative diseases known as the transmissible spongiform encephalopathies (TSEs), also called the prion diseases. There can be a variety of conformations, and each conformation is associated with a specific disease as well as a strain variation (Collinge, 2005). Soto, Estrada, and Castilla (2006) refer to prion disorders as one of the protein misfolding disorders. They include the TSEs and Alzheimer, Parkinson, and Huntington diseases in this group. TSEs include inherited (also called familial), sporadic, and acquired forms.

The gene that encodes the prion protein, *PRNP*, has been located on chromosome 20p. In the normal population, polymorphisms or variations are noted in the human prion protein gene. Persons who are homozygous for either methionine or valine at codon 129 of the gene may be predisposed to developing sporadic or acquired CJD, while heterozygosity at that locus seems to have a somewhat protective effect, but this picture is still evolving. It has been noted that in two other prion diseases with genetic forms, fatal familial insomnia and Gerstmann–Straüssler–Scheinker disease, persons who are homozygous at codon 129 of the prion protein gene and who possess the specific mutant allele for the particular disease have an earlier onset than those who are heterozygous (Online Mendelian Inheritance in Man, OMIM™, 2007).

Despite advances in knowledge about prions and their transmission, there are still some uncertainties regarding the mechanism(s) explaining pathology, transmission, tissue affinity, and variations in the clinical pictures. These uncertainties have resulted in questioning of the prion hypothesis by some investigators (Hopkin, 2006).

TRANSMISSIBLE SPONGIFORM ENCEPHALOPATHIES (TSEs)

TSEs occur in both animals and humans. These have in common spongiform brain changes resembling a "swiss cheese" appearance, as well as the accumulation of amyloidal aggregates of the abnormal prions and long incubation periods. Therefore, TSEs may not be clinically manifested during a given person's or animal's lifetime (Mabbott & MacPherson, 2006). Scrapie, a TSE in sheep, had long been known and described and was believed for many years to be caused by a slow-acting virus before it was realized that abnormal prions were the etiologic agents. TSEs occur in many animal species. Besides the ones in nature, they have been identified in pets and in captive animals of at least 17 species in zoos and in animal laboratories (Blakeslee, 1999a; Brown et al., 2001; Daszak, Cunningham, & Hyatt, 2000). Transmissible spongiform encephalopathies can arise through germline mutations that can be inherited, through acquisition of infection such as via infected blood or tissue or ingestion of contaminated foodstuff, and through other events (many unclear) resulting in accumulation of PrP^{SC} (Wadsworth, Hill, Beck, & Collinge, 2003). The known animal and human prion diseases are shown in Tables 21.1 and 21.2, and selected ones are discussed in detail below.

Scrapie

Scrapie can be transmitted from ewe to lamb. Its name comes from affected animals trying to scrape or rub their fleece off their sides. Affected animals become wasted and ataxic. The incubation period for scrapie is about 3 years. Some scientists believe that the agent that causes scrapie crossed the species barrier to cows as BSE (Brown, 2001). In the United States, scrapie was identified in Vermont sheep, and two flocks were quarantined and then euthanized under a declaration of extraordinary emergency (U. S. Department of Agriculture, 2001).

Bovine Spongiform Encephalopathy (BSE)

Bovine spongiform encephalopathy, commonly known as mad cow disease, was first formally identified in cattle in the United Kingdom in 1986 (Wells et al., 1987). It resembled scrapie, a TSE affecting sheep in England

Table 21.1. Human Transmissible Spongiform Encephalopathies

Type of Encephalopathy	Characteristics
Creutzfeldt–Jakob disease: iatrogenic/infectious, inherited, variant, sporadic	Discussed in this chapter.
Fatal familial insomnia	Genetically determined. Inherited in an autosomal dominant manner. Associated with a mutation on codon 178 of the prion protein gene (*PRNP*) but requires the normal methionine codon at position 129 for expression. Appears between ages 40 and 60 years often between 45 and 51 years. Signs and symptoms include restlessness; marked reduction in sleep time; specific polysomnographic changes; and alteration of autonomic functions such as hypothermia, tachycardia, hypertension, ataxia, myoclonus, dysarthria, and endocrine disturbances. May also see decreased attention, hallucinations, confusion, and memory impairment. Progresses rapidly, with death occurring at a mean of 13 months after presentation.
Gerstmann–Sträussler— Scheinker syndrome	First described in 1936. Genetically determined. Most have autosomal dominant inheritance. Much heterogeneity. Very rare, with only about 2 dozen families known. Certain specific gene mutations appear associated with certain clinical features. Symptoms include progressive cerebellum degeneration with ataxia and, later, dementia.
Sporadic fatal insomnia	Recently identified. Have normal *PRNP* but same symptoms as familial form. Rare.

Sources: Montagna, 2005; Online Mendelian Inheritance in Man, OMIM™, 2007; Tyler, 2005.

for more than 200 years. Until 1988, cattle, other ruminants, and other animals were fed a meat and bonemeal product as a supplement that was made from the rendered carcasses of livestock including sheep. Around 1980, the rendering process was changed in a way that may have allowed the etiologic agent to survive, contaminate the supplement, and thus infect cattle. Cattle carcasses were also recycled through the rendering plants, eventually causing a large-scale BSE epidemic in the United Kingdom. This accounting of BSE originating from scrapie in this way is not universally accepted, and another theory is that it arose from unrecognized endemic BSE (Brown et al., 2001). In experiments, brain homogenates from BSE-infected cattle were fed to goats, who developed BSE, demonstrating that

Table 21.2. Transmissible Spongiform Encephalopathies (TSEs) in Animals

TSE	Hosts	Comments
Bovine spongiform encephalopathy	Cattle	Discussed in this chapter. Signs and symptoms include kicking, abnormal gait, nervousness, and pelvic limb ataxia.
Chronic wasting disease of deer and elk	Wild deer, elk	Endemic in northeast Colorado and Wyoming. Estimated to affect 1–15% of deer and 17% of elk in this area. Reported from Illinois, Wisconsin and West Virginia. Humans are warned to avoid contacting brain, spinal cord, eyes, spleen, or lymph nodes of any deer or elk they kill and to use rubber gloves to cut up carcasses. Found/reported in mid-1960s at Wildlife Research Station in Ft. Collins, Colorado, and in the wild in 1981. Present in game farms in South Dakota, Nebraska, Oklahoma, and Saskatchewan. Symptoms include excessive drooling, staggering, and weight loss. Represents prion exposure threat to humans handling or consuming infected meat.
Exotic ungulate encephalopathy	Ruminants such as eland, greater kudu, Arabian oryx, bison, and others	So far only identified in captive populations beginning in 1986.
Feline spongiform encephalopathy	Domestic cats, cheetahs, pumas, ocelots, tigers	Found to date in captive animals, beginning in 1990 with the domestic cat.
Scrapie	Sheep, goats	First prion strain to be identified. Enzootic in the United Kingdom. Recognized as a distinct disorder in 1738. Affected animals develop ataxia and scrape fleece off sides of body. Can be transmitted from ewe to lamb. Placenta can contaminate the environment. Many strains of agent are known. Worldwide distribution. Relatively common.
Transmissible mink encephalopathy	Mink	Vary rare. Occurs in mink farms in the United States.

Sources: Angers et al., 2006; Blakeslee, 1999b, 2000; Enserink, 2001; Ironside, 1997; Lueck, McIlwain, & Zeidler, 2000; Patterson & Painter, 1999; Sigurdson & Miller, 2003.

transmission from ingestion could occur (Foster, Hope, & Fraser, 1993). Beef might also be contaminated by contact with nervous system tissue during processing (Brown et al., 2001). Although other countries used rendering processes similar to the United Kingdom's around the same time, it is theorized that the proportion of sheep and the proportion of scrapie in the carcasses used in rendering in the United Kingdom was higher than in other countries or that a pathogenic mutation occurred in cattle (Brown et al., 2001). Imported cases in other countries have resulted from importation of either live animals or of food supplements. Nonimported cases of BSE have been described in many other countries.

In 1988, the United Kingdom took action that included making BSE a notifiable disease; conducting BSE surveillance with brain histologic examination; banning ruminant protein in ruminant feed; banning the export of U.K. cattle born before the July 1988 feed ban; instituting compulsory slaughter of nearly 200,000 BSE-infected cattle; and destroying milk from affected cattle. Countries in the European Union as well as the United States also took action in 1989 and 1990 by banning U.K. cattle importation. Other measures to prevent the spread of BSE are found in Brown and colleagues (2001). An economic impact, not only on British beef but on related industries such as gelatin and tallow for candles, was also felt with the various bans on export and import. Within weeks after the identification of BSE in the United Kingdom, concern was raised about the possibility of human infection, and in May 1990, a CJD Surveillance Unit was established in Scotland. Its activities were later extended to other countries in Europe (Brown et al., 2001). Ironically, at the same time, the British agriculture minister claimed that beef was "completely safe" and appeared on TV encouraging his 4-year-old daughter to bite into a hamburger ("Timeline," 2000). Consumer reaction was intense, at times bordering on panic (Cowley, 2001; Daley, 2000). Various other recommendations related to trade and animal health were developed through the World Health Organization (WHO) and other worldwide agencies (WHO, 2001a). Economic effects continue to be felt. It was not until March of 2006 that the European Union lifted the ban on British beef imports.

North America has not been immune to BSE. In Canada, a BSE-infected cow was discovered in Alberta in May 2003, and two more were confirmed in 2005. The United States confirmed BSE in a dairy cow in Washington that had been imported from Canada, and in June 2005, BSE was confirmed in a cow in Texas born in the United States. In March 2006, another case was confirmed in a native-born cow in Alabama. All were born before the 1997 feed regulations were put in place. The trade repercussions varied in severity and time (Mathews, Vandeveer, & Gustafson, 2006). At the end of 2006, researchers reported using transgenic techniques to develop cattle deficient in normal cellular prion protein which could be models for research and provide bovine products free of prion proteins (Richt et al., 2007).

Kuru

Among the Fore women of New Guinea (and, rarely, men), ritualistic cannibalism was formerly practiced in what was described by Rhodes (1997) as "a mortuary feast of love." In this cultural tradition, when kin died, a ceremony was held that involved the cooking and eating of virtually the entire body, during which women would share the feast with their children. Often those who were dying assigned certain body parts in advance of their death to specific relatives to eat after they died. By the early 1950s, kuru, a progressive, fatal neurological disorder, came to Western attention. It is thought, but not known, that kuru may have originated as a sporadic case of CJD, and that cannibalism of an infected person facilitated its spread. None of the Fores born since the government mandated cessation of cannibalism have been known to have acquired the disease, but observation has indicated that the incubation period could be as long to 50 years (Alter, 2000; Collinge et al., 2006). There are also questions raised as to whether endocannibalism might still be discretely practiced, especially in remote areas (Focosi, 2006).

The Fore described kuru in three stages, translated to "walk-about yet" (still ambulatory), "sit down finish" (no longer able to walk), and "sleep finish" (stupor), the final phase (Rhodes, 1997). It occurred mainly in women and children and was investigated by a team led by D. Carleton Gajdusek (Gajdusek & Zigas, 1957), who ultimately received a Nobel prize in 1976 for his work demonstrating that kuru was infectious. Persons homozygous for the *PRNP* codon 129 methionine/methionine genotype are preferentially infected (OMIM, 2007), and those who were heterozygous at codon 129 had longer incubation times and increased resistance to disease (Collinge et al., 2006). Part of the significance of kuru is that the long incubation periods of infection with prions can exceed 50 years and that various estimates of the extent of the vCJD epidemic might be underestimates (Collinge et al., 2006).

Creutzfeldt–Jakob Disease (CJD)

Classification of CJD is as sporadic, inherited or familial (about 10%), and acquired, which includes iatrogenic or variant (Bratosiewicz-Wasik, Liberski, Golanska, Jansen, & Wasik, 2007; Glatzel, Stoeck, Seeger, Lührs, & Aguzzi, 2005). The WHO developed a revised subtype definition for CJD that is shown in Table 21.3. The so-called classical form of CJD was first described in the 1920s independently by two German neurologists, Creutzfeldt and Jakob. The overall incidence is about 1 in

Table 21.3. Revised World Health Organization Definition of
Creutzfeldt–Jakob Disease Subtypes

Subtype	Symptoms	
Sporadic CJD	Definite	Diagnosed by standard neuropathological techniques, immunocytochemically, Western blot-confirmed protease-resistant PrP, and/or presence of scrapie-associated fibrils
	Probable	Progressive dementia and at least two out of the following four clinical features:
		• myoclonus • visual or cerebellar disturbance • pyramidal/extrapyramidal dysfunction • akinetic mutism
		and
		• typical EEG during an illness of any duration and/or a positive 14-3-3 CSF assay and a clinical duration to death <2 years • routine investigations should not suggest an alternative diagnosis
	Possible	Progressive dementia and at least two out of the following four clinical features:
		• myoclonus • visual or cerebellar disturbance • pyramidal/extrapyramidal dysfunction • akinetic mutism
		and
		No EEG or atypical EEG and a duration <2 years
Iatrogenic CJD		Progressive cerebellar syndrome in a recipient of human cadaveric-derived pituitary hormone or sporadic CJD with a recognized exposure risk, e.g., antecedent neurosurgery with dura mater graft
Familial CJD		Definite or probable CJD plus definite or probable CJD in a first-degree relative and/or neuropsychiatric disorder plus disease-specific PrP gene mutation

CJD = Creutzfeldt–Jakob Disease; CSF = cerebrospinal fluid; EEG = electroencephalogram.
Source: World Health Organization (1998).

1–2 million persons per year. The mean age of onset is between 55 and
65 years, but it has occurred in persons as young as 14 years and in
a person 92 years of age. Approximately 85% of classic CJD cases are
sporadic (Collinge, 2005). In sporadic CJD, neurodegeneration is rapidly
progressive, and signs and symptoms include progressive dementia and

cognitive decline, behavioral changes, myoclonus, cerebellar ataxia, visual symptoms, delusions, speech abnormalities, and other signs. No cure is known. Pathology may include neuronal cell death with spongiform changes and vacuolation in the central nervous system, reactive astrocytosis, and, in some cases, amyloid plaques. Onset may be sudden or insidious over weeks (Glatzel et al., 2005). A prodrome may occur with nonspecific symptoms such as anxiety, sleep disturbances, and weight loss (Collins, Lawson, & Masters, 2004). The forms and variations that occur might ultimately be related to varying prion strains or to varying prion gene mutations. Those with methionine/methionine homozygosity at the *PRNP* codon 129 are overrepresented among persons with sporadic CJD (Glatzel et al., 2005). In the genetic or familial form, onset is typically earlier with a longer duration, and there are multiple known mutations in the *PRNP* gene. Inheritance is autosomal dominant (Lashley, 2005, 2007; OMIM, 2007).

The first reported case of iatrogenic CJD was in a woman who received a corneal transplant (Duffy et al., 1974). Iatrogenic CJD is believed to account for only about 5% of all CJD cases. The implications of these cases, however, are frightening. Iatrogenic CJD cases have been documented following dura mater graft transplants in neurosurgery such as for aneurysm repair (over 80 reports, many from a single manufacturer, LYODURA), corneal transplants, liver transplants, the use of contaminated neurosurgical instruments or stereotactic depth electroencephalographic electrodes during surgery, and the administration of cadaveric human pituitary hormones. In the latter case, inadvertent CJD transmission occurred in some patients who received intramuscular injections of human growth hormone for treating short stature, and a few cases occurred in women treated for infertility using human pituitary gonadotrophin. There were over 100 reports of CJD via human pituitary hormone transmission (Lueck, McIlwaine, & Zeidler, 2000), but the use of recombinant pituitary hormone therapy instead of pooled human tissue has largely eliminated this source of infection. Of great concern has been the possible transmission of CJD through blood or blood product transfusion. To date, two documented cases and one subclinical case of CJD in humans acquired via transfusion of blood or blood products have been reported (Hewitt, Llewelyn, MacKenzie, & Will, 2006; Llewelyn et al., 2004; Peden, Head, Ritchie, Bell, & Ironside, 2004). CJD has been transmitted from humans to animals via blood, however, and blood can transmit scrapie between animals (Brown, 2005). The prion is highly resistant to disinfection and sterilization processes. Prion diseases can be transmitted via stainless steel surgical instruments, and infective prions have shown resistance to the usual sterilization procedures, although recommendations for sterilization have been developed (Belay & Schonberger, 2005;

Head & Ironside, 2007; Sutton, Dickinson, Walker & Raven, 2006; Wadsworth et al., 2007). Other reusable instruments such as angioplasty catheters have been scrutinized as potential vehicles for CJD transmission, as have certain procedures involving lymphoid tissue such as appendectomy and tonsillectomy and procedures such as electromyography. In some areas such as Great Britain, disposable instruments are used in all adenotonsillectomy procedures. A recent study indicated that a proportion of surgical instruments ready for use had protein levels that could pose a risk of infection via prions (Murdoch et al., 2006). A review of recommendations regarding disinfection and sterilization methods may be found in Sutton et al. (2006).

Variant Creutzfeldt–Jakob Disease (vCJD)

In 1995, the CJD Surveillance Unit received notification about three cases of CJD. These patients were young (16, 19, and 29 years of age) and had amyloid plaques that were usually found in only 5% to 10% of sporadic cases of CJD (Bateman et al., 1995; Britton, Al-Sarraj, Shaw, Campbell, & Collinge, 1995; Brown et al., 2001). By December 1995, the unit had been informed of 10 suspected cases of CJD in persons under 50 years of age, some of whom were ultimately found to have sporadic or familial CJD. By early 1996, a distinct clinical syndrome was identified in 10 cases and led to the conclusion that a previously unrecognized variant of CJD was "probably due to exposure to BSE." This was named new variant CJD and then variant CJD (vCJD) (Brown et al., 2001; Will et al., 1996). Neurologists in the United Kingdom were contacted in an effort to try to identify additional cases. More cases continue to be reported. Foodborne transmission of BSE to humans, or in some cases transmission through contaminated blood or tissues, is still believed to be the cause of vCJD (Collinge, 2005; Ludlam & Turner, 2006). As of February 2007, the number of definitive and probable vCJD cases in the United Kingdom was 165, with 158 deaths (National Creutzfeldt-Jakob Disease Surveillance Unit, 2006). Relatively few cases have been reported outside the United Kingdom. The country with the next highest number of cases is France. Three U.S. cases have been identified, one in a 30-year-old man who lived in Houston, one in a 25-year-old Florida woman, and one in a Saudi Arabian native who had lived in the United States since 2005. The first two had previously lived in the United Kingdom, and the third was thought to have been infected as a child in Saudi Arabia (Center for Infectious Disease and Research Policy, 2005; Centers for Disease Control and Prevention, 2006).

In contrast to sporadic CJD, vCJD cases have an earlier age of onset with a mean age of 26 years (range of 12 to 74 years) and tend to

Table 21.4. New World Health Organization Variant Creutzfeldt–Jakob Disease Case Definition (17 May 2001)

Subtype		Characteristics
I	A	Progressive neuropsychiatric disorder
	B	Duration of illness >6 months
	C	Routine investigations do not suggest an alternative diagnosis
	D	No history of potential iatrogenic exposure
	E	No evidence of a familial form of TSE
II	A	Early psychiatric symptoms[a]
	B	Persistent painful sensory symptoms[b]
	C	Ataxia
	D	Myoclonus or chorea or dystonia
	E	Dementia
III	A	EEG does not show the typical appearance of sporadic CJD[c] (or no EEG performed)
	B	Bilateral pulvinar high signal on MRI
IV	A	Positive tonsil biopsy[d]
Definite vCJD		IA and neuropathological confirmation of vCJD[e]
Probable vCJD		I, 4/5 of II, and IIIA plus IIIB or IA plus IVA
Possible vCJD		I, 4/5 of II, and IIIA

EEG = electroencephalogram; MRI = magnetic resonance imaging; TSE = transmissible spongiform encephalopathies.
[a] Depression, anxiety, apathy, withdrawal, delusions.
[b] This includes both frank pain and/or dysaesthesia.
[c] Generalized triphasic periodic complexes at approximately 1 per second.
[d] Tonsil biopsy is not recommended routinely, nor in cases with EEG appearances typical of sporadic CJD, but may be useful in suspect cases in which the clinical features are compatible with vCJD and MRI does not show bilateral pulvinar high signal.
[e] Spongiform change and extensive PrP deposition, with florid plaques throughout the cerebrum and cerebellum.
Source: World Health Organization, 2001b.

present with behavioral changes or psychiatric symptoms such as agitation, aggression, anxiety, depression, and poor concentration. Sensory disturbances such as pain and parasthesias may also appear early. The median duration of illness is about 14 months (Tyler, 2005). Overt neurological signs, usually appearing about 6 months after the onset of illness, signal rapid progression, and cerebellar ataxia often appears early. This may be followed by cognitive impairment, involuntary movements, and incontinence of urine. Neurologic deterioration progresses, and the patient may become mute, immobile, and unresponsive (Will, 2003). Neuropathologically, extensive "florid" amyloid plaques are seen in the brain with surrounding spongiform changes (Glatzel et al., 2005). A revised and still current case definition for vCJD was released on May 17, 2001, by the WHO and is found in Table 21.4.

IMPLICATIONS

The outbreak of vCJD raised many questions and issues. Major concerns at the time included what the magnitude of the outbreak would ultimately be—in other words, how many people would be affected; what the geographic distribution would be because, since 2001, about 99% of known cases were in the United Kingdom; and what would be the length of the incubation period. Some of the more drastic predictions regarding the numbers of people who would be affected have not materialized. The knowledge that persons may be infected with abnormal prions and be clinically asymptomatic for long periods of time leads to questions about the potential transmission of vCJD by blood or blood product transfusion, or during medical/surgical procedures on such individuals who would not be recognized as subclinically infected. These procedures would include endoscopies, vascular catheterizations, surgical operations, and blood and organ donations. In vCJD, prions may concentrate in lymphoid tissue such as tonsils and the appendix. In persons with vCJD, biopsy of the tonsils may be used to detect characteristic prion proteins by immunostaining and Western blot. In other forms of CJD, these characteristic prion proteins are not detectable in tonsils, and no screening test is currently available (Collinge, 2005).

Various countries have issued recommendations excluding donors with certain characteristics and risks relating to vCJD from donating blood. The FDA Food and Drug Administration implemented a blood donor deferral policy in 1999. This policy excluded donors who had spent specified periods of time in the United Kingdom and other areas (Belay & Schonberger, 2005; Gottlieb, 1999). In the United Kingdom, all blood from U.K. donors is filtered to eliminate leukocytes since they have been implicated as carriers of infectivity. Prevention also extends to appropriate disinfection and sterilization processes, to revision of guidelines for transfusion of blood, and for modifications to surgical procedures such as appendectomies to minimize risk of transmission. In early 2001, it came to light that more than 1,500 Spaniards had apparently been treated with a drug made from the blood of multiple donors, one of whom died of vCJD, setting off anger at Britain over its "failure to control" BSE ("Exposure to CJD," 2001). Protection of health care workers and morticians from inadvertent infection has also been raised as an issue, and groups such as WHO have published guidelines available on the Internet (WHO, 2003).

Breaches in infection control in hospitals have come to light and posed ethical dilemmas. In one instance, in the United Kingdom, a baby was born to a mother by cesarean section. The mother had vCJD. The instruments were used on other such births with sterilization procedures that would not have killed prions, and there was a delay in notification of those families. The baby in the original case was found to have vCJD in February 2000. In another instance, a Melbourne, Australia, hospital notified nine neurosurgical patients that they might have been exposed to CJD. Surgical equipment used on an elderly person with CJD was used again with routine sterilization not adequate to destroy abnormal prions if present (Zinn, 2000). On May 9, 2006, a patient in Colorado who died after neurosurgery in March 2006 was confirmed as having classic CJD. Because instruments used on this person might have been used in neurosurgeries performed on six other patients, these people were notified about potential risk (Squires, 2006). Because CJD can take years to be manifested, actual disease transmission in these individuals will not be known for some time.

SUMMARY

Many uncertainties exist about the most worrisome human prion disease—vCJD. The concept of a conformationally altered protein causing transmissible disease is a relatively recent one. Attention brought to the BSE epidemic and the connection to the development of vCJD in humans has been intense. Social, economic, and political consequences and consumer reactions, sometimes bordering on hysteria, have occurred. Because the incubation period can be long, a test for detection of infection with abnormal prions before symptoms appear would be very desirable. To date, definitive diagnosis of vCJD is usually made through pathological examination of the brain, although altered prions can now be detected through pathological study of lymphoid tissue such as the tonsils. In the case of genetic forms, direct gene testing is available, and it is possible to do presymptomatic testing in at-risk family members. Such testing has many social and psychological implications for the person or family, and genetic counseling is required (Collinge, 2005; Lashley, 2005). Those at risk should be counseled to inform physicians and dentists prior to any procedures and to refrain from donation of blood or organs (Collinge, 2005). Rational policies for preventing infection by blood transfusion and other means are being developed. A rapid diagnostic test and successful treatment approaches are needed. In the United States, officials state that no one has been known to have contracted vCJD from eating U.S. beef, and the vCJD cases reported to date had previously lived, and presumably became infected, outside the United States. The transgenic development of prion-free cattle holds promise for the future (Richt et al., 2007).

REFERENCES

Alter, M. (2000). How is Creutzfeldt-Jakob disease acquired? *Neuroepidemiology*, *19*, 55–61.

Angers, R. C., Browning, S. R., Seward, T. S., Sigurdson, C. J., Miller, M. W., Hoover, E. A., et al. (2006). Prions in skeletal muscles of deer with chronic wasting disease. *Science, 311*, 1117.

Bateman, D., Hilton, D., Love, S., Zeidler, M., Beck, J., & Collinge, J. (1995). Sporadic Creutzfeldt-Jakob disease in an 18-year-old in the UK. *Lancet, 346*, 1155–1156.

Belay, E. D., & Schonberger, L. B. (2005). The public health impact of prion diseases. *Annual Review of Public Health, 26*, 191–212.

Blakeslee, S. (1999a, March 30). "Mad cow disease" seen in French zoos. *New York Times* [Electronic version]. Retrieved December 15, 2006, from http://www.nytimes.com.science/033099scilemur-madcow.html

Blakeslee, S. (1999b, February 23). Weighing 'mad cow' risks in American deer and elk. *New York Times* [Electronic version]. Retrieved December 15, 2006, from http://www.nytimes.com/library/national/science/022399sci-mad-elk.html

Blakeslee, S. (2000, October 31). Biologists say hunters should beware of brain disease. *New York Times* [Electronic version]. Retrieved from http://www.nytimes.com/2000/I0/31/science/31HUNT.html

Bratosiewicz-Wasik, J., Liberski, P. P., Golanska, E., Jansen, G. H., & Wasik, T. J. (2007). Regulatory sequences of the *PRNP* gene influence susceptibility to sporadic Creutzfeldt-Jakob disease. *Neuroscience Letters, 411*, 163–167.

Britton, T. C., Al-Sarraj, S., Shaw, C., Campbell, T., & Collinge, J. (1995). Sporadic Creutzfeldt-Jakob disease in a 16-year-old in the UK. *Lancet, 346*, 1155.

Brown, P. (2001). Bovine spongiform encephalopathy and variant Creutzfeldt-Jakob disease. *British Medical Journal, 322*, 841–844.

Brown, P. (2005). Blood infectivity, processing and screening tests in transmissible spongiform encephalopathy. *Vox Sanguinis, 89*, 63–70.

Brown, P., Will, R. G., Bradley, R., Asher, D. M., & Detwiler, L. (2001). Bovine spongiform encephalopathy and variant Creutzfeldt-Jakob disease: Background, evolution, and current concerns. *Emerging Infectious Diseases, 7*, 6–16.

Center for Infectious Disease and Research Policy. (2005, November 22). *Briton has second vCJD case found in US*. Retrieved June 3, 2006, from http://www.cidrap.umn.edu/cidrap/content/other/bse/news/nov2205vcjd.html

Centers for Disease Control and Prevention. (2006, August 14). Fact sheet: Variant Creutzfeldt–Jakob disease. Retrieved December 19, 2006, from http://www.cdc.gov/ncidod/dvrd/vcjd/factsheet_nvcjd.htm

Collinge, J. (2005). Molecular neurology of prion disease. *Journal of Neurology, Neurosurgery and Psychiatry, 76*, 906–919.

Collinge, J., Whitfield, J., McKintosh, E., Beck, J., Mead, S., Thomas, D. J., et al. (2006). Kuru in the 21st century—An acquired human prion disease with very long incubation periods. *Lancet, 367*, 2068–2074.

Collins, S. J., Lawson, V. A., & Masters, C. L. (2004). Transmissible spongiform encephalopathies. *Lancet, 363,* 51–61.

Cowley, G. (2001, March 12). Cannibals to cows: The path of a deadly disease. *Newsweek,* p. 52–61.

Daley, S. (2000, December 1). As mad cow disease spreads in Europe, consumers panic. *New York Times* [Electronic version]. Retrieved December 19, 2006, from http://www.nytimes.com/2000/12/Ol/world/01COW.html

Daszak, P., Cunningham, A. A., & Hyatt, A. D. (2000). Emerging infectious diseases of wildlife—Threats to biodiversity and human health. *Science, 287,* 443–449.

Duffy, P., Wolf, J., Collins, G., DeVoe, A. G., Streeten, B., & Cowen, D. (1974). Possible person-to-person transmission of Creutzfeldt-Jakob disease. *New England Journal of Medicine, 290,* 692–693.

Exposure to CJD from blood product? (2001). *ProMED Digest, 29,* unpaginated.

Focosi, D. (2006). Incubation period of human prion disease. *Lancet, 368,* 913–914.

Foster, J. D., Hope, J., & Fraser, H. (1993). Transmission of bovine spongiform encephalopathy to sheep and goats. *Veterinary Record, 128,* 119–203.

Gajdusek, D. C., & Zigas, V. (1957). Degenerative disease of the central nervous system in New Guinea: The endemic occurrence of "kuru" in the native population. *New England Journal of Medicine, 257,* 974–981.

Glatzel, M., Stoeck, K., Seeger, H., Lührs, T., & Aguzzi, A. (2005). Human prion diseases. *Archives of Neurology, 62,* 545–552.

Gottlieb, S. (1999). FDA bans blood donation by people who have lived in UK. *British Medical Journal, 319,* 535.

Head, M. W., & Ironside, J. W. (2007). vCJD and the gut: Implications for endoscopy. *Gut, 56,* 9–11.

Hewitt, P. A., Llewelyn, C. A., Mackenzie, J., & Will, R. G. (2006). Creutzfeldt-Jakob disease and blood transfusion: Results of the UK Transfusion Medicine Epidemological Review study. *Vox Sang, 91,* 221–230.

Hopkin, M. (2006). Sheep study calls for closer look at prion hypothesis. *Nature Medicine, 12,* 484.

Lashley, F. R. (2005). *Clinical genetics in nursing practice* (3rd ed.). New York: Springer.

Lashley, F. R. (2007). *Essentials of clinical genetics in nursing practice.* New York: Springer.

Llewelyn, C. A., Hewitt, P. E., Knight, R. S., Amar, K., Cousens, S., Mackenzie, J., et al. (2004). Possible transmission of variant Creutzfeldt-Jakob disease by blood transfusion. *Lancet, 363,* 417–421.

Ludlam, C. A., & Turner, M. L. (2006). Managing the risk of transmission of variant Creutzfeldt Jakob disease by blood products. *British Journal of Haematology, 132,* 13–24.

Lueck, C. J., Mcllwaine, G. G., & Zeidler, M. (2000). Creutzfeldt-Jakob disease and the eye. *Eye, 14,* 263–290.

Mabbott, N. A., & MacPherson, G. G. (2006). Prions and their lethal journey to the brain. *Nature Reviews Microbiology, 4,* 201–211.

Mathews, K. H., Jr., Vandeveer, M., & Gustafson, R. A. (2006, June). *An economic chronology of bovine spongiform encephalopathy in North America* (LDP-M-1143-01, pp. 1–19). Washington, DC: U.S. Department of Agriculture.

Mead, S. (2006). Prion disease genetics. *European Journal of Human Genetics, 14,* 273–281.

Montagna, P. (2005). Fatal familial insomnia: A model disease in sleep pathology. *Sleep Medicine Reviews, 9,* 339–353.

Murdoch, H., Taylor, D., Dickinson, J., Walker, J. T., Perrett, D., Raven, N. D., et al. (2006). Surface decontamination of surgical instruments: An ongoing dilemma. *Journal of Hospital Infection, 63,* 432–438.

National Creutzfeldt-Jakob Disease Surveillance Unit. (2007). *CJD Statistics.* Retrieved February 13, 2007, from http://www.cjd.ed.ac.uk/figures.htm

Online Mendelian Inheritance in Man, OMIM™. McKusick–Nathans Institute for Genetic Medicine, Johns Hopkins University, (Baltimore, MD), and the National Center for Biotechnology Information, National Library of Medicine, (Bethesda, MD). (2007). Retrieved January 2, 2007, from http://www.ncbi.nlm.nih.gov/omim/

Peden, A. H., Head, M. W., Ritchie, D. L., Bell, J. E., & Ironside, J. W. (2004). Preclinical CJD after blood transfusion in a PRNP codon 129 heterozygous patient. *Lancet, 364,* 529–531.

Prusiner, S. B. (1982). Novel proteinaceous infectious particles cause scrapie. *Science, 216,* 136–144.

Prusiner, S. B. (2001). Shattuck lecture-neurodegerative diseases and prions. *New England Journal of Medicine, 344,* 1516–1524.

Rampton, S., & Stauber, J. (1997). *Mad cow USA. Could the nightmare happen here?* Monroe, ME: Common Courage Press.

Rhodes, R. (1997). *Deadly feasts.* New York: Simon & Schuster.

Richt, J. A., Kasinathan, P., Hamir, A. N., Castilla, J., Sathiyaseelan, T., Vargas, F., et al. (2007). Production of cattle lacking prion protein. *Nature Biotechnology, 25,* 132–138.

Sigurdson, C. J., & Miller, M. W. (2003). Other animal prion diseases. *British Medical Bulletin, 66,* 199–212.

Soto, C., Estrada, L., & Castilla, J. (2006). Amyloids, prions and the inherent infectious nature of misfolded protein aggregates. *Trends in Biochemical Science, 31,* 150–155.

Squires, C. (2006). *Colo. patient dies of rare brain disease.* Retrieved May 19, 2006, from http://cnn.netscape.cnn.com/newstory.jsp?idq=/ff/story/0001/20060518/2241402611.htm

Sutton, J. M., Dickinson, J., Walker, J. T., & Raven, N. D. H. (2006). Methods to minimize the risks of Creutzfeldt-Jakob disease transmission by surgical procedures: Where to set the standard? *Clinical Infectious Diseases, 43,* 757–764.

Timeline: How the crisis unfolded. (2000, October 25). *CNN.com* [Electronic version]. Retrieved December 16, 2006, from wysiwyg://26/http://europe.cnn.com

Tyler, K. L. (2005). Prions and prion diseases of the central nervous system (transmissible neurodegenerative diseases). In G. L. Mandell, J. Bennett, & R.

Dolin. (Eds.), *Mandell, Douglas, and Bennett's principles and practice of infectious diseases* (6th ed., pp. 2219–2235). Philadelphia: Churchill Livingstone Elsevier.

U.S. Department of Agriculture. (2001, 23 March). *USDA removes quarantined sheep from second Vermont farm* (News Release No. 0053.01). Washinton, DC: Author.

Wadsworth, J. D. F., Hill, A. F., Beck, J. A., & Collinge, J. (2003). Molecular and clinical classification of human prion disease. *British Medical Bulletin, 66,* 241–254.

Wadsworth, J. D. F., Joiner, S., Fox, K., Linehan, J. M., Desbruslais, M., Brandner, S., et al. (2007). Prion infectivity in variant Creutzfeldt—Jacob disease rectum. *Gut, 56,* 90–94.

Wells, G. H., Scott, A. C., Johnson C. I., Gunning, R. F., Hancock, R. D., & Jeffrey, M. (1987). A novel progressive spongiform encephalopathy in cattle. *Veterinary Record, 121,* 419–420.

Will, R. G. (2003). Acquired prion disease: Iatrogenic CJD, variant CJD, kuru. *British Medical Bulletin, 66,* 255–265.

Will, R. G., Ironside, J. W., Zeidler, M., Cousens, S. N., Estibeiro, K., Alperovitch, A., et al. (1996). A new variant of Creutzfeldt-Jakob disease in the U.K. *Lancet, 347,* 921–925.

World Health Organization. (1998). Human transmissible spongiform encephalopathies. *Weekly Epidemiological Record, 73,* 361–366.

World Health Organization. (2000). *WHO infection control guidelines for transmissible spongiform encephalopathies. Report of a WHO consultation, Geneva, Switzerland, 23–26 March 1999* (WHO/CDS/CSR/APH/2000.3). Retrieved December 19, 2006, from http://www.who.int/emc/diseases/bse/index.html

World Health Organization. (2001a, June 14). *Joint WHO/FAO/OIE technical consultation on BSE: Public health, animal health and trade* (Press Release WHO/28). Retrieved December 19, 2006, from http://www.who.int/inf-pr-2001/en/pr2001-28.html

World Health Organization. (2001b, May 17). New case definition for variant Creutzfeldt-Jakob disease (vCJD). *Communicable Disease Surveillance and Response (CSR).* Retrieved December 19, 2006, from http://www.who.int/emc/diseases/bse/index.html

World Health Organization. (2003). Infection control guidelines for transmissible spongiform encephalopathies. Retrieved December 19, 2006, from http://www.who.int/csr/resources/publications/bse/whocdscraph2003.pdf.

Zinn, C. (2000). Nine hospital patients may have been exposed to CJD. *British Medical Journal, 320,* 1296.

CHAPTER TWENTY-TWO

SARS

From Zoonosis to Pandemic Threat

Bart L. Haagmans and Albert D. M. E. Osterhaus

Severe acute respiratory syndrome (SARS), characterized by a rapidly progressive atypical pneumonia, emerged in southern China in November 2002. Subsequent outbreaks occurred in early 2003 in Hong Kong, Hanoi, Toronto, and Singapore and could be directly traced back to one index patient who acquired the infection in Guangdong and travelled to Hong Kong. The index patient for each of the above clusters had stayed at the same hotel in Hong Kong as the initial (Case A) patient, a physician (Parashar & Anderson, 2004). The World Health Organization (WHO) issued a global alert in February 2003 (Skowronski et al., 2005). Overall, 30 countries have reported a total of 8,098 probable cases of SARS. Eventually, the cause of the illness was revealed to be a SARS-associated coronavirus (SARS-CoV).

The clinical symptoms of SARS patients were those of lower respiratory tract disease. Upon admission the clinical features included fever, nonproductive cough, myalgia, and dyspnea, whereas only few patients reported rhinorrhea (Peiris, Lai, et al., 2003; Wang et al., 2004). Besides these symptoms, affected individuals had peripheral T-cell lymphocytopenia, thrombocytopenia, prolonged coagulation profiles, and mildly elevated serum hepatic enzymes.

The clinical course of SARS follows two phases: one in which there is active viral replication and the patients experience the systemic symptoms and one in which there is immunopathological injury and progression of pneumonia. Chest radiography reveals infiltrates with subpleural consolidation or "ground-glass" changes compatible with viral pneumonitis. Around 20–30% of individuals with SARS require management in intensive care units, and the overall fatality rate reaches approximately 10%. In typical cases, which are largely confined to adult and elderly individuals, SARS presents with acute respiratory distress syndrome (ARDS), characterized by the presence of diffuse alveolar damage (DAD) and multiorgan dysfunction (MOD) upon autopsy (Franks et al., 2003). The pathological changes in lung alveoli most likely follow a common pathway characterized by an acute phase of protein-rich alveolar fluid influx into the alveolar lumina as a consequence of the injury to the alveolar wall (Nicholls et al., 2003). Subsequently, Type 2 pneumocyte hyperplasia takes place to replace the loss of infected Type 1 pneumocytes and to cover the denuded epithelial basement membrane, resulting in restoration of the normal alveolar architecture. Severe alveolar injury may lead to fibrosis with loss of alveolar function in more protracted cases. In the acute phase, there is a strong inflammatory response characterized by the production of several cytokines, including interleukin (IL)-6, IL-8, and interferon (IFN)-γ-inducible protein 10 (IP-10; Wong, Lam, et al., 2004). This strong host response may be involved in the complications of SARS.

Although the main clinical symptoms are those of severe respiratory illness, SARS-CoV actually also causes a gastrointestinal and urinary tract infection: SARS-CoV was detected in the feces and urine of patients (Chan et al., 2004). Fecal transmission proved to be important in at least one major community outbreak in Hong Kong (Amoy Gardens), in which over 300 patients were infected within a few days.

Transmission of the virus may have been affected by several factors. Unlike the situation with several other respiratory viral infections, viral load of SARS-CoV in the upper respiratory tract increased progressively to peak at around day 10 after disease onset (Peiris, Chu, et al., 2003). Therefore, virus transmission is lower in the first days of illness, a finding supported by epidemiological observations. Second, the viral load in the nasopharyngeal aspirate may vary quite significantly (Hung et al., 2004). Finally, a progressive association between age and disease severity was observed in SARS patients, and none of the SARS-CoV-infected children required intensive care (Peiris, Chu, et al., 2003). So far, no satisfactory explanation for this finding has been reported, but it may point to the importance of comorbid factors. Interestingly, age dependence in severity of DAD, ARDS, MOD, and mortality has also been observed in other (nonviral) causes of ARDS (Rubenfeld et al., 2005). Overall, the transmissibility of SARS-CoV as indicated by the reproductive number (R_0) has been estimated to be relatively low (2–3; Lipsitch et al., 2003; Riley et al., 2003). In these analyses, superspreading events have not been taken into account; therefore dissemination by patients (such as the person who traveled from Guangdong to Hong Kong and spread the infection to at least 16 hotel guests in Hong Kong and the subsequent infection of 138 patients by the same patient after admission) may have been crucial in the subsequent global spread of SARS-CoV. Factors associated with superspreading events are not well understood but may include coinfection with other viruses as well as host factors such as immunosuppression and/or environmental factors.

Although several infectious agents, including a *Chlamydia* and human metapneumovirus, were considered as the causative agent, the clinical progression, lack of response to antibiotics, and/or the inability to confirm these findings in the majority of patients argued against their role. Moreover, fatal severe disease due to human metapneumovirus infection previously had been observed only in immunosuppressed patients. Three groups independently reported the isolation of a previously undiscovered CoV from clinical specimens of SARS patients (Drosten et al., 2003; Ksiazek et al., 2003; Peiris, Lai, et al., 2003). Through electron microscopy, serology, and reverse transcription polymerase chain reaction (RT-PCR) with consensus and random primers and subsequent sequencing of the whole genome, its identity could be revealed (Marra et al., 2003, Rota et al., 2003). This virus was consistently found in clinical specimens from patients with the disease and not in healthy controls.

A crucial requirement for the fulfillment of Koch's postulates to establish the cause of an infectious disease is reproduction of the disease in a relevant animal model. Infection of cynomolgus macaques (*Macaca fascicularis*) with a SARS-CoV isolate led to disease for which the pathology was similar to that seen in human patients with SARS, with epithelial necrosis, serosanguinous alveolar exudates, hyaline membranes, Type 2 pneumocyte hyperplasia, and the presence of syncytia (Fouchier et al., 2003; Kuiken et al., 2003). The virus was successfully reisolated from these lesions and detected in Type 1 and Type 2 pneumocytes, and an antibody response to the virus was shown in the infected animals. By contrast, infection of macaques with human metapneumovirus did not result in the same pathology and produced a mild suppurative rhinitis in some animals with erosions in the infected airways. Since the presence of SARS-CoV was confirmed in the majority of patients with suspected SARS, since the pathology caused by SARS-CoV infection in macaques was pathologically similar to that seen in human patients with SARS, since the virus was successfully reisolated from lung lesions of these animals, and since a specific antibody response to the virus was shown in the infected animals, scientists concluded that SARS-CoV is the causative agent of this infectious disease entity.

SARS-CoV is a positive-stranded RNA virus, related to CoVs from Group 2 despite the fact that it does not encode a hemagglutinin-esterase

Table 22.1. Clinical Evidence for SARS for Surveillance Purposes

---

A clinical case of SARS is an individual with

1. A history of fever or documented fever >38° C (100.4° F),
   AND

2. One or more symptoms of lower respiratory tract illness (cough, difficulty breathing, shortness of breath),
   AND

3. Radiographic evidence of lung infiltrates consistent with pneumonia or ARDS or autopsy findings consistent with the pathology of pneumonia or ARDS without an identifiable cause,
   AND

4. No alternative diagnosis can fully explain the illness.

Source: World Health Organization, 2004, p. 13.

protein (Snijder et al., 2003). The genome contains nine open reading frames (ORFs), which encode two large polyproteins with diverse enzymatic activities needed for efficient replication, several structural proteins, and accessory proteins with unknown function (ORF3a/b, ORF6, ORF7a/b, ORF8a/b, and ORF9b). ORFs 2–8 are encoded in subgenomic messenger RNAs synthesized as a nested set of 3' coterminal molecules. The genome is packaged together with the nucleocapsid protein, several membrane proteins (M, E, and ORF3a), and the spike protein. These spike proteins form the typical "corona" as seen by electron microscopy and constitute the major antigenic determinants, mediate receptor association, and fusion of viral and cellular membranes. Wong, Li, Moore, Choe, and Farzan (2004) demonstrated that a 193-amino acid fragment of the S protein (corresponding to residues 318–510) located in the S1 region interacts with the viral receptor, angiotensin-converting enzyme 2 (ACE2; Li et al., 2003). Angiotensin-converting enzyme 2 is expressed in the lung and in the gastrointestinal tract (Hamming et al., 2004). In addition, diverse members of the DC-SIGN family of proteins (such as DC-SIGN and L-SIGN) may enhance infection of ACE2-expressing cells (Jeffers et al., 2004). After engagement with ACE2 and proteolysis mediated by cathepsin L in an endosomal or lysosomal compartment (Simmons et al., 2005), SARS-CoV fuses with host cell membranes after conformational changes of the two heptad regions located in the S2 region, HR-1 and HR-2 (Bosch et al., 2004; Liu et al., 2004).

Clinical symptoms of acute respiratory disease, together with epidemiological data, may lead to the suspicion that a patient suffers from SARS. The WHO developed clinical evidence to be used for public health surveillance purposes as shown in Table 22.1. Other definitions are available from other agencies such as the Centers for Disease Control and Prevention (CDC) at http://www.cdc.gov/ncidod/sars. Although seroconversion usually occurs in Weeks 2 or 3 of illness, serodiagnosis represents the gold standard for confirmation of a SARS diagnosis. Real-time PCR assays, however, usually detect SARS-CoV during the first week in specimens of the lower respiratory tract (e.g., bronchoalveolar lavage, sputum, endotracheal aspirates), nasopharyngeal aspirate, throat swabs, and/or serum (Chan et al., 2004). Fecal samples may show very high viral loads toward the end of the first week and second week of illness. In the event that SARS returns, laboratories will be faced with significant challenges to diagnose SARS because of other respiratory viruses circulating and a range of assays to detect SARS-CoV in clinical samples that have been tested on few clinical samples thus far. Testing of multiple respiratory and nonrespiratory specimens from the same patient and conformation by a reference laboratory should be considered.

The fact that many of the early SARS patients in Guangdong had epidemiological links to the live-animal market trade was consistent with the hypothesis that an animal virus had become transmissible from human to human. Sampling of several animal species found in one of the live-game markets in Guangdong revealed that some of them had been exposed to a virus genetically and antigenically related to the human SARS-CoV. In particular, a SARS-like coronavirus was detected by RT-PCR in the nasal and fecal swabs of palm civets (*Paguma larvata*) and a raccoon dog (*Nyctereutes procyonoides*; Guan et al., 2003). Several lines of evidence suggest that these animals served as intermediate hosts for the virus as the vast majority of civets on farms were found negative for SARS-CoV (Tu et al., 2004) and viruses isolated from palm civets genetically evolved quite rapidly in these animals (He et al., 2004, Kan et al., 2005). Although subsequent studies suggested horseshoe bats (*Rhinolophus* spp.) as a possible natural reservoir for SARS-CoV-like viruses, sequence comparison of the spike genes from bat SARS-like CoV and palm civet SARS-like CoV revealed only 64% genetic homology (Lau et al., 2005; Li, Shi, et al., 2005). More recent studies have demonstrated that approximately 6% of bats sampled in China were positive for CoVs (Tang et al., 2006). Interestingly, these CoVs are genetically diverse, and many bat CoVs clustered with existing Group 1 viruses, while others formed a separate lineage that included only viruses from bats (putative Group 5). Other SARS-CoV-like viruses clustered in a putative Group 4 consisting of two subgroups, one of bat CoVs and another of SARS-CoVs from humans and other mammalian hosts. However, from these studies the direct progenitor of the SARS-CoV isolated from palm civets has not been determined.

Genetic sequencing of the CoVs found in palm civets revealed more than 99% homology with human SARS-CoV, but a 29-nucleotide deletion in ORF8 (Song et al., 2005). In addition, viruses with a 415-nucleotide deletion resulting in the loss of the whole ORF8 region were found at the late phase of the outbreak. These results indicated that the expression of ORF8 is dispensable for SARS-CoV infection of humans. In addition, it was demonstrated that spike proteins from isolates of palm civets utilized civet ACE2 more efficiently than human ACE2, whereas late-phase isolates such as TOR2 utilized both receptors with equal efficiency (Li, Zhang, et al., 2005). These differences could be explained by specific amino acid differences in the spike protein region that interacts with ACE2. Precursors of SARS-CoV in animals are thus likely to be less pathogenic to humans, and exposure to such viruses may have led to antigenic stimulation that results in a serological response. This was observed when SARS-CoV reemerged in four patients in Guangdong in December 2003, causing a milder clinical disease (Liang et al., 2004). Similarly, animal traders working with live animals had high seroprevalence for both the human and animal SARS coronavirus, although they did not have a history of SARS.

Possible options for the reemergence of SARS include the undetected continued transmission of the virus from the outbreak in the summer of 2003, escape of the virus from laboratories that handle live SARS coronavirus (Lim et al., 2004), or the reemergence of SARS-CoV or a related virus from an animal reservoir. There is no evidence at present that the virus has persisted in the human population. Although the virus may be detected by RT-PCR in the feces for months after the onset of disease, virus isolation is rarely possible after the third week of illness, and there is no evidence for disease transmission by patients in late convalescence. The reemergence of SARS-CoV or related viruses from animal reservoirs remains possible, given that SARS-CoV is detectable in the feces and respiratory secretions of small mammals within live-animal markets in southern China. Reemergence in four patients with SARS in Guangdong in December 2003 and January 2004, along with molecular epidemiological linkage to viruses isolated from animals in live-game markets, prompted the wholesale cull of palm civets and other small mammals in these markets in January 2004. No further human cases of SARS acquired from animals have since been reported.

The major sources of transmission in humans are droplets that deposit on the respiratory epithelium. Later in the outbreak, it was shown that isolation, quarantine, and personal protective equipment significantly decreased nosocomial infections and played a significant role in outbreak management. The first efforts to treat SARS patients were mainly based on the use of ribavirin and corticosteroids. Ribavirin, which targets inosine monophosphate dehydrogenase, has been known for a long time as a broad-spectrum antiviral agent. However, current data do not support the use of ribavirin for SARS treatment as in vitro studies did not show significant antiviral activity and ribavirin enhanced the infectivity of SARS-CoV in mice (Barnard et al., 2006). Corticosteroids significantly reduced IL-8 and IP-10 serum levels 5–8 days after treatment; however, when given in the earlier phase they may prolong viremia (Lee et al., 2004). On the other hand, a protective effect of IFN-α has been obtained in a preliminary study during the SARS outbreak (Loutfy et al., 2003). These results are in concordance with several studies that noted antiviral activity in vitro (Cinatl et al., 2003) and animal studies showing that pegylated IFN-α effectively reduced SARS-CoV replication and excretion, viral antigen expression by Type 1 pneumocytes, and the pulmonary damage in cynomolgus macaques that were infected experimentally with SARS-CoV (Haagmans et al., 2004). Because IFNs are used clinically to treat viral infections, these drugs could be considered for off-label use in SARS prophylactic or early postexposure treatment of SARS if it should reemerge.

In SARS patients who recover, high levels of spike glycoprotein-specific antibody responses are observed, suggesting that antibody responses play a role in determining the ultimate disease outcome of SARS-CoV-infected patients (Zhang et al., 2006). The protective efficacy of SARS-CoV-neutralizing human antibodies was demonstrated in vitro and in several animal models. Prophylactic administration of a human monoclonal antibody at 10 mg/kg reduced replication of SARS-CoV in the lungs of infected ferrets by 3 logs, completely prevented the development of SARS-CoV-induced macroscopic lung pathology, and abolished shedding of virus in pharyngeal secretions (Ter Meulen et al., 2004). Other monoclonal antibodies were evaluated for their efficacy in mouse and hamster models (Roberts et al., 2006; Sui et al., 2005; Traggiai et al., 2004). Although enhanced entry of certain SARS-CoV pseudotyped viruses in Vero cells was observed in the presence of antibodies directed against the spike protein (Yang et al., 2005), its relevance in vivo still awaits further investigation. So far there is no evidence for antibody-dependent enhancement of infection as described earlier for feline coronavirus, in which case passive and active immunization against feline coronavirus enhanced feline coronavirus infection and caused early death (Vennema et al., 1990).

These results provided evidence that vaccines able to elicit neutralizing antibodies are likely to be effective against SARS. Less than a year after the first SARS outbreak, a range of candidate vaccines was developed and early in 2006 some companies in China and the United States initiated Phase I trials, and several other candidate SARS vaccines are at various stages of preclinical and clinical development. Although much effort has been focused on developing a SARS vaccine, the commercial viability of developing a vaccine for SARS-CoV will ultimately depend on whether the virus reemerges in the near future. It is not clear whether future outbreaks should be expected, but vaccines, antivirals, or passive immunization would be relevant in the context of protecting high-risk individuals such as laboratory and health care workers. Future vaccines may be generated from the full-length infectious complementary DNA clone of SARS-CoV. This clone may provide a source for genetic manipulation of the genome (Yount, Roberts, Lindesmith, & Baric, 2006). Once the viral virulence factors are understood, attenuated strains may be obtained through manipulation of the SARS-CoV genome and may be considered as attenuated live vaccines.

REFERENCES

Barnard, D. L., Day, C. W., Bailey, K., Heiner, M., Montgomery, R., Lauridsen, L., et al. (2006). Enhancement of the infectivity of SARS-CoV in BALB/c mice by IMP dehydrogenase inhibitors, including ribavirin. *Antiviral Research, 71,* 53–63.

Bosch B. J., Martina, B. E. E., Van der Zee, R., Lepault, J., Haijema, B. J., Versluis, C., et al. (2004). Severe acute respiratory syndrome coronavirus (SARS-CoV) infection inhibition using spike protein heptad repeat-derived peptides. *Proceedings of the National Academy Sciences, USA, 101,* 8455–8460.

Chan, K. H., Poon, L. L., Cheng, V. C., Guan, Y., Hung, I. F., Kong, J., et al. (2004). Detection of SARS coronavirus in patients with suspected SARS. *Emerging Infectious Diseases, 10,* 294–299.

Cinatl, J., Morgenstern, B., Bauer, G., Chandra, P., Rabenau, H., & Doerr, H. W. (2003). Treatment of SARS with human interferons. *Lancet, 362,* 293–294.

Drosten, C., Gunther, S., Preiser, W., van der Werf, S., Brodt, H. R., Becker, S., et al. (2003). Identification of a novel coronavirus in patients with severe acute respiratory syndrome. *New England Journal of Medicine, 348,* 1967–1976.

Fouchier, R. A., Kuiken, T., Schutten, M., van Amerongen, G., van Doornum, G. J., van den Hoogen, et al. (2003). Aetiology: Koch's postulates fulfilled for SARS virus. *Nature, 423,* 240.

Franks, T. J., Chong, P. Y., Chui, P., Galvin, J. R., Lourens, R. M., Reid, A. H., et al. (2003). Lung pathology of severe acute respiratory syndrome (SARS): A study of 8 autopsy cases from Singapore. *Human Pathology, 34,* 743–748.

Guan, Y., Zheng, B. J., He, Y. Q., Liu, X. L., Zhuang, Z. X., Cheung, C. L., et al. (2003). Isolation and characterization of viruses related to the SARS coronavirus from animals in southern China. *Science, 302,* 276–278.

Haagmans, B. L., Kuiken, T., Martina, B. E., Fouchier, R. A., Rimmelzwaan, G. F., van Amerongen, G., et al. (2004). Pegylated interferon-alpha protects type 1 pneumocytes against SARS coronavirus infection in macaques. *Nature Medicine, 10,* 290–293.

Hamming, I., Timens, W., Bulthuis, M. L., Lely, A. T., Navis, G. J., & van Goor, H. (2004). Tissue distribution of ACE2 protein, the functional receptor for

SARS coronavirus. A first step in understanding SARS pathogenesis. *Journal of Pathology, 203,* 631–637.

He, J. F., Peng, G. W., Min, J., Yu, D. W., Liang, W. J., Zhang, S. Y., et al. (2004). Molecular evolution of the SARS coronavirus during the course of the SARS epidemic in China. *Science, 303,* 1666–1669.

Hung, I. F., Cheng, V. C., Wu, A. K., Tang, B. S., Chan, K. H., Chu, C. M., et al. (2004). Viral loads in clinical specimens and SARS manifestations. *Emerging Infectious Diseases, 10,* 1550–1557.

Jeffers, S. A., Tusell, S. M., Gillim-Ross, L., Hemmila, E. M., Achenbach, J. E., Babcock, G. J., et al. (2004). CD209L (L-SIGN) is a receptor for severe acute respiratory syndrome coronavirus. *Proceedings National Academy Sciences, USA, 101,* 15748–15753.

Kan, B., Wang, M., Jing, H., Xu, H., Jiang, X., Yan, M., et al. (2005). Molecular evolution analysis and geographic investigation of severe acute respiratory syndrome coronavirus-like virus in palm civets at an animal market and on farms. *Journal of Virology, 79,* 11892–11900.

Ksiazek, T. G., Erdman, D., Goldsmith, C. S., Zaki, S. R., Peret, T., Emery, S., et al. (2003). A novel coronavirus associated with severe acute respiratory syndrome. *New England Journal of Medicine, 348,* 1953–1966.

Kuiken, T., Fouchier, R. A., Schutten, M., Rimmelzwaan, G. F., van Amerongen, G., van Riel, D., et al. (2003). Newly discovered coronavirus as the primary cause of severe acute respiratory syndrome. *Lancet, 362,* 263–270.

Lau, S. K., Woo, P. C., Li, K. S., Huang, Y., Tsoi, H. W., Wong, B. H., et al. (2005). Severe acute respiratory syndrome coronavirus-like virus in Chinese horseshoe bats. *Proceedings National Academy Sciences, USA, 102,* 14040–14045.

Lee, N., Allen Chan, K. C., Hui, D., Ng, E., Wu, A., Chiu, R., et al. (2004). Effects of early corticosteroid treatment on plasma SARS-associated coronavirus RNA concentrations in adult patients. *Journal of Clinical Virology, 31,* 304–309.

Li, W., Moore, M. J., Vasilieva, N., Sui, J., Wong, S. K., Berne, M. A., et al. (2003). Angiotensin-converting enzyme 2 is a functional receptor for the SARS coronavirus. *Nature, 426,* 450–454.

Li, W., Shi, Z., Yu, M., Ren, W., Smith, C., Epstein, J. H., et al. (2005). Bats are natural reservoirs of SARS-like coronaviruses. *Science, 310,* 676–679.

Li, W., Zhang, C., Sui, J., Kuhn, J. H., Moore, M. J., Luo, S., et al. (2005). Receptor and viral determinants of SARS coronavirus adaptation to human ACE2. *The EMBO Journal, 24,* 1634–1643.

Liang, G., Chen, Q., Xu, J., Liu, Y., Lim, W., Peiris, J. S., et al. (2004). Laboratory diagnosis of four recent sporadic cases of community-acquired SARS, Guangdong province, China. *Emerging Infectious Diseases, 10,* 1774–1781.

Lim, P. L., Kurup, A., Gopalakrishna, G., Chan, K. P., Wong, C. W., Ng, L. C., et al. (2004). Laboratory-acquired severe acute respiratory syndrome. *New England Journal of Medicine, 350,* 1740–1745.

Lipsitch, M., Cohen, T., Cooper, T. Robins, J. M., Ma, S., James L., et al. (2003) Transmission dynamics and control of severe acute respiratory syndrome. *Science, 300,* 1966–1970.

Liu, S., Xiao, G., Chen, Y., He, Y., Niu, J., Escalante, C. R., et al. (2004). Interaction between heptad repeat 1 and 2 regions in spike protein of SARS associated coronavirus: Implications for virus fusogenic mechanism and identification of fusion inhibitors. *Lancet, 363,* 938–947.

Loutfy, M. R., Blatt, L. M., Siminovitch, K. A., Ward, S., Wolff, B., Lho, H., et al. (2003). Interferon alfacon-1 plus corticosteroids in severe acute respiratory syndrome: A preliminary study. *Journal of the American Medical Association, 290,* 3222–3228.

Marra, M. A., Jones, S. J., Astell, C. R., Holt, R. A., Brooks-Wilson, A., Butterfield, Y. S., et al. (2003). The genome sequence of the SARS-associated coronavirus. *Science, 300,* 1399–1404.

Nicholls, J. M., Poon, L., Lee, K., Ng, W., Lai, S., Leung, C., et al. (2003). Lung pathology of fatal severe acute respiratory syndrome. *Lancet, 361,* 1773–1178.

Parashar, U. D., & Anderson, L. J. (2004). Severe acute respiratory syndrome: Review and lessons of the 2003 outbreak. *International Journal of Epidemiology, 33,* 628–634.

Peiris, J. S., Lai, S. T., Poon, L. L., Guan, Y., Yam, L. Y., Lim, W., et al. (2003). Coronavirus as a possible cause of severe acute respiratory syndrome. *Lancet, 361,* 1319–1325.

Peiris, J. S. M., Chu, C. M., Cheng, V. C., Chan, K. S., Hung, I. F., Poon, L. L., et al. (2003). Clinical progression and viral load in a community outbreak of coronavirus-associated SARS pneumonia: A prospective study. *Lancet, 361,* 1767–1772.

Riley, S., Fraser, C., Donnelly, C. A., Ghani, A. C., Abu-Raddad, L. J., Hedley A. J., et al. (2003). Transmission dynamics of the etiological agent of SARS in Hong Kong: Impact of public health interventions. *Science, 300,* 1961–1966.

Roberts, A., Thomas, W. D., Guarner, J., Lamirande, E. W., Babcock, G. J., Greenough, T. C., et al. (2006). Therapy with a severe acute respiratory syndrome–associated coronavirus-neutralizing human monoclonal antibody reduces disease severity and viral burden in golden syrian hamsters. *Journal of Infectious Diseases, 193,* 685–692.

Rota, P. A., Oberste, M. S., Monroe, S. S., Nix, W. A., Campagnoli, R., Icenogle, J. P., et al. (2003). Characterization of a novel coronavirus associated with severe acute respiratory syndrome. *Science, 300,* 1394–1399.

Rubenfeld, G. D., Caldwell, E., Peabody, E., Weaver, J., Martin, D. P., Neff, M., et al. (2005). Incidence and outcomes of acute lung injury. *New England Journal of Medicine, 353,* 1685–1693.

Simmons, G., Gosalia, D. N., Rennekamp, A. J., Reeves, J. D., Diamond, S. L., & Bates, P. (2005). Inhibitors of cathepsin L prevent severe acute respiratory syndrome coronavirus entry. *Proceedings of the National Academy Sciences, USA, 102,* 11876–11881.

Skowronski, D. M., Astell, C., Brunham, R. C., Low, D. E., Petric, M., Roper, R. L., et al. (2005). Severe acute respiratory syndrome (SARS): A year in review. *Annual Review of Medicine, 56,* 357–381.

Snijder, E. J., Bredenbeek, P. J., Dobbe, J. C., Thiel, V., Ziebuhr, J., Poon, L. L., et al. (2003). Unique and conserved features of genome and proteome of SARS-coronavirus, an early split-off from the coronavirus group 2 lineage. *Journal Molecular Biology, 331,* 991–1004.

Song, H. D., Tu, C. C., Zhang, G. W., Wang, S. Y., Zheng, K., Lei, L. C., et al. (2005). Cross-host evolution of severe acute respiratory syndrome coronavirus in palm civet and human. *Proceedings of the National Academy Sciences, USA, 102,* 2430–2435.

Sui, J., Li, W., Roberts, A., Matthews, L. J., Murakami, A., Vogel, L., et al. (2005). Evaluation of human monoclonal antibody 80R for immunoprophylaxis of severe acute respiratory syndrome by an animal study, epitope mapping, and analysis of spike variants. *Journal of Virology, 79,* 5900–5906.

Tang, X. C., Zhang, J. X., Zhang, S. Y., Wang, P., Fan, X. H., Li, L. F., et al. (2006). Prevelance and genetic diversity of coronaviruses in bats from China. *Journal of Virology, 80,* 7481–7490.

Ter Meulen, J., Bakker, A. B., van den Brink, E. N., Weverling, G. J., Martina, B. E., Haagmans, B. L., et al. (2004). Human monoclonal antibody as prophylaxis for SARS coronavirus infection in ferrets. *Lancet, 363,* 2139–2141.

Traggiai, E., Becker, S., Subbarao, K., Kolesnikova, L., Uematsu, Y., Gismondo, M. R., et al. (2004). An efficient method to make human monoclonal antibodies from memory B cells: Potent neutralization of SARS coronavirus. *Nature Medicine, 10,* 871–875.

Tu, C., Crameri, G., Kong, X., Chen, J., Sun, Y., Yu, M., et al. (2004). Antibodies to SARS coronavirus in civets. *Emerging Infectious Diseases, 10,* 2244–2248.

Vennema, H., De Groot, R. J., Harbour, D. A., Dalderup, M., Gruffydd-Jones, T., Horzinek, M. C., et al. (1990). Early death after feline infectious peritonitis virus challenge due to recombinant vaccinia virus immunization. *Journal of Virology, 64,* 1407–1409.

Wang J. T., Sheng, W. H., Fang, C. T., Chen, Y. C., Wang, J. L., Yu, C. J., et al. (2004). Clinical manifestations, laboratory findings, and treatment outcomes of SARS patients. *Emerging Infectious Diseases, 10,* 818–824.

Wong, C. K., Lam, C. W., Wu, A. K., Ip, W. K., Lee, N. L., Chan, I. H., et al. (2004) Plasma inflammatory cytokines and chemokines in severe acute respiratory syndrome. *Clinical Experimental Immunology, 136,* 95–103.

Wong, S. K., Li, W., Moore, M. J., Choe, H., & Farzan, M. (2004). A 193-amino acid fragment of the SARS coronavirus S protein efficiently binds angiotensin-converting enzyme 2. *Journal of Biological Chemistry, 279,* 3197–3201.

World Health Organization. (2004, October). *WHO guidelines for the global surveillance of severe acute respiratory syndrome (SARS). Updated recommendations.* Geneva, Switzerland: World Health Organization Department of Communicable Disease, Surveillance, and Response.

Yang, Z. Y., Werner, H. C., Kong, W. P., Leung, K., Traggiai, E., Lanzavecchia, A., et al. (2005). Evasion of antibody neutralization in emerging severe acute respiratory syndrome coronaviruses. *Proceedings National Academy Sciences, USA, 102,* 797–801.

Yount, B., Roberts, R. S., Lindesmith, L., & Baric, R. S. (2006). Rewiring the severe acute respiratory syndrome coronavirus (SARS-CoV) transcription circuit: Engineering a recombination-resistant genome. *Proceedings of the National Academy Sciences, USA, 103,* 12546–12451.

Zhang, L., Zhang, F., Yu, W., He, T., Yu, J., Yi, C. E., et al. (2006). Antibody responses against SARS coronavirus are correlated with disease outcome of infected individuals. *Journal of Medical Virology, 78,* 1–8.

CHAPTER TWENTY-THREE

West Nile Virus

Felissa R. Lashley

Glaser (2004) called it the "perfect microbial storm" (p. 557). On August 23, 1999, a physician from Queens, a borough of New York City, reported two cases of unusual encephalitis to the New York City Department of Health. Investigators identified a cluster of six patients with encephalitis, four of whom required respiratory support. Initial antibody testing was positive for St. Louis encephalitis virus. The first group of cases resided in a 2-mile square area in Queens. Active surveillance was initiated on September 3, 1999, and a clinical case was defined as "a presumptive diagnosis of viral encephalitis with or without muscle weakness or acute flaccid paralysis, Guillain-Barré syndrome, aseptic meningitis, or presence of the clinical syndrome characterizing the initial cluster of cases in a patient presenting after August 1st" (Centers for Disease Control and Prevention [CDC], 1999a, p. 845).

At the same time, local health officers had noted an increase in fatalities among New York City birds, especially crows, and the Bronx zoo reported deaths in several exotic birds including Chilean flamingos, an Asian pheasant, and a cormorant. Testing of autopsy specimens from the birds revealed meningoencephalitis and myocarditis as well as the presence of a West Nile-like virus sequence found by genomic analysis. Further testing on the human tissue revealed West Nile-like viral presence as well (CDC, 1999a, 1999b). Thus, the first identification of West Nile virus (WNV) in humans in North America was made. Some responses bordered on panic. A Brazilian airline, for example, sprayed flights arriving from New York with insecticide before arrival to kill any possible infected mosquitoes on board ("West Nile Virus—USA," 1999), and there was even speculation that the outbreak represented a bioterrorist attack (Preston, 1999).

West Nile virus is an arbovirus of the *Flaviviridae* family. It is a member of the Japanese encephalitis serocomplex, which also includes Japanese encephalitis virus, Murray Valley (in Australia) encephalitis virus, St. Louis encephalitis virus, and the Kunjin virus, which appears to be a subtype of WNV (van der Meulen, Pensaert, & Nauwynck, 2005; Watts, Granwehr, Shope, Solomon, & Tesh, 2006). Various strains of the virus exist. West Nile virus was first isolated from a woman in the West Nile province of Uganda in 1937 (Smithburn, Hughes, Burke, & Paul, 1940).

Endemic disease exists in many countries, predominately in Africa (e.g., South Africa, Uganda, Nigeria, and Botswana), the Middle East, and Eurasia, including Israel, Azerbaijan, Egypt, Ukraine, Portugal, Pakistan, India, and other countries (Hubalek & Halouzka, 1999). Antibody seroprevalence varies across geography and age groups and can be difficult to detect because of nonspecificity and cross-reactivity with other flaviviruses and because the antibodies can wane over time. The New York outbreak was the first detected in the Western hemisphere (Hayes & Gubler, 2006). Since then, WNV has spread across North America (Watts et al., 2006). In the United States, cases have been reported from all 48 contiguous states.

The principal vectors of WNV are mosquitoes, usually those species that feed on birds such as *Culex* (especially *C. pipiens*), but also others such as *Aedes*, and occasionally ticks (Watts et al., 2006). Birds are the principal host, but other vertebrates and especially horses can also harbor the virus at moderate to high levels. Some of the vertebrates that may become infected are lemurs, bears, rabbits, dogs, camels, sheep, goats, and crocodiles (van der Meulen et al., 2005). High levels of the virus in birds may persist for long periods of time (20–100 days); thus, migratory birds are implicated in the introduction of WNV. There is usually a bird—mosquito cycle, although bird—tick cycles or frog—mosquito cycles occur (CDC, 1999a; Hubálek & Halouzka, 1999). In the New York outbreak described above, the principal birds affected were crows, but deaths in many species occurred, and a large number of bird species are now known to harbor the virus, including bluejays, bald eagles, American robins, sandhill cranes, yellow-billed cuckoos, house sparrows, owls, mallards, and red-tailed and broad-winged hawks (CDC, 1999b).

Transmission generally occurs from the bite of an infected mosquito. Transmission may also occur through blood transfusion, tissue and organ transplantation, transplacentally from mother to child, and probably through breast-feeding as well as through direct inoculation, for example, in the laboratory (Alpert, Fergerson, & Noel, 2003; Alter, Stramer, & Dodd, 2007; CDC, 2002a, 2002b; Hayes & Gubler, 2006). There was the suspicion of transmission of WNV among farm workers at a turkey breeding farm, possibly via aerosol (CDC, 2003). Nonviremic transmission with horizontal transmission of the virus can occur (Higgs, Schneider, Vanlandingham, Klingler, & Gould, 2005). Routine screening of blood for WNV RNA began in June 2003, but there are some questions whether this is a cost-effective approach (Korves, Goldie, & Murray, 2006; Lee & Biggerstaff, 2006). It has been recommended that gamete donors who have WNV infection defer donation until 14 days after resolution or 28 days from symptom onset (Practice Committee of the Society for Assisted Reproductive Technology and Practice Committee of the American Society for Reproductive Medicine, 2005). Further studies are needed to more clearly delineate outcomes after WNV infection in pregnancy (O'Leary et al., 2006).

The incubation period for the onset of symptoms after infection is about 2 to 14 days (Hayes & Gubler, 2006). Clinically, there are three basic outcomes following infection with WNV:

- No discernable symptoms. This outcome occurs in the majority. About 80% of infections with WNV are asymptomatic and self-limiting.
- West Nile fever, a self-limited illness occuring in about 20% of infections. Symptoms are those of a febrile, flu-like illness, including sudden onset of moderate to high fever, anorexia, fatigue, malaise, weakness, headache, myalgia, lymphadenopathy, and sore throat. A maculopapular or roseolar rash may be present on the trunk, extremities, and head in about half of the cases, particularly in children. Vomiting and diarrhea may occur in up to one third. Most cases resolve within 1 week but symptoms such as weakness and fatigue may persist for as long as 1 month or more.
- Development of central nervous system infection, usually manifested as encephalitis, meningitis, or flaccid paralysis, sometimes called neuroinvasive disease. This outcome usually occurs in less than 1% of those infected, although in a few outbreaks, a greater percentage of those infected have had neurological effects. Signs and symptoms include headache, high fever, vomiting, diarrhea, stiff neck, alterations in consciousness and mental status such as lethargy, seizures, weakness, focal neurological deficits, movement disorders, and others. This outcome occurs more often in those over the age of 50 years and/or those who are immunosuppressed. Neurologic deficits and symptoms can persist for months or years (Dean & Palermo, 2005; Hayes & Gubler, 2006; Lashley, 2006). Some outbreaks have been particularly severe, with about 30% of those infected developing neuroinvasive disease.

Hepatosplenomegaly, hepatitis, pancreatitis, myocarditis, and anterior myelitis are sometimes seen, more often in tropical countries. Chorioretinitis and other eye diseases such as uveitis and optic neuritis may also be seen (Hayes & Gubler, 2006). The fatality rate is highest for those who develop acute encephalitis, which is more likely in those over 60 years of age. Relatively common long-term problems of somatic complaints, motor skill and executive function abnormalities and tremors have been reported even in those who had West Nile fever as well as those who had neuroinvasive disease. This has led to the suggestion that the milder form of West Nile virus infection may not be as benign as has been thought, and that a subclinical encephalitis may be present even in mildly affected patients (Carson et al., 2006). There is no specific treatment. Supportive therapy for those with severe disease includes symptomatic treatment and maintenance of fluid and electrolytes.

In 1996, a major outbreak of West Nile fever occurred in Bucharest and the lower Danube valley of Romania. With about 500 clinical cases of illness (393 confirmed), thousands of antibody conversions, and a case fatality rate of nearly 10%, this outbreak was the largest arboviral illness in Europe since the epidemics caused by the Sindbis virus in the 1980s (Hubálek & Halouzka, 1999; Petersen & Roehrig, 2001). Investigators from the National Center for Infectious Diseases were called in to investigate the Romanian outbreak further. Through case—control studies, investigators concluded that meningoencephalitic illness was associated with age over 70 years, residence in a house as opposed to an apartment, seeing presence of mosquitoes in the home, the person recalling being bitten by a mosquito five or more times per day, and spending more time outdoors (Han et al., 1999; "NCID Investigates West Nile," 1997). Important aspects of this outbreak were the emergence of West Nile fever in epidemic form in a temperate climate as well as its emergence in an urban area in addition to the surrounding rural one.

Investigators have speculated about various factors that may contribute to West Nile fever outbreaks, including heavy rain, flooding, irrigation, and higher than usual temperatures, possibly related to global warming. West Nile virus appears able to overwinter in an adverse climate. Various possibilities include persistence in hibernating female mosquitos or chronically infected birds or frogs, or reintroduction by chronically infected birds from tropical or subtropical climates who migrated into the area. In the case of the Romanian outbreak, phylogenetic studies indicated that the virus might have been introduced from birds migrating from sub-Saharan Africa to north Africa to southern Europe (Savage et al., 1999). In 1997, a central European outbreak occurred in the Czech republic (Hubálek, Halouzka, & Juricova, 1999). In 1997 and 1998, sporadic infections continued in Romania, and in two cases the original diagnosis was measles (Cernescu, Nedelcu, Tardei, Ruta, & Tsai, 2000). An outbreak also occurred in the Volgograd region of Russia from July through September 1999, with a varying reported number of suspected cases (826 in one report and 942 in another), of which 84 developed meningoencephalitis and 40 were fatal (Petersen & Roehrig, 2001; Platonov et al., 2001).

In the 1999 New York outbreak, 62 human cases were identified, with 7 deaths. Most occurred in New York City, but cases were detected in counties surrounding New York City and in one Canadian citizen who visited New York City in late August and developed ultimately fatal encephalitis on September 5 (CDC, 1999b; Enserink, 2000). The wane in reported cases by the end of October was attributed to both cooler weather and the mosquito control programs undertaken. New York City conducted intensive programs of aerial and ground spraying to control mosquitos and did door-to-door surveys to look for antibody seroprevalence and find those who did not become ill in order to understand better the components of infection. Hotlines were set up and mosquito repellents distributed through local firehouses. Public education about avoiding mosquito exposure and about remaining inside during pesticide spraying took place through the media including the Internet (CDC, 1999b).

As with the Romanian outbreak, questions were raised about how WNV emerged in an urban, temperate area such as New York City. Ideas included those mentioned earlier as well as the illegal importation of one or more exotic infected birds, entry to the United States through hurricane winds of infected tropical bird(s), entry of an infected traveler from Africa or another endemic area, transportation of an infected mosquito by jet from an endemic area, or even a bioterrorist attack. Of course, even within New York City, green areas and pooled water abide, providing a friendlier environment for vectors (Giladi et al., 2001; Lanciotti et al., 1999). At the end of October 1999, dead crows and other birds elsewhere on the Atlantic coast (e.g., in Baltimore) were found to harbor WNV. Scientists concluded that either the virus had spread south with migrating birds or the virus had been in the area for a period of time and had just been recognized ("West Nile Virus: Migrating," 1999). There was also concern that the virus might overwinter in vectors living in subway tunnels or basements (Cowley & Kalb, 1999). By February 2000, New York was proactively preparing for the possibility of another outbreak and hiring additional health department staff who had expertise in arboviral infections. And another outbreak did come. At the end of 2000, there were 21 confirmed cases from Connecticut, New York, and New Jersey and 5 deaths (CDC, 2001; "West Nile Virus," 1999).

In Israel, a human outbreak occurred in 1999 that affected 2 persons and in 2000 that affected 417 persons, of whom 38 died (Giladi et al., 2001). Also in 2000, France experienced an epizootic outbreak in horses, goats, camels, and other animals that lead to some import restrictions on these animals from other countries ("West Nile Virus, Horses," 2001). Economic consequences follow both human and animal outbreaks. In France, the 2000 outbreak in horses resulted in the cancellation of many equestrian events, job layoffs, and other loss of income (Murgue et al., 2001). Other WNV epidemics/epizootics than those mentioned in this chapter have included Israel (1951–1954, 1957, humans; 1997, 1998, 1999, geese), South Africa (1974, humans), Morocco (1996, horses), Tunisia (1997, humans), Italy (1998, horses), Russia (1999, humans, birds), and the United States (1999, 2000, horses). Since the initial outbreak in New York, WNV has moved across the United States, eventually establishing itself as endemic (Glaser, 2004). Between 1999 and 2005, more than 8,000 cases of neuroinvasive WNV disease were reported (Debiasi & Tyler, 2006). New cases are reported each year.

The 1999 New York outbreak called into question how prepared the United States was to handle a large vectorborne disease outbreak. The CDC and the U.S. Department of Agriculture convened a meeting in November 1999 to establish guidelines to monitor and prevent future outbreaks (CDC, 2000). A study by the CDC revealed that extensive surveillance, prevention, and control activities appeared present nationally. The most recent guidelines for these are available online from the CDC's Web site at http://www.cdc.gov/ncidod/dvbid/westnile/resources/wnv-guidelines-aug-2003.pdf.

SUMMARY

The emergence of WNV as an epidemic illness in temperate and urban climates is an example of how circumstances can broaden the scope and impact of an endemic disease when new territory is affected. Its emergence resulted in a major U.S. public health endeavor, particularly in the northeastern states. West Nile virus has established itself as endemic and enzootic in the United States within a few short years. Large avian die-offs may forecast human epidemics. Thus, health care professionals in such areas need to be alert for febrile patients who might be infected with WNV. However, for every obvious infection, there may be 120 to 160 inapparent infections since the majority of WNV infections are asymptomatic (Craven & Roehrig, 2001). Long-term problems of somatic complaints, motor skill and executive function abnormalities, and tremors have been reported as relatively common occurrences even among patients with West Nile fever, who are more mildly affected than those with neuroinvasive disease. This has led to speculation that there is more pathologic damage to areas of the brain than formerly thought (Carson, et al., 2006). Clinicians should be alert for such sequelae. Because no specific treatment is available, although ribavirin has been used in a small number of persons, the development of an efficacious, safe vaccine especially for use in immunosuppressed persons might be useful. Interferon α-2b is being used for treatment of neuroinvasive disease in clinical trials (Kramer, Li, & Shi, 2007). Surveillance needs to be continued along with appropriate mosquito control measures (see Appendix C, Table C.5) and public education.

REFERENCES

Alpert, S. G., Fergerson, J., & Noel, L. P. (2003). Intrauterine West Nile virus: Ocular and systemic findings. *American Journal of Ophthamology, 136,* 733–735.

Alter, H. J., Stramer, S. L., & Dodd, R. Y. (2007). Emerging infectious diseases that threaten the blood supply. *Seminars in Hematology, 44,* 32–41.

Carson, P. J., Konewko, P., Wold, K. S., Mariani, P., Goll, S., Bergloff, P., et al. (2006). Long-term clinical and neuropsychological outcomes of West Nile virus infection. *Clinical Infectious Diseases, 43,* 723–730.

Centers for Disease Control and Prevention. (1999a). Outbreak of West Nile-like viral encephalitis—New York, 1999. *Morbidity and Mortality Weekly Report, 48,* 845–849.

Centers for Disease Control and Prevention. (1999b). Update: West Nile virus encephalitis—New York, 1999. *Morbidity and Mortality Weekly Report, 48,* 944–946, 955.

Centers for Disease Control and Prevention. (2000). Guidelines for surveillance, prevention, and control of West Nile virus infection—United States. *Morbidity and Mortality Weekly Report, 49,* 25–28.

Centers for Disease Control and Prevention. (2001). Serosurveys for West Nile virus infection—New York and Connecticut counties, 2000. *Morbidity and Mortality Weekly Report, 50,* 37–39.

Centers for Disease Control and Prevention. (2002a). Laboratory-acquired West Nile virus infections—United States, 2002. *Morbidity and Mortality Weekly Report, 51,* 1133–1135.

Centers for Disease Control and Prevention. (2002b). Possible West Nile virus transmission to an infant through breastfeeding—Michigan, 2002. *Morbidity and Mortality Weekly Report, 51,* 877–878.

Centers for Disease Control and Prevention. (2003). West Nile virus infection among turkey breeder farm workers—Wisconsin, 2002. *Morbidity and Mortality Weekly Report, 52,* 1017–1019.

Cernescu, C., Nedelcu, N. I., Tardei, G., Ruta, S., & Tsai, T. F. (2000). Continued transmission of West Nile Virus to humans in southeastern Romania, 1997–1998. *Journal of Infectious Diseases, 181,* 710–712.

Cowley, G., & Kalb, C. (1999, October 11). Anatomy of an outbreak. *Newsweek,* 76–78.

Craven, R. B., & Roehrig, J. T. (2001). West Nile virus. *Journal of the American Medical Association, 286,* 651–653.

Dean, J. L., & Palermo, B. J. (2005). West Nile virus encephalitis. *Current Infectious Disease Reports, 7,* 292–296.

Debiasi, R. L., & Tyler, K. L. (2006). West Nile virus meningoencephalitis. *Nature Clinical Practce Neurology, 2,* 264–275.

Enserink, M. (2000). The enigma of West Nile. *Science, 290,* 1482–1484.

Giladi, M., Matzkor-Cotter, E., Martin, D. A., Siegman-Igra, Y., Korczyn, A. D., Rosso, R., et al. (2001). West Nile encephalitis in Israel, 1999: The New York connection. *Emerging Infectious Diseases, 7,* 659–661.

Glaser, A. (2004). West Nile virus and North America: An unfolding story. *Scientific and Technical Review, 23,* 557–568.

Han, L. L., Popovici, F., Alexander, J. P., Jr., Laurentia, V., Tengelsen, L. A., Cernescu, C., et al. (1999). Risk factors for West Nile virus infection and meningoencephalitis, Romania, 1996. *Journal of Infectious Diseases, 179,* 230–233.

Hayes, E. B., & Gubler, D. J. (2006). West Nile virus: Epidemiology and clinical features of an emerging epidemic in the United States. *Annual Review of Medicine, 57,* 181–194.

Higgs, S., Schneider, B. S., Vanlandingham, D. L., Klingler, K. A., & Gould, E. A. (2005). Nonviremic transmission of West Nile virus. *Proceedings of the National Academy of Sciences, USA, 102,* 8871–8874.

Hubálek, Z., & Halouzka, J. (1999). West Nile fever—A reemerging mosquito borne viral disease in Europe. *Emerging Infectious Diseases, 5,* 643–650.

Hubálek, Z., Halouzka, J., & Juricova, Z. (1999). West Nile fever in Czechland. *Emerging Infectious Diseases, 5,* 594–595.

Korves, C. T., Goldie, S. J., & Murray, M. B. (2006). Cost-effectiveness of alternative blood-screening strategies for West Nile virus in the United States. *PLoS Medicine, 3*(2), 211–223.

Kramer, L. D., Li, J., & Shi, P. Y. (2007). West Nile virus. *Lancet Neurology, 6,* 171–181.

Lanciotti, R. S., Roehrig, J. T., Deubel, V., Smith, J., Parker, M., Steele, K., et al. (1999). Origin of the West Nile virus responsible for an outbreak of encephalitis in the northeastern United States. *Science, 286,* 2333–2337.

Lashley, F. R. (2006). Emerging infectious diseases at the beginning of the 21st century. *Online Journal of Issues in Nursing, 11*(1), 2–16.

Lee, B. Y., & Biggerstaff, B. J. (2006). Screening the United States blood supply for West Nile virus: A question of blood, dollars, and sense. *PLoS Medicine, 3,* 168–169.

Murgue, B., Murri, S., Zientara, S., Durand, B., Durand, J.-P., & Zeller, H. (2001). West Nile outbreak in horses in southern France, 2000: The return after 35 years. *Emerging Infectious Diseases, 7,* 692–696.

NCID investigates West Nile fever outbreak in Romania. (1997). *NCID Focus, 6*(1), unpaginated.

O'Leary, D. R., Kuhn, S., Kniss, K. L., Hinckley, A. F., Rasmussen, S. A., Pape, W. J., et al. (2006). Birth outcomes following West Nile virus infection of pregnant women in the United States: 2003–2004. *Pediatrics, 117,* 537–545.

Petersen, L. R., & Roehrig, J. T. (2001). West Nile virus: A reemerging global pathogen. *Emerging Infectious Diseases, 7,* 611–614.

Platonov, A. E., Shipulin, G. A., Shipulina, O. Y., Tyutyunnik, E. N., Frolochkina, T., Lanciotti, R. S., et al. (2001). Outbreak of West Nile virus infection, Volgograd region, Russia, 1999. *Emerging Infectious Diseases, 7,* 128–132.

Practice Committee of the Society for Assisted Reproductive Technology and Practice Committee of the American Society for Reproductive Medicine. (2005). American Society for Reproductive Medicine/Society for Assisted Reproductive Technology position statement on West Nile virus. *Fertility and Sterility, 83,* 527–528.

Preston, R. (1999, October 18 and 25). West Nile mystery. *The New Yorker,* p. 90–95.

Savage, H. M., Ceianu, C., Nicolescu, G., Karabatsos, N., Lanciotti, R., Vladimiresch, A., et al. (1999). Entomologic and avian investigations of an epidemic of West Nile fever in Romania in 1996, with serologic and molecular characterization of a virus isolate from mosquitoes. *American Journal of Tropical Medicine and Hygiene, 61,* 600–611.

Smithburn, K. C., Hughes, T. P., Burke, A. W., & Paul, J. H. (1940). A neurotropic virus isolated from the blood of a native of Uganda. *American Journal of Tropical Medicine, 20,* 471–492.

van der Muelen, K. M., Pensaert, M. B., & Nauwynck, H. J. (2005). West Nile virus in the vertebrate world. *Archives of Virology, 150,* 637–657.

Watts, D. M., Granwehr, B. P., Shope, R. E., Solomon, T., & Tesh, R. B. (2006). Japanese encephalitis and West Nile and other flavivirus infections. In R. L. Guerrant, D. H. Walker, & P. F. Weller (Eds.), *Tropical infectious diseases: Principles, pathogens, and practice* (2nd ed., pp. 823–830). Philadelphia: Churchill Livingstone Elsevier.

West Nile virus, horses—France. (2001, January 13). *ProMED Digest,* unpaginated.

West Nile virus: Migrating birds: Request for information. (1999). *ProMED Digest 99*(241), unpaginated.

West Nile virus—USA. (1999). *ProMED Digest 99*(272), unpaginated.

PART III

Special Considerations

CHAPTER TWENTY-FOUR

The Role of Infection in Some Cancers and Chronic Diseases

Felissa R. Lashley

The headlines read "FDA Licenses New Vaccine for Prevention of Cervical Cancer and Other Diseases in Females Caused by Human Papillomavirus" (U.S. Food and Drug Administration, 2006). With those headlines came a major advance in the prevention of cervical cancer, a cancer known to be due to certain human papillomavirus (HPV) types. This association and the availability of a vaccine is discussed further below.

Relatively recently, the association has been made between infection with a microbial agent and the development of a cancer or chronic disease, particularly one for which no cause had been established. For some of these conditions, the causative involvement of microbes has been established, for others the association is very strong, and for the rest evidence is suggestive but definitive association is lacking. Drs. Barry J. Marshall and J. Robin Warren were awarded the 2005 Nobel Prize in Physiology or Medicine for their work in establishing the connection between *Helicobacter pylori* infection and gastritis, which can lead to peptic ulcer disease (Zetterström, 2006). Difficulties in establishing microbial etiology include the following: The disease condition is rare, characteristics of the microbe make it difficult to detect, technologies for detection are not advanced enough to detect the microbe, there is failure to consider an infectious etiology for a specific disease, technology is not being appropriately applied, the disease is not in fact due to an infectious agent, an organism may trigger a host immune response that continues even when the viable organism is no longer present or persists at low levels that are difficult to detect (Fredricks & Relman, 1998), or it may produce a toxin that in turn causes the chronic condition. Clinical, epidemiological, and pathological characteristics may suggest a microbial etiology for certain cancers and chronic diseases. These include seasonality, occurrence in case clusters or epidemic curve, diseases associated with high fever or leukemoid reaction, pathological changes suggestive of an infectious process, response to antimicrobial therapy (Fredricks & Relman, 1998), and similarities with animal diseases known to be caused by an infectious agent.

Another way to consider the relationship between infectious agents and chronic disease is as follows:

1. Chronic disease is produced through direct effects leading to tissue pathology or organ decompensation. An example is hepatitis B virus and chronic liver diseases as well as hepatocellular carcinoma.
2. Initial infection causes permanent deficits or disabilities. An example is poliovirus infection causing paralysis, which can be permanent.
3. Infection has an indirect effect by predisposing to chronic sequelae. For example, intrauterine infection in pregnancy can lead to spontaneous preterm births, thus indirectly increasing the child's risk of various neurological and other deficits (Klein & Gibbs, 2005; O'Connor, Taylor, & Hughes, 2006).

Some of the microbes associated with a given cancer or chronic disease have recently been identified and are therefore considered emerging; others have been known for a long period of time. In all cases, the effects and sequelae of any microbial infection are influenced by host factors such as genetic susceptibility, resistance, and immune response; factors related to the microorganism such as virulence; and environmental factors such as crowding and cleanliness of the environment (Lashley, 2005, 2006, 2007). The best rationale for seeking to demonstrate a microbial etiology is the potential for successful prevention and treatment.

LINKING SPECIFIC MICROBIAL ORGANISMS WITH CANCERS AND CHRONIC DISEASES

Worldwide, it is estimated that infection may be responsible overall for 17.8% of the global cancer burden. If infection leading to cancer were prevented, there would be 7.7% and 26.3% fewer cancers in the developed and developing world, respectively (Parkin, 2006). Cancers may arise after infection through the following mechanisms: persistence of the microbe causing chronic inflammation, direct transformation of cells, or immunosuppression (Kuper, Adami, & Trichopoulos, 2000). In addition to the link between certain infectious agents and cancer, there are links between such agents and other chronic diseases. For example, dilated cardiomyopathy, a cause of heart failure and the need for heart transplantation, can result from cardiotropic viruses that include adenovirus, Epstein–Barr virus, cytomegalovirus, hepatitis C virus, and parvovirus B19 (Cooper et al., 2006). Table 24.1 lists some cancers and chronic diseases for which a microbial etiology is established or strongly suspected. The human T-cell lymphotropic virus 1 (HTLV-1), *H. pylori*, human herpesvirus 8 (HHV-8), *Chlamydophila* (formerly *Chlamydia*) *pneumoniae*, and human papillomaviruses are discussed below as examples of specific known associations between emerging microbes and disease. Prion diseases such as variant Creutzfeldt–Jakob disease, a neurological condition, are discussed in chapter 21. Recently it has been suggested that Crohn disease might be due to a combination of genetic predisposition and multiple interacting microorganisms (Eckburg & Relman, 2007). Other associations are under investigation. For examples, see Table 24.1.

Human T-Lymphotropic Virus Type 1 (HTLV-1)

Human T-cell lymphotropic virus 1 is a complex human oncogenic retrovirus first described in 1980 (Gallo, 2005; Poiesz et al., 1980). It causes adult T-cell leukemia/lymphoma (ATL) and an HTLV-1-associated myelopathy/tropical spastic paraparesis (HAM/TSP), and it has also been linked with uveitis, infective dermatitis syndrome, polymyositis, Sjögren syndrome, arthritis, idiopathic thrombocytopenic purpura, and invasive cervical cancer (Blattner & Charurat, 2005; Jarrett, 2006; Matsushita, Ozaki, Arima, & Tei, 2005). Human T-cell lymphotropic virus 1 was the first human retrovirus to be associated with a malignancy, and it is still believed that the entire disease spectrum of HTLV-1 is not yet known. The cumulative lifetime risk in HTLV-1-infected people for developing ATL or HAM/TSP is about 5% (Proietti, Carneiro-Proietti, Catalan-Soares, & Murphy, 2005). Infection with *Strongyloides stercoralis* may be a cofactor in the development of ATL (Blattner & Charurat, 2005). Other recently identified important retroviruses that cause human disease include HTLV-2, associated with hairy cell leukemia and a neurological disorder resembling HAM/TSP, and human immunodeficiency virus (HIV) 1, and HIV-2, which cause the immunodeficiency leading to the spectrum of conditions comprising acquired immunodeficiency syndrome (AIDS). Human T-cell lymphotropic virus 3 and HTLV-4 were recently identified in central Africa, where it is believed that transmission to humans occurred through contact with infected primates through hunting, butchering, and keeping

Table 24.1. Selected Chronic Diseases for Which Microbial Etiology Is Known or Suggested

Disease(s)	Putative or Established Microbial Agent(s)	Comments
Adult T-cell leukemia/lymphoma HTLV-1-associated myelopathy/tropical spastic paraparesis (HAM/TSP)	Human T-lymphotropic virus (HTLV) type 1	Discussed in text.
Arthritis	Varies, unknown for most types.	Joint neutrophilia and reports of some response to antibiotic agents have suggested microbial etiology. Viral, bacterial, fungal, and parasitic agents have all been associated with specific types of arthritis. For example, the Ross River virus can cause polyarthritis as part of its manifestations. *Borrelia burgdorferi*, the agent of Lyme disease, can cause chronic arthritis. *Bartonella henselae* has been suggested as a cause of juvenile rheumatoid arthritis. A type of arthritis also follows parvovirus B19 infection.
Bladder cancer	*Schistosoma haematobium*	Schistosomiasis from a trematode parasite leads to urinary tract lesions that may result in bladder carcinoma (squamous cell), probably from prolonged irritation leading to hyperplasia and malignancy. Prevalent in Africa.
Burkitt lymphoma Hodgkin disease Leiomyosarcoma Nasopharyngeal carcinoma	Human herpesvirus 4 (Epstein–Barr virus; EBV)	EBV has been linked to a variety of human cancers and is considered a Group 1 carcinogen. Other genetic or environmental conditions may play cofactor roles. It also causes infectious mononucleosis.
Cardiomyopathy, inflammatory	Parvovirus B19, EBV, adenovirus, cytomegalovirus, hepatitis C virus	Major cause of cardiac failure and transplant.
Castleman disease (multicentric)	Human herpesvirus 8 (HHV-8)	Discussed in text.

Table 24.1. *(continued)*

Disease(s)	Putative or Established Microbial Agent(s)	Comments
Cervical carcinoma and less strong association for vulvar intraepithelial neoplasia, vaginal intraepithelial neoplasia, penile intraepithelial neoplasia, and anal carcinomas	Human papillomaviruses (HPVs)	HPVs include more than 100 types, each with a particular tissue preference. HPV types 16, 18, 31, and 33 are associated with anogenital malignancy. HPVs have been implicated in progression from premalignancy for penile, vulvar, and anal carcinomas. Molecular techniques indicate an association between oral cancer and HPV-16. Also see text.
Cholangiocarcinoma	*Opisthorchis viverrini*	Parasitic liver fluke. Endemic in Thailand and Laos. Chronic infection is usually asymptomatic unless heavy infestation is present.
Cholangiocarcinoma	*Clonorchis sinensis*	Parasitic liver fluke. Endemic in China, Japan, Korea, Taiwan, and Vietnam. Known as a Group 2 carcinogen.
Coronary artery disease	*Chlamydophila pneumoniae*	Discussed in text.
Creutzfeldt–Jakob disease	Altered prions	Several slowly progressive fatal neurodegenerative diseases with long incubation periods are due to altered prions. See chapter 21 for discussion.
Crohn disease	Unknown	Chronic inflammatory enteritis (pathologically similar to mycobacterial enteritis) causing abdominal pain, fever, and diarrhea. Extraintestinal manifestations include uveitis and arthritis. Suggestion has been made that multiple microbial interactions may be involved in etiology.
Gallbladder cancer	*Salmonella typhi* *Salmonella paratyphi* *Helicobacter pylori*	All are associated with a higher relative risk for development of gallbladder cancer.
Guillain–Barré syndrome (GBS)	*Campylobacter spp.*	May follow *Campylobacter* enteritis. Establishing causal relationship difficult due to rarity of GBS.

(continued)

Table 24.1. *(continued)*

Disease(s)	Putative or Established Microbial Agent(s)	Comments
Hairy cell leukemia	HTLV-2	Relationship not firmly established. Also may result in neurological syndrome resembling HAM/TSP. HTLV-2 found more frequently in injecting drug users and certain Caribbean and South American Indian groups.
Hepatocellular carcinoma (HCC)	Chronic hepatitis B virus infection Chronic hepatitis C virus infection	HCC is the result of cirrhosis often secondary to chronic hepatitis B and C viral infections. About two thirds of HCC occurs in Asia. Prevention by hepatitis B vaccine is possible but is not available for hepatitis C. Treatment of chronic hepatitis such as by interferon alfa may decrease long-term risk. See chapter 12.
Kaposi sarcoma	HHV-8	Discussed in text.
Multiple sclerosis (MS)	HHV-6 implicated	Neurotropic virus. MS is a progressive CNS demyelination disease. HHV-6 DNA sequences and antigens have been associated with MS lesions, but association is speculative.
Peptic ulcer Gastric lymphoma Gastric adenocarcinoma Rheumatoid arthritis	*H. pylori*	Discussed in text.
Sarcoidosis	Unknown *Mycobacterium*	Multisystem inflammatory disorder. Higher incidence in winter and spring. Can be acute or chronic. Apparent transmission by organ transplantation possible.
Tropical sprue	Unknown bacteria	Chronic diarrhea, malabsorption, weight loss, fever, fatigue. Endemic and epidemic in tropical countries.
Progressive multifocal leukoencephalopathy	JC virus	This polyomavirus may reactivate in the immunosuppressed.

Table 24.1. *(continued)*

Disease(s)	Putative or Established Microbial Agent(s)	Comments
Whipple disease	*Tropheryma whipplei* (formerly *whippelii*)	Systemic disease featuring abnormal fat deposits in intestinal tissue and lymph nodes. Findings include lymphadenopathy, polyarthritis, weight loss, diarrhea, and malabsorption. Extraintestinal disease can involve the heart and central nervous system. The causative organism is difficult to cultivate. There are many unknowns about the source and route of infection, pathogenesis, host susceptibility, full clinical spectrum, and therapy. See Fenollar, Puéchal, & Raoult, 2007 for review and current therapeutic recommendations.

Sources: Calabrese & Naides, 2005; Cesarman & Mesri, 2007; Cooper et al., 2006; Eash, Manley, Gasparovic, Querbes, & Atwood, 2006; Eckburg & Relman, 2007; Fenollar, Puéchal, & Raoult, 2007; Feuer & Green, 2005; Glatzel, Stoeck, Seeger, Lührs, & Aguzzi, 2005; Guerrant, Walker, & Weller, 2006; Herrera, Benítez-Bribiesca, Mohar, & Ostrosky-Wegman, 2005; IARC Working Group on the Evaluation of Carcinogenic Risks to Humans, 1994; Kumar, Kumar, & Kumar, 2006; Mager, 2006; Mandell, Bennett, & Dolin, 2005; Otasevic et al., 2007; Randi, Franceschi, & La Vecchia, 2006; Richie, 2005; Schottenfeld & Beebe-Dimmer, 2005; Thacker, Mirzaei, & Ascherio, 2006.

them as pets (Feuer & Green, 2005; Wolfe, Daszak, Kilpatrick, Burke, 2005). Close contact with blood and body fluids allowed emergence of simian retroviruses that crossed the species barrier to humans (Wolfe et al., 2005). Retroviruses are enveloped RNA viruses that have an enzyme known as reverse transcriptase, which allows them to make a DNA copy that is integrated into the host's DNA (Blattner & Charurat, 2005; Proietti et al., 2005).

Human T-cell lymphotropic virus 1 has a worldwide distribution and is considered endemic in southern Japan, East Asia, Papua New Guinea, the Caribbean basin, several Latin American countries, and parts of sub-Sarahan Africa. The prevalence is also high in the southeastern United States and in central Brooklyn, where there is a large Caribbean population. About 20 million people worldwide are believed to be infected. In endemic areas such as Okinawa, the prevalence rate is as high as 35% (Araujo & Silva, 2006; Levine et al., 1999; Proietti et al., 2005; Reynolds, Bessong, & Quinn, 2006). Seroprevalence in women is higher than in men after 20 to 30 years of age. In most of Europe and the United States, the incidence is low, about 0.05% overall, although higher levels have been reported in persons from endemic population groups who settled in other countries. Higher seroprevalence is also found in injecting drug users, their sexual contacts, sex workers, and affected families (Proietti et al., 2005). Human T-cell lymphotropic virus 1 is transmitted through sexual contact, parenterally through transfusion of infected blood and blood products including contaminated needles, and vertically from mother to child through breast milk and during pregnancy. The transplacental route is considered rare. Transmission through saliva is possible, but there is no definitive evidence (Proietti et al., 2005; Ravandi et al., 2005). Detection in blood is by enzyme immunosorbent assay for screening, with positive detection followed by Western blot for confirmation, and proviral detection by polymerase chain reaction (PCR) is also used (Stramer, Foster, & Dodd, 2006; Vitone et al., 2006)

Adult T-cell leukemia/lymphoma was first described in Japan in 1977, and the etiologic connection to HTLV-1 was made a few years later (Poiesz et al., 1980; Uchiyama, Yodoi, Sagawa, Takatsuki, & Uchino, 1977; Yoshida, Miyoshi, & Hinuma, 1982; Yoshida, Seiki, Yamaguchi, & Takatsuki, 1984). In Japan, the lifetime risk for developing ATL among HTLV-1 carriers is 6.6% for men and 2.1% for women (Jarrett, 2006). There are four clinical subtypes: acute ATL, chronic ATL, smoldering ATL, and the lymphoma type ATL. Acute ATL is seen in 55% to 75% of patients. Disease usually occurs 20 to 30 years after infection, and a typical age of onset is in the fourth or fifth decade of life (Proietti et al., 2005). Clinical features include leukemia, hypercalcemia, lymphadenopathy, hepatosplenomegaly, and skin and bone lesions. Strongyloidiasis is a very common opportunistic infection. In the acute and lymphomatous subtypes, the lymphocytes may show polylobulated nuclei, or a "flower cell" appearance. Adult T-cell leukemia/lymphoma is rapidly progressive, and 4-year survival times are 5% for acute, about 5.7% for lymphoma, 26.9% for chronic, and 62.8% for smoldering types (Ravandi et al., 2005). Death may be due to hypercalcemia or infection (Jarrett, 2006). Treatment approaches using antiretroviral agents and cancer chemotherapeutic agents as well as interferon have been tried, and bone marrow transplantation has also been used (Taylor & Matsuoka, 2005).

HAM/TSP develops in about 4% of HTLV-1-infected people and is more frequent in females. It typically occurs in adulthood, usually in the fourth or fifth decade of life. HAM/TSP is a chronic neurodegenerative disease with white matter degeneration and fibrosis, and it may be due to the immune system response to HTLV-1. The typical pattern is that of slow onset and chronicity. It often begins with a stiff gait and slow progression to leg weakness, increasing spasticity, back pain, urinary incontinence, paresthesias, and impotence. About one third have upper limb weakness.

HAM/TSP can be rapidly progressive in older people or in those who receive HTLV-1 contaminated blood but is more typically progressive over a period of about 10 years. Treatment generally consists of supportive therapy, immunosuppression, corticosteroids, interferon, and antiretroviral agents (Araujo & Silva, 2006; Blattner & Charurat, 2005; Proietti et al., 2005). Diagnostic guidelines have been developed (De Castro-Costa et al., 2006). Because HAM/TSP is the most common but not the only neurological manifestation of HTLV-1 infection, the term HTLV-1 neurological complex has been suggested in order to better describe the full neurological spectrum (Araujo & Silva, 2006).

In an effort to prevent transmission through blood transfusion, screening of blood donors for HTLV-1 began in 1988 in the United States and is in place in some other countries such as Japan. However, lookback recipient tracing has a low yield in the United States (Stramer et al., 2006). Counseling regarding risk and ways to prevent transmission (such using latex condoms for sexual relationships, not sharing needles, and avoiding the breast-feeding of infants in developed countries) should be provided to those found to harbor HTLV-1 and are similar to those in place for HIV infection. Health care workers are at risk through parenteral exposure to infected blood, but that risk is thought to be low and has been reported for both HTLV-1 and -2 (Menna-Barreto, 2006).

Helicobacter pylori

H. pylori is causally associated with gastritis, primary peptic ulcer disease both gastric and duodenal, gastric adenocarcinoma, and gastric mucosa-associated lymphoid tissue (MALT) lymphoma (Chiba, Seno, Marusawa, Wakatsuki, & Okazaki, 2006). Learning the nature of these associations changed therapy for these disorders and allowed cures through the use of antimicrobial agents. Because of its association with gastric cancer, *H. pylori* has been called a Class I carcinogen by the World Health Organization (IARC Working Group on the Evaluation of Carcinogenic Risks to Humans, 1994), and it was the first bacterial agent so designated.

It was not until 1982 that this organism was isolated (Marshall, 1983). It was originally named as a member of the *Campylobacter* genus and was given its present name in 1989. *H. pylori* is a gram-negative rod-shaped, urease-producing, microaerophilic bacterium that has multiple flagella on only one end and is thus motile (Marshall & Gillman, 2006). It is usually spiral shaped. Its urease enzyme allows it to colonize the gastric epithelium, where it causes gastric inflammation (Sgouros & Bergele, 2006).

H. pylori is said to be one of the most common infections worldwide, affecting more than 70% in developing countries and about 30% of people in developed countries. In developing areas, infection occurs early in childhood, while in developed areas infection occurs later. While *H. pylori* infection occurs worldwide, the prevalence varies across populations and increases with age. For example, in the United States, prevalence is under 20% at 20 years of age and about 50% at 50 years of age, while it is less than 20% under 20 years of age in Japan but 70% to 80% at 40 years of age. In Korea, the prevalence is 50% at 5 years of age and 90% at 20 years (Ando et al., 2006). *H. pylori* infection is seen most commonly in conjunction with crowded living conditions and lower socioeconomic status (Schottenfeld & Beebe-Dimmer, 2005). In the EUROGAST study of 3,000 subjects in 13 countries, the prevalence of *H. pylori* infection for the lowest, middle, and higher socioeconomic groups were, respectively, 85%, 52%, and 11% (EUROGAST Study Group, 1993). Poor sanitation, overcrowded conditions, and contaminated water facilitate infection. Other factors may contribute to *H. pylori* infection that are specific to the host (such as genetic factors including *HLA-DQB1*0401* association with increased susceptibility to gastric cancer, immune status, and sociocultural factors), the organism (such as the strain of organism, colonization factors, evasion of the host immune system, virulence factors, and degree of infectivity), and the environmental factors mentioned (Chiba et al., 2006; Watanabe et al., 2006). The cytotoxin-associated gene A (CagA) positive strain is more virulent (Hatakeyama & Higashi, 2005).

There is uncertainty about how *H. pylori* is transmitted. In humans it is present in vomitus and in stools. Gastroenteritis facilitates exposure to stool and vomitus, perhaps even by aerosolized material that may aid in transmission, especially in countries where such illness is common (Parsonnet, Shmuely, & Haggerty, 1999). The mode of transmission is believed to be person to person by the fecal—oral, gastrointestinal—oral (documented spread iatrogenically by endoscopy), and possibly by the oral–oral routes. The evidence for the latter is inferred by the findings of the organism in dental plaque and saliva; however, there is little concordance between spouses, and patients are not usually reinfected by their spouses. Intrafamilial clustering does occur, and there is an association with low socioeconomic status (with such factors as overcrowding and inadequate sanitation) and with higher income areas with increased use of antibiotics, perhaps leading to eradication (Gisbert, 2005; Kivi & Tindberg, 2006). In Pennsylvania, one study found that drinking water from wells and other sources containing *H. pylori* was associated with a risk of developing peptic ulcers ("*Helicobacter pylori*," 1999), but the importance of contaminated water is unsettled (Kivi & Tindberg, 2006).

The method of detection and diagnosis depends on the level of specificity necessary. Techniques can be invasive (usually endoscopic) or noninvasive. Invasive techniques depend on biopsy, histological findings, culture of the organism, and/or the rapid urease test for diagnosis. Noninvasive techniques include the urea breath test, based on the characteristic of *H. pylori* to be urease producing, and stool antigen tests (O'Morain, 2006).

Not all who are colonized with *H. pylori* develop chronic infection and disease. Initial infection may be associated with a self-limited illness of epigastric discomfort, nausea, burping, vomiting, and sometimes fever or may be asymptomatic. Hypochlorhydria may develop. In childhood, there may be clearing and then reinfection over a period of time. But in most persons, after acquisition, *H. pylori* persists, often without symptoms for a period of time, and leads to changes in gastric physiology and mucosa (Ando et al., 2006; Peek & Crabtree, 2006). Many factors are thought to interact in terms of the outcome of *H. pylori* acquisition, as delineated above, to determine subsequent outcomes. Colonization may lead to inflammation and chronic gastritis, eventually often resulting in gastric cancer. The risk of gastric cancer that has been ascribed to *H. pylori* infection is 60% to 80% (Blaser, 2005). Gastric cancer is the fourth most common cancer in the world and the second most common cancer-related death with a less than 20% survival rate (Matysiak-Budnik & Mégraud, 2006). Another outcome can be peptic ulcer disease, both gastric and duodenal. *H. pylori* is found in 85% to 95% of persons with peptic ulcer disease (O'Morain, 2006). Another outcome is functional dyspepsia, which refers to chronic discomfort or pain in the upper abdomen.

The recommendation of the American Gastroenterological Association (2005) is that *H. pylori* testing be part of the management, and, if positive, treatment for eradication therapy can be given with or without proton pump inhibitor (PPI) therapy. Eradication therapy is typically done for 10 days with a PPI and two antibiotics or with the addition of a fourth agent, usually bismuth. Compliance and resistance compromise eradication rates (McLoughlin, O'Morain, & O'Connor, 2005). Eradication in nonulcerative disease is still controversial (Blaser, 2005), but other general recommendations include elimination of *H. pylori* for ulcers and uninvestigated dyspepsia under certain circumstances, and, if *H. pylori* infection is detected—for example, through community "screen and treat" programs—especially in populations with a high incidence of *H. pylori*-associated diseases, a test and treat strategy for first-degree relatives of persons with gastric cancer. The screen and treat strategy approach could reduce *H. pylori*-associated death by 15% (Malfertheiner et al., 2005).The third Maastricht Consensus conference has a detailed update on management of *H. pylori* including the recommendation that unexplained recurrent abdominal pain in children is an indication for a test and treat strategy (Malfertheiner et al., in press).

H. pylori has also been associated in the literature with MALT lymphomas. Eradication of *H. pylori* has led to regression in some, and treatment also includes chemotherapy (Chiba et al., 2006). Usually, relapse is associated with recolonization (Montalban & Norman, 2006). It has also been speculated that *H. pylori* might be associated with nongastrointestinal chronic conditions such as respiratory disorders, possibly including bronchiectasis, lung cancer and other cancers, acute anterior uveitis, coronary artery disease, certain autoimmune disorders, and chronic urticaria (Kanbay, Kanbay, & Boyacioglu, 2007; Otasevic et al., 2007). The evidence for these associations has been carefully reviewed and has not been found to be convincing when subjected to appropriate controls and evaluated for design flaws. A weak association for CagA-positive strains has been found in some studies of ischemic heart disease (Pasceri et al., 2006), but more prospective studies are needed to confirm such an association. Leontiadis, Sharma, and Howden (1999) established nine criteria by which to judge such studies: "Is the evidence from true experiments in humans? Is the association strong? Is the association consistent from study to study? Is the temporal relationship correct? Is there a dose-response relationship? Does the association make epidemiological sense? Does the association make biological sense? Is the association specific? Is the association analogous to a previously proven causal association?" (p. 926).

Human Herpesvirus Type 8 (HHV-8)

Experience with Kaposi sarcoma (KS) in the context of the HIV epidemic led to the suspicion that an infectious agent was responsible for the disease because of epidemiological observations about the spread and transmission. Human herpesvirus type 8 (HHV-8) is also known as KS-associated herpesvirus (KSHV), and was discovered in material from a KS lesion in a patient with AIDS in 1994 (Chang et al., 1994). HIV/AIDS-associated KS was first reported in 1981 in the United States as a forecaster of the HIV epidemic and in recent years has been declining in frequency for unknown reasons. Some believe that the decline is due to decreased viral loads due to highly active antiretroviral therapy (HAART). Human herpesvirus type 8 was quickly linked to a causal relationship with KS. Since that time, it has also been linked to primary effusion lymphoma, which is a non-Hodgkin lymphoma occurring more frequently in HIV-infected persons, and multicentric Castleman disease, which is a hyperplastic B-cell lymphoproliferative disorder (Carbone et al., 2005; Cesarman & Mesri, 2007; Schulz, 2006). However, the mechanism by which causation occurs has not yet been elucidated, nor is whether or not other conditions or cofactors are necessary for malignancy development in addition to HHV-8.

Human herpesvirus type 8 is one of eight herpesviruses known to infect humans. One other, HHV-4 or Epstein–Barr virus, has also been closely linked to malignancy development. Human herpesvirus type 8 is classified in the herpesvirus family in the Gammaherpesvirinae subfamily as a rhadinovirus (Kaye, 2005). There are several variants or types. In endemic countries in childhood, transmission occurs horizontally by nonsexual transmission among children (Kaye, 2005; Schulz, 2006). Sexual transmission is prevalent in persons with multiple sexual partners and men who have sex with men. There have been a few cases described of parenteral transmission from transplantation and transfusion as well as vertical transmission from mother to child. Human herpesvirus type 8 has been found in saliva, and saliva may be involved in both sexual and nonsexual transmission (Kaye, 2005). There are still some unknowns regarding transmission. The question of whether or not to screen donors pretransplant for HHV-8 is debated (Marcelin, Calvez, & Dussaix, 2007).

Kaposi sarcoma is considered an endothelial cell tumor that occurs in four epidemiological groups: (a) classic KS, which occurs in older men of Mediterranean and Eastern European Jewish origin and has an indolent course; (b) endemic KS, which occurs in equatorial Africa across age groups but mainly in children and adults under 40 years of age and which can be aggressive; (c) iatrogenic KS, which is seen in immunosuppressed non-AIDS patients, mainly those who are organ transplant recipients; and (d) HIV/AIDS-associated KS. In all age and epidemiological groupings, men are preferentially affected (Kaye, 2005), and the reason for this is unknown. Kaposi sarcoma lesions may appear on the skin as reddish, purple, or brown patches, plaques, or nodules and are often multiple. When associated with HIV infection, they may affect the oral cavity, lymphatics, gastrointestinal tract, lung, liver, adrenal glands, and heart, and they may be disseminated. Complications can arise because of the size of the tumor. In the classical form, the disease is only slowly progressive and is usually confined to the legs. Treatment is palliative and may be with radiation or chemotherapy, and newer approaches such as antiangiogenesis compounds are underway (Kaye, 2005). Reduction in immunosuppression can lead to remission, and HAART can be used in treating epidemic KS because of the boosting of the immune response (Kaye, 2005). Information about HHV-8 in Castleman disease and in primary effusion lymphomas is sparse because of the relative rarity of these conditions (Cesarman & Masri, 2007).

Chlamydophila pneumoniae

Known cardiovascular risk factors such as smoking do not fully explain noted geographical and temporal variations in coronary heart disease (CHD). Thus, microbial agents have been suspected of playing a role in etiology, and attention has focused on cytomegalovirus, *H. pylori*, *C. pneumoniae*, and more recently frequent or chronic enterovirus infections (Pesonen et al., in press). The most attention has centered upon *C. pneumoniae*, which has been suspected of playing a causative role in the development of atherosclerosis and CHD, both major causes of morbidity and mortality. The basis for this suspicion has been the recovery of the organism in atherosclerotic plaques, and the long-held idea that an infectious agent might trigger the inflammation that occurs during the development of atherosclerosis (Ridker, Kundsin, Stampfer, Poulin, & Hennekens, 1999).

C. pneumoniae is a unique bacterium because it is an obligate intracellular organism that is more characteristic of a virus. It persists in tissues and relies on the host cell for energy. The genus Chlamydophila is currently known to contain three species that cause disease in humans, one of which, Chlamydophila trachomatis, is responsible for the eye disease trachoma. Only one strain of C. pneumoniae is known (Jackson, 2005). In fact, it was during a trachoma study in Taiwan in 1965 that C. pneumoniae was first found, and it was not until 1983 that its occurrence in a college student with pharyngitis led to the recognition of its major causative niche (Grayston, Kuo, Wang, & Altman, 1986). C. pneumoniae is a common cause of acute respiratory infection including bronchitis, sinusitis, and community-acquired pneumonia. Connections with Alzheimer disease, asthma, and reactive arthritis have also been proposed (Gerard et al., 2005; Martin, 2006; Ozgul, Dede, Taskaynatan, Aydogan, & Kalyon, 2006). The majority of the population is exposed to the organism after 5 years of age, and by early adulthood about 50% are seropositive. This rises to about 75% in elderly persons. Infection is often subclinical and unrecognized (Jackson, 2005). Transmission is person to person via respiratory secretions (Centers for Disease Control and Prevention, 2005)

Ways that infection might contribute to the development of atherosclerosis include damage to endothelial cells by the microbe or its endotoxins or immune complexes; possible binding of endotoxin to lipoproteins, causing disturbances including alterations of cholesterol metabolism; activation of macrophages leading to cytokine production; up-regulation of the major histocompatibility complex; increased synthesis of acute phase proteins such as fibrinogen; enhanced activity of procoagulant mediators leading to a hypercoagulable state; and heat shock protein expression (Gupta & Camm, 1999; Pesonen et al., in press).

Evidence for the involvement of C. pneumoniae in atherosclerosis includes seroepidemiologic studies finding elevated antibodies and immune complexes containing C. pneumoniae antigen in patients with acute myocardial infarctions and CHD, after controlling for confounding factors (Saikku et al., 1988); the presence of C. pneumoniae in atherosclerotic plaques observed through electron microscopy studies, immunocytochemical staining, and PCR testing; and in situ hybridization studies. It has been observed that the organism can infect and replicate within macrophages, smooth muscle, and endothelial cells and can be transported to coronary arteries from the respiratory tract. Furthermore, animal model experiments have shown that rabbits infected with *C. pneumoniae* who develop pneumonia can develop atherosclerotic lesions. Other evidence comes from the response to antibiotics. The organism is present in many atherosclerotic lesions in viable form and in early lesions associated with pathological changes. The secretion and expression of heat shock proteins (HSPs) after *C. pneumoniae* infection may be involved in vascular lesion formation (Mussa et al., 2006).

Experimental studies using antibiotics to treat or prevent CHD have been conducted, but most have not been prospective and have used a small sample size. In the ROXIS pilot study using roxithromycin to treat patients with non-Q-wave myocardial infarctions and angina, results appeared promising (Gurfinkel et al., 1999). More recently, Grayston and colleagues (2005) reported the results of the Azithromycin and Coronary Event Study trial in which 4,012 patients with stable coronary artery disease received either 600 mg of azithromycin or placebo weekly for 1 year and were followed for 3.9 years. They concluded that the risk of cardiac events among these patients was not altered by the administration of azithromycin. Cannon and colleagues (2005) enrolled 4,162 patients who had been hospitalized with acute coronary syndrome in a double-blind study in which one group received gatifloxacin and the other a placebo. No statistically significant difference was seen in the end points including death, myocardial infarction, unstable angina, and stroke between the two groups.

At this time, it can be said that there is a strong association between *C. pneumoniae* and atherosclerosis but that all criteria for causality have not been completely fulfilled (Shor & Phillips, 1999). If *C. pneumoniae* causes, substantially contributes to, or exacerbates CHD, it opens new avenues for both prevention and treatment in at least some cases.

Human Papillomaviruses

Human papillomaviruses (HPVs) are nonenveloped, double-stranded DNA viruses that preferentially infect epithelial cells (Bonnez & Reichman, 2005; Hebner & Laimins, 2006). They can cause various lesions that run the gamut from warts to cervical neoplasms, depending on the HPV type. More than 100 types have been identified to date, and among these some are considered high risk for cancer development. These include types 16, 18, 31, 33, 45, and 51, which are the types most frequently associated with cervical cancer, while types 6 and 11 cause about 90% of genital warts (Gravitt & Jamshidi, 2005; Hebner & Laimins, 2006; U.S. Food and Drug Administration, 2006). HPVs have been linked to both internal and external anogenital warts or condyloma acuminata, common warts, plantar warts, intraepithelial neoplasia, cervical carcinoma, respiratory papillomatosis, and other manifestations. Human papillomavirus infections may be clinically evident, asymptomatic, or latent (Bonnez & Reichman, 2005). Anogenital warts may occur in males and females and are common among men who have sex with men. The association of HPV infection and anorectal cancer was first identified in this population, and receptive anal intercourse increases the risk of transmission (Frazer et al., 2006). Approximately 90% or more of cervical cancer and more than 50% of other anogenital cancers result from HPV (de Martel & Parsonnet, 2006). Transmission of genital HPVs is through sexual contact and infrequently from an infected mother to her infant in the perinatal period, usually manifesting as respiratory papillomatosis. Skin-to-skin contact is another means of transmission as are fomites, but in nongenital HPV infections the latter is less efficient. Genital HPV infection is considered a frequent consequence of sexual activity and is most commonly seen in younger women who have recently begun sexual activity, with another rise around menopause, and in most cases is self-limiting with no overt manifestations (Gravitt & Jamshidi, 2005).

Cervical cancer is the second most common cancer found in women worldwide, and it develops from cervical intraepithelial neoplasias (Hebner & Laimins, 2006; Snijders, Steenbergen, Heideman, & Meijer, 2006). The HPV types most commonly associated with cervical cancers are types 16 and 18. Type 16 alone is the cause of more than half of invasive cervical cancers (Frazer et al., 2006). In regard to cervical HPV infection, there appear to be two major patterns. In the first, cytologic changes may occur after infection, but clearance of the virus and these cytologic changes occur in about 85%. In those whose infection persists for a year or more, progression to malignancy is more likely (Gravitt & Jamshidi, 2005). Overall, however, progression to malignancy is relatively rare and may take years to develop. Progression to invasive cervical cancer also depends on various host factors such as genetic susceptibilities, nutrition, increased parity, smoking, viral variants, viral load, the presence of other sexually transmitted diseases, oral contraceptive use, and other factors (Frazer et al., 2006). Various screening tests have been used for detection including the Pap test, liquid-based cytology, and, in high-risk women, HPV testing (Sheary & Dayan, 2005). Treatment depends on stage of cancer and other factors and may include surgery, radiation, and chemotherapy (most recently with a combination of cisplatin and topotecan; Moore, 2006).

Gardasil, the first vaccine to prevent cervical cancer, precancerous genital lesions, and genital warts due to HPV 6, 11, 16, and 18 was approved by the FDA on June 8, 2006, in the United States. It is recommended for women 9 to 26 years of age, and it is important to administer before sexual activity. It contains no live virus and is given in a series of three injections over a 6-month period (U.S. Food and Drug Administration, 2006). Effective use worldwide will also depend on various sociocultural factors. For example, in some Asian cultures, there is fear that if girls and young women are vaccinated, it is tantamount to an admission of promiscuity, leading to various consequences (MacKenzie, 2005). In addition, there is an objection that giving the vaccine would undermine abstinence education ("Rolling Out HPV Vaccines," 2006).

SUMMARY

Links between chronic diseases and microbial agents have been clearly established in a few instances. Many of these agents are newly emergent, having been recognized in the past 30 years. Further work is needed to delineate more clearly other causative relationships. Such work holds promise for new approaches to prevention and treatment.

REFERENCES

American Gastroenterological Association. (2005). American Gastroenterological Association medical position statement: Evaluation of dyspepsia. *Gastroenterology, 129*, 1753–1755.

Ando, T., Goto, Y., Maeda, O., Watanabe, O., Ishiguro, K., & Goto, H. (2006). Causal role of *Helicobacter pylori* infection in gastric cancer. *World Journal of Gastroenterology, 12*, 181–186.

Araujo, A. Q. C., & Silva, M. T. T. (2006). The HTLV-1 neurological complex. *Lancet Neurology, 5*, 1068–1075.

Blaser, M. (2005). *Helicobacter pylori* and other gastric *Helicobacter* species. In G. L. Mandell, J. E. Bennett, & R. Dolin (Eds.), *Mandell, Douglas, and Bennett's principles and practice of infectious diseases* (6th ed., pp. 2098–2118). Philadelphia: Elsevier Churchill Livingstone.

Blattner, W., & Charurat, M. (2005). Human T-cell lymphotropic virus types I and II. In G. L. Mandell, J. E. Bennett, & R. Dolin (Eds.), *Mandell, Douglas, and Bennett's principles and practice of infectious diseases* (6th ed., pp. 1862–1873). Philadelphia: Elsevier Churchill Livingstone.

Bonnez, W., & Reichman, R. C. (2005). Papillomaviruses. In G. L. Mandell, J. E. Bennett, & R. Dolin, R. (Eds.), *Mandell, Douglas, and Bennett's principles and practice of infectious diseases* (6th ed., pp. 1841–1856). Philadelphia: Elsevier Churchill Livingstone.

Calabrese, L. H., & Naides, S. J. (2005). Viral arthritis. *Infectious Disease Clinics of North America, 19*(4), 963–980.

Cannon, C. P., Braunwald, E., McCabe, C. H., Grayston, J. T., Muhlestein, B., Giugliano, R. P., et al. (2005). Antibiotic treatment of *Chlamydia pneumoniae* after acute coronary syndrome. *New England Journal of Medicine, 352,* 1646–1652.

Carbone, A., Gloghini, A., Vaccher, E., Cerri, M., Gaidano, G., Dalla-Favera, R., et al. (2005). Kaposi's sarcoma-associated herpesvirus/human herpesvirus type 9-positive solid lymphomas: A tissue-based variant of primary effusion lymphoma. *Journal of Molecular Diagnosis, 7,* 17–27.

Centers for Disease Control and Prevention. (2005, October 6). *Chlamydia pneumoniae.* Retrieved July 15, 2006, from http://www.cdc.gov/ncidod/dbmd/diseaseinfo/chlamydiapneumonia_t.htm

Cesarman, E., & Mesri, E. A. (2007). Kaposi sarcoma-associated herpesvirus and other viruses in human lymphomagenesis. *Current Topics in Microbiology and Immunology, 312,* 263–287.

Chang, Y., Cesarman, E., Pessin, M. S., Lee, F., Culpepper, J., Knowles, D., et al. (1994). Identification of herpesvirus-like DNA sequences in AIDS-associated Kaposi's sarcoma. *Science, 266,* 1865–1869.

Chiba, T., Seno, H., Marusawa, H., Wakatsuki, Y., & Okazaki, K. (2006). Host factors are important in determining clinical outcomes of *Helicobacter pylori* infection. *Journal of Gastroenterology, 41,* 1–9.

Cooper, L. T., Virmani, R., Chapman, N. M., Frustaci, A., Rodeheffer, R. J., Cunningham, M. W., et al. (2006). National Institutes of Health-sponsored workshop on inflammation and immunity in dilated cardiomyopathy. *Mayo Clinic Proceedings, 81,* 199–204.

De Castro-Costa, C. M., Araujo, A. Q., Barreto, M. M., Takayanagui, O. M., Sohler, M. P., da Silva, E. L., et al. (2006). Proposal for diagnostic criteria of tropical spastic paraparesis/HTLV-I-associated myelopathy (TSP/HAM). *AIDS Research and Human Retroviruses, 22,* 931–935.

de Martel, C., & Parsonnet, J. (2006). Tropical infectious diseases and malignancy. In R. L. Guerrant, D. H. Walker, & P. F. Weller (Eds.), *Tropical infectious diseases* (2nd ed., pp. 135–141). Philadelphia: Churchill Livingstone Elsevier.

Eash, S., Manley, K., Gasparovic, M., Querbes, W., & Atwood, W. J. (2006). The human polyomaviruses. *Cellualaar and Molecular Life Sciences, 63,* 865–876.

Eckburg, P. B., & Relman, D. A. (2007). The role of microbes in Crohn's disease. *Clinical Infectious Diseases, 44,* 256–262.

EUROGAST Study Group. (1993). Epidemiology of, and risk factors for, *Helicobacter pylori* infection among 3194 asymptomatic subjects in 17 populations. *Gut, 34,* 1672–1676.

Fenollar, F., Puéchal, X., & Raoult, D. (2007). Whipple's disease. *New England Journal of Medicine, 356,* 55–66.

Feuer, G., & Green, P. L. (2005). Comparative biology of human T-cell lymphotropic virus type 1 (HTLV-1) and HTLV-2. *Oncogene, 24,* 5996–6004.

Frazer, I. H., Cox, J. T., Mayeaux, E. J., Jr., Franco, E. L., Moscicki, A. B., Palefsky J. M., et al. (2006). Advances in prevention of cervical cancer and other human papillomavirus-related diseases. *Pediatric Infectious Disease Journal,* *25*(2 Suppl.), S65–81.

Fredricks, D. N., & Relman, D. A. (1998). Infectious agents and the etiology of chronic idiopathic diseases. *Current Clinical Topics in Infectious Diseases,* *18,* 180–200.

Gallo, R. C. (2005). History of the discoveries of the first human retroviruses: HTLV-1 and HTLV-2. *Oncogene, 24,* 5926–5930.

Gerard, H. C., Wildt, K. L., Whittum-Hudson, J. A., Lai, Z., Ager, J., & Hudson, A. P. (2005). The load of *Chlamydia pneumoniae* in the Alzheimer's brain varies with APOE genotype. *Microbial Pathogenesis, 39,*19–26.

Gisbert, J. P. (2005). The recurrence of *Helicobacter pylori* infection: Incidence and variables influencing it. A critical review. *American Journal of Gastroenterology, 100,* 2083–2099.

Glatzel, M., Stoeck, K., Seeger, H., Lührs, T., & Aguzzi, A. (2005). Human prion diseases. *Archives of Neurology, 62,* 545–552.

Gravitt, P. E., & Jamshidi, R. (2005). Diagnosis and management of oncogenic cervical human papillomavirus infection. *Infectious Disease Clinics of North America, 19,* 439–458.

Grayston, J. T., Kuo, C. C., Wang, S. P., & Altman, J. (1986). A new *Chlamydia psittaci* strain, TWAR, isolated in acute respiratory tract infections. *New England Journal of Medicine, 315,* 161–168.

Guerrant, R. L., Walker, D. H., & Weller, P. F. (Eds.). (2006). *Tropical infectious diseases* (2nd ed.). Philadelphia: Churchill Livingstone Elsevier.

Gupta, S., & Camm, A. J. (1999). Chronic infection, *Chlamydia,* and heart disease. *Developments in Cardiovascular Medicine, 218,* 1–127.

Gurfinkel, E. P., Bozovich, G., Beck, E., Testa, E., Livellara, B., & Mautner, B. (1999). Treatment with the antibiotic roxithromycin in patients with acute non-Q-wave coronary syndromes: The final report of the ROXIS study. *European Heart Journal, 20,* 121–127.

Hatakeyama, M., & Higashi, H. (2005). *Helicobacter pylori* CagA: A new paradigm for bacterial carcinogenesis. *Cancer Science, 96,* 835–843.

Hebner, C. M., & Laimins, L. A. (2006). Human papillomaviruses: Basic mechanisms of pathogenesis and oncogenicity. *Reviews in Medical Virology, 16,* 83–97.

Helicobacter pylori, ulcers and drinking water—USA. (1999). *ProMED Digest,* *99*(133), unpaginated.

Herrera, L. A., Benítez-Bribiesca, L., Mohar, A., & Ostrosky-Wegman, P. (2005). Role of infectious diseases in human carcinogenesis. *Environmental and Molecular Mutagenesis, 45,* 284–303.

IARC Working Group on the Evaluation of Carcinogenic Risks to Humans. (1994). *Schistosomes, liver flukes and* Helicobacter pylori: *Views and expert opinions of an IARC Working Group on the Evaluation of Carcinogenic Risks in Humans, Monograph 61.* Lyon, France: International Agency for Research on Cancer.

Jackson, L. A. (2005). *Chlamydophila (Chlamydia) pneumoniae.* In G. L. Mandell, J. E. Bennett, & R. Dolin (Eds.), *Mandell, Douglas, and Bennett's principles and practice of infectious diseases* (6th ed., pp. 2258–2268). Philadelphia: Elsevier Churchill Livingstone.

Jarrett, R. F. (2006). Viruses and lymphoma/leukaemia. *Journal of Pathology, 208,* 176–186.

Kanbay, M., Kanbay, A., & Boyacioglu, S. (2007). *Helicobacter pylori* infection as a possible risk factor for respiratory system disease: A review of the literature. *Respiratory Medicine, 101,* 203–209.

Kaye, K. M. (2005). Kaposi's sarcoma-associated herpesvirus (human herpesvirus type 8). In G. L. Mandell, J. E. Bennett, & R. Dolin (Eds.), *Mandell, Douglas, and Bennett's principles and practice of infectious diseases* (6th ed., pp. 1827–1832). Philadelphia: Elsevier Churchill Livingstone.

Kivi, M., & Tindberg, Y. (2006). *Helicobacter pylori* occurrence and transmission: A family affair? *Scandinavian Journal of Infectious Diseases, 38,* 407–417.

Klein, L. L., & Gibbs, R. S. (2005). Infection and preterm birth. *Obstetric and Gynecologic Clinics of North America, 32,* 397–410.

Kumar, S., Kumar, S., & Kumar, S. (2006). Infection as a risk factor for gallbladder cancer. *Journal of Surgical Oncology, 93,* 633–639.

Kuper, H., Adami, H.-O., & Trichopoulos, D. (2000). Infections as a major preventable cause of human cancer. *Journal of Internal Medicine, 248,* 171–183.

Lashley, F. R. (2005). *Clinical genetics in nursing practice* (3rd ed.). New York: Springer.

Lashley, F. R. (2006). Emerging infectious diseases at the beginning of the 21st century. *Online Journal of Issues in Nursing, 11*(1), 2–16.

Lashley, F. R. (2007). *Essentials of clinical genetics in nursing practice.* New York: Springer.

Leontiadis, G. I., Sharma, V. K., & Howden, C. W. (1999). Non-gastrointestinal tract associations of *Helicobacter pylori* infection. *Archives of Internal Medicine, 159,* 925–940.

Levine, P. H., Dosik, H., Joseph, E. M., Felton, S., Bertoni, M. A., Cervantes, J., et al. (1999). A study of adult T-cell leukemia/lymphoma incidence in central Brooklyn. *International Journal of Cancer, 80,* 662–666.

MacKenzie, D. (2005, April 18). Will cancer vaccine get to all women? *New Scientist, 2495,* 8.

Mager, D. L. (2006). Bacteria and cancer: Cause, coincidence or cure? A review. *Journal of Translational Medicine, 4,* 14.

Malfertheiner, P., Mégraud, F., O'Morain, C., Bazzoli, F., El-Omar, E., Graham, D., et al. (in press). Current concepts in the management of *Helicobacter pylori* infection – The Maastricht III Consensus Report. *Gut.*

Malfertheiner, P., Sipponen, P., Naumann, M., Moayyedi, P., Mégraud, F., Xiao, S. D., et al. (2005). *Helicobacter pylori* eradication has the potential to prevent gastric cancer: A state-of-the-art critique. *American Journal of Gastroenterology, 100,* 2100–2115.

Mandell, G. L., Bennett, J. E., & Dolin, R. (Eds.). (2005). *Mandell, Douglas, and Bennett's principles and practice of infectious diseases* (6th ed.). Philadelphia: Elsevier Churchill Livingstone.

Marcelin, A. G., Calvez, V., & Dussaix, E. (2007). KSHV after an organ transplant: Should we screen? *Current Topics in Microbiology and Immunology*, *312*, 245–262.

Marshall, B. J. (1983). Unidentified curved bacilli on gastric epithelium in active chronic gastritis. *Lancet*, *1*, 1273–1275.

Marshall, B. J., & Gilman, R. H. (2006). *Helicobacter pylori* infections. In R. L. Guerrant, D. H. Walker, & P. F. Weller (Eds.), *Tropical infectious diseases* (2nd ed., pp. 300–309). Philadelphia: Churchill Livingstone Elsevier.

Martin, R. J. (2006). Infections and asthma. *Clinics in Chest Medicine*, *27*, 87–98.

Matsushita, K., Ozaki, A., Arima, N., & Tei, C. (2005). Human T-Lymphotropic virus type I infection and idiopathic thrombocytopenic purpura. *Hematology*, *10*, 95–99.

Matysiak-Budnik, T., & Mégraud, F. (2006). *Helicobacter pylori* infection and gastric cancer. *European Journal of Cancer*, *42*, 708–716.

McLoughlin, R. R., O'Morain, C. A., & O'Connor, H. J. (2005). Eradication of *Helicobacter pylori*: Recent advances in treatment. *Fundamentals in Clinicl Pharmacology*, *19*, 421–427.

Menna-Barreto, M. (2006). HTLV-II transmission to a health care worker. *American Journal of Infection Control*, *34*, 158–160.

Montalban, C., & Norman, F. (2006). Treatment of gastric mucosa-associated lymphoid tissue lymphoma: *Helicobacter pylori* eradication and beyond. *Expert Reviews in Anticancer Therapy*, *6*, 361–371.

Moore, D. H. (2006). Cervical cancer. *Obstetrics & Gynecology*, *107*, 1152–1161.

Mussa, F. F., Chai, H., Wang, X., Yao, Q., Lumsden, A. B., & Chen, C. (2006). *Chlamydia pneumoniae* and vascular disease: An update. *Journal of Vascular Surgery*, *43*, 1301–1307.

O'Connor, S. M., Taylor, C. E., & Hughes, J. M. (2006). Emerging infectious determinants of chronic diseases. *Emerging Infectious Diseases*, *12*, 1051–1057.

O'Morain, C. (2006). Role of *Helicobacter pylori* in functional dyspepsia. *World Journal of Gastroenterology*, *12*, 2677–2680.

Otasevic, L., Zlatanovic, G., Stanojevic-Paovic, A., Miljkovic-Selimovic, B., Dinic, M. et al. (2007). *Helicobacter pylori*: An underestimated factor in acute anterior uveitis and spondyloarthropathies? *Ophthalmologica*, *221*, 6–13.

Ozgul, A., Dede, I., Taskaynatan, M. A., Aydogan, H., & Kalyon, T. A. (2006). Clinical presentations of chlamydial and non-chlamydial reactive arthritis. *Rheumatology International*, *26*, 879–885.

Parkin, D. M. (2006). The global health burden of infection-associated cancers in the year 2002. *International Journal of Cancer*, *118*, 3030–3044.

Parsonnet, J., Shmuely, H., & Haggerty, T. (1999). Fecal and oral shedding of *Helicobacter pylori* from healthy infected adults. *Journal of the American Medical Association*, *282*, 2240–2245.

Pasceri, V., Patti, G., Cammarota, G., Pristipino, C., Richichi, G., & DiSciascio, G. (2006). Virulent strains of *Helicobacter pylori* and vascular diseases: A meta-analysis. *American Heart Journal*, *151*, 1215–1222.

Peek, R. M., Jr., & Crabtree, J. E. (2006). *Helicobacter* infection and gastric neoplasia. *Journal of Pathology, 208,* 233–248.

Pesonen, E., Andsberg, E., Öhlin, H., Puolakkainen, M., Rautelin, H., Sarna, S., et al. (in press). Dual role of infections as risk factors for coronary heart disease. *Atherosclerosis.*

Poiesz, B. J., Ruscetti, F. W., Gazdar, A. F., Bunn, P. A., Minna, J. D., & Gallo, R. C. (1980). Detection and isolation of type C retrovirus particles from fresh and cultured lymphocytes of a patient with cutaneous T-cell lymphoma. *Proceedings of the National Academy of Sciences, USA, 77,* 7415–7419.

Proietti, F. A., Carneiro-Proietti, A. B. F., Catalan-Soares, B. C., & Murphy, E. L. (2005). Global epidemiology of HTLV-I infection and associated diseases. *Oncogene, 24,* 6058–6068.

Randi, G., Franceschi, S., & La Vecchia, C. (2006). Gallbladder cancer worldwide: Geographical distribution and risk factors. *International Journal of Cancer, 118,* 1591–1602.

Ravandi, F., Kantarjian, H., Jones, D., Dearden, C., Keating, M., & O'Brien, S. (2005). Mature T-cell leukemias. *Cancer, 104,* 1808–1818.

Reynolds, S. J., Bessong, P. O., & Quinn, T. C. (2006). In R. L. Guerrant, D. H. Walker, & P. F. Weller (Eds.), *Tropical infectious diseases* (2nd ed., pp. 852–883). Philadelphia: Churchill Livingstone Elsevier.

Richie, R. C. (2005). Sarcoidosis: A review. *Journal of Insurance Medicine, 37,* 283–294.

Ridker, P. M., Kundsin, R. B., Stampfer, M. J., Poulin, S., & Hennekens, C. H. (1999). Prospective study of *Chlamydia pneumoniae*, IgG seropositivity and risks of future myocardial infarction. *Circulation, 99,* 1161–1164.

Rolling out HPV vaccines worldwide. (2006). *Lancet, 367,* 2034.

Saikku, P., Leinonen, M., Mattila, K., Ekman, M. R., Nieminen, M. S., Makela, P. H., et al. (1988). Serological evidence of an association of a novel *Chlamydia*, TWAR, with chronic coronary heart disease and acute myocardial infarction. *Lancet, 2*(8618), 983–986.

Schottenfeld, D., & Beebe-Dimmer, J. (2005). Advances in cancer epidemiology: Understanding causal mechanisms and the evidence for implementing interventions. *Annual Review of Public Health, 26,* 37–60.

Schulz, T. F. (2006). The pleiotropic effects of Kaposi's sarcoma herpesvirus. *Journal of Pathology, 208,* 187–198.

Sgouros, S. N., & Bergele, C. (2006). Clinical outcome of patients with *Helicobacter pylori* infection: The bug, the host, or the environment? *Postgraduate Medical Journal, 82,* 338–342.

Sheary, B., & Dayan, L. (2005). Cervical screening and human papillomavirus. *Australian Family Physician, 34,* 578–580.

Shor, A., & Phillips, J. I. (1999). *Chlamydia pneumoniae* and atherosclerosis. *Journal of the American Medical Association, 282,* 2071–2073.

Snijders, P. F., Steenbergen R., Heideman D., Meijer C. (2006). HPV-mediated cervical carcinogenesis: Concepts and clinical applications. *Journal of Pathology, 208*(2), 152-164.

Stramer, S. L., Foster, G. A., & Dodd, R. Y. (2006). Effectiveness of human T-lymphotropic virus (HTLV) recipient tracing (lookback) and the current HTLV-I and -II confirmatory algorithm, 1999–2004. *Transfusion, 46,* 703–707.

Taylor, G. P., & Matsuoka, M. (2005). Natural history of adult T-cell leukemia/ lymphoma and approaches to therapy. *Oncogene, 24,* 6047–6057.

Thacker, E. L., Mirzaei, F., & Ascherio, A. (2006). Infectious mononucleosis and risk for multiple sclerosis: A meta-analysis. *Annals of Neurology, 59,* 499–503.

Uchiyama, T., Yodoi, J., Sagawa, K., Takatsuki, K., & Uchino, H. (1977). Adult T-cell leukemia: Clinical and hematologic features of 16 cases. *Blood, 50,* 481–492.

U.S. Food and Drug Administration. (2006, June 8). FDA licenses new vaccine for prevention of cervical cancer and other diseases in females caused by human papillomavirus. *FDA News, P06-77,* unpaginated.

Vitone, F., Gibellini, D., Schiavone, P., D'Antuono, A., Gianni, L., Bon, I., et al. (2006). Human T-lymphotopic virus type I (HTLV-I) prevalence and quantitative detection of DNA proviral load in individuals with indeterminate/positive serological results. *BMC Infectious Diseases, 6,* 41.

Watanabe, Y., Aoyama, N., Sakai, T., Shirasaka, D., Maekawa, S., Kuroda, K., et al. (2006). *HLA-DQB1* locus and gastric cancer in *Helicobacter pylori* infection. *Journal of Gastroenterology and Hepatology, 21,* 420–424.

Wolfe, N. D., Daszak. P., Kilpatrick, A. M., & Burke, D. S. (2005). Bushmeat hunting, deforestation, and prediction of zoonoses emergence. *Emerging Infectious Disease, 11,* 1822–1837.

Yoshida, M., Miyoshi, I., & Hinuma, Y. (1982). A retrovirus from human leukemia cell lines: Its isolation, characterization, and implication in human adult T-cell leukemia (ATL). *Princess Takamatsu Symposium, 12,* 285–294.

Yoshida, M., Seiki, M., Yamaguchi, K., & Takatsuki, K. (1984). Monoclonal integration of human T-cell leukemia provirus in all primary tumors of adult T-cell leukemia suggests causative role of human T-cell leukemia virus in the disease. *Proceedings of the National Academy of Sciences, USA, 81,* 2534–2537.

Zetterström, R. (2006). The Nobel Prize in 2005 for the discovery of *Helicobacter pylori*: Implications for child health. *Acta Paediatrica, 95,* 3–5.

CHAPTER TWENTY-FIVE

Travel, Recreation, and Emerging Infectious Diseases

Felissa R. Lashley

Healing drumbeats were heard throughout St. Mark's church in the Bowery section of New York City in March 2006. The occasion was a celebration of solidarity for the African dance and drumming community and their supporters as part of a healing ceremony for Vado Diomande (Rosenstock, 2006). Vado Diomande, who was 44 years old at the time, is a djembe drummer and dancer who was performing at a university in Pennsylvania when he collapsed with shortness of breath, malaise, and a dry cough. He was diagnosed with inhalation anthrax caused by *Bacillus anthracis*. A few months earlier, Mr. Diomande had traveled to his country of origin, Côte d'Ivoire in Africa. He brought back untreated goat skins as these are said to be necessary for the full-bodied sound of an authentic African drum (Centers for Disease Control and Prevention [CDC], 2006b; Newman, 2006). He had close contact with these skins by repeated soaking of them, scraping the hair with a razor, stretching the hides over the bases of the drums without the use of protective clothing or masks, and working in a poorly ventilated space. This was the first case of naturally acquired inhalation anthrax since 1976 in the United States, but cases of cutaneous anthrax from a goat hide drum bought in Haiti were described in 1974. Investigation revealed anthrax spores in Mr. Diomande's work area but not in his home (CDC, 1974, 2006b). Mr. Diomande has made a full recovery, and in June he began performing again. The rarity of inhalation anthrax in the United States suggested the possibility of bioterrorism, which was ruled out. Bioterrorism and anthrax are described in chapter 27.

As illustrated in the above example, and in chapters 3 and 16, both travel and the seeking of recreational pursuits have increasingly resulted in exposure of persons to emerging infectious diseases they might not otherwise encounter. To some extent, travel and recreation overlap because many engage in recreational activities as part of their travel, and many travel for the specific purpose of recreational pursuits. In regard to travel, tourists increasingly seek more exotic destinations such as tropical rainforests, and business travelers may visit more remote areas for their activities, which can include private business initiatives, religious or missionary activities, or work on behalf of the government, including the armed services. Virtually any destination can be reached in 36 hours of travel, and many in far less time. This time frame allows for the unrecognized global spread of microbes from one place to another. Ostroff and Kozarsky (1998) state that the "global village of the late 20th century provides global opportunities for disease emergence and transmission" (p. 231). Travel may be daily as in commuting; periodic or seasonal for leisure, tourism, or recreation; or long term for colonization or migration (Martens & Hall, 2000). Longer term residents in developing countries are at higher risk for acquiring endemic diseases, which may be detected when they return to their home countries. Increasingly, travel is between developed and developing countries, and vice versa.

It is estimated that among short-term travelers to tropical or subtropical destinations, 50% to 75% report some health impairment as a consequence, often to an infectious agent (Keystone, Steffen, & Kozarsky, 2006). Diarrhea, ranging from self-limited to life threatening, affects 20% to 70% of travelers to tropical and subtropical countries. The organisms involved vary according to geographic region, with the highest risks for those visiting the Middle East, Southeast Asia, Latin America/Carribbean, and sub-Saharan Africa. The etiology may be bacterial, such as enterotoxigenic *Escherichia coli*, enteroaggressive *E. coli*, *Campylobacter* spp., *Shigella* spp., or nontyphoid *Salmonella*; viral such as noroviruses and rotavirus; and parasitic such as *Cyclospora*, *Giardia lamblia*, or *Cryptosporidium* (see chapter 3; Gascon, 2006; Yates, 2005). Some infectious diseases linked to travel are not considered emerging or reemerging in the context of this book and will not be considered here.

TRAVEL

The risk of travel-associated emerging or reemerging infectious diseases is due to several factors:

- New emerging diseases may appear in areas frequented by travelers, providing the first information about a new agent outside that region.
- Travelers may encounter infections endemic to where they are visiting that are nonendemic for their country of origin, which they then transport back.
- Travelers may seek adventure such as engaging in strenuous or unusual outdoor activities including cave exploration; eat unusual or local foods such as bushmeat, sometimes from street vendors; use recreational drugs; come into close contact with animals, both in relatively protected environments such as aquariums or more exposed ones such as when on a safari; or engage in sexual adventures, thus increasing the opportunity to encounter emerging infectious diseases.
- They may decide to adapt local customs such as walking barefoot, acquiring cutaneous larva migrans; sleeping in exposed areas without mosquito nets and being exposed to mosquitos carrying malaria or dengue; or sleeping in accommodations allowing exposure to rodents carrying the vectors or agents of hemorrhagic fevers or plague.

Millions of Muslims embark on a religious pilgrimage to Mecca called the Hajj, which according to Islam should be undertaken once in the able-bodied Muslim's lifetime (Ahmed, Arabi, & Memish, 2006). People from Asia making the religious pilgrimage to Mecca in 1987 brought an epidemic strain of Group A *Neisseria meningitidis* that was transmitted to other pilgrims, who brought it back to sub-Saharan Africa, where it caused epidemics (Moore, Reeves, Schwartz, Gellin, & Broome, 1989). Such epidemics also occurred in 2000 and 2001 and affected thousands. The conditions at the Mecca sites in Saudi Arabia have been described as an "amplifying chamber" in relation to infectious disease risks. International collaboration is an approach for addressing disease potential during the Hajj, and given the huge scope, there are relatively few actual problems despite the potential (Ahmed et al., 2006).

Migrants and immigrants also represent a type of traveler, and at times of turmoil or disaster, large numbers of migrants may be suddenly admitted from developing to developed countries, or they may enter more gradually, possibly bringing with them endemic infectious diseases from their countries that are not endemic to their new locale (Gushulak & MacPherson, 2000). The number of global migrants has increased from 84 million in 1975 to 175 million in 2000 (Maloney, Ortega, & Cetron, 2006). The CDC categorizes foreign-born persons who enter the United States as immigrants; refugees/asylees; nonimmigrants, which includes those on a temporary visa for pleasure, business or work, students, and visitors as well as their families; and unauthorized aliens.

In 1992, 27% of the tuberculosis (TB) cases in the United States occurred in foreign-born persons, and this increased to 53.3% in 2003. Moreover, these cases of TB tended to be due to drug-resistant strains of *Mycobacterium tuberculosis* (CDC, 2005a). A person does not necessarily have to personally travel to be exposed to infectious diseases that are travel-related. In one report, a woman in Georgia with no risk factors or relevant travel history acquired malaria. It was postulated that resident *Anopheles quadrimaculatus* mosquitoes acted as vectors and that transmission was related to the woman's housing proximity to that of the housing of seasonal migrant workers who were natives of malaria-endemic countries and who were potentially gametocytemic (MacArthur et al., 2001). Some of these diseases may be acquired en route, for example, if migrating persons must traverse or ingest contaminated water to reach their destinations. Frequently, they will then seek unskilled work in restaurants in the developed nation, where the infectious agent they have acquired or harbor is transmitted to residents via a foodborne route (Niler, 2000). An example of serious effects of illegal immigration was in the case of a group of illegal stowaways who were in a shipboard cargo container for 2 weeks. Three contracted viral myocarditis due to Coxsackie B virus that was exacerbated by malnutrition, dehydration, and gastroenteritis (Li, Beck, Shi, & Harruff, 2004). Migrants or immigrants may be reexposed to endemic diseases not only when they return to visit their native country (Keystone et al., 2006) but also when they associate with newly arrived persons from their country or ethnic group.

Those migrating or immigrating because of civil unrest or adverse environmental conditions are at high risk for the emergence of disease because they may be malnourished, stressed, exposed to crowded and unsanitary living conditions where clean water and food may not be available, or vulnerable to sexual predators leading to the acquisition of sexually transmitted diseases. They may not be sheltered from exposure to vectors and animals. An example was the movement in 1994 of Rwandan refugees into Zaire, where outbreaks such as cholera swept through refugee camps (Wilson, 1995).

Travelers are both potential victims of an emerging infectious disease and vehicles for further spread, particularly when they return home. When people travel they bring with them pathogens that are in or on their bodies (these can be in an incubation period, latent, or chronic); their normal microbiological flora, which may or may not be similar to the flora in the new locale; their own vulnerability to infection; their cultural preferences, customs, and behaviors that may make them vulnerable to disease; and their baggage, which may also transport organisms, vectors, or contaminated foods (Cookson, Carballo, Nolan, Keystone, & Jong, 2001; Wilson, 1995). Indeed, returning travelers have been referred to as "canary birds" for disease outbreaks (Jelinek & Muhlberger, 2005). In July 2006, a 68-year-old man traveling from Sierra Leone via Abidjan via Belgium en route to Frankfurt, Germany, was diagnosed with Lassa fever, a hemorrhagic fever (see chapter 8), soon after his arrival. An alert seeking passengers who traveled with him as well as for the flight crew and the plane cleaning crew was issued by public health authorities but no secondary cases were identified ("Lassa Fever," 2006). Some pathogens can only be transmitted under certain circumstances. For example, if a person infected with schistosomiasis contaminates water in a new region, it still requires a certain kind of snail to establish a disease cycle. Changing weather and climactic conditions are increasing the geographic range of some disease vectors and allowing emergence in new areas.

Travelers may also be at risk for acquiring infectious disease during transport to or from their destinations. Outbreaks of emerging infectious diseases occurring in persons who have traveled together (such as on the same aircraft) are often difficult to detect once the affected persons have scattered to various geographic locales. Examples of these include malaria, TB, severe acute respiratory syndrome (SARS), and legionellosis. More than one billion persons travel by air each year (Mangili & Gendreau, 2005). Exposure of both passengers and flight crews to TB have been described on commercial aircraft. Those at greatest risk were on longer flights, seated in closer proximity to the source person, or seated in the same section as the source person (Mangili & Gendreau, 2005). Malaria may be acquired by travelers who have visited endemic areas as well as by those who become infected during brief stops at airports in endemic malarial areas (sometimes known as "runway malaria") or who are bitten in flight by infected mosquitos (Isaacson, 1989; Isaacson & Frean, 2001). The term *airport malaria* is used to describe malaria that is acquired through the bite of a mosquito that had been imported to a nonendemic malarial country by air. The first described case was in France in the late 1970s. In a review of the comparatively rare airport malarial cases, a number of them occurred in persons associated occupationally with airports such as cargo handlers and customs officers. Other cases occurred, however, in those who lived or visited near an international airport. In one case, the landlord of a public house near Gatwick Airport in London developed malaria, and it was thought that an imported infected mosquito was brought into the pub through a vehicle carrying the aircrew there from the airport (Isaacson, 1989). Live mosquitos were detected in 12 of 67 airplanes that arrived at Gatwick Airport in London in one study. And in 27 airplanes arriving at Nairobi airport in 1986, 150 adult mosquitos were detected. A study conducted in 2000 also found mosquitos on flights from Africa (Karch, Delile, Guillet, & Mouchet, 2001). Mosquitos are carried not only in the passenger or cargo hold, but also in the wheel bays. Various disinfection is recommended for vector control, but this does not eliminate all risk (Isaacson, 1989; Karch et al., 2001). Travelers often acquire malaria because of inadequate chemoprophylaxis, especially during travel to areas where the malarial parasite is resistant to chloroquine (CDC, 2001b), or because the traveler has not taken the appropriate precautions. However, even appropriate chemoprophylaxis may not be 100% effective. In long-term travelers, risks may be accentuated, and conditions such as pregnancy may influence prophylaxis (Chen, Wilson & Schlagenhauf, 2006). It is believed the risks for the transport of *Anopheles* mosquitoes carrying malaria from Africa to developed countries will increase as more air routes from Africa are added, thus giving rise to cases of local transmission of malaria in nonendemic areas (Tatem, Rogers, & Hay, 2006). Malaria is considered in detail in chapter 17.

Severe acute respiratory syndrome (SARS), a recently emerged disease due to the SARS coronavirus (see chapter 22), was associated with onboard transmission aboard various airplane flights. In one instance, a flight carrying 120 passengers from Hong Kong to Beijing resulted in laboratory-confirmed SARS in 16 people, with 2 probable cases and 4 reported others (Olsen et al., 2003). Even mumps (a vaccine-preventable viral disease) has been spread during an airline flight. A total of 11 potentially infected people traveled by air in a 1-month period between March and April 2006. Two cases of mumps were found after follow-up of passengers possibly exposed on the flight (CDC, 2006a). Foodborne outbreaks have also been reported. In one case, during a flight from South America to Los Angeles that coincided with a cholera epidemic in South America, a cold seafood appetizer resulted in cholera developing in 75 passengers with 1 fatality (Eberhart-Phillips et al., 1996). In the last few years, no foodborne outbreaks resulting from transmission during air travel have been reported (Mangili & Gendreau, 2005). Ventilation rates on aircraft may be higher than some other enclosed forms of transportation, and the risk of TB transmission is relatively low but is higher on flights from TB-endemic regions such as Africa and parts of Asia (Byrne, 2007).

Outbreaks of infectious diseases may also occur on cruise ships. Gastroenteritis from various sources have been reported to occur on cruise ships from both contaminated water and food because sometimes these ships purchase local foodstuff or water that is contaminated. Before 1996, however, there were no confirmed reports of waterborne outbreaks of *E. coli* on cruise ships. Today, *E. coli* is called an emerging waterborne pathogen on cruise ships. Outbreaks are believed to occur from water that is taken on in foreign ports. Recommendations have been made to ensure improved handling practices, careful disinfection, and monitoring of water quality to prevent future outbreaks. Ships docking in U.S. ports are also supposed to report the number of passengers or crew members who have visited the ship's physician for diarrhea 24 hours before arrival. This surveillance is under the auspices of the Vessel Sanitation Program of the CDC (Daniels et al., 2000). The semiclosed air systems on cruise ships have also led to outbreaks of influenza, and the CDC has recommended that travelers at high risk for complications should consider receiving an influenza vaccine before travel with a large tourist group, to the tropics, or in the Southern hemisphere from April through September. They also suggest that crew members have at least an 80% vaccination rate (CDC, 2001a). Norovirus gastroenteritis outbreaks on cruise ships have increased in recent years and have been particularly resistant to sanitary procedures. In many of these outbreaks, multiple modes of transmission occurred including foodborne, person-to-person, and environmental contamination (Isakbaeva et al., 2005).

Travel-related Legionnaires disease has also been reported. Legionnaires disease is caused by *Legionella pneumophila*, a bacterium, and first was noticed among those attending an American Legion convention in Philadelphia in July 1976. Retrospective studies indicated at least two prior outbreaks. Aerosols from the cooling system were identified as the source of the organism in that outbreak (Breiman & Butler, 1998). Today, about 21% of all reported cases of Legionnaires disease are travel associated (CDC, 2005b). Recent reports have described outbreaks among cruise ship passengers who used or spent time near a whirlpool spa. These outbreaks often are undetected because travelers disperse after disembarking. In another outbreak, the water supply system was the source of infection (Castellani Pastoris et al., 1999). In one instance in 1994, a New Jersey physician notified the health department that three patients with atypical pneumonia all had been passengers on the same cruise ship. This led to an investigation that detected 50 passengers from that ship with Legionnaires disease. The investigation of this outbreak led to new CDC guidelines for prevention of Legionnaires disease aboard cruise ships (Jernigan et al., 1996). In another instance, *L. pneumophila* was found in porous stones used in a spa filter that was the source of two cases of Legionnaires disease aboard a cruise ship (Kura et al., 2006), and the organism has been recovered in water samples from showers and washbasins on ferries and cruise ships (Azara et al., 2006) In another travel-related occurrence, a multistate outbreak of Legionnaire disease occurred among nine members of tour groups staying at lodges in Vermont, where they had gone to observe fall foliage. Most of those affected were senior citizens, who presumably were more vulnerable because of immunocompromise and underlying illnesses (Mamolen et al., 1993). In fact, in many of these outbreaks, elderly persons are particularly vulnerable. Legionnaires disease is considered in detail in chapter 15.

Souvenirs may be an unwitting source of infection. In one particular instance, a traveler brought home a camel hair saddle from Pakistan. It was given to a 12-year-old girl. Later, she developed a large carbuncle that turned out to be cutaneous anthrax, a rare disease in developed countries but still a problem in countries such as Iran, Turkey, Pakistan, and the Sudan (Smith, 1995).

Food- and waterborne illnesses are a very frequent consequence of travel. Travel to developing countries may put the traveler into contact with contaminated food and water, often by the fecal–oral route. Contamination may occur during growing, harvesting, handling, transporting, storing, or preparation of the foods. When abroad, travelers may wish to try local foods including bushmeat, and buy samples from street vendors whose hygienic practices are unknown. Cholera, cryptosporidiosis, and other infectious agents causing diarrhea have been acquired by travelers in this way. Some travel, especially to southern China, is specifically for unusual experiences that may include eating exotic animals as a delicacy. A concern is that the civet cat, a popular exotic food delicacy, has also been shown to be the source of the 2002–2003 SARS outbreak in China (Cheng, 2007). Gnathostomosis (gnathostomiasis), caused by a nematode, has been acquired in Acapulco, Mexico, after eating poorly cooked or raw fish, particularly as ceviche, in which fish salad is "cooked" only in lime juice (Rojas-Molina, Pedraza-Sanchez, Torres-Bibiano, Meza-Martinez, & Escobar-Gutierrez, 1999). Both recreational and drinking water may be contaminated in developing countries. Many of those who participated in the Eco-Challenge in Borneo in the fall of 2000 acquired leptospirosis, which developed after their return home. Participants noted that in the course of their participation, they acquired open sores and leech bites that might have contributed to acquiring infection ("Leptospirosis," 2001). Food- and waterborne infections are considered in more detail in chapter 3 and with discussions of specific diseases such as cholera, cryptosporidiosis, cyclosporiasis, and *E. coli* (see chapters 4, 5, 6, and 9).

Risks from emerging infectious agents may also result from the need for medical treatment in developing countries where equipment, needles, and syringes may not be sterile. There may also be a risk from blood transfusions, especially where endemic transmissible infections are prevalent in the blood donor population (see chapter 3). For example, a case of human immunodeficiency virus (HIV) infection was acquired by a tourist in Africa by a transfusion received after a bus accident (Hill, 1989). More than 5% of European travelers to tropical countries reported accidents

(Rack et al., 2005). Endemic diseases in local areas pose a risk to travelers. In two recent instances, one in a group from Pennsylvania and one from Washington, coccidioidomycosis was acquired while in Mexico, presumably from dust exposure (Cairns et al., 2000; CDC, 2000a). Dengue (see chapter 7) is endemic in tropical and subtropical regions, and in 2005, 96 cases of travel-associated dengue were reported to the CDC (CDC, 2006d).

RECREATION

Increasingly, recreational activities both close to home and at near and far distances bring people into greater contact with animals and vectors of emerging infectious diseases. These may occur when people pursue hobbies that expose them to zoonoses such as by close contact with wild animals or pets, during cave exploration, hiking in wilderness areas, hunting, camping, and pursuing recreational water activities such as swimming, boating, or white-water rafting. Even swallowing a small amount of water while engaging in these activities might prove hazardous. Acquisition of infectious diseases through recreational activities involving water and food are discussed also in chapter 3.

In one instance, a female veterinary ophthalmologist fell off her raft during a white-water excursion in a Costa Rican rain forest. She returned home to Utah, where 4 days later she developed fever, shaking chills, diaphoresis, headache, muscle and eye aches, and renal and liver involvement. It was determined that she had acquired leptospirosis, considered to be a reemerging disease in the United States (Levett, 2001). Leptospirosis is caused by the spirochete *Leptospira interrogans*. Humans become infected with the spirochetes when they enter microabrasions in skin or via intact mucous membranes (Meites et al., 2004). Leptospirosis was also responsible for an outbreak involving triathletes who became ill after swimming in a lake in Springfield, Illinois (CDC, 1998). Another example was an outbreak in the Yaeyama Islands of Japan in which 71% of the leptospirosis cases were associated with recreational water sports (Narita, Fujitani, Haake, & Paterson, 2005). Leptospirosis can be acquired closer to home as well. In 1996, three inner city residents of Baltimore, Maryland, who had flu-like illnesses were determined actually to have leptospirosis. It was postulated that they contracted leptospirosis by walking barefoot through alleys contaminated by infected animal urine (Ault, 2000). In California, leptospirosis is still a reportable disease, and most of the cases tend to occur in previously healthy adult White males with exposure to contaminated freshwater while engaging in various recreational activities (Meites et al., 2004).

Animals can be a source of infectious disease. Close contact between animals and people occurs during visits to places such as petting zoos and animal farms. Cases of *E. coli* O157:H7 may result from such contact. In some instances, *E. coli* infection results in the more serious hemolytic uremic syndrome (HUS), such as occurred recently in North Carolina, Florida, and Arizona. In these 3 outbreaks, there was close contact with animals at petting zoos or as part of fairs (CDC, 2005c). Many people keep exotic pets such as reptiles including turtles, snakes, lizards, and iguanas. Sometimes these are illegally imported. Over 90% of reptiles may carry *Salmonella enterica*, which can cause gastroenteritis, which in children may lead to more severe illnesses such as septicemia or meningitis. It is believed that salmonellosis from pet reptiles is underreported. There has been a resurgence of keeping small turtles as pets, and this has been associated with cases of salmonellosis. In several cases, the turtles were purchased as souvenirs while on vacation (CDC, 2005d). In the 1970s, several outbreaks associated with small turtle pets occurred, but regulations put in place diminished the spread. Those who are immunosuppressed need to exert caution with reptilian pets, avoid close contacts with animals, and take other precautions (CDC, 2002). There has been a trend toward more exotic pets. In May 2003, the first cases of monkeypox were reported among members of a family in Wisconsin. These cases were found to be associated with two prairie dogs that were purchased as pets. The prairie dogs had been housed at the distributor with an infected Gambian giant rat from Ghana and other exotic rodent species. In all, 72 people were infected in this outbreak (CDC, 2003b). Monkeypox is discussed in chapter 19.

Expansion of walking in forested areas and the expansion of housing into areas formerly inhabited only by wildlife have exposed persons to closer proximity with the vectors of emerging infectious diseases. The most well-known examples are Lyme disease, resulting from the tickborne rickettsia *Borrelia burgdorferi*, as well as ehrlichiosis and anaplasmosis, discussed in detail in chapter 16. Leisure travel adventures are becoming increasingly exotic including game safaris. Such adventures have resulted in the acquisition of African tickborne fever, caused by a rickettsia, usually diagnosed when the traveler returns home (Chomel, Belotto, & Meslin, 2007). Even lying or walking on the beach in a tropical or subtropical country may result in disease. Cutaneous larva migrans is the most frequent skin disease among travelers returning from tropical countries. This hookworm may be shed by dogs or cats that shed the eggs via feces on sandy beaches or soils where the relaxing tourist who goes barefoot on the sand or who lies on it may acquire the disease (Caumes, 2000; Tremblay, MacLean, Gyorkos, & MacPherson, 2000). Closer to home, cryptosporidiosis can be acquired from swimming pools and other recreational waters including water parks and fountains (White, 2005). Home gardening can occasionally be hazardous. *Legionella longbeachae*-associated pneumonia has been traced to contaminated potting soil in California, Oregon, Washington, Japan, the Netherlands, and Australia (CDC, 2000b; den Boer, et al., 2007). Possible modes of transmission might be inhalation and ingestion due to exposure to aerosolized *L. longbeachae* or poor gardening hygiene, and were associated with underlying illness, smoking, poor hand washing after gardening and being near dripping hanging flower pots (O'Connor, et al., 2007). Malaria may also be acquired during recreational pursuits in the United States, albeit rarely, since there have been a number of cases reported from Suffolk County, New York, acquired during hiking and camping (CDC, 2000c).

In Sweden, a popular sport is orienteering, in which running participants use a compass and map to find the fastest route. Between 1979 and 1992, there were a number of sudden unexpected cardiac deaths among orienteers aged 18 to 32 years. Investigation revealed the presence of subacute myocarditis, probably induced by *Bartonella* spp. infections, which might have been acquired because of exposure and because intense training can affect immune function. After research, a series of recommendations for prevention were issued (McGill et al., 2001; Wesslen et al., 2001).

An example of a reemerging disease associated with travel and/or recreational activity is plague caused by a gram-negative bacteria, *Yersinia pestis*. It is considered an emerging or reemerging infectious disease because its geographic boundary contacts with humans have expanded. Humans may encounter plague-carrying fleas when hiking, hunting, or camping in endemic areas. It is transmitted by fleas that primarily infect domestic rats and other rodents and can affect other small mammals including dogs and cats (Butler & Dennis, 2005). Plague is usually inapparent in its natural reservoir hosts in its enzootic state. This type of transmission is of low risk to humans. However, epizootic plague with rapid spread may occur, resulting in widespread die-offs of infected rodents and natural hosts. When this happens, their fleas disperse; thus, this type poses more of a threat to humans. Other mammals can become incidentally infected, and rabbits have occasionally been a source of infection for hunters. Ungulates such as deer, camel, and goats can become infected, and eating undercooked infected goat and camel meat has been documented as a source of plague outbreaks in northern Africa, the Middle East, and central Asia (Christie, Chen, & Elberg, 1980; Dennis & Mead, 2006). In Rocky Mountain National Park, near Estes Park, Colorado, there are signs warning visitors not to handle the friendly ground squirrels since they may carry plague. Despite the fact that they go on to explain what plague is, many tourists continue to disregard the warnings and feed and handle the ground squirrels.

Currently, plague is more of a rural or suburban fringe illness in the United States, and the last known urban outbreak was in Los Angeles in 1924–1925. Y. *pestis*-infected rats have been found in recent decades, however, in cities such as Tacoma, Washington; San Francisco; Los Angeles; and Dallas. Worldwide, 80% of cases are found in Africa. In the United States, about 80% of cases occur in Colorado, New Mexico, and Arizona with 10% in California. Transmission is usually through handling infected animals, typically as a result of being bitten by infected fleas, or through inhalation of infected respiratory droplets (pneumonic plague), which can be tranmitted from person to person (Dennis & Mead, 2006). Travel-associated plague has been called peripatetic plague. Outcomes may be poorer because the person might delay seeking treatment or the diagnosis might not be considered if health care providers do not consider plague as a potential diagnosis. In one case of peripatetic plague in November 2002, a husband and wife became ill in New York City, where they sought emergency care in a hospital where plague was not usually seen. They both were from New Mexico, and because they had contacted their New Mexico physician, diagnosis of bubonic plague was not delayed. Subsequent investigation demonstrated infected wood rat fleas on their property in New Mexico (CDC, 2003a). Because plague is considered a Category A agent for bioterrorism (see chapter 27), this type of outbreak was intensively investigated.

Major outbreaks of pneumonic and bubonic plague occurred in India in 1994, and travelers entering the United States were observed for symptoms although no plague cases were identified in the United States. However, many travelers who were ill were not detected at entry points but came to attention after return to their community physician (CDC, 1994). This has implications for containment of infectious diseases, particularly those that are easily spread from person to person often by airborne or respiratory droplet transmission.

CONCLUSION

Travel and leisure time and recreational pursuits bring people into greater contact with the vectors and agents of emerging infectious diseases, especially if travel is to developing countries or exotic locales. Depending on the mode of spread, there are a variety of preventive measures that can be taken. These include chemotherapy prophylaxis such as for malaria and immunization recommendations that are specific to country of travel or special situations. Other precautions are summarized in Appendix C, Tables C.1–C.6. Information may be obtained from organizations such as the following: the CDC Traveler's Health Web site at http://www.cdc.gov/travel, the World Health Organization Web site at http://www.who.int/ith, and the Travel Medicine Program Health Canada Web site at http://www.hc-sc.gc.ca/hpblcdc/osh/mp_e.html as well as local and regional traveler's health clinics.

A variety of questionnaires asking travelers at airports in Johannesburg, various European airports, and New York City about prophylaxis revealed a higher knowledge of risk than actual precautions (Hamer & Connor, 2004; Toovey, Jamieson, & Holloway, 2004; Van Herck et al., 2004). But sometimes, knowledge is incomplete. In one instance, 5 cases of malaria due to *Plasmodium falciparum* occurred in a family near Chicago, Illinois. They were traveling to the native country of the parents and one child, Nigeria. They sought information and assumed that the antimalarial drugs were for treatment and not prophylaxis, so they did not obtain a prescription (CDC, 2006c). This points out the importance of thoroughly assessing the pretravel needs as well as being alert to the possibility of a travel-related febrile episode or infectious disease and asking the appropriate questions. Emergency department assessments of persons presenting with fever require evaluation including travel history and consideration of uncommon pathogenic agents (Pigott, 2007; Woodrow et al., 2007).

REFERENCES

Ahmed, Q. A., Arabi, Y. M., & Memish, Z. A. (2006). Health risks at the Hajj. *Lancet, 367,* 1008–1015.

Ault, A. (2000, October 10). Deadly infection re-emerges as people get adventurous. *New York Times* [Electronic version]. Retrieved December 15, 2006, from http://www.nytimes.com/2000/10/10/science/10WORM.html

Azara, A., Plana, A., Sotgiu, G., Dettori, M., Deriu, M. G., Masia, M. D., et al. (2006). Prevalence study of *Legionella* spp contamination in ferries and cruise ships. *BMC Public Health, 6,* 100.

Breiman, R. F., & Butler, J. C. (1998). Legionnaires' disease: Clinical epidemiological, and public health perspectives. *Seminars in Respiratory Infection, 13*(2), 84–89.

Butler, T., & Dennis, D. T. (2005). *Yersinia* species, including plague. In G. L. Mandell, J. E. Bennett, & R. Dolin (Eds.), *Mandell, Douglas, and Bennett's principles and practice of infectious diseases* (6th ed., pp. 2691–2701). Philadelphia: Elsevier Churchill Livingstone.

Byrne, N. (2007). Low prevalence of TB on long-haul aircraft. *Travel Medicine and Infectious Disease, 5,* 18–23.

Cairns, L., Blythe, D., Kao, A., Pappagianis, D., Kaufman, L., Kobayashi, J., et al. (2000). Outbreak of coccidioidomycosis in Washington state residents returning from Mexico. *Clinical Infectious Diseases, 30*, 61–64.

Castellani Pastoris, M., Lo Monaco, R., Goldoni, P., Mentore, B., Balestra, G., Ciceroni, L., et al. (1999). Legionnaires' disease on a cruise ship linked to the water supply system: Clinical and public health implications. *Clinical Infectious Diseases, 28*, 33–38.

Caumes, E. (2000). Treatment of cutaneous larva migrans. *Clinical Infectious Diseases, 30*, 811–814.

Centers for Disease Control and Prevention. (1974). Cutaneous anthrax acquired from imported Haitian drums—Florida. *Morbidity and Mortality Weekly Report, 23*, 142, 147.

Centers for Disease Control and Prevention. (1994). International notes update: Human plague—India, 1994. *Morbidity and Mortality Weekly Report, 43*, 689–691.

Centers for Disease Control and Prevention. (1998). Update: Leptospirosis and unexplained acute febrile illness among athletes participating in triathlons—Illinois and Wisconsin, 1998. *Morbidity and Mortality Weekly Report, 47*, 673–676.

Centers for Disease Control and Prevention. (2000a). Coccidioidomycosis in travelers returning from Mexico—Pennsylvania, 2000. *Morbidity and Mortality Weekly Report, 49*, 1004–1006.

Centers for Disease Control and Prevention. (2000b). Legionnaires' disease associated with potting soil—California, Oregon and Washington May–June 2000. *Morbidity and Mortality Weekly Report, 49*, 777–778.

Centers for Disease Control and Prevention. (2000c). Probable locally acquired mosquito-transmitted *Plasmodium vivax* infection—Suffolk county, New York, 1999. *Morbidity and Mortality Weekly Report, 49*, 495–498.

Centers for Disease Control and Prevention. (2001a). Influenza B virus outbreak on a cruise ship—Northern Europe, 2000. *Morbidity and Mortality Weekly Report, 50*, 137–140.

Centers for Disease Control and Prevention. (2001b). Malaria deaths following inappropriate malaria chemoprophylaxis—United States, 2001. *Morbidity and Mortality Weekly Report, 50*, 597–599.

Centers for Disease Control and Prevention. (2002). Guidelines for the prevention of opportunistic infections among HIV-infected persons—2002. Recommendations of the United States Public Health Service and the Infectious Disease Society of America. *Morbidity and Mortality Weekly Report, 51*(RR-8), 1–52.

Centers for Disease Control and Prevention. (2003a). Imported plague—New York City, 2002. *Morbidity and Mortality Weekly Report, 52*, 725–728.

Centers for Disease Control and Prevention. (2003b). Update: Multistate outbreak of monkeypox—Illinois, Indiana, Kansas, Missouri, Ohio, Wisconsin, 2003. *Morbidity and Mortality Weekly Report, 52*, 642–646.

Centers for Disease Control and Prevention. (2005a). Controlling tuberculosis in the United States. Recommendations from the American Thoracic Society, CDC, and the Infectious Diseases Society of America. *Morbidity and Mortality Weekly Report, 54*(RR-12), 1–82.

Centers for Disease Control and Prevention. (2005b). Cruise-ship associated Legionnaires disease, November 2003–May 2004. *Morbidity and Mortality Weekly Report, 54,* 1153–1155.

Centers for Disease Control and Prevention. (2005c). Outbreaks of *Escherichia coli* O157:H7 associated with petting zoos–North Carolina, Florida, and Arizona, 2004 and 2005. *Morbidity and Mortality Weekly Report, 54,* 1277–1280.

Centers for Disease Control and Prevention. (2005d). Salmonellosis associated with pet turtles—Wisconsin and Wyoming, 2004. *Morbidity and Mortality Weekly Report, 54,* 223–225.

Centers for Disease Control and Prevention. (2006a). Exposure to mumps during air travel—United States, April, 2006. *Morbidity and Mortality Weekly Report, 55,* 401–402.

Centers for Disease Control and Prevention. (2006b). Inhalation anthrax associated with dried animal hides—Pennsylvania and New York City, 2006. *Morbidity and Mortality Weekly Report, 55,* 280–282.

Centers for Disease Control and Prevention. (2006c). Malaria in multiple family members—Chicago, Illinois, 2006. *Morbidity and Mortality Weekly Report, 55,* 645–648.

Centers for Disease Control and Prevention. (2006d). Travel-associated dengue—United States, 2005. *Morbidity and Mortality Weekly Report, 55,* 700–702.

Chen, L. H., Wilson, M. E., & Schlagenhauf, P. (2006). Prevention of malaria in long-term travelers. *Journal of the American Medical Association, 296,* 2234–2244.

Cheng, M. H. (2007). SARS source back on the menu. *Lancet Infectious Diseases, 7,* 14.

Chomel, B. B., Belotto, A., & Meslin, F.-X. (2007). Wildlife, exotic pets, and emerging zoonoses. *Emerging Infectious Diseases, 13,* 6–11.

Christie, A. B., Chen, T. H., & Elberg, S. S. (1980). Plague in camels and goats: Their role in human epidemics. *Journal of Infectious Diseases, 141,* 724–726.

Cookson, S. T., Carballo, M., Nolan, C. M., Keystone, J. S., & Jong, E. C. (2001). Migrating populations—A closer view of who, why, and so what. *Emerging Infectious Diseases, 7*(3, Suppl.), 551.

Daniels, N. A., Neimann, J., Karpati, A., Parashar, U. D., Greene, K. D, Wells, J. G., et al. (2000). Traveler's diarrhea at sea: Three outbreaks of waterborne enterotoxigenic *Escherichia coli* on cruise ships. *Journal of Infectious Diseases, 181,* 1491–1495.

Den Boer, J. W., Yzerman, E. P., Jansen, R., Bruin, J. P., Verhoef, L. P., Neve, G., et al. (2007). Legionnaires' disease and gardening. *Clinical Microbiology and Infection, 13,* 88–91.

Dennis, D. T., & Mead, P. S. (2006). Plague. In R. L. Guerrant, D. H. Walker, & P. F. Weller (Eds.), *Tropical infectious diseases* (2nd ed., pp 471–481). Philadelphia: Churchill Livingstone Elsevier.

Eberhart-Phillips, J., Besser, R. E., Tormey, M. P., Koo, D., Feikin, D., Araneta, M. R., et al. (1996). An outbreak of cholera from food served on an international aircraft. *Epidemiology and Infection, 118,* 9–13.

Gascon, J. (2006). Epidemiology, etiology and pathophysiology of traveler's diarrhea. *Digestion, 73*(Suppl. 1), 102–108.

Gushulak, B. D., & MacPherson, D. W. (2000). Population mobility and infectious diseases. *Clinical Infectious Diseases, 31,* 776–780.

Hamer, D. H., & Connor, B. A. (2004). Travel health knowledge, attitudes and practices among United States travelers. *Journal of Travel Medicine, 11,* 23–26.

Hill, D. R. (1989). HIV infection following motor vehicle trauma in central Africa. *Journal of the American Medical Association, 261,* 3282–3283.

Isaacson, M. (1989). Airport malaria: A review. *Bulletin of the World Health Organization, 67,* 737–743.

Isaacson, M., & Frean, J. A. (2001). African malaria vectors in European aircraft. *Lancet, 357,* 235.

Isakbaeva, E. T., Widdowson, M.-A., Beard, R. S., Bulens, S. N., Mullins, J., Monroe, S. S., et al. (2005). Norovirus transmission on cruise ship. *Emerging Infectious Diseases, 11,* 154–157.

Jelinek, T., & Muhlberger, N. (2005). Surveillance of imported diseases as a window to travel health risks. *Infectious Disease Clinics of North America, 19,* 1–13.

Jernigan, D. B., Hofmann, J., Cetron, M. S., Genese, C. A., Nuorti, J. P., Fields, B. S., et al. (1996). Outbreak of Legionnaires' disease among cruise ship passengers exposed to a contaminated whirlpool spa. *Lancet, 347,* 494–499.

Karch, S., Delile, M.-F., Guillet, P., & Mouchet, J. (2001). African malaria vectors in European aircraft. *Lancet, 357,* 235.

Keystone, J. S., Steffen, R., & Kozarsky, P. E. (2006). Health advice for international travel. In R. L. Guerrant, D. H. Walker, & P. F. Weller (Eds.), *Tropical infectious diseases* (2nd ed., pp. 1400–1424). Philadelphia: Churchill Livingstone Elsevier.

Kura, F., Amemura-Maekawa, J., Yagita, K., Endo, T., Ikeno, M., Tsuji, H., et al. (2006). Outbreak of Legionnaires' disease on a cruise ship linked to spa-bath filter stones contaminated with *Legionella pneumophila* serogroup 5. *Epidemiology and Infection, 134,* 385–391.

Lassa fever—Europe ex Sierra Leone (02). (2006). *ProMED Digest, 329,* unpaginated.

Levett, P. N. (2001). Leptospirosis. *Clinical Microbiology Reviews, 14,* 296–326.

Leptospirosis, Eco-Challenge race—Borneo: 2000. (2001). *ProMED Digest, 19,* unpaginated.

Li, M. K., Beck, M. A., Shi, Q., & Harruff, R. C. (2004). Unexpected hazard of illegal immigration: Outbreak of viral myocarditis exacerbated by confinement and deprivation in a shipboard cargo container. *American Journal of Forensic Medical Pathology, 25,* 117–124.

MacArthur, J. R., Holtz, T. H., Jenkins, J., Newell, J. P., Koehler, J. E., Parise, M. E., et al. (2001). Probable locally acquired mosquito-transmitted malaria in Georgia, 1999. *Clinical Infectious Diseases, 32,* E124–128.

Maloney, S. A., Ortega, L. S., & Cetron, M. S. (2006). Migrant, immigrant, and refugee health. In R. L. Guerrant, D. H. Walker, & P. F. Weller (Eds.), *Tropical infectious diseases* (2nd ed., pp. 1425–1435). Philadelphia: Churchill Livingstone Elsevier.

Mamolen, M., Breiman, R. F., Barbaree, J. M., Gunn, R. A., Stone, K. M., Spika, J. S., et al. (1993). Use of multiple molecular subtyping techniques to investigate a Legionnaires' disease outbreak due to identical strains at two tourist lodges. *Journal of Clinical Microbiology, 31,* 2584–1401.

Mangili, A., & Gendreau, M. A. (2005). Transmission of infectious diseases during commercial air travel. *Lancet, 365,* 989–996.

Martens, P., & Hall, L. (2000). Malaria on the move: Human population movement and malaria transmission. *Emerging Infectious Diseases, 6,* 103–109.

McGill, S., Wesslen, L., Hjelm, E., Holmberg, M., Rolf, C., & Friman, G. (2001). Serological and epidemiological analysis of the prevalence of *Bartonella* spp antibodies in Swedish elite orienteers. *Scandinavian Journal of Infectious Diseases, 33,* 423–428.

Meites, E., Jay, M. T., Deresinski, S., Shieh, W.-J., Zaki, S. R., Tompkins, L., et al. (2004). Reemerging leptospirosis, California. *Emerging Infectious Diseases, 10,* 406–412.

Moore, P. S., Reeves, M. W., Schwartz, B., Gellin, B. G., & Broome, C. V. (1989). Intercontinental spread of an epidemic group A *Neisseria meningitidis* strain. *Lancet, 2,* 260–263.

Narita, M., Fujitani, S., Haake, D. A., & Paterson, D. L. (2005). Leptospirosis after recreational exposure to water in the Yaeyama islands, Japan. *American Journal of Tropical Medicine and Hygiene, 73,* 652–656.

Newman, A. (2006, February 24). *Drum maker in Brooklyn has no fear of anthrax.* Retrieved July 7, 2006, from http://firedrumcircle.tribe.net/thread/409cc0b0-73c0-4c7c-8ab5-a90c67047eld

Niler, E. (2000). Diseased passage. *Scientific American, 383*(1), 23–24.

O'Connor, B. A., Carman, J., Eckert, K., Tucker, G., Givney, R., & Cameron, S. (2007). Does using potting mix make you sick? Results from a *Legionella longbeachae* case-control study in South Australia. *Epidemiology and Infection, 135,* 34–39.

Olsen, S. J., Chang, H. L. Cheung, T. Y., Tang, A., Fisk, T. L., Ooi, S. P., et al. (2003). Transmission of the severe acute respiratory syndrome on aircraft. *New England Journal of Medicine, 349,* 2416–2422.

Ostroff, S. M., & Kozarsky, P. (1998). Emerging infectious diseases and travel medicine. *Infectious Disease Clinics of North America, 12,* 231–241.

Pigott, D. C. (2007). Emergency department evaluation of the febrile traveler. *Journal of Infection, 54,* 1–5.

Rack, J., Wichmann, O., Kamara, B., Gunther, M., Cramer, J., Schonfeld, C., et al. (2005). Risk and spectrum of diseases in travelers to popular tourist destinations. *Journal of Travel Medicine, 12,* 248–253.

Rojas-Molina, N., Pedraza-Sanchez, S., Torres-Bibiano, B., Meza-Martinez, H., & Escobar-Gutierrez, A. (1999). Gnathostomosis, an emerging foodborne zoonotic disease in Acapulco, Mexico. *Emerging Infectious Diseases, 5,* 264–266.

Rosenstock, B. (2006, March 15–21). Healing drumbeats at St. Marks for anthrax victim. *The Villager, 75*(43), 1.

Smith, L. (1995). The case of the camel hair carbuncle. *Patient Care, 29*(10), 138–139.

Tatem, A. J., Rogers, D. L., & Hay, S. I. (2006). Estimating the malaria risk of African mosquito movement by air travel. *Malaria Journal, 5,* 57.

Toovey, S., Jamieson, A., & Holloway, M. (2004). Travelers' knowledge, attitudes and practices on the prevention of infectious diseases: Results from a study at Johannesburg International Airport. *Journal of Travel Medicine, 11,* 16–22.

Tremblay, A., MacLean, J. D., Gyorkos, T., & MacPherson, D. W. (2000). Outbreak of cutaneous larva migrans in a group of travellers. *Tropical Medicine and International Health, 5,* 330–334.

Van Herck, K., Van Damme, P., Castelli, F., Zuckerman, J., Nothdurft, H., Dahlgren, A. L., et al. (2004). Knowledge, attitudes and practices in travel-related infectious diseases: The European airport survey. *Journal of Travel Medicine, 11,* 3–8.

Wesslen, L., Ehrenborg, C., Holmberg, M., McGill, S., Hjelm, E., Lindquist, O., et al. (2001). Subacute *Bartonella* infection in Swedish orienteers succumbing to sudden unexpected cardiac death or having malignant arrhythmias. *Scandinavian Journal of Infectious Diseases, 33,* 429–438.

White, A. C., Jr. (2005). Cryptosporidiosis (*Cryptosporidium hominis, Cryptosporidium parvum,* and other species). In G. L. Mandell, J. E. Bennett, & R. Dolin (Eds.), *Mandell, Douglas, and Bennett's principles and practice of infectious diseases* (6th ed., pp. 3215–3228). Philadelphia: Elsevier Churchill Livingstone.

Wilson, M. E. (1995). Travel and the emergence of infectious diseases. *Emerging Infectious Diseases, 1,* 39–46.

Woodrow, C. J., Eziefula, A. C., Agranoff, D., Scott, G. M., Watson, J., Chiodini, P. L., et al. (2007). Early risk assessment for viral haemorrhagic fever: Experience at the Hospital for Tropical Diseases, London, UK. *Journal of Infection, 54,* 6–11.

Yates, J. (2005). Traveler's diarrhea. *American Family Physician, 71,* 2095–2100.

CHAPTER TWENTY-SIX

Immunocompromised Persons and Emerging Infectious Diseases

Victoria Davey

Immunocompromised persons have one or more conditions that lead to defective immune system function. Impaired immune system function can range from temporary and mild immunosuppression to permanent and life-limiting immunodeficiency diseases. More than a decade has passed since the first Institute of Medicine report noted that immunocompromised persons are a group at particular risk for emerging infections (Lederberg, Shope, & Oaks, 1992) and this opinion was reiterated in a subsequent report (Smolinski, Hamburg, & Lederberg, 2003). Increasing numbers of people are living with defects in immune system function for many reasons: life-prolonging treatment of inherited or acquired immunodeficiency diseases, therapies for malignancies and related diseases that result in short- or long-term immunosuppression, increased stem cell and organ transplantation, and an aging population experiencing immune system decline. Emerging and reemerging pathogens present new risks to this diverse group that will require special vigilance and development of treatment strategies (Lashley, 2004, 2006; Trevejo, Barr, & Robinson, 2005).

Primary immunodeficiency diseases, such as common variable immunodeficiency and severe combined immunodeficiency, occur in as many as 1/2,000 births; many have a specific genetic defect defined (Bonilla & Geha, 2006). More than 100 such diseases have been described. Primary immunodeficiency diseases have become manageable when expert multidisciplinary teams apply prophylactic antibiotic regimens, aggressive treatment of infections, and administration of immunoglobulin replacement and immunomodulatory agents. Human stem cell transplantation has, in some cases, proven effective (for a comprehensive review, see Bonilla et al., 2005). Gene therapy is being cautiously approached as an option for some of these disorders (Bonilla & Geha, 2006).

Acquired immunodeficiency may also be called secondary immunodeficiency. The best known infectious type is the acquired immunodeficiency syndrome (AIDS), caused by the human immunodeficiency virus (HIV) types 1 and 2. Other reasons for secondary immunodeficiency are part of day-to-day life, such as pregnancy, aging, and splenectomy after trauma. Still others are caused by an accumulation of host defense defects such as those observed in diabetes mellitus and chronic renal failure. Immune system suppression is a well-described side effect of many drugs, such as cancer chemotherapy and corticosteroids. Deliberate drug-induced immune system suppression is employed as part of a treatment strategy for malignancies and autoimmune diseases and to prevent rejection of transplanted cells and organs. The prevalence of persons living with organ transplantation, HIV infection, and cancer has been roughly estimated to be over 9.5 million in the United States (3.6% of the population; Kemper, Davis, & Freed, 2002). The proportion of the U.S. population that is over 65 years old is increasing rapidly and is estimated to be 80 million by 2050 (White, Henretig, & Dukes, 2002). The magnitude of the immunocompromised population at risk from emerging infections is large and growing (Smolinski et al., 2003, Weber & Rutala, 2003).

Human interactions with the environment seen with global travel (see chapter 25); changes in food and water acquisition and distribution; new, aggressive medical therapies; longer life spans; and changes in social patterns, such as urbanization, lead to the likelihood that previously undescribed pathogens may cause human disease in the susceptible immunocompromised hosts, as they do in the normal host (Fenton & Pedersen, 2005; Lashley, 2004). Protective measures to decrease risk of food- and waterborne infections are found in Appendix B.

Organisms that cause disease in immunocompromised persons may also be pathogenic in the immunocompetent individual. However, infections seen in those who are immunosuppressed, especially in HIV infection, tend to have certain defining characteristics, including differences in presentation, atypical location, wider dissemination, more rapid progression, and greater severity, and they are more difficult to treat (Georgiev, 1998; Trevejo et al., 2005).

All of these reasons—increasing survivability of persons with inherited and acquired defects, treatments that employ immune system manipulation, changing interactions of the immunocompromised person with the environment, and dire consequences—heighten the need for vigilance for emerging pathogens particular to the immunocompromised person. This chapter will describe various causes of immunocompromise and delineate known or potential emerging infectious agents that may pose a threat to this growing population.

THE SUPPRESSED OR DEFICIENT IMMUNE SYSTEM

The immune system exhibits remarkable orchestration of its molecular, cellular, and chemical components. Primary or secondary immunodeficiency may result from failure of a single component, but it is important to remember that the resultant immune defects are usually multiple. Table 26.1 delineates some of the major human immunodeficiency diseases and conditions or events that lead to immunosuppression. Of these, the most frequently encountered are in the secondary immune defect category: (a) immune dysfunction resulting from cancer therapies, preparation for bone marrow or stem cell transplantation, or immunosuppression after organ transplantation (see Table 26.2); (b) HIV infection; (c) diabetes mellitus; (d) pregnancy; and (e) aging. The immunosuppression that results from these entities will be discussed in more detail below. Table 26.3 lists recently reported emerging pathogens in these immunocompromised populations.

Immune Suppression Caused by Cancer and Cancer Therapy

Patients with cancer experience immune system dysfunction as a result of their malignancies and from immunosuppressive effects of treatment. Leukemias and lymphomas may lead to physical replacement of normal bone marrow stem cells with malignant cells. Solid tumors can obstruct blood flow and fluid drainage, become necrotic, or grow into oral or gastrointestinal cavities, predisposing to infection (Segal, Walsh, Gea-Banacloche, & Holland, 2005). Defects in production of antibodies occur with multiple myeloma and chronic lymphocytic leukemia, and lymphomas and are associated with diminished cellular immunity. Chemotherapy with cytotoxic drugs can cause B- and T-lymphocyte dysfunction (Segal et al., 2005; van Burik & Freifeld, 2004), although the most frequently encountered deleterious effect of cytotoxic drugs and therapeutic radiation is neutropenia and neutrophil dysfunction.

Table 26.1. Causes of Immunocompromise and Major Susceptibilities

Cause of Immunocompromise	Recognized Diseases or Risks	Major Susceptibilities
Barrier or mechanical defects of skin	Major surgery, burns, trauma Dermatologic conditions Decubitus, vascular, or diabetic ulcers Catheter or stent-related	Coagulase negative staphylococci, *Staphylococcus aureus*, *Stenotrophomonas maltophilia*, *Pseudomonas aeruginosa*, *Acinetobacter* spp., *Corynebacterium* and *Bacillus* spp., *Candida* spp., mucormycosis
Defects of mucous membranes	Radiation- or chemotherapy-induced mucositis Inhalation injuries Endotracheal intubation	Viridans streptococci, *Enterococcus* spp., *Capnocytophaga* spp., *Stomatococcus mucilaginosus*, *Candida* spp., herpes simplex
Obstruction/structural alterations	Tumors Cystic fibrosis, chronic obstructive pulmonary disease	Gram-negative and anaerobic bacteria, fungi including *Aspergillus* and *Candida* spp.
Primary Primary humoral immunodeficiency diseases	X-linked and autosomal recessive agammaglobulinemia IgA deficiency IgG subclass deficiency Hyper-IgM syndromes Common variable immunodeficiency	Chronic sinopulmonary infections, meningitis, bacteremia with encapsulated organisms; *Streptococcus pneumoniae*; *Hemophilus influenzae*; enterovirus infections
Primary cellular immunodeficiency	Defects of IL-12/interferon axis	*Mycobacteria* spp., *Salmonella* spp.
Combined immunodeficiency diseases	Severe combined immunodeficiency Adenosine deaminase deficiency Purine nucleoside phosphorylase deficiency Major histocompatability complex (MHC) Class II deficiency DiGeorge anomaly Hereditary ataxia telangiectasia Wiskott–Aldrich syndrome	Bacteria: *Mycobacteria* Fungi: *Aspergillus Cryptococcus*, *Histoplasma*, *Coccidioides*, *Pneumocystis jiroveci* (formerly *carinii*) Protozoa: *Toxoplasma* Viruses: cytomegalovirus, herpes simplex, Helminths: *Strongyloides stercoralis*

Table 26.1. *(continued)*

Cause of Immunocompromise	Recognized Diseases or Risks	Major Susceptibilities
Complement protein defects	Hereditary angioedema	Encapsulated bacteria, especially meningococci
Defects in phagocyte number or function	Chronic granulomatous disease; Job syndrome or hyper-IgE recurrent infection syndrome; Chediak–Higashi syndrome; leukocyte adhesion deficiency 1, 2; cyclic neutropenia	*S. aureus,* coagulase negative staphylococci, Viridans streptococci, *Enterococcus* spp., *Escherichia coli, P. aeruginosa, Klebsiella pneumoniae, Enterobacter* and *Citrobacter* spp., *Serratia* spp., *Paecilomyces lilacinus, Aspergillus* spp., *Fusarium* spp.
Secondary or acquired Defects in phagocyte number or function	Cancer chemotherapy or irradiation Acute leukemia	*S. aureus,* coagulase negative staphylococci, *Viridans* streptococci, *Enterococcus* spp., *E. coli, P. aeruginosa, K. pneumoniae, Enterobacter* and *Citrobacter* spp., *Aspergillus* spp., *Fusarium* spp.
Drug induced	Glucocorticoids Cytotoxic agents Antiproliferative/ antimetabolite drugs Calcineurin inhibitors Antilymphocyte agents Monoclonal/polyclonal antibodies	Can result in phagocyte, B-cell, and T-cell defects; adenoviruses; *Listeria, Nocardia, Mucor* spp.; *Legionella*; respiratory syncytial virus; parvovirus B19; West Nile virus
Environmental/ treatment induced	Malnutrition Pregnancy Malignancy Solid organ transplantation Bone marrow or hematopoietic stem cell transplantation	

(continued)

Table 26.1. *(continued)*

Cause of Immunocompromise	Recognized Diseases or Risks	Major Susceptibilities
Infectious	HIV-1, HIV-2	Bacteria: *Mycobacteria*, *Pneumococcus*, *Pseudomonas* spp. Fungi: *Aspergillus*, *Cryptococcus*, *Histoplasma*, *Coccidioides*, *P. jiroveci* Protozoa: *Toxoplasma* Viruses: adenoviruses, cytomegalovirus, herpes simplex Helminths: *S. stercoralis*
	Cytomegalovirus (CMV)	*Pneumocystis* pneumonia, *Aspergillus fumigatus*, *Candida* spp.
	Human herpesvirus 6	May activate Epstein–Barr virus; CMV, HIV

HIV = human immunodeficiency syndrome; Ig = immunoglobulin; IL = interleukin.
Sources: Ader et al., 2005; Bartlett & Gallant, 2005; Bonilla et al., 2005; Bonilla & Geha, 2006; CDC, 2005a; Corcoran & Doyle, 2004; Costa & Alexander, 2005; Kotloff, Ahya, & Crawford, 2004; Leen & Rooney, 2004; Segal, Walsh, Gea-Banacloche, & Holland, 2005; Sims, Ostrosky-Zeichner, & Rex, 2005.

Chemotherapy and radiation decrease phagocytic activity of neutrophils, decrease their ability to move and gather at the site of inflammation (chemotaxis), and decrease intracellular killing. In addition, these agents can alter skin and mucosal integrity, which are important defenses against infection (Freifeld, Kalil, & Rubinstein, 2004; Segal et al., 2005). The past two decades have seen gram-positive organisms replace gram-negative organisms as a common cause of infection in the neutropenic host (Segal et al., 2005), an effect thought to have been caused by improved treatment and prophylaxis for gram-negative organisms, long-term indwelling intravenous access lines, and shifts in antibiotic usage patterns. Bacterial infections predominate in the first days postchemotherapy or postradiation, but with persistent neutropenia, invasive and cutaneous fungal infections also occur (Freifeld et al., 2004; van Burik & Freifeld, 2004).

The use of aggressive cytotoxic chemotherapy and prophylactic antimicrobial drugs during cancer treatment has led to the recognition that new pathogens and newly resistant pathogens are constant foes. Included are viral infections, such as those caused by parvovirus B19 and BK

Table 26.2. Drugs Used for Immunosuppression

Drug Name	Use	Immunologic Effects
Glucocorticoids	Maintenance of immunosuppression posttransplant; anti-inflammatory agents	Inhibit inflammation, inhibit cellular immunity, alter lymphocyte trafficking
Cytotoxic agents		
Cyclophosphamide, busulfan, fludarabine, methotrexate	Myeloablation/ conditioning preparation for hematopoietic stem cell transplantation; treatment for malignancies and autoimmune diseases	Act directly on lymphocytes as well as other immune system cells
Antiproliferative/antimetabolite drugs		
Sirolimus	Prevention of organ transplant rejection	Inhibits T-cell activation
Everolimus	Prevention of organ transplant rejection	Inhibits T-cell activation
Azathioprine	Posttransplant and treatment of autoimmune disease	Inhibits nucleoside synthesis
Mycophenolate mofetil	Posttransplant and autoimmune disease immunosuppression	Interrupts development of activated T and B cells
Calcineurin inhibitors		
Cyclosporine A	Posttransplant immunosuppression; treatment of acute rejection; treatment of autoimmune diseases	Interrupts T-cell activation
Tacrolimus	Posttransplant immunosuppression; prevention of acute rejection	Inhibits various pathways of T cell activation
Antilymphocyte preparations		
Antithymocyte globulin	Reversal of acute rejection	Opsonizes (a process of making cells susceptible to destruction) and modulates T- and B-cell activities

(continued)

Table 26.2. *(continued)*

Drug Name	Use	Immunologic Effects
Monoclonal or polyclonal antibodies		
OKT3	Reversal of acute rejection	Reduces CD3 marked T lymphocytes that are important to rejection pathways
Daclizumab	Prevention of acute rejection	Blocks IL-2 receptors
Infliximab	Treatment of autoimmune diseases (rheumatoid arthritis and Crohn disease)	Blocks TNF pathways
Alemtuzumab	Treatment of chronic lymphocytic leukemia	Induces apoptosis of lymphocytes
Rituximab	Treatment of non-Hodgkin lymphoma; other lymphomas; idiopathic thrombocytic purpura; and prevention of rejection in renal transplant	Induces destruction of B cells

IL = interleukin; TNF = tumor necrosis factor.
Sources: Blaes, Peterson, Bartlett, Dunn, & Morrison, 2005; Kahan, 2003; Krensky, Vincenti, & Bennett, 2006; Resnick, Shapira, & Slavin, 2005; Ringden & Le Blanc, 2005; Segal, Walsh, Gea-Banacloche, & Holland, 2005; Valantine & Zuckermann, 2005.

polyomavirus (Corcoran & Doyle, 2004; Galan, Rauch & Otis, 2005). Case reports of emerging bacterial infections in cancer patients include nontyphoidal salmonellosis, *Escherichia coli* O157:H7, *Bacillus cereus*, *Bordetella bronchiseptica*, multidrug-resistant *Pseudomonas aeruginosa*, and *Roseomonas mucosa* (Elshibly et al., 2005; Ohmagari et al., 2005; Saleeby, Howard, Hayden, & McCullers, 2005; Trevejo et al., 2005). Threats from non-*albicans Candida* species and other fungal or yeast infections such as *Trichosporon* species, *Malassezia* species, and *Hansenula anomala* are reported in the literature as well (Fleming, Walsh, & Anaissie, 2002; Sims, Ostrosky-Zeichner, & Rex, 2005). In patients with hematological malignancies and hematopoietic stem transplants, *Aspergillus*, *Scedosporium*, and *Fusarium* infections are replacing *Candida* infection as a common, serious invasive pathogen, linked to improved diagnosis and effective prophylaxis for *Candida* (Patterson, 2005; Walsh et al., 2004). Table 26.1 provides an overview of pathogens associated with malignancies and their treatment effects.

Table 26.3. Emerging Infections in Immunocompromised Persons Recently Reported

Agent	Reported Sites	Underlying Immune Defect/Risk Factors	References
Bacteria			
Acinetobacter spp.	Wound infections, osteomyelitis, cutaneous	Severe trauma/prolonged hospitalization (wounded Iraq campaign soldiers)	Davis, Moran, McAllister, & Gray, 2005
Anaplasma phagocytophilum	Systemic	Elderly, immunosuppressed	Dumler et al., 2005
Bacillus cereus	Bloodstream, meningitis	Immunosuppressive drugs, injection drug users, neonates, ventriculoperitoneal shunts	El Saleeby, Howard, Hayden, & McCullers, 2004
Multidrug-resistant *Pseudomonas aeruginosa*	Bloodstream	Prolonged hospitalization, HIV	Obritsch, Fish, MacLaren, & Jung, 2005
Roseomonas mucosa	Line-related sepsis	Large B-cell non-Hodgkin lymphoma	Elshibly et al., 2005
Fungi			
Aspergillus spp.	Systemic	COPD	Ader et al., 2005
Cladophialophora bantiana	Brain abscess	Heart and lung transplant	Levin, Baty, Fekete, Truant, & Suh, 2004
Fusarium spp.	Bloodstream, pulmonary	HSCT, solid organ transplant	Costa & Alexander, 2005; Walsh et al., 2004
Scedosporium spp.	Bloodstream, pulmonary	HSCT, solid organ transplant	Costa & Alexander, 2005; Walsh et al., 2004
Penicillium marneffei	Bloodstream, pulmonary	Renal transplant	Costa & Alexander, 2005
Phialemonium obovatum and other spp.	Peritonitis, endocarditis, osteomyelitis, cutaneous, catheter and prosthetic valve related	HSCT, burn patients	Scott, Sutton, & Jagirdar, 2005

(continued)

Table 26.3. *(continued)*

Agent	Reported Sites	Underlying Immune Defect/Risk Factors	References
Trichoderma longibrachiatum	Pulmonary	HSCT, solid organ transplant	Costa & Alexander, 2005; Walsh et al., 2004
Trichosporon spp.	Pulmonary	Hematologic malignancy, HSCT, solid organ transplant	Ahmad, Al-Mahmeed, & Khan, 2005; Costa & Alexander, 2005
Viruses			
Adenovirus	Serious systemic illness	HSCT, immuno-suppressive therapy, GVHD	Leen & Rooney, 2004
BK polyomavirus	Pneumonia	Chemotherapy	Galan, Rauch, & Otis, 2005
Influenza A, H5N1	Respiratory	Case reported in a pregnant woman; deaths reported in immunocompetent persons also	Shu, Yu, & Li, 2006
Parvovirus B19	Fetal loss, fetal hydrops, severe anemia, hepatitis, transient aplastic crisis	Pregnancy, chemotherapy, im-munosuppressive drugs, HIV	Corcoran & Doyle, 2004
Poliovirus, vaccine derived	Paralytic illness	Child with undiagnosed immunodeficiency	Cherkasova et al., 2005
Metapneumovirus	Respiratory	Elderly, other im-munocompromised	Fouchier, Rimmelzwaan, Kuiken, & Osterhaus, 2005
West Nile virus	Neurologic disease	Transmitted via transplant of organs from infected person	CDC, 2005a

COPD = chronic obstructive pulmonary disease; GVHD = graft-versus-host disease; HSCT = hematopoietic stem cell transplant.

Immune Suppression After Hematopoietic Stem Cell Transplantation

Autologous (from self), syngeneic (from an identical twin), or allogeneic (from a nonidentical sibling or unrelated donor) hematopoietic stem cell transplantation (HSCT) of bone marrow, growth factor-stimulated peripheral blood, and cord blood has been employed as a treatment for leukemias, lymphomas, aplastic anemia, solid tumors, congenital immunodeficiency diseases, autoimmune diseases, and inborn errors of metabolism (Alaez et al., 2006; Petropoulos & Chan, 2005; Ringden & Le Blanc, 2005). Preparative or conditioning regimens ablate or partially ablate the recipient's marrow with radiation or a variety of cytotoxic and immunomodulatory agents, the choice of which is influenced by the underlying disease and the age and health of the recipient (see Table 26.2; Resnick, Shapira, & Slavin, 2005). In the immediate posttransplant period, there is generally severe pancytopenia lasting 2 to 4 weeks that may require aggressive supportive care, including red cell transfusion; administration of hematologic growth factors; administration of prophylactic and therapeutic antibiotics, antifungals, and antiviral drugs; hyperalimentation; and, in some cases, a protective environment (Ringden & Le Blanc, 2005). Gram-positive and gram-negative bacteremias and sepsis can occur, particularly when the neutrophil count falls below $500/mm^3$. Among gram-positive organisms, coagulase-negative staphylococci and streptococci often predominate, and among gram-negative organisms, *Escherichia coli*, *Klebsiella*, *Enterobacter*, and *Pseudomonas* species are commonly seen. Ten percent of patients may develop invasive fungal infections. As neutropenia reverses with donor marrow engraftment, infections with viruses such as respiratory syncytial virus, adenovirus, and reactivation of dormant herpes simplex virus or cytomegalovirus (CMV) become more prevalent as humoral, cellular, and pulmonary alveolar macrophage function may be impaired for a year or more (Gandhi & Khanna, 2004; Ringden & LeBlanc, 2005; Segal et al., 2005).

Acute and chronic graft-versus-host disease (GVHD) occurs frequently in patients who undergo HSCT. This condition, in which donor T lymphocytes recognize the recipient's cells as foreign and mount an immune response directed against them, can cause severe damage to multiple organs. Graft-versus-host disease is treated with immunosuppressive drugs, including corticosteroids, cyclosporine, thalidomide, tacrolimus, sirolimus, and anti-B-cell antibodies or total body radiation. Any of these agents may further delay immune recovery from HSCT and increase risks for infectious complications (Blazar & Murphy, 2005; Ferrara & Yanik, 2005; Horwitz & Sullivan, 2006).

Techniques to restore the immune system or enhance recovery after HSCT are being studied and include administration of cytokines, CMV or Epstein–Barr virus-specific cytotoxic T cells, and monoclonal antibodies (Ringden & Le Blanc, 2005).

Immune Suppression After Solid Organ Transplantation

There were over 28,000 organ transplantation operations performed in the United States in 2005. Included in this figure are kidney, kidney–pancreas, pancreas, heart, heart–lung, liver, and intestine transplants (Organ Procurement and Transplantation Network, 2006). Infection after transplantation is a major complication, ranking third in incidence after surgical events and graft rejection (Dummer, 2005). Factors important in the development of infection and the types of infection are (a) the patient's underlying illness(es) (e.g., diabetes mellitus or hepatitis C [see chapter 12] confer their own infection risks); (b) surgical factors (e.g., the type of anastomoses required, amount of time spent in the operating room, and/or development of lymphoceles from inadequate lymphatics drainage); (c) susceptibility of the grafted organ to CMV, which results in direct organ damage and increased immunosuppression; (d) the type and duration of immunosuppression required (Dummer, 2005); and (e) infectious agents transmitted from the donor to recipient, such as West Nile virus and rabies (Centers for Disease Control and Prevention [CDC], 2005a; Srinivasan et al., 2005). In the early posttransplant period (days to weeks), the patient is most at risk from bacterial infection (commonly gram-negative bacteria), reflecting the general postoperative state and nosocomial transmission risk. From the second to sixth months, opportunistic infections, including fungal infections, *Pneumocystis jiroveci* (formerly *carinii*), and *Nocardia*, tend to occur. After 6 months, community-acquired infections and latent viral infections are seen. Prophylactic regimens can anticipate and prevent many of these infections (Candel et al., 2005; Guaraldi et al., 2005; Kotloff, Ahya, & Crawford, 2004).

Posttransplant immunosuppression required for graft retention is accomplished by a variety of drugs. Most of these blunt cell-mediated immunity, but they can also cause decreased antibody production and neutropenia. The goal of transplanted graft maintenance is immunologic tolerance—allowing the recipient to retain the functioning organ, without incurring too high a risk of infection from immunosuppression (Table 26.2; Haberal & Dalgic, 2004).

Eligibility for solid organ transplant has broadened and survival has increased due to improved surgical techniques, immunosuppressive regimens that maintain grafts yet preserve some immune function, and prophylactic antimicrobials that prevent many infections. Infections with new or unusual organisms will appear in the diverse population that comprises solid organ transplant patients as recipients resume active lives. Awareness, vigilance, and patient education can help protect this vulnerable immunocompromised population (Levin, Baty, Fekete, Truant, & Suh, 2004; Medeiros, Chen, Kendall, & Hillers, 2004; Roland, 2004; Strippoli, Hodson, Jones, & Craig, 2006).

Immunocompromise in HIV/AIDS

The HIV/AIDS epidemic was recognized in 1981 when unusual cases of *P. jiroveci* formerly *carinii* pneumonia and Kaposi sarcoma were seen in homosexual men from New York and California (CDC, 1981). Because of the average 10-year period between infection and development of AIDS, the epidemic's beginnings had actually occurred years earlier. The global spread of HIV has been assisted by a profusion of human and environmental factors. They include ecologic changes that brought humans and animals into close contact; social patterns and behavior changes like urban migration, sexual practices, drug use, and transfusion of blood products; increased international travel; and viral factors, including the long period of asymptomatic illness that allows HIV to be transmitted before the host is debilitated by AIDS (Lederman, Rodriquez, & Sieg, 2006). The cumulative number of persons, adults and children, living with AIDS is estimated by the World Health Organization (WHO) as 40.3 million. More than 20 million persons have died from the disease (WHO, 2005). At the end of December 2004, there were 916,997 cumulative reported cases of AIDS in the United States (CDC, 2006). HIV/AIDS provides a model of the potential devastation of an emerging infectious disease, but with its huge number of victims it is also responsible for a substantial percentage of the population of immunocompromised persons at risk for other emerging infections. In fact, many infections that now fit the definition of "emerging" have been identified in people with HIV/AIDS.

HIV causes dysfunction of nearly all components of the immune system. After infection with HIV, the immune system mounts a vigorous response, as it would to any invading microorganism, but untreated HIV eventually overcomes the normal host's defenses, ultimately leading to death, usually from opportunistic infections and cancers (Lederman et al., 2006). Human immunodeficiency virus preferentially infects $CD4^+$ lymphocytes, as well as monocytes and macrophages. The progressive decline in numbers and the dysfunction of the $CD4^+$ lymphocyte that accompanies infection constitute the cornerstones of the immune system dysfunction caused by HIV. Human immunodeficiency virus causes death or dysfunction of the $CD4^+$ lymphocytes through a variety of mechanisms: direct infection (use of the $CD4^+$ lymphocyte to produce new viral particles), clumping of infected and uninfected CD4$^+$ lymphocytes (syncytia formation), changing the normal "programmed" cell life cycle (apoptosis), and possibly causing an autoimmune phenomenon in which the activated immune system kills uninfected CD4$^+$ lymphocytes as well as those infected with HIV. Human immunodeficiency virus is not as lethal to macrophages—they remain a chronically infected reservoir of HIV that is less susceptible to any of the currently available antiviral medications (Dybul, Connors, & Fauci, 2005). Other effects of HIV on immune system elements lead to broad dysfunction: B lymphocytes have decreased ability to respond to antigens, neutrophils experience dysregulation, and cytokine/lymphokine production and activity are disrupted. There is a progressive loss of ability to produce interleukin 2 (IL-2) and IL-12, which stimulate proliferation and lytic activity of cytotoxic T lymphocytes and natural killer cells (Lederman et al., 2006).

Human immunodeficiency virus-infected persons with advanced disease are susceptible to a variety of bacterial, viral, fungal, and parasitic infections as a consequence of their broad immune system defects. Without treatment with highly active antiretroviral therapy that protects against HIV/AIDS-associated infections by preserving or returning a degree of immune system function, patients present with characteristic infections associated with specific levels of immune system decline in HIV infection. These include *P. jiroveci* pneumonia, recurrent oral candidiasis, perirectal herpes simplex, and *Mycobacterium avium* complex bacteremia. Other infections that occur frequently are tuberculosis, cerebral toxoplasmosis, *Cryptococcus neoformans*, persistent cryptosporidiosis, and microsporidiosis. Many were formerly rare disorders in humans, having mostly been zoonotic or of limited prevalence. These uncommon infections include isosporiasis and progressive multifocal encephalopathy caused by JC virus, *Rhodococcus equi*, *Bartonella* spp., non-*albicans Candida*, *Penicillium marneffei*, and *Sporothrix schenckii* (Bartlett & Gallant, 2005). Table 26.1 lists some of the emerging pathogens of particular concern in HIV-infected patients. Also see Appendix A and chapter 13 on HIV.

Immunosuppression in Diabetes Mellitus

According to the CDC, 7% of people in the United States have Type 1 or Type 2 diabetes mellitus, leading government public health experts to call diabetes mellitus an unfolding epidemic. This increase has been attributed primarily to an epidemic of obesity; national data indicate that two thirds of U.S. adults are overweight or obese. Approximately 1.5 million new cases of diabetes mellitus were diagnosed in U.S. adults in 2005. Diabetes mellitus is the sixth leading cause of death in this country and a major contributor to serious health problems (CDC, 2005b; National Center for Health Statistics [NCHS], 2006). Newly diagnosed cases crossed ethnic and age groups but were greatest among people aged 40–59 years. Diabetes mellitus is more prevalent in African Americans, Hispanics, certain Native Americans, and other ethnic minority groups than in White Americans (NCHS, 2006).

Diabetes mellitus causes suppression of cell-mediated immunity and phagocyte function as well as altered vascularization. Hyperglycemia aids growth and colonization of some organisms, including *Candida* spp. Susceptibility to infection appears to lessen with better glycemic control (Powers, 2005). Immunosuppression in diabetes mellitus leads to an increase in common infections like urinary tract and wound infections, as well as more serious infections. Rhinocerebral mucormycosis, a devastating fungal infection originating in the nasal mucosa, occurs classically after an episode of diabetic ketoacidosis (Powers, 2005). A 22-year review of 40 cases of intracranial fungal infections demonstrated that 40% of patients had diabetes as a risk factor (Dubey et al., 2005). Malignant external otitis, often caused by *P. aeruginosa*, tends to occur in older diabetics (Handzel & Halperin, 2003). *Coccidioides immitis*, an increasingly reported human pathogen, is a fungus endemic to desert areas of California, Arizona, New Mexico, and western Texas. In diabetics, it has been reported to cause pulmonary infection characterized by multiple thin-walled pulmonary cavities, but there is disagreement as to whether diabetes constitutes a specific risk factor for *C. immitis* infection (Kirkland & Fierer, 1996; Snyder, 2005). Several studies show that diabetics have increased rates of disease from *Mycobacterium tuberculosis* (Coker et al., 2006; Ponce-de-Leon et al., 2004; Wang, Lee, & Hsueh, 2005).

Immunosuppression in Pregnancy

Pregnancy results in a mild state of immunosuppression, leaving pregnant women potentially vulnerable to emerging infections (Jamieson, Theiler & Rasmussen, 2006; Rasmussen & Hayes, 2005). Hormonal changes brought about by the pregnant uterus, including elevated serum levels of endogenous corticosteroids and progesterone, can lead to poor lymphocyte function. Decreased levels of the immunoglobulin G have been described (Claman, 1995), and, in general, pregnancy may produce an immune response directed more toward T_H2-like functions (regulation of B-cell functions) rather than T_H1 activity (regulation of T-cell functions; Kaaja & Greer, 2005). Infections reported to be particularly severe in the pregnant woman include hepatitis (see chapter 12), influenza (see chapter 14), cholera (see chapter 4), scarlet fever, malaria (see chapter 17), gonorrhea, typhoid, leprosy, psittacosis, and listeriosis (see chapter 3; Cunningham et al., 2006; Jorgensen, 1997; Laibl & Sheffield, 2006; Siegmann-Igra et al., 2002). The 2003–2004 global outbreak of severe acute respiratory syndrome (SARS) was reported to cause marked morbidity in pregnant women and their fetuses, including increased requirement for mechanical ventilation and disseminated intravascular coagulopathy, fetal loss, and intrauterine fetal growth retardation. Mortality was also greater in pregnant women than nonpregnant women in a case—control study (Lam et al., 2004; Wong, Chow, & Leung, 2004). Death of a pregnant woman with avian influenza A type H5N1 has been reported (Shu & Yu, 2006).

Immune System Decline in Aging

The human immune system deteriorates with aging, a process known as immunosenescence. Both cellular and humoral immunity decline, but a great deal of recent research focuses on changes in T-cell immunity as a primary factor (Eaton, Burns, Kusser, Randall, & Haynes, 2004; Nikolich-Zugich, 2005. One theory suggests that a lifetime of exposure to infectious agents and ongoing chronic, subclinical viral infections such as CMV may interfere with balance and function of naive and memory T cells, leading to a spectrum of immune dysfunction, including poor response to vaccinations (Nikolich-Zugich, 2005; Pawelec, 2005). Poor T- and B-cell functions combined with impairment of certain mechanical aspects of host defense (e.g., normal blood circulation, a vigorous cough reflex, and normal wound healing), leaves the elderly susceptible to a variety of infections. For example, bacteriuria and urinary tract infections are seen with high frequency in men with obstructed urine flow as a consequence of prostatic hypertrophy. Pneumonias from all causes are 50 times more common in persons over 75 years old than in teenagers. Institutionalized elderly persons are at greater risk for person-to-person transmitted nosocomial infections, such as tuberculosis and diarrheal disease from enteric pathogens, many of which may be resistant strains. The physiologic response to infection can also be diminished, with less fever, less leukocytosis, and blunted clinical signs and symptoms (Crossley & Peterson, 2005; Dieffenbach & Tramont, 2005). SARS and West Nile virus are two emerging infections that have been shown to have severe effects in the elderly (Nikolich-Zugich, 2005).

CONCLUSION

The immunocompromised state includes a wide range of inherited and acquired immune system defects. There is a growing body of knowledge concerning susceptibility to infection in this diverse group, but there is also increasing recognition that the person with a defective or suppressed immune system may be at risk for infections from an untold number of unrecognized organisms. These include animal and plant pathogens, organisms thought to be nonpathogenic, and recurrence of latent infections. Recognition and study of the types of infections that occur in the immunocompromised person have led to a greater understanding of the workings of the human immune system and may also enhance our ability to protect and treat this vulnerable population from infection with emerging organisms.

REFERENCES

Ader, F., Nseir, S., Le Berre, R., Leroy, S., Tillie-Leblond, I., Marquette, C. H., et al. (2005). Invasive pulmonary aspergillosis in chronic obstructive pulmonary disease: An emerging fungal pathogen. *Clinical Microbiology and Infection, 11,* 427–429.

Ahmad, S., Al-Mahmeed, M., & Khan, Z. U. (2005). Characterization of trichosporon species isolated from clinical specimens in Kuwait. *Journal of Medical Microbiology, 54*(Pt. 7), 639–646.

Alaez, C., Loyola, M., Murguia, A., Flores, H., Rodriguez, A., Ovilla, R., et al. (2006). Hematopoietic stem cell transplantation (HSCT): An approach to autoimmunity. *Autoimmunity Reviews, 5,* 167–169.

Bartlett, J. G., & Gallant, J. E. (2005). *2005–2006 medical management of HIV infection.* Baltimore: Johns Hopkins Medicine Health Publishing Business Group.

Blaes, A. H., Peterson, B. A., Bartlett, N., Dunn, D. L., & Morrison, V. A. (2005). Rituximab therapy is effective for posttransplant lymphoproliferative disorders after solid organ transplantation. *Cancer, 104,* 1661–1667.

Blazar, B. R., & Murphy, W. J. (2005). Bone marrow transplantation and approaches to avoid graft-versus-host disease (GVHD). *Philosophical Transactions of the Royal Society of London. Series B, Biological Sciences, 360,* 1747–1767.

Bonilla, F. A., Bernstein, I. L., Khan, D. A., Ballas, Z. K., Chinen, J., Frank, M. M., et al. (2005). Practice parameter for the diagnosis and management of primary immunodeficiency. *Annals of Allergy, Asthma & Immunology, 94,* S1–63.

Bonilla, F. A., & Geha, R. S. (2006). Update on primary immunodeficiency diseases. *Journal of Allergy and Clinical Immunology, 117,* S435–441.

Candel, F. J., Grima, E., Matesanz, M., Cervera, C., Soto, G., Almela, M., et al. (2005). Bacteremia and septic shock after solid-organ transplantation. *Transplantation Proceedings, 37,* 4097–4099.

Centers for Disease Control. (1981). Kaposi's sarcoma and pneumocystis pneumonia among homosexual men—New York and California. *Morbidity and Mortality Weekly Report, 31,* 507–515.

Centers for Disease Control and Prevention. (2005a). West Nile virus infections in organ transplant recipients—New York and Pennsylvania, August–September, 2005. *Morbidity and Mortality Weekly Report, 54,* 1021–1023.

Centers for Disease Control and Prevention. (2005b). *National diabetes fact sheet, 2005*. Retrieved April 21, 2006, from http://www.diabetes.org/uedocuments/NationalDiabetesFactSheetRev.pdf

Centers for Disease Control and Prevention. (2006). Table 15. *Reported AIDS cases and annual rates (per 100,000 population) by metropolitan area of residence and age category, cumulative through 2004—United States*. Retrieved April 11, 2006, from http://www.cdc.gov/hiv/topics/surveillance/resources/reports/2004report/table15.htm

Cherkasova, E. A., Yakovenko, M. L., Rezapkin, G. V., Korotkova, E. A., Ivanova, O. E., Eremeeva, T. P., et al. (2005). Spread of vaccine-derived poliovirus from a paralytic case in an immunodeficient child: An insight into the natural evolution of oral polio vaccine. *Journal of Virology, 79*, 1062–1070.

Claman, H. N. (1995). Immunology of reproduction and infertility. In M. M. Frank, F. K. Austen, H. N. Claman, & E. R. Unanue (Eds.), *Samter's immunologic diseases* (Vol. 11, pp. 999–1007). Boston: Little, Brown.

Coker, R., McKee, M., Atun, R., Dimitrova, B., Dodonova, E., Kuznetsov, V., et al. (2006). Risk factors for pulmonary tuberculosis in Russia: Case-control study. *British Medical Journal, 332*, 85–87.

Corcoran, A., & Doyle, S. (2004). Advances in the biology, diagnosis, and host-pathogen interactions of parvovirus B19. *Journal of Medical Microbiology, 53*, 459–475.

Costa, S. F., & Alexander, B. D. (2005). Non-aspergillus fungal pneumonia in transplant recipients. *Clinical Chest Medicine, 26*, 675–690, vii.

Crossley, K. B., & Peterson, P. K. (2005). Infections in the elderly. In G. L. Mandell, J. E. Bennett, & R. E. Dolin (Eds.), *Mandell, Douglas, and Bennett's principles and practice of infectious diseases* (6th ed., pp. 3517–3523). Philadelphia: Churchill Livingstone Elsevier.

Cunningham, F. G., Leveno, K. L., Bloom, S. L., Hauth, J. C., Gilstrap, L. C., & Wenstrom, K. D. (Eds.). (2006). *Williams obstetrics* (22nd ed.). New York: McGraw-Hill.

Davis, K. A., Moran, K. A., McAllister, C. K., & Gray, P. J. (2005). Multi-drug resistant *Acinetobacter* extremity infections in soldiers. *Emerging Infectious Diseases, 11*, 1218–1224.

Dieffenbach, C. W., & Tramont, E. C. (2005). Innate (general or nonspecific) host defense mechanisms. In G. L. Mandell, J. E. Bennett, & R. E. Dolin (Eds.), *Mandell, Douglas, and Bennett's principles and practice of infectious diseases* (6th ed., pp. 34–41). Philadelphia: Churchill Livingstone Elsevier.

Dubey, A., Patwardhan, R. V., Sampth, S., Santosh, V., Kolluri, S., & Nanda, A. (2005). Intracranial fungal granuloma: Analysis of 40 patients and review of the literature. *Surgical Neurology, 63*, 254–260.

Dumler, J. S., Choi, K.-S., Garcia-Garcia, J. C., Barat, N. S., Scorpio, D. G., Garyu, J. W., et al. (2005). Human granulocytic anaplasmosis and *Anaplasma phagocytophilum*. *Emerging Infectious Diseases, 11*, 1828–1834.

Dummer, J. S. (2005). Risk factors and approaches to infections in transplant recipients. In G. L. Mandell, J. E. Bennett, & R. E. Dolin (Eds.), *Mandell, Douglas, and Bennett's principles and practice of infectious diseases* (6th ed., pp. 3477–3486). Philadelphia: Churchill Livingstone Elsevier.

Dybul, M., Connors, M., & Fauci, A. S. (2005). The immunology of human immunodeficiency virus infection. In G. L. Mandell, J. E. Bennett, & R. E. Dolin (Eds.), *Mandell, Douglas, and Bennett's principles and practice of infectious diseases* (6th ed., pp. 1527–1545). Philadelphia: Churchill Livingstone Elsevier.

Eaton, S. M., Burns, E. M., Kusser, K., Randall, T. D., & Haynes, L. (2004). Age-related defects in CD4 T cell cognate helper function lead to reductions in humoral responses. *Journal of Experimental Medicine, 200,* 1613–1622.

El Saleeby, C. M., Howard, S. C., Hayden, R. T., & McCullers, J. A. (2004). Association between tea ingestion and invasive *Bacillus cereus* infection among children with cancer. *Clinical Infectious Diseases, 39,* 1536–1539.

Elshibly, S., Xu, J., McClurg, R. B., Rooney, P. J., Millar, B. C., Alexander, H. D., et al. (2005). Central line-related bacteremia due to *Roseomonas mucosa* in a patient with diffuse large B-cell non-Hodgkin's lymphoma. *Leukemia and Lymphoma, 46,* 611–614.

Fenton, A., & Pedersen, A. B. (2005). Community epidemiology framework for classifying disease threats. *Emerging Infectious Diseases, 11,* 1815–1821.

Ferrara, J. L., & Yanik, G. (2005). Acute graft versus host disease: Pathophysiology, risk factors, and prevention strategies. *Clinical Advances in Hematology and Oncology, 3,* 415–419, 428.

Fleming, R. V., Walsh, T. J., & Anaissie, E. J. (2002). Emerging and less common fungal pathogens. *Infectious Disease Clinics of North America, 16,* 915–933.

Fouchier, R. A., Rimmelzwaan, G. F., Kuiken, T., & Osterhaus, A. D. (2005). Newer respiratory virus infections: Human metapneumovirus, avian influenza virus, and human coronaviruses. *Current Opinions in Infectious Disease, 18,* 141–146.

Freifeld, A. G., Kalil, A., & Rubenstein, E. (2004). Fever in the neutropenic cancer patient. In M. D. Abeloff (Ed.), *Clinical oncology* (3rd ed., pp. 925–940). New York: Churchill Livingstone.

Galan, A., Rauch, C. A., & Otis, C. N. (2005). Fatal BK polyoma viral pneumonia associated with immunosuppression. *Human Pathology, 36,* 1031–1034.

Gandhi, M. K., & Khanna, R. (2004). Human cytomegalovirus: Clinical aspects, immune regulation, and emerging treatments. *Lancet Infectious Diseases, 4,* 725–738.

Georgiev, V. S. (1998). *Infectious diseases in immunocompromised hosts.* Boca Raton, FL: CRC Press.

Guaraldi, G., Cocchi, S., Codeluppi, M., Di Benedetto, F., De Ruvo, N., Masetti, M., et al. (2005). Outcome, incidence, and timing of infectious complications in small bowel and multivisceral organ transplantation patients. *Transplantation, 80,* 1742–1748.

Haberal, M., & Dalgic, A. (2004). New concepts in organ transplantation. *Transplantation Proceedings, 36,* 1219–1224.

Handzel, O., & Halperin, D. (2003). Necrotizing (malignant) external otitis. *American Family Physician, 68,* 309–312.

Horwitz, M. E., & Sullivan, K. M. (2006). Chronic graft-versus-host-disease. *Blood Reviews, 20,* 15–27.

Jamieson, D.J., Theiler, R.N., & Rasmussen, S.A. (2006). Emerging infections and pregnancy. *Emerging Infectious Diseases, 12*(11), 1638–1643.

Jorgensen, D. M. (1997). Gestational psittacosis in a Montana sheep rancher. *Emerging Infectious Diseases, 3*, 191–194.

Kaaja, R. J., & Greer, I. A. (2005). Manifestations of chronic disease during pregnancy. *Journal of the American Medical Association, 294*, 2751–2757.

Kahan, B. D. (2003). Mechanisms of pharmacologic immune suppression. In L. A. Doughty & P. Linden (Eds.), *Immunology and infectious disease* (pp. 79–113). Norwell, MA: Kluwer Academic Publishers.

Kemper, A. R., Davis, M. M., & Freed, G. L. (2002). Expected adverse events in a mass smallpox vaccination campaign. *Effective Clinical Practice, 5*, 84–90.

Kirkland, T. N., & Fierer, J. (1996). Coccidioidomycosis: A reemerging infectious disease. *Emerging Infectious Diseases, 2*, 192–199.

Kotloff, R. M., Ahya, V. N., & Crawford, S. W. (2004). Pulmonary complications of solid organ and hematopoietic stem cell transplantation. *American Journal of Respiratory and Critical Care Medicine, 170*, 22–48.

Krensky, A. M., Vincenti, F., & Bennett, W. M. (2006). Chapter 52. Immunosuppressants, tolerogens, and immunostimulants. In L. L. Brunton, J. S. Lazo, & K. L Parker (Eds.), *Goodman & Gilman's the pharmacologic basis of therapeutics*. Retrieved May 3, 2006, from http://www.accessmedicine.com/content.aspx?aID=951722&searchStr=951722#searchTerm

Laibl, V., & Sheffield, J. (2006). The management of respiratory infections during pregnancy. *Immunology and Allergy Clinics of North America, 26*, 155–172.

Lam, C. M., Wong, S. F., Leung, T. N., Chow, K. M., Yu, W. C., Wong, T. Y., et al. (2004). A case-controlled study comparing clinical course and outcomes of pregnant and non-pregnant women with severe acute respiratory syndrome. *British Journal of Obstetrics and Gynaecology, 111*, 771–774.

Lashley, F. R. (2004). Emerging infectious diseases: Vulnerabilities, contributing factors and approaches. *Expert Review of Anti-Infective Therapy, 2*, 299–316.

Lashley, F. R. (2006). Emerging infectious diseases at the beginning of the 21st century. *Online Journal of Issues in Nursing, 11*, 2–16.

Lederberg, J., Shope, R., & Oaks, S. C. (1992). Report: Institute of Medicine. *Emerging infections: Microbial threats to health in the United States*. Washington, DC: National Academy Press.

Lederman, M. M., Rodriguez, B., & Sieg, S. (2006). *Immunopathogenesis of HIV infection. HIVInSite Knowledge Base Chapter*. Retrieved April 11, 2006, from http://hivinsite.ucsf.edu/InSite?page=kb-02-01-04#S5X

Leen, A. M., & Rooney, C. M. (2004). Adenovirus as an emerging pathogen in immunocompromised patients. *British Journal of Haematology, 128*, 135–144.

Levin, T. P., Baty, D. E., Fekete, T., Truant, A. L., & Suh, B. (2004). *Cladophialophora bantiana* brain abscess in a solid-organ transplant recipient: Case report and review of the literature. *Journal of Clinical Microbiology, 42*, 4374–4378.

Medeiros, L. C., Chen, G., Kendall, P., & Hillers, V. N. (2004). Food safety issues for cancer and organ transplant patients. *Nutrition and Clinical Care, 7*(4), 141–148.

National Center for Health Statistics. (2006). *Prevalence of overweight and obesity among adults: United States 2003–2004.* Retrieved April 21, 2006, from http://www.cdc.gov/nchs/products/pubs/pubd/hestats/obese03_04/overwght_adult_03.htm

Nikolich-Zugich, J. (2005). T cell aging: Naive but not young. *Journal of Experimental Medicine, 201,* 837–840.

Obritsch, M. D., Fish, D. N., MacLaren, R., & Jung, R. (2005). Nosocomial infections due to multidrug-resistant *Pseudomonas aeruginosa:* Epidemiology and treatment options. *Pharmacotherapy, 25,* 1353–1364.

Ohmagari, N., Hanna, H., Graviss, L., Hackett, B., Perego, C., Gonzalez, V., et al. (2005). Risk factors for infections with multidrug-resistant *Pseudomonas aeruginosa* in patients with cancer. *Cancer, 104,* 205–212

Organ Procurement and Transplantation Network. (2006). *The organ procurement and transplantation network database.* Retrieved April 30, 2006, from http://www.optn.org/latestData/rptData.asp

Patterson, T. F. (2005). Advances and challenges in management of invasive mycoses. *Lancet, 366,* 1013–1025.

Pawelec, G. (2005). Immunosenescence and vaccination. *Immunity and Aging,* 2(16). Retrieved April 30, 2006, from http://www.immunityageing.com/content/2/1/16

Petropoulos, D., & Chan, K. W. (2005). Umbilical cord blood transplantation. *Current Oncology Reports, 7,* 406–409.

Ponce-de-Leon, S., Garcia-Garcia, M. D., Garcia-Sancho, M. C., Gomez-Perez, F. J., Valdespino-Gomez, J. L., Olaiz-Fernandez, G., et al. (2004). Tuberculosis and diabetes in southern Mexico. *Diabetes Care, 27,* 1584–1588.

Powers, A. C. (2005). Chronic complications of diabetes mellitus. In D. L. Kasper, E. Braunwald, A. S. Fauci, S. L. Hauser, D. L. Longo, J. L. Jameson, et al. (Eds.), *Harrison's on-line* (16th ed.). New York: McGraw-Hill. Retrieved August 20, 2006, from http://www.accessmedicine.com/content.aspx?aID=99213&searchStr=99213#searchTerm

Rasmussen, S. A., & Hayes, E. B. (2005). Public health approach to emerging infections in pregnant women. *American Journal of Public Health, 95,* 1942–1944.

Resnick, I. B., Shapira, M. Y., & Slavin, S. (2005). Nonmyeloablative stem cell transplantation and cell therapy for malignant and non-malignant diseases. *Transplant Immunology, 14,* 207–219.

Ringden, O., & Le Blanc, K. (2005). Allogeneic hematopoietic stem cell transplantation: State of the art and new perspective. *APMIS, 113,* 813–830.

Roland, M. E. (2004). Solid-organ transplantation in HIV-infected patients in the potent antiretroviral era. *Topics in HIV Medicine, 12*(3), 73–76.

Saleeby, C. M., Howard, S. C., Hayden, R. T., & McCullers, J. A. (2004). Association between tea ingestion and invasive *Bacillus cereus* infection among children with cancer. *Clinical Infectious Diseases, 39,* 1536–1539.

Scott, R. S., Sutton, D. A., & Jagirdar, J. (2005). Lung infection due to opportunistic fungus, *Phialemonium obovatum,* in a bone marrow transplant recipient: An emerging infection with fungemia and Crohn disease-like involvement of the gastrointestinal tract. *Annals of Diagnostic Pathology, 9,* 227–230.

Segal, B. H., Walsh, T. J., Gea-Banacloche, J. C., & Holland, S. M. (2005). Infections in the cancer patient. In V. T. DeVita, S. Hellman, & S. A. Rosenberg (Eds.), *Cancer: Principles & practice of oncology* (7th ed.). Philadelphia: Lippincott Williams & Wilkins.

Shu, Y., Yu, H., & Li, D. (2006). Lethal avian influenza A (H5N1) infection in a pregnant woman in Anhui province, China. *New England Journal of Medicine, 354,* 1421–1422.

Siegman-Igra, Y., Levin, R., Weinberger, M., Golan, Y., Schwartz, D., Samra, Z., et al. (2002). *Listeria monocytogenes* infection in Israel and review of cases worldwide. *Emerging Infectious Diseases, 8,* 305–310.

Sims, C. R., Ostrosky-Zeichner, L., & Rex, J. H. (2005). Invasive candidiasis in immunocompromised hospitalized patients. *Archives of Medical Research, 36,* 660–671.

Smolinski, M. S., Hamburg, M. A., & Lederberg, J. (Eds.). (2003). *Microbial threats to health: Emergence, detection and response.* Washington, DC: Institute of Medicine, National Academy Press.

Snyder, C. H. (2005). Coccidiodal meningitis presenting as memory loss. *Journal of the American Academy of Nurse Practitioners, 17,* 181–186.

Srinivasan, A., Burton, E. C., Kuehnert, M. J., Rupprecht, C., Sutker, W. L., Ksiazek, T. G., et al.(2005). Transmission of rabies virus from an organ donor to four transplant recipients. *New England Journal of Medicine, 352,* 1103–1111.

Strippoli, G. F. M., Hodson, E. M., Jones, C., & Craig, J. C. (2006). Pre-emptive treatment for cytomegalovirus viremia to prevent cytomegalovirus disease in solid organ transplant recipients. *Transplantation, 81,* 139–145.

Trevejo, R. T., Barr, M. C., & Robinson, R. A. (2005). Important emerging bacterial zoonotic infections affecting the immunocompromised. *Veterinary Research, 36,* 493–506.

Valantine, H., & Zuckermann, A. (2005). From clinical trials to clinical practice: An overview of certican (everolimus) in heart transplantation. *Journal of Heart and Lung Transplantation, 24,* S185–190.

van Burik, J.-A. H., & Freifeld, A. G. (2004). Infection in the severely immunocompromised patient. In M. D. Abeloff (Ed.), *Clinical oncology* (3rd ed., pp. 941–956). New York: Churchill Livingstone.

Walsh, T. J., Groll, A., Hiemenz, J., Fleming, R., Roilides, E., & Anaissie, E. (2004). Infections due to emerging and uncommon medically important fungal pathogens. *Clinical Microbiology and Infection, 10*(Suppl. 1), 48–66.

Wang, J. Y., Lee, L. N., & Hsueh, P. R. (2005). Factors changing the manifestation of pulmonary tuberculosis. *International Journal of Tuberculosis and Lung Disease, 9,* 777–783.

Weber, D. J., & Rutala, W. A. (2003). Immunization of immunocompromised persons. *Immunology and Allergy Clinics of North America, 23,* 605–634.

White, S. R., Henretig, F. M., & Dukes, R. G. (2002). Medical management of vulnerable populations and co-morbid conditions of victims of bioterrorism. *Emergency Medicine Clinics of North America, 20,* 365–392.

Wong, S. F., Chow, K. M., & Leung, T. N. (2004). Pregnancy and perinatal outcomes of women with severe acute respiratory syndrome. *American Journal of Obstetrics and Gynecology, 191,* 292–297.

World Health Organization. (2005). *AIDS epidemic update, December 2005. Global estimates for adults and children, 2005.* Retrieved April 14, 2006, from http://www.unaids.org/en/default/asp

CHAPTER TWENTY-SEVEN

Bioterrorism in the Context of Infectious Diseases

Miriam Cohen

A FICTIONAL BUT PLAUSIBLE SCENARIO

It had been a hard-fought victory. The candidate came from behind to beat the incumbent, and now it was time to celebrate and thank thousands of supporters that made her bid for political office a success. Nearly 12,000 thousand campaign workers, supporters, family, and friends were in Memorial Auditorium to witness the beginning of a new political era.

Preparations had been underway for this gala event for weeks, and a large number of workers had set the final touches for the stage, the entertainment, the banquet, and the speeches. Unnoticed among the hundreds of busy workers were four individuals who seemed to focus their attention on the air-conditioning system.

As the gala event reached the grand finale, the revelers witnessed hundreds of colorful balloons being released from the auditorium ceiling. What they did not notice was an ultra-fine powder simultaneously released from four parts of the auditorium air-handling system, creating an invisible cloud that enveloped the jubilant crowd. An hour later, the last of the crowd had left, and an hour after that, the four air-conditioning workers were crossing the state line.

Later that week, hospitals throughout the region began to see an alarming influx of patients presenting with malaise, high fever, chills, headache, cough with production of bloody sputum, and toxemia. Radiographic examination revealed patchy or consolidated bronchopneumonia. This pneumonia clinically progressed into dyspnea, stridor, and cyanosis.

In the cases that first arrived, death was due to respiratory failure, circulatory collapse, and a bleeding diathesis. This course was seen in nearly every patient presenting in this fashion. They were now arriving in ever-increasing numbers. Makeshift morgues to handle the growing number of dead were established in refrigerated trailers. No one knew with what they were dealing.

Epidemiologists determined that there was one event in common among all the cases, and that was attendance at the political gala. Yersinia pestis, the etiologic agent of plague, was identified by immunofluorescent staining of material from sputum of a dozen of the first patients. Microbiologists ran their tests three times to make sure of their unprecedented results.

By the end of the second week, nearly all of the 4,000 persons who did not receive appropriate antibiotic therapy in time had died. A small number of nurses, physicians, and other health care providers exposed in the beginning of the epidemic also died. Many died before the diagnosis of primary pneumonic plague was established. The state police and Federal Bureau of Investigation, despite 10 days of intensive investigation, had no leads identifying the perpetrators of this act of biological terrorism.

INTRODUCTION

The bombings of the World Trade Center in New York City and the Alfred P. Murrah Federal Building in Oklahoma City catalyzed an awakening of American society to the reality of terrorism on its own soil. The September 11, 2001, airplane hijackings and subsequent suicide attacks on the World Trade Center and the Pentagon brought home the possibility of terrorism on American soil with tragic punctuation. The 1995 nerve agent attack in the Tokyo subway system by the Aum Shinrikyo, an apocalyptic religious cult, added a new and frightening dimension to terrorism—the use of chemical and biological weapons as agents of mass destruction. In the fall of 2001, the United States experienced its first multistate bioterrorism event with the delivery of anthrax spores in a powdered form through the mail, an act for which the perpetrators are still unknown. Franz et al. (1997) note that international changes, including the breakup of the Soviet Union and the perceived dominance of the United States as a conventional military world power, have raised concerns about the use of biological weapons as a new tool of warfare and terrorism against civilians.

A BRIEF HISTORY OF BIOLOGICAL WEAPON USE

The use of pathogenic microorganisms as weapons is not a 20th century phenomenon. For centuries, militaries developed and used crude methods for dispersing these agents as weapons of warfare. The Center for Non-proliferation Studies (1999a) has chronicled major uses of these agents in warfare. In 1346–1347, the Mongols reportedly catapulted corpses of plague victims over the walls into Kaffa (now in the Ukraine), forcing the weary Genoans to flee. Christopher, Cieslak, Pavlin, and Eitzen (1999) related that during the French and Indian Wars, Sir Jeffrey Amherst, a British commander in North America, suggested the deliberate use of smallpox against hostile Indian tribes. On June 24, 1763, an officer under Amherst's direction gave blankets and a handkerchief from the smallpox hospital to Indians as "gifts." Smallpox epidemics in the immunologically naive tribes followed, though other contacts with Europeans may have also served to transmit smallpox to the tribes.

In 1932, the Imperial Japanese Army began systematic development and testing of biological agents at Ping Fan in Manchuria. Harris (1997) thoroughly examined the activities of the infamous Unit 731, responsible for the majority of these activities. During the years up to the end of World War II, the leaders of Unit 731 conducted an extensive array of live human experiments, including exposures to cold and to a long list of highly toxic agents, including *Y. pestis*, *Bacillus anthracis*, *Vibrio cholerae*, and *Neisseria meningitides*. Over the course of the program, an estimated 3,000 prisoners, mostly Chinese, died in these experiments.

Two more recent incidents illustrate the potential use of biological weapons. In April 1979, within the city of Sverdlovsk (now Yekaterinburg) in Russia's Ural Mountains, a mysterious outbreak of anthrax took the lives of nearly 70 local citizens. Russian officials attributed the outbreak to consumption of tainted meat sold on the black market. U.S. officials thought differently, believing that the epidemic was due to an explosion at the nearby Soviet Institute of Microbiology and Virology, believed to be a military biological weapons plant. In 1992, Boris Yeltsin, then president of Russia, admitted that there had been an accident at the Institute that resulted in the release of spores of weaponized *B. anthracis*. Meselson et al. (1994), using exquisite epidemiologic reasoning and evidence, convincingly concluded that the escape of an aerosol of anthrax bacilli from the military facility caused the outbreak.

In 1978, Bulgarian Secret Police agents reportedly assassinated Georgi Markov, a Bulgarian in exile in London. As described by Simon (1999), Markov was attacked by an unknown assailant with a weapon disguised as an umbrella. A pellet, no larger than the head of a pin, was discharged into the subcutaneous tissue of his leg while he waited for a bus. He died 3 days later and, upon autopsy, the pellet was found. The pellet was machined to contain a toxin (in this case, ricin) that would be released when body heat melted the coat of wax encasing the toxin. A similar assassination was attempted just weeks later, but fortunately the toxin was not released as planned.

Following the first Gulf War it was learned that Iraq had a large biological weapons program. The Center for Nonproliferation Studies notes that Iraq acknowledged the testing of biological agents between March of 1988 and January of 1991 (Center for Non Proliferation Studies, 1999b).

TERRORISM

O'Neill (1995) defines terrorism as "the unlawful use of force against persons or property to intimidate or coerce a government, the civilian population, or any segment thereof, in the furtherance of political or social objectives" (p. 120). Extrapolating to chemical or biological terrorism, Perrotta, Rawlings, and Eckman (1998) suggested that the use of harmful chemicals, pathogenic microbes, or plant or microbial toxins as weapons of terrorism should be known as bioterrorism. That the act is executed in the furtherance of political or social objectives serves to differentiate it from criminal assault.

It is important to understand the variety of categories of terrorist groups because such knowledge helps predict the kind and size of weapons such groups are generally likely to use or are capable of using. Generally, terrorist groups are classified as foreign, domestic, or religious. Foreign terrorist groups may be state supported or independent (Fainberg, 1997). It is clear that the government of the former Soviet Union supported an enormous offensive biological weapons program as detailed by Alibek (Alibek & Handelman, 1999), who, before his defection to the United States, was among the top leaders of that program. A variety of pathogens including *Francisella tularensis* (tularemia), variola virus (smallpox), and *B. anthracis* (anthrax) were weaponized and made ready for missiles aimed at American targets. It is unclear if terrorists were provided with biological weapons from the Soviet Union's sizeable arsenal. International intelligence information, as described by Cole (1997), suggests that 17 countries are suspected of having active biological weapons research programs.

There is a plethora of domestic antigovernment, neo-Nazi groups within the United States that have already made attempts to acquire biological agents and toxins. Tucker (1999) reported that in 1995 Larry Wayne Harris, a purported laboratory technician from Ohio, ordered three vials of *Y. pestis* (plague bacillus) from a Maryland biomedical supply firm. Concerned about his impatience and apparent unfamiliarity with laboratory techniques, the company notified federal authorities.

Upon investigation, authorities found the vials in the glove compartment of his car. He was arrested and was later identified as a member of a White Supremacy organization. He pleaded guilty to federal charges of mail fraud. Tucker (1999) further recounted that later, in 1998, Mr. Harris was again arrested in possession of what he described as "enough military-grade anthrax to wipe out Las Vegas" (p. 284). The vials were later determined to contain harmless veterinary vaccine against anthrax.

O'Neill (1995) reported that the quasi-militia, antitax group, the Patriots Council, headquartered in Minneapolis, was planning to assassinate a deputy U.S. marshal and a local sheriff using ricin, a protein toxin derived from the castor plant, *Ricinus communism*. Plans were progressing until four individuals were caught and convicted of violating the Biological Weapons Anti-Terrorism Act of 1989.

Religious cults vary in sophistication and resources, but at least one group, the Rajneesh, successfully carried out what most consider the first biological terrorism attack on American soil. Török et al. (1997) investigated a large community-wide outbreak of salmonellosis in Dalles, Oregon, in 1984. More than 750 individuals became ill after eating from salad bars in 10 area restaurants. This exhaustive epidemiologic examination initially failed to identify any plausible, naturally occurring source for the contamination. It was not until 1 year later that a law enforcement and public health investigation identified the source as a clinical laboratory operated by the Rajneesh. The cult had intentionally seeded area salad bars to influence voter turnout in an upcoming election.

The March 1995 release of the organophosphate nerve agent sarin in the Tokyo subway system is generally regarded as the wake-up call regarding the use of chemical or biological agents against civilian populations. Olsen (1995) investigated the incident perpetrated by members of the Aum Shinrikyo and noted that the cult had previously tested a variety of biological agents such as *B. anthracis* and the toxin that causes botulism on unsuspected civilian populations in Japan. In the sarin release, 12 persons died and nearly 5,500 injuries were reported. While most intelligence sources indicate that only foreign state-supported groups would have the resources to execute a credible bioterrorism event, the Rajneesh and Aum Shinrikyo appear to serve as exceptions to that belief.

To date, no comprehensive assessment of the threat and risks of bioterrorism has been conducted for the United States (U.S. General Accounting Office, 1999). Osterholm (1999) suggests, "It is not a matter of if a bioterrorism event will occur in the United States, but rather when, where, and how large" (p. 462). Hughes (1999) considers bioterrorism an emerging infectious disease threat since an attack will manifest as a sizeable epidemic, and the resources necessary to mount an effective response will include the same disease surveillance, epidemiology, and laboratory components as does a naturally occurring outbreak. McDade and Franz

(1998) note that partnerships among health care providers, state and local health agencies, and the Centers for Disease Control and Prevention (CDC) are essential for preparedness. This chapter focuses on the use of pathogenic microbes and their toxins as weapons of terrorism.

REQUIREMENTS FOR AN IDEAL BIOLOGICAL AGENT

Nearly any pathogenic microorganism could be used to cause disease in humans on a limited or small scale. Fortunately, relatively few would be effective if employed as a weapon of terrorism against a large population. Sidell, Takafuji, and Franz (1997) outlined six key factors that make a pathogen or toxin suitable for large-scale biological warfare attack and therefore attractive to terrorists:

- readily available or easy to produce in large quantities;
- highly virulent for lethal or incapacitating effects in humans, with appropriate particle size in aerosol;
- easy to disseminate with proper technology;
- stable, able to withstand harsh environmental conditions, and likely to affect only the target population, not the terrorists.

While the cultivation and growth of pathogenic microbes for these purposes is a relatively simple operation, there remain significant barriers to implementing a biologic weapon of mass destruction. Hinton, in his testimony before the U.S. Senate, observed that a terrorist group would need "a relatively high degree of sophistication to successfully and effectively process, improvise a weapon, and disseminate biological agents to cause mass casualties" ("Combating Terrorism," 1999, p. 3). One such technological impediment is the fact that the respiratory system is the most likely target of a widespread attack, and particles must be in the range of 1–5 micrometers in diameter in order to reach the alveolar spaces where damage first occurs. It has been technologically difficult to meet these specifications. Osterholm and Schwartz (2000) relate discussions with an expert on particle technology who believes the technology is readily available.

The intentional dissemination of *B. anthracis*, the biological agent of anthrax, through the U.S. mail beginning in September 2001 was the first successful bioterrorism attack in the United States in the 21st century. The still unidentified terrorists used the U.S. mail delivery system to infect 22 persons with anthrax (Lucey, 2005). There were 11 confirmed cases of inhalational anthrax with 5 deaths; 11 confirmed or probable cases of cutaneous anthrax (Inglesby et al., 2002). Postexposure prophylaxis was recommended for more than 10,000 people (Gerberding, Hughes, &

Koplan, 2002). Prior to the events of 2001, the expertise of health care professionals with anthrax in the clinical and public health sectors was limited (Lucey, 2005). Since then much has been learned, and there is an increased body of knowledge and expertise about anthrax.

Potential Biologic Agents

The CDC (1999) convened a panel of experts to identify biological agents considered to be of greatest potential concern to civilians as well as review those biological threat agents that were previously identified by the military and the Working Group on Civilian Biodefense (Rotz, K., Khan, A., Lillibridge, S., Ostroff, S., & Hughes, J., 2002). Applying a variety of criteria, three categories of agents emerged, A, B, & C. The highest priority for preparedness was assigned to Category A agents while efforts for Category B agents will focus in increasing awareness and improving surveillance and laboratory diagnosis. Those agents in Category C will continue to be assessed for threats posed to the public as information about their epidemiology and pathogenesis becomes more available (Rotz, et al., 2002). All categories are reviewed regularly by the CDC. Other organizations such as the World Health Organization (WHO) may list various other agents as having the potential for use by bioterrorists. The agents included in each category are listed in Table 27.1. The definitions of the categories are as follows (CDC, 2001a):

Category A

- Can be disseminated or transmitted easily from person to person
- Result in high mortality rates and have the potential for major public health impact
- Cause possible public panic and social disruption
- Require special action for public health preparedness

Category B

- Are moderately easy to disseminate
- Result in moderate morbidity and low mortality rates
- Require specific enhancements of CDC's diagnostic capacity as well as enhanced disease surveillance

Category C

- Are available
- Have ease of production and dissemination
- Have potential for high morbidity and mortality rates and major health impact

Table 27.1. Critical Biological Agent Categories for Public Health Preparedness

Biologic Agent	Disease(s)
Category A Agents	
Variola virus	Smallpox
Bacillus anthracis	Anthrax
Yersinia pestis	Plague
Clostridium botulinum toxin	Botulism
Francisella tularensis	Tularemia
Ebola virus	Ebola hemorrhagic fever
Marburg virus	Marburg hemorrhagic fever
Lassa virus	Lassa fever
Junin virus	Argentine hemorrhagic fever
Other arenaviruses	
Category B Agents	
Coxiella burnetti	Q fever
Brucella species	Brucellosis
Burkholderia mallei	Glanders
Venezuelan equine encephalitis virus	Venezuelan encephalomyelitis
Eastern equine encephalitis virus	Eastern equine encephalomyelitis
Western equine encephalitis virus	Western equine encephalomyelitis
Others include:	
Ricin toxin from *Ricinus communis*	*Salmonella* species
Epsilon toxin of *Clostridium*	*Shigella dysenteriae*
perfringens	*Escherichia coli* O157:H7
Staphylococcus enterotoxin B	*Vibrio cholerae*
	Cryptosporidium parvum
	(now *hominis*)
Category C Agents	
• Nipah virus	
• Hantaviruses	
• Tickborne hemorrhagic fever viruses	
• Tickborne encephalitis viruses	
• Yellow fever	
• Multidrug-resistant tuberculosis	

Source: Centers for Disease Control and Prevention, 2000a, pp. 5–6.

SELECTED BIOLOGICAL AGENTS AND THEIR DISEASES

The intent of the terrorist may not be immediately evident, but experience suggests that striking fear, panic, and dread in a society is at the heart of their actions. To that end, the use of agents with high public recognition value might cause the desired social disruption, even if no one becomes ill. The evidence for this lies in the fears and concerns expressed by the public whenever a threat of the release of a high profile biological agent is reported. Because these high profile agents are well-suited for the desires of the terrorist, brief descriptions of three Category A agents and their diseases—smallpox, anthrax, plague, botulism, and tularemia—are presented. The hemorrhagic fevers (Ebola, Lassa, Marburg, and others) are discussed in chapter 8.

Smallpox

Recognized as a clinical entity since biblical times, smallpox was eradicated from the globe in 1980 as the result of decades of exhaustive planning and fieldwork (Fenner, Henderson, Arita, Jezel, & Ladnyi, 1988). Since that time, stocks of variola virus were consolidated into two WHO-approved repositories. Recently, Alibek and Handelman (1999) expressed concern that other clandestine virus stockpiles, as well as expertise and equipment, may have been recruited from the enormous Soviet biological warfare program, which has sharply declined in recent years due to the dissolution of that union and the severe financial environments in the remaining countries. It is this concern that resurrects the specter of the use of variola virus as a biological weapon. Such a release would have dire consequences for the planet, since nearly all immunity against variola infection has waned in the more than 20 years since the last individual was immunized.

Variola is a member of the virus genus *Orthopoxvirus* and is nearly indistinguishable from the other members—monkeypox, vaccinia, and cowpox (see chapter 19; Moore, Seward, & Lane, 2006). This DNA virus infects only humans, although the origins of human disease are unknown. The Institute of Medicine (1999a) observed that from the time smallpox was first described as a human illness until the end of the 19th century, it was considered a uniformly severe disease with case-fatality rates of up to 40% in unvaccinated individuals. Throughout the remaining 80 years of the virus's uncontrolled existence, case-fatality rates were approximately 30%.

Franz and colleagues (1997) outline the pathogenesis of smallpox as beginning with a small aerosol exposure. From the respiratory system, the virus travels to regional lymph nodes, where it replicates, produces a viremia, and results in viral multiplication in the spleen, bone marrow, and lymph nodes. By the eighth day after infection, a second viremia occurs, this time followed by fever and toxemia. At the end of a 12–14-day incubation period, an abrupt onset of systemic toxicity with serious malaise, high fever, rigors, vomiting, headache, and backache occurs. A maculopapular rash first appears on the oral and pharyngeal mucosa. The oropharyngeal lesions ulcerate quickly and release large amounts of virus into the saliva, as first described by Sarkar, Mitra, Mukherjee, and

De (1973). Respiratory secretions that contain virus from these lesions are the most important source of exposure to contacts. This step occurs during the first week of illness and corresponds with the period during which patients are most contagious.

The rash progresses to the face and forearms, followed by spread to the lower extremities and then centrally to the trunk. Lesions quickly progress from macules to papules and eventually to pustular vesicles. They are more abundant on the extremities and the face, and this centrifugal distribution is an important, although unexplained, clinical feature. During the second week, the pustules form scabs that leave depressed depigmented scars upon healing. Since the virus can be easily recovered from scabs throughout convalescence, patients should be isolated until all scabs separate (Mitra, Sarkar, & Mukherjee, 1974).

Should the victim succumb to the effects of viral infection, death usually occurs during the second week of illness, most likely as the result of toxemia associated with circulating immune complexes and soluble variola antigens (Fenner et al., 1988). There have been two irregularly observed variations of smallpox disease, flat type and hemorrhagic type. Both of these clinical forms were seen in less than 5% of patients, but they were characterized by severe systemic toxicity and high mortality.

While testing of antiviral drugs is an active field of research and development, few, if any, antiviral agents are suitable for use against smallpox (Institute of Medicine, 1999a). Cidofovir, initially developed as a DNA polymerase inhibitor for the treatment of cytomegalovirus retinitis, was found to have inhibitory properties against variola infection in cell culture. Because of potential renal toxicity and low oral bioavailability, however, cidofovir is of limited utility for treating or preventing variola infection in humans. Other strategies are being examined, but they suffer from a lack of a clinically meaningful animal model and from the inaccessibility of virus stocks for testing of drug effectiveness (Moore et al., 2006).

The vaccine used in the historic WHO Smallpox Eradication Program did not contain variola virus. The vaccine, prepared on a large scale by inoculating the shaved abdomens of calves, contained vaccinia virus, another member of the *Orthopox* genus that has little pathogenicity for immunocompetent humans (McClain, 1997). This vaccine was administered through a process called scarification that used a bifurcated needle to intradermally inoculate susceptible populations. Vaccination, targeted by intensive, active surveillance, was the linchpin of the smallpox eradication program. After the eradication program was complete, there was no incentive for vaccine manufacturers to continue to formulate smallpox vaccine, so stores of usable vaccine were diminished. In September 2000, the CDC entered into an agreement with OraVax to manufacture smallpox vaccine (LeDuc & Jahrling, 2001). As of late 2001, the U.S. smallpox vaccine supply was considered to be adequate for the vaccination of 50 million people (Henderson, D., Inglesby, T. & O'Toole T., 2002).

The WHO had planned to destroy all stocks of variola virus by 1999, but concerns about terrorist organizations possessing the virus for nefarious purposes resulted in the postponement of this action for reevaluation in 2002 (LeDuc & Jahrling, 2001). The Institute of Medicine (1999a) conducted an assessment of the future scientific needs for live variola virus and concluded that there are legitimate scientific circumstances that support keeping the virus stocks intact. No further action has been taken. The airborne spread, high communicability, nearly complete sensitivity of human populations, and high lethality of this virus make it an excellent candidate for use as a weapon of mass destruction (Henderson et al., 1999). Following the intentional release of anthrax spores in fall 2001, there were sharpened fears about smallpox and other potential agents that might be used in bioterrorist attacks. Because of its potential for use in a bioterrorist attack, an interim smallpox release plan, guidelines, and a revision of vaccine recommendations from the Advisory Committee on Immunization Practices were issued in November 2001 (available from the CDC Web site at http://www.cdc.gov/). The federal government initiated a smallpox vaccination program directed at establishing smallpox response teams in each and every state in the United States. The goal of this voluntary vaccination program was to form a cadre of vaccinated health care professionals in each state who would be prepared to respond immediately to the health needs of citizens in the event of a smallpox attack. A total of 32,644 individuals were vaccinated during the civilian vaccination program (CDC, (2005a). Because of its potential for use in a bioterrorist attack, the Advisory Committee on Immunization Practices issued a statement in June, 2003 restating its support for the continuation of smallpox preparedness planning within the broader context of emergency preparedness planning at all levels of government,(available from the CDC Web site at http://www.cdc.gov/agent/smallpox/vaccination/acipjun2003.asp).

For additional information about smallpox and smallpox vaccination, including adverse events, see CDC, 2003, or visit the CDC Web site at www.cdc.bt.gov. One suspect case of smallpox is a public health emergency and requires immediate reporting to local and state officials. All health care professionals must be aware of the reporting requirements for smallpox and have current contact information for their health department. Health professionals are encouraged to become current in the diagnosis and treatment of smallpox as well as the smallpox vaccination technique.

Anthrax

Described first in biblical times, this zoonotic disease is caused by the gram-positive, spore-forming rod *B. anthracis*. Anthrax occurs primarily in herbivores, such as goats, sheep, cattle, and horses. Humans are most often infected by contact with infected animals or contaminated animal products (Friedlander & Longfield, 2000). Outbreaks of anthrax during the 16th and 18th centuries occurred with devastating agricultural consequences. The majority of cases of human anthrax reported in the United States are natural and cutaneous. In one case, doing field autopsies of dead sheep, later culture positive for *B. anthracis,* was the suspected exposure (Taylor, Dimmitt, Ezzel, & Whitford, 1993). In the summer of 2000, one such sporadic case of cutaneous anthrax occurred in North Dakota. The 67-year-old infected man had participated in the disposal of cows that had died of anthrax. He became ill 4 days later, initially noticing a bump on his cheek. He was treated with ciprofloxacin and recovered (CDC, 2001b). A recent case of inhalational anthrax occurred in a New York City resident who had traveled to Côte d'Ivoire, Africa (CDC, 2006). Anthrax is reported in domestic and wild animals in the United States. The first use of *B. anthracis* in warfare is suggested by substantial evidence indicating that Germany used this organism, and others, during World War I (Christopher et al., 1999). The Germans reportedly infected Romanian sheep that were being exported to Russia, in an apparent attempt to infect Russian soldiers.

 B. anthracis is a relatively large gram-positive bacillus that is nonmotile and forms spores (Walker, 2006). Microscopic examination shows a jointed bamboo-rod cellular appearance of the organism when grown on common laboratory media. The virulence of *B. anthracis* is attributed to four known factors: three protein exotoxin components called the protective antigen, lethal factor, and edema factor and an antiphagocytic capsule (Dixon, Meselson, Guillemin, & Hanna, 1999). The exotoxin components, which are individually without biologic activity, combine in binary form to create two toxins. Edema factor joins with protective antigen to form edema toxin, which is responsible for increased cellular levels of cyclic adenosine monophosphate that lead to the massive edema observed in anthrax-affected tissues and organs. Lethal toxin consists of lethal factor and protective antigen and is responsible for increasing macrophage release of tumor necrosis factor and interleukin 1, both of which play a role in the sudden death (shock) observed in the systemic phase of inhalational anthrax (Hanna, Acosta, & Collier, 1993).

 There are three clinical manifestations of *B. anthracis* in humans: inhalational, gastrointestinal, and cutaneous anthrax (Heymann, 2004). However, Lucey (2005) believes that meningitis should also be listed as a distinct clinical manifestation of *B. anthracis* in humans. Lucey (2005) notes that meningitis was the presenting symptom in the first diagnosed case of anthrax in the 2001 anthrax event; the high case-fatality rate makes it a medical emergency requiring immediate aggressive treatment. Additionally, a diagnosis of anthrax meningitis should trigger a rapid public health response (Lucey, 2005). Before October 2001, inhalational anthrax was rarely seen but was known as Woolsorter disease because workers in industrial mills were at the highest risk of exposure from the hides, wool, and hair of contaminated animals (Brachman, 1980). A case of cutaneous anthrax from wool exposure occurred in 1987 in the United States. A textile worker contracted Anthrax. The source of exposure is thought to have been imported cashmere (CDC, 1988). The most recent case of naturally occurring inhalational anthrax occurred in February 2006. A New York City drum maker developed inhalational anthrax as a direct result of hand cleaning and finishing of imported untanned animal hides (CDC, 2006). Gastrointestinal anthrax results from ingestion of contaminated meat that has not been sufficiently cooked. This manifestation is not seen in the United States; it was inaccurately reported to be the cause of the 1979 Sverdlovsk outbreak previously described.

In late 2001, 11 cases of inhalational anthrax occurred as a result of the intentional distribution of *B. anthracis* spores in letters delivered by the U.S. Postal Service (CDC, 2001b). Cases occurred in media workers, postal workers, a woman who worked in a nonpatient care area of a hospital, and a 94-year-old woman in rural Connecticut. The exposure source for the latter two is unknown (CDC, 2001b).

The vast majority of reported cases of anthrax have been cutaneous anthrax, where pathogenic endospores of *B. anthracis* have been introduced by cut or abrasion (Friedlander & Longfield, 2000). Within 36 hours of development of a painless, pruritic papule, a vesicle forms and undergoes central necrosis. The black eschar is often surrounded by edema and remains painless. Complications are rare; most cases of cutaneous anthrax are self-limiting, but dissemination can occur in about 20% of cases, so antibiotic treatment is indicated (Dixon et al., 1999; Friedlander & Longfield, 2000). Eleven cases (seven confirmed and four suspected) of cutaneous anthrax resulting from deliberate distribution of anthrax spores occurred in the United States in the fall of 2001 (Jernigan, DB, Raghunathan, PL, Bell, BP, Brechner R B, Butler JC, et, al, 2001).

The intentional airborne spread of anthrax endospores is of great public health concern. In this case, spore-bearing particles are deposited in the alveolar spaces where macrophages phagocytize and transport them to regional lymph nodes. Vegetative anthrax bacilli multiply there and are spread by blood and lymph systems throughout the body, leading to severe septicemia. Concentrations of exotoxins increase rapidly and result in severe local effects, thoracic hemorrhagic necrotizing lymphadenitis, hemorrhagic necrotizing mediastinitis, and toxemia (Abramova, Grinberg, Yampolskaya, & Walker, 1993). This rapid onset of shock and respiratory distress is followed by death within 36 hours in nearly all untreated victims.

The 22 cases of anthrax occurring in fall 2001 led to additional information on clinical signs and symptoms, management and progress, as well as dissemination and spread (Jernigan et al., 2001; Swartz, 2001). Clinically, patients first present with flu-like symptoms including fever, dyspnea, cough, headache, vomiting, weakness, and chest pain that persist for 2–3 days (Lucey, 2005). In previous reports (Friedlander, 1997), the incubation period for inhalational anthrax was between 1 and 6 days, but the investigation of the Sverdlovsk release by Meselson et al. (1994) suggests cases occurred from 2 to 43 days after exposure. Nearly all of the cases of inhalational anthrax in Sverdlovsk resulted from the initial release of the anthrax bacillus. Neither secondary aerosols nor person-to-person spread of the organism appear to play a role in spread of the disease. These observations about incubation period and the lack of person-to-person spread have important implications for the public health response to an epidemic of inhalational anthrax. Those individuals exposed to anthrax are not contagious, and quarantine is not required (Heymann, 2004). Standard precautions are used for patients with inhalational or cutaneous anthrax (Heymann, 2004). However, those workers responsible for disinfection of anthrax-contaminated areas must use personal protective equipment (Heymann, 2004).

The patient may experience a period of clinical improvement for 1–2 days but rapidly deteriorates with the sudden onset of respiratory distress, dyspnea, cyanosis, chest pain, and diaphoresis. The radiographic observation of a widened mediastinum is an important clue to making the diagnosis of inhalational anthrax. Without suspicion from public health or law enforcement sources, it is unlikely that such a diagnosis will otherwise be made in emergency rooms, clinics, or physicians' offices. Autopsy results indicating thoracic hemorrhagic necrotizing lymphadenitis, hemorrhagic necrotizing mediastinitis, or hemorrhagic meningitis should raise strong suspicions of anthrax infection (Inglesby et al., 1999) and may provide the first clue to the identity of the epidemic disease.

Treatment of anthrax is complicated by a lack of clinical trials of treatments for inhalational anthrax, contraindications for use of selected antibiotics in subgroups (children, pregnant women), the extended presence of anthrax spores in the lungs, and the logistic issues of treating very large population groups (Inglesby et al., 1999). Intravenous administration of penicillin and doxycycline has most often been recommended, although intravenous ciprofloxacin has been recommended by a consensus group (Dixon et al., 1999; Inglesby et al., 1999). This group, recognizing that there is great risk of recurrence in survivors of inhalational anthrax due to the possibility of delayed germination of spores remaining in alveolar spaces, recommends that treatment continue for 60 days, with oral therapy replacing intravenous therapy as soon as the patient's clinical condition improves. Postexposure prophylaxis may include the use of oral doxycycline or ciprofloxacin. Another approach to treatment for anthrax that is in the exploratory stages is the use of an agent to block the action of bacterial virulence factors (Sellman, Mourez, & Collier, 2001). The most current treatment guidelines for anthrax are available from the CDC.

A vaccine that protects against anthrax is available, but supplies are currently severely limited, due, in part, to the demand for the vaccine by the U.S. military, which inoculated all military personnel. The capacity to make more vaccine is quite modest, and supplies are expected to remain limited for the foreseeable future. If supplies were available, administration of vaccine would require concurrent antibiotic administration to protect individuals exposed to anthrax spores from a bioterrorist attack. The Advisory Committee on Immunization Practices (ACIP) does not recommend routine vaccination with anthrax vaccine of civilian U.S. populations who do not have an occupational risk of exposure to *B. anthracis* (CDC, 2002).

The Department of Defense (DoD) surveyed vaccinated military personnel to assess the occurrence of adverse events from anthrax vaccine. According to the *Morbidity and Mortality Weekly Report* report covering the years 1998–2000 no unusual or unexpected local or systemic reactions to the vaccine occurred. (CDC, 2000b). In 1999, the CDC released interim guidelines for the management of exposure to and decontamination of those individuals exposed to anthrax (CDC, 1999). According to Heymann (2004), individuals who may have been exposed and may be contaminated require only showering with copious amounts of water and soap. Routine laundering of clothes is sufficient. Physical surfaces may be cleaned with a 0.5% hypochlorite solution following a crime scene investigation. Additional recommendations for avoiding exposure and for decontamination may be found in CDC, 2001c.

Plague

Few human diseases generate as much fear and emotion as plague does, and much has been written about its impact on human populations. This zoonotic infection is caused by *Y. pestis,* a relatively small gram-negative coccobacillus that does not form spores. This organism has been the cause of three great pandemics in the 6th, 14th, and 20th centuries. The second pandemic, known as the Black Death, took the lives of more than 40 million people from 1346 through the end of the 14th century (Butler & Dennis, 2005; Dennis & Mead, 2006).

In more modem times, nearly 700 persons with plague, including 56 fatal cases, were reported from India in a 2-month period in 1994 (CDC, 1994a, 1994b). In 1997, a plague patient in Madagascar transmitted pneumonic plague to 18 persons, including 8 persons who died (Ratsitorahina, Chanteau, Rahalison, Rastisofasoamanana, & Biosier 2000). During the period from 1971–1995 there were 1–40 cases of human infection (average 13 cases) reported yearly from 13 western states (CDC, 2005a).

There are three clinical presentations of plague: bubonic, septicemic, and pneumonic. Naturally occurring plague is most commonly transmitted by the bite of a flea infected with Y. pestis and results in bubonic plague. This happens usually when humans encroach on the mostly rural habitat of rats of the genus Rattus, where they are likely to come into contact with infected fleas from those rats. Other animals such as ground squirrels or chipmunks can also harbor fleas that are infected. Infection causes a severe febrile illness that generally includes headache, chills, myalgia, malaise, prostration, and gastrointestinal symptoms. Bubonic plague is characterized by acute regional lymphadenopathy that manifests as a bubo, most often in the inguinal, axillary, or cervical regions, depending upon where the infected flea inoculates the plague bacilli. These buboes, which are extremely painful to touch or movement, appear within 24 hours of the onset of systemic symptoms (Butler & Dennis, 2005; Dennis & Mead, 2006). Septicemic plague can occur secondarily to bubonic plague or can develop without detectable lymphadenopathy. The case-fatality rate for untreated bubonic plague is 50–60%; septicemic plague is virtually invariably fatal (Heymann, 2004).

The pneumonic form of plague is the most dangerous in terms of public health threat and is the form most likely to occur after the airborne release of a plague biological weapon (Inglesby et al., 2000). Primary pneumonic plague is characterized by a severe pneumonia, high fever, dyspnea, and hemoptysis, which occur within 1–3 days of the infective aerosol exposure from a biological weapon or another pneumonic plague patient (secondary spread). Secondary pneumonic plague, which may follow the bubonic or septicemic forms, results from hematogenous spread of the plague bacilli to the lungs. Without effective treatment, the case-fatality rate for pneumonic plague is essentially 100% but with treatment about 40–50% (Butler & Dennis, 2005; Dennis & Mead, 2006).

Upon introduction into the human host, Y. pestis synthesizes a variety of virulence factors, including an antiphagocytic capsule that allows the organism to resist phagocytosis and to replicate unimpeded (Dennis &

Mead, 2006). The endotoxin of *Y. pestis* contributes to the development of septic shock in manners similar to those seen with other gram-negative organisms. As might be expected, complications of gram-negative sepsis could include disseminated intravascular coagulation, adult respiratory distress syndrome, and multiple organ system failure.

Inglesby and associates (2000), in their consensus work on the management of plague used as a biological weapon, suggest that the first indication of a covert attack with plague might be a sudden outbreak of illness presenting as severe pneumonia and sepsis. Since this would be primary pneumonic plague, buboes would rarely be seen. Autopsy findings would include areas of profound lobular exudation and bacillary aggregation (Dennis & Meier, 1997) since *Y. pestis* is believed to be the only gram-negative bacterium capable of causing fulminant pneumonia with blood-tinged sputum in an otherwise healthy individual.

It was previously recommended by public health officials that strict isolation be maintained for close contacts of patients with pneumonic plague who have refused prophylaxis. Isolation of close contacts is no longer recommended (Henderson, Inglesby, & O'Toole, 2002). Individuals living or working in close proximity to patients with plague, confirmed or suspected, and have not had prophylaxis should use droplet precautions and wear a surgical mask. Transmission by droplet nuclei has also not been proved (Henderson, et al., 2002), so it is recommended that disposable surgical masks be used to prevent the transmission of plague (Henderson et al., 2002). The use of standard respiratory droplet precautions for patients is recommended until the first 48 hours of treatment is completed and the onset of clinical improvement has occurred. Plague is a reportable condition in nearly all 50 states; proven or suspect cases must be reported to state or local health authorities immediately (Rousch, Birkhead, Koo, Cobb, & Fleming, 1999).

There are little modern data that support clear recommendations for the best treatment of plague. Since the 1950s, intramuscular streptomycin has been used to treat plague (Perry & Featherston, 1997), but streptomycin is uncommonly found in the United States. Gentamicin has been used as an alternative to streptomycin as it is widely available and inexpensive (American Hospital Formulary Service, 2000). A critical review and development of consensus recommendations for therapies were conducted by Inglesby and colleagues (2000). They make two general recommendations based on the size of the population likely to require treatment. For treating a modest number of patients, parenteral administration of streptomycin or gentamicin is recommended. In a large casualty situation, intravenous or intramuscular therapy is not logistically feasible. In those situations, oral administration of doxycycline (or tetracycline) or ciprofloxacin is recommended. Presumptive treatment of persons in the exposed area with fever and cough should occur immediately. The special situations of treating children, immunocompromised persons, and pregnant women are also outlined in these recommendations. Asymptomatic close contacts of persons with pneumonic plague should receive a 7-day course of antibiotics as well.

The plague bacillus, in contrast to the anthrax bacillus, does not survive for extended periods of time outside of the host, nor does it form environmentally hardy spores. No special decontamination of environmental surfaces, other than normal hospital cleaning, is indicated.

Botulism

Botulism results from toxins of the bacteria *Clostridium botulinum*. These toxins are designated by letters from A through G, and most human cases result from Types A, B, and E. Botulinum toxins are among the most potent known, with extremely tiny amounts sufficient to cause symptoms. The bacteria are found in soil and have the ability to form spores that under the appropriate conditions of anaerobic environment, nonacidic pH, and low salt and sugar content can germinate and produce toxin. Botulism occurs naturally, but rarely, most frequently by ingestion of foods containing botulinum toxin, wound botulism resulting from wound colonization by *C. botulinum* with in situ toxin production, and infant botulism resulting from intestinal colonization by *C. botulinum*, with toxin production (Sobel, 2005; Villar, Elliott, & Davenport, 2006). Cases have also been described in injection drug users who "skin pop" drugs such as cocaine or black tar heroin (which may be considered a type of wound botulism), and botulism following the inhalation of adulterated cocaine (Roblot et al, 2006) and inhalation botulism among laboratory workers in Germany have been described. The toxin has been weaponized in military and terrorist programs.

Foodborne botulism is rare as a result of eating commercially processed foods and is more often seen in home-canned foods; however, there have been unusual vehicles such as sautéed onions served on a patty melt sandwich, which affected 28 people in Peoria, Illinois, in 1984 (Cohen et al., 1988). Other food vehicles have been garlic in oil, smoked fish, canned asparagus, canned clams, and in September 2006, bottled carrot juice in Georgia and Florida ("Botulism, Carrot Juice," 2006). Outbreaks tend to be small. Some believe that unless a cause such as a food safety failure has occurred, botulism should be treated as a potential bioterror occurrence.

The clinical picture may begin in a nonspecific manner, which may include constipation, but soon, bilateral cranial nerve palsies manifesting as ptosis, blurred vision, dysphagia, and dysarthria are seen with dry mouth and throat. A descending flaccid symmetric bilateral voluntary muscle paralysis occurs, which can cause paralysis of the diaphragm and accessory respiratory muscles, leading to respiratory arrest. Signs result from the toxin binding to nerve terminals and blocking neuromuscular junctions. Progression will occur, the extent of which is variable. It can be irreversible if botulism antitoxin is not quickly administered, ideally within 24 hours or less. Patients often require supportive intensive care and mechanical ventilation, and if botulism were used as a bioterror weapon this would cause massive strain on available medical equipment and personnel. Botulism may have significant long-lasting physical and psychosocial effects (Cohen et al., 1988; Hardin & Cohen, 1988).

Tularemia

Tularemia is caused by the gram-negative non-spore-forming bacteria *F. tularensis*. *F. tularensis* is a zoonotic agent that has many small mammal hosts such as rabbits and muskrats. It is spread by direct contact with animal fluids or tissues, especially rabbits; ingestion of, or direct contact with, contaminated food, water, or soil; the bite of infected arthropods such as ticks or deer flies; and inhalation of infectious aerosols such as contaminated dust or feces or in the lab (Eliasson, Broman, Forsman, & Bäck, 2006). Person-to-person spread is not documented. Tularemia is considered an occupational risk for professional landscapers, hunters, trappers, and others who handle infected animal carcasses It is endemic on Martha's Vineyard, where a pneumonic outbreak occurred in 2000 that was associated with lawn mowing and brush cutting, especially among professional landscapers for whom exposure to aerosolized organisms was presumed (Feldman et al., 2003). It is also prevalent in Arkansas, Missouri, Oklahoma, Kansas, South Dakota, and Montana. For many years tularemia was not a nationally notifiable disease, but it was reinstated in 2000 (CDC, 2002).

There are various subspecies. Type A is more common in North America, and it is more virulent than others. *F. tularensis* is considered a potential agent of bioterrorism because it is highly infective, extremely virulent, and easy to disseminate via aerosol, and it has a low infectious dose. As few as 10 colony-forming units can cause human disease, and without treatment it can have a 30–60% mortality rate (McLendon, Apicella, & Allen, 2006). Clinical manifestations are highly variable depending on type, route of infection, and dose, and it occurs in six recognized clinical forms: pneumonic, typhoidal, ulceroglandular, glandular, oculoglandular, and oropharyngeal. In the context of bioterrorism, aerosol release would be most likely. Incubation would be 3 to 5 days, and pneumonic presentation would include fever, fatigue, chills, headache, and malaise. Typically, a nonproductive cough would be seen with dyspnea and chest pain. A rash may appear. Respiratory failure may occur, requiring mechanical ventilation and straining resources, and systemic inflammatory response syndrome can develop. Diagnosis requires a high index of suspicion and may include serological tests and polymerase chain reaction techniques. Peribronchial cuffing may be seen on x-ray. A rapid, inexpensive diagnostic test would be desirable. Treatment in adults usually consists of parenteral streptomycin or gentamicin (Mitchell & Penn, 2005).

OTHER CONSIDERATIONS

Depending on the scope of an intentional release of a pathogenic microbe, a potentially larger epidemic of psychological and psychiatric disorders will quickly follow the infectious disease threat. Holloway, Norwood, Fullerton, Engel, and Ursano (1997) point out that a significant number of psychological factors can be associated with the use of biological agents. These include horror, anger, panic, magical thinking about microbes, fear of invisible agents, fear of contagion, attribution of arousal symptoms to infection, and others. A study of the adult survivors of the anthrax events of 2001 was conducted 1 year after they were infected. The authors concluded that the survivors of anthrax had continuing health problems and suffered from psychological distress from the bioterrorism-caused illness (Reissman, 2004). Clearly humans have deep-seated fear of infection and death. Mental health issues are receiving attention on both a local and national level. Resources are available for health care practitioners and the general public from the CDC Web site. The fear, panic, and dread can spread, perhaps even faster than the microbial threat, with hyperbolic media coverage (Smith, Veenhuis & Mc Cormack, 2000). Thus the provision of mental health services must be a priority, concomitant with provision of medical services (DiGiovanni, 1999).

Much of the work toward understanding the impact of microbiological agents has been conducted in military settings. The populations exposed and studied have most often been predominantly young adult males in good physical condition. In the case of a release of a pathogenic microbe in the general population, the entire population spectrum of a city or region might be affected. This would include subpopulations with special vulnerabilities or needs, and these populations must be considered in preparedness planning. Examples of these special populations include children; the frail elderly, whether at home or in a long-term care facility; and those individuals who are dependent on medical devices such as ventilators and portable oxygen devices. The American Academy of Pediatrics' Committee on Environmental Health and Infectious Diseases (2000) point out the special needs and concerns of the pediatric population with regard to exposure to chemical or biological terrorism. The standard public health model of primary prevention is of limited utility to the health care community as it relates to bioterrorism. Prevention of a bioterrorism act falls mostly into the purview of law enforcement and criminal intelligence and lies outside the realm of most nurses, physicians, and health officials. Therefore, prevention of as many cases of disease as possible in the face of an intentional release is a reasonable goal of bioterrorism response and preparedness planners. Kaufmann, Meltzer, and Schmid (1997) evaluated the economic impact of bioterrorist attacks using three different classic biological agents. The range was estimated at from $477.7 million per 100,000 persons for their brucellosis scenario, to $26.2 billion per 100,000 persons exposed to the anthrax bacillus. Their study, using an insurance analogy, clearly indicated that postattack prophylaxis and response is the single most important means of reducing the losses. Importantly, they suggest that the presence of a well-designed, implemented, and exercised response utilizing postattack prophylaxis may act as a deterrent to those who would execute such an attack for maximum impact.

BIOTERRORISM PREPAREDNESS AND RESPONSE

To prepare for a possible bioterrorist attack, hospitals, managed care organizations, federally qualified health centers, home health organizations, and other health care providers and/or agencies should participate in the bioterrorism preparedness activities in their community and state. Hospitals and other health care institutions must be prepared for the surge of patients as well as the "worried well patient." They will need to provide for medical and nursing care, security, possibly decontamination, and infection control.

Recommendations of a CDC Strategic Planning Workgroup on Biological and Chemical Terrorism Preparedness and Response (CDC, 2000a) provide excellent background information and a sound foundation for development of a national response capacity but do not provide direction at the local or facility level. Macintyre and associates (2000) point out that most health care facilities are poorly prepared to mount an effective response to the great influx of patients and their infections. The authors propose a concept of operation for civilian hospital settings that highlights prompt recognition, staff and facility protection, patient decontamination and triage, medical therapy, and external coordination with emergency response and public health agencies. The use of the Incident Command System and the National Incident Management System as tools for incident management is recommended.

The Association of Professionals in Infection Control and Epidemiology, Inc. (2000) has developed a bioterrorism readiness plan template for health care facilities that focuses on infection control and prophylaxis considerations in hospitals and other institutions. The plan fails, however, to detail the vital role infection control nurses play in the surveillance and reporting of communicable diseases. Timely detection and reporting of the first signals of an unusual (potentially intentionally caused) outbreak is crucial to the best possible response outcome (Institute of Medicine, 1999b).

Many of the nursing, medical, and public health aspects of bioterrorism preparedness and response are new to emergency response planners. Therefore, public health agencies are now being included in the planning process. This is a relatively new development and one that will benefit preparedness and response efforts. An additional partner in this effort is law enforcement. Acts of bioterrorism are considered criminal acts. Therefore, health care institutions must establish working relationships with law enforcement officials. It is vital that health care institutions work with their community partners at a state and local level to assure that an effective preparedness and response plan is developed for their institution and community. State agencies including, but not limited to, health departments and offices of emergency management are working with local health authorities in preparedness efforts including detecting and responding to an intentionally caused epidemic. In most cases, the office of the state epidemiologist will serve as a contact for information for each state's plan. The CDC has a 24-hour emergency phone number (770-488-1700) for information and assistance, but all callers should first contact their local and state health departments for direct assistance. Local law enforcement agencies have a similar communications procedure that ensures that the Federal Bureau of Investigation is notified of a potential crime. More information about the federal government's emergency response and preparedness can be found at www.bt.cdc.gov.

Nurses and other frontline health care providers have a variety of opportunities to participate in planning and preparing for a bioterrorist attack. It is commonly understood that a well-executed plan will not guarantee that all morbidity and mortality will be prevented, but it is guaranteed that many more will die in the absence of such a plan. One opportunity for health care providers to be prepared for a bioterror attack and to be of service to the community is the Medical Reserve Corps. Medical Reserve Corps are being established in local jurisdictions throughout the United States. These are state-initiated volunteer organizations of health professionals established to provide another resource for communities in the event of a bioterror attack. Drills and exercises are an important component of the preparedness and response efforts at every level and jurisdiction. TOPOFF is a national exercise program that has examined the response to a potential attack. For example, the TOPOFF 3 exercise in New Jersey in April 2005 used the release of weaponized *Y. pestis* with resulting pneumonic plague to test response systems in selected communities and hospitals. Nurses, physicians, and other health care providers should when possible participate in these activities. The lessons learned provide a framework for educational and logistical needs.

REFERENCES

Abramova, F. A., Grinberg, L. M., Yampolskaya, O. V., & Walker, D. H. (1993). Pathology of inhalational anthrax in 42 cases from the Sverdlovsk outbreak of 1979. *Proceedings of the National Academy of Sciences, USA, 90,* 2291–2294.

Alibek, K., & Handelman, S. (1999). *Biohazard.* New York: Random House.

American Academy of Pediatrics, Committee on Environmental Health and Committee on Infectious Diseases. (2000). Chemical-biological terrorism and its impact on children: A subject review. *Pediatrics, 105,* 662–670.

American Hospital Formulary Service. (2000). AHFS *drug information.* Bethesda, MD: American Society of Health System Pharmacists.

Association for Professionals in Infection Control and Epidemiology, Inc. (2000). *Bioterrorism readiness plan: A template for healthcare facilities.* Retrieved December 15, 2006, from http://www.apic.org/html/educ/readinow.html

Botulism, carrot juice—USA (Multistate) (02). (2006). *ProMED, 453,* unpaginated.

Brachman, P. S. (1980). Inhalation anthrax. *Annals of the New York Academy of Sciences, 353,* 83–93.

Butler, T., & Dennis, D. T. (2005). *Yersinia* species including plague. In G. L. Mandell, J. E. Bennett, & R. Dolin (Eds.), *Mandell, Douglas, and Bennett's principles and practice of infectious diseases* (6th ed., pp. 2691–2701). Philadelphia: Churchill Livingstone Elsevier.

Center for Nonproliferation Studies. (1999a). *Chronology of state use and biological and chemical weapons control. Chemical & Biological Weapons Resource.* Retrieved December 26, 2006, from http://cns.miis.edu/research/cbw/pastuse.htm

Center for Nonproliferation Studies (1999b). Iraq Nuclear Biological, Chemical and Missiles Capabilities Program. Retrieved December 27, 2006, from http://.cns.miis.edu/research/wmdme/iraq.htm

Centers for Disease Control. (1988). Human cutaneous anthrax—North Carolina, 1987. *Morbidity and Mortality Weekly Report, 37, (26).* Retrieved December 27, 2006, from http://www.cdc.gov/mmwr/preview/mmwrhtml/00001063.htm

Centers for Disease Control and Prevention. (1994a). Human plague—United States, 1993–1994. *Morbidity and Mortality Weekly Report, 43,* 242–246.

Centers for Disease Control and Prevention. (1994b). Update—Human plague India, 1994. *Morbidity and Mortality Weekly Report, 43*, 761–762.

Centers for Disease Control and Prevention. (1999). Bioterrorism alleging use of anthrax and interim guidelines for management—United States, 1998. *Morbidity and Mortality Weekly Report, 48*, 69–74.

Centers for Disease Control and Prevention. (2000a). Biological and chemical terrorism: Strategic plan for preparedness and response. Recommendations of the CDC Strategic Planning Workgroup. *Morbidity and Mortality Weekly Report, 49*(RR-4), 5–6.

Centers for Disease Control and Prevention. (2000b). Surveillance for adverse events associated with anthrax vaccination—U.S. Department of Defense, 1998–2000. *Morbidity and Mortality Weekly Report, 49*, 341–345.

Centers for Disease Control and Prevention. (2002). Notice to readers: Use of anthrax vaccine in response to terrorism: Supplemental recommendations of the Advisory Committee on Immunization Practices. *Morbidity and Mortality Weekly Report, 51(45)*. Retrieved December 27, 2006, from http://www.cdc.gov/mmwr/preview/mmwrhtml/mm5145a4.htm

Centers for Disease Control and Prevention. (2001a). *Potential agents of bioterror categories.* Retrieved August 24, 2006, from http://www.bt.cdc.gov/agent/agentlist-category.asp

Centers for Disease Control and Prevention. (2001b). Update. Investigation of anthrax associated with intentional exposure and interior health guidelines, October 2001. *Morbidity and Mortality Weekly Report, 50*, 889–893.

Centers for Disease Control and Prevention. (2001c). Update: Investigation of bioterrorism-related anthrax—Connecticut 2001. *Morbidity and Mortality Weekly Report, 50*, 1077–1079.

Centers for Disease Control and Prevention. (2002). Tularemia—United States, 1990–2000. *Morbidity and Mortality Weekly Report, 51*, 182–184.

Centers for Disease Control and Prevention. (2003). Smallpox vaccination and adverse reactions: Guidance for clinicians. *Morbidity and Mortality Weekly Report, 52*(RR-04), 1–28.

Centers for Disease Control and Prevention. (2005a, January 7). *Plague fact sheet.* Retrieved December 27, 2006, from http://www.cdc.gov/ncidod/dvbid/plague

Centers for Disease Control and Prevention. (2005b). Update adverse events following civilian smallpox vaccination United States, 2003. *Morbidity and Mortality Weekly Report 52(15)*. Retrieved December 27, 2006, from http://www.cdc.gov/mmwr/preview/mmwrhtml/mm521a5.htm

Centers for Disease Control and Prevention. (2006). Inhalation anthrax associated with dried animal hides—Pennsylvania and New York City, 2006. *Morbidity and Mortality Weekly Report, 55*, 280–282.

Christopher, G. W., Cieslak, T. J., Pavlin, J. A., & Eitzen, E. M. (1999). Biological warfare: A historical perspective. In J. Lederberg (Ed.), *Biological weapons: Limiting the threat* (pp. 18–19). Cambridge, MA: MIT Press.

Cohen, F. L., Hardin, S. B., Nehring, W., Keough, M. A., Laurenti, S., McNabb, J., et al. (1988). Physical and psychosocial health status 3 years after catastrophic illness—Botulism. *Issues in Mental Health Nursing, 9,* 387–398.

Cole, L. (1997). *The eleventh plague* (pp. 4–6). New York: W. H. Freeman.

Combating terrorism observations on biological terrorism and public health initiatives: Testimony before the Committee on Veterans Affairs and the Subcommittee on Labor, Health and Human Services, Education and Related Agencies, Committee on Appropriations, U.S. Senate, GAO/T-NSIAD- 99-112. (1999). (statement of Henry L. Hinton, Jr.).

Dennis, D., & Meier, F. (1997). Plague. In C. R. Horsburgh & A. M. Nelson (Eds.), *Pathology of emerging infections* (pp. 21–47). Washington, DC: American Society of Microbiology Press.

Dennis, D. T., & Mead, P. S. (2006). Plague. In R. L. Guerrant, D. H. Walker, & P. F. Weller (Eds.), *Tropical infectious diseases* (2nd ed., pp. 471–481). Philadelphia: Churchill Livingstone Elsevier.

DiGiovanni, C., Jr. (1999). Domestic terrorism with chemical or biological agents: Psychiatric aspects. *American Journal of Psychiatry, 156,* 1500–1505.

Dixon, T. C., Meselson, M., Guillemin, J., & Hanna, P. C. (1999). Medical progress: Anthrax. *New England Journal of Medicine, 341,* 815–826.

Eliasson, H., Broman, T., Forsman, M., & Bäck, E. (2006). Tularemia: Current epidemiology and disease management. *Infectious Disease Clinics of North America, 20,* 289–311.

Fainberg, A. (1997). Debating policy priorities and implications. In B. Roberts (Ed.), *Terrorism with chemical and biological weapons: Calibrating risks and responses* (pp. 75–94). Alexandria, VA: Chemical and Biological Arms Control Institute.

Feldman, K. A., Stiles-Enos, D., Julian, K., Matyas, B. T., Telford, S. R., III, Chu, M. C., et al. (2003). Tularemia on Martha's Vineyard: Seroprevalence and occupational risk. *Emerging Infectious Diseases, 9,* 350–354.

Fenner, F., Henderson, D. A., Arita, I., Jezel, Z., & Ladnyi, L. D. (1988). *Smallpox and its eradication* (p. 1460). Geneva, Switzerland: World Health Organization.

Franz, D. R., Jahrling, P. B., Friedlander, A. M., McClain, D. J., Hoover, D. L., Byrne, W. R., et al. (1997). Clinical recognition and management of patients exposed to biological warfare agents. *Journal of American Medical Association, 278,* 399–411.

Friedlander, A. M. (1997). Anthrax. In F. R. Sidell, E. T. Takafuji, & D. R. Franz (Eds.), *Medical aspects of chemical and biological warfare* (pp. 468–478). Washington, DC: Borden Institute.

Friedlander, A. M., Jr., & Longfield, R. N. (2000). Anthrax. In G. T. Strickland (Ed.), *Hunter's tropical medicine and emerging infectious diseases* (8th ed., pp. 384–388). Philadelphia: W. B. Saunders.

Hanna, P. C., Acosta, D., & Collier, R. J. (1993). On the role of macrophages in anthrax. *Proceedings of the National Academy of Sciences, USA, 90,* 10198–10201.

Hardin, S. B., & Cohen, F. L. (1988). Psychosocial effects of a catastrophic botulism outbreak. *Archives of Psychiatric Nursing, 2,* 173–184.

Harris, S. H. (1997). *Factories of death.* New York: Routledge.

Henderson, D. A., Inglesby, T. V., Bartlett, J. G., Ascher, M. S., Eitzen, E., Jahrling, P. B., et al. (2002). Smallpox as a biological weapon. In D. V. Henderson, T. V. Inglesby & T. O'Toole (Eds.) *Bioterrorism guidelines for medical and public health management.*

Heymann, D. (2004). Anthrax. In D. Heymann (Ed.), *Control of communicable diseases manual* (pp. 20–25). Washington, DC: American Public Health Association.

Holloway, H. C., Norwood, A. E., Fullerton, C. S., Engel, D., & Ursano, R. J. (1997). The threat of biological weapons: Prophylaxis and mitigation of psychological and social consequences. *Journal of the American Medical Association, 278,* 425–427.

Hughes, J. M. (1999). The emerging threat of bioterrorism. *Emerging Infectious Diseases, 5,* 494–495.

Inglesby, T. V., Dennis, D. T., Henderson, D. A., Bartlett, J. G., Ascher, M. S., Eitzen, E., et al. (2000). Plague as a biological weapon: Medical and public health management. *Journal of the American Medical Association, 283,* 2281–2295.

Inglesby, T. V., Henderson, D. A., Bartlett, J. G., Ascher, M. S., Eitzen, E., Jahrling, P. B., et al. (1999). Anthrax as a biological weapon: Medical and public health management. *Journal of the American Medical Association, 281,* 1735–1745.

Inglesby, T. V., O'Toole, T., Henderson, Bartlett, J. G., Eitzen, E., Friedlander, A. J., et al. (2002). Anthrax as a biological weapon updated recommendations for management. In D. Henderson, T. Inglesby, & T. O'Toole (Eds.), *Bioterrorism: Guidelines for medical and public health management* (pp. 63–97). Chicago: AMA.

Institute of Medicine. (1999a). *Assessment of future scientific needs for live variola virus* (pp. 20–86). Washington, DC: National Academy Press.

Institute of Medicine. (1999b). *Chemical and biological terrorism. Research and development to improve civilian medical response* (pp. 65–77). Washington, DC: National Academy Press.

Jernigan, J. A., Stephens, D. S., Ashford, D. A., Omenaca, C., Topiel, M. S., Galbraith, M., et al. (2001). Bioterrorism-related inhalational anthrax: The first 10 cases reported in the United States. *Emerging Infectious Diseases, 7,* 993–944.

Kaufmann, A. F., Meltzer, M. I., & Schmid, G. P. (1997). The economic impact of a bioterrorist attack. Are prevention and post-attack intervention programs justifiable? *Emerging Infectious Diseases, 3,* 83–94.

LeDuc, J. W., & Jahrling, P. B. (2001). Strengthening national preparedness for smallpox: An update. *Emerging Infectious Diseases, 7,* 155–157.

Lucey, D. (2005). Anthrax. In G. L. Mandell, J. E. Bennett & R. Dolin (Eds.), *Principles and practice of infectious diseases* (6th ed., pp. 3618–3623). Elsevier Churchill Livingstone.

Macintyre, A. G., Christopher, G. W., Eitzen, E., Gum, R., Weir, S., DeAtley, C., et al. (2000). Weapons of mass destruction events with contaminated casualties: Effective planning for health care facilities. *Journal of the American Medical Association, 283,* 242–249.

McClain, D. J. (1997). Smallpox. In F. R. Sidell, E. T. Takafuji, & D. R. Franz (Eds.), *Medical aspects of chemical and biological warfare* (pp. 543–548). Washington, DC: Borden Institute.

McDade, J. E., & Franz, D. (1998). Bioterrorism as a public health threat. *Emerging Infectious Diseases, 4,* 493–494.

McGovern, T. W., & Friedlander, A. M. (1997). Plague. In F. R. Sidell, E. T. Takafuji, & D. R. Franz (Eds.), *Medical aspects of chemical and biological warfare* (pp. 479–502). Washington, DC: Borden Institute.

McLendon, M. K., Apicella, M. A., & Allen, L.-A. H. (2006). *Francisella tularensis*: Taxonomy, genetics, and immunopathogenesis of a potential agent of biowarfare. *Annual Review of Microbiology, 60,* 167–185.

Meselson, M., Guillemin, J., Hugh-Jones, M., Langmuir, A., Popova, I., Shelokov, A., et al. (1994). The Sverdlovsk anthrax outbreak of 1979. *Science, 26*(6), 1202–1208.

Mitchell, C. L., & Penn, R. L. (2005). *Francisella tularensis* (tularemia) as an agent of bioterrorism. In G. L. Mandell, J. E. Bennett, & R. Dolin (Eds), *Mandell, Douglas, and Bennett's principles and practice of infectious diseases* (6th ed., pp. 3607–3612). Philadelphia: Churchill Livingstone Elsevier.

Mitra, A. C., Sarkar, J. K., & Mukherjee, M. K. (1974). Virus content of smallpox scabs. *Bulletin of the World Health Organization, 51,* 106–107.

Moore, Z. S., Seward, J. F., & Lane, J. M. (2006). Smallpox. *Lancet, 367,* 425–435.

Olsen, K. B. (1995). Overview: Recent incidents and responder implications. In *Proceedings of the seminar on responding to the consequences of chemical and biological terrorism* (No. 1996-416-003, pp. 2.36–2.93). Washington, DC: U.S. Government Printing Office.

O'Neill, J. P. (1995). Terrorism briefing. In *Proceedings of the seminar on responding to the consequences of chemical and biological terrorism* (No. 1996-416-003, pp. 1.20–1.23), Washington, DC: U.S. Government Printing Office.

Osterholm, M. T. (1999). Bioterrorism: Media hype or real potential nightmare? *American Journal of Infection Control, 27,* 461–462.

Osterholm, M. T., & Schwartz, J. (2000). *Living terrors* (pp. 113–117). New York: Delacorte Press.

Perrotta, D. M., Rawlings, J., & Eckman, M. (1998). The specter of chemical and biological terrorism. *Disease Prevention News, 58*(8), 1–6.

Perry, R. D., & Featherston, J. D. (1997). *Yersinia pestis*—Etiologic agent of plague. *Clinical Microbiology Reviews, 10,* 35–66.

Ratsitorahina, M., Chanteau, S., Rahalison, L., Ratisofaoamanana, L., & Boisier, P. (2000). Epidemiological and diagnostic aspects of the outbreak of pneumonia plague in Madagascar. *Lancet, 355,* 111–113.

Reissman, D. B., Whitney, E. A., Taylor, T. H. Jr., Hayslett, J. A., Dull, P. M., Arias, I. et al. (2004). One-year health assessment of adult survivors of

Bacillus anthracis infection. *Journal of the American Medical Association, 291*, 1994–1998.

Roblot, F., Popoff, M., Carlier, J. P., Godet, C., Abbadie, P., Matthis, S., et al. (2006). Botulism in patients who inhale cocaine: The first cases in France. *Clinical Infectious Diseases, 43*, e51–e52.

Roush, S., Birkhead, G., Koo, D., Cobb, A., & Fleming, D. (1999). Mandatory reporting of diseases and conditions by health care professionals and laboratories. *Journal of the American Medical Association, 282*, 164–170.

Sarkar, J. K., Mitra, A. C., Mukherjee, M. K., & De, S. K. (1973). Virus excretion in smallpox. 2. Excretion in the throat of household contacts. *Bulletin of the World Health Organization, 48*, 523–527.

Sellman, B. R., Mourez, M., & Collier, R. J. (2001). Dominant-negative mutants of a toxin subunit: An approach to therapy of anthrax. *Science, 292*, 695–697.

Sidell, F. R., Takafuji, E. T., & Franz, D. R. (Eds.). (1997). *Medical aspects of chemical and biological warfare*. Washington, DC: Borden Institute.

Simon, J. D. (1999). Biological terrorism: Preparing to meet the threat. In J. Lederberg (Ed.), *Biological weapons: Limiting the threat* (p. 238). Cambridge, MA: MIT Press.

Sobel, J. (2005). Botulism. *Clinical Infectious Diseases, 41*, 1167–1173.

Smith, C. G., Veenhuis, P. E., & McCormack, J. N. (2000). Bioterrorism: A new threat with psychological and social sequelae. *North Carolina Medical Journal, 6*(3) 150–165.

Swartz, M. N. (2001). Recognition and management of anthrax—An update. *New England Journal of Medicine, 345*, 1621–1626.

Taylor, J. P., Dimmitt, D. C., Ezzell, J. W., & Whitford, H. (1993). Indigenous human cutaneous anthrax in Texas. *Southern Medical Journal, 86*(1), 1–4.

Török, T. J., Tauxe, R. V., Wise, R. P., Livengood, J. R., Sokolow, R., Mauvais, S., et al. (1997). A large community outbreak of salmonellosis caused by intentional contamination of restaurant salad bars. *Journal of American Medical Association, 278*, 389–398.

Tucker, J. B. (1999). Bioterrorism: Threats and responses. In J. Lederberg (Ed.), *Biological weapons: Limiting the threat* (pp. 283–285). Cambridge, MA: MIT Press.

U.S. General Accounting Office. (1999). *Combating terrorism: Need for comprehensive threat and risk assessments of chemical and biological attacks* (GAO/NSIAD-99-163). Washington, DC: U.S. Government Printing Office.

Villar, R. G., Elliott, S. P., & Davenport, K. M. (2006). Botulism: The many faces of botulinum toxin and its potential for bioterrorism. *Infectious Disease Clinics of North America, 20*, 313–327.

Walker, D. H. (2006). Anthrax. In R. L. Guerrant, D. H. Walker, & P. F. Weller (Eds.), *Tropical infectious diseases* (2nd ed., pp. 448–453). Philadelphia: Churchill Livingstone Elsevier.

CHAPTER TWENTY-EIGHT

Behavioral and Cultural Aspects of Transmission and Infection

Barbara Jeanne Fahey

A transmissible emerging or re-emerging infectious disease can occur at any given location with potential to spread rapidly through portals such as travel, trade, environmental conditions, migratory activity, and socio-political–economic activity. There is an exquisite interrelationship of behavior and culture with both acquisition and spread of emerging and reemerging infectious diseases. The emergence and resurgence of infectious diseases is the culmination of multiple inter-connecting factors—often influenced by human behavior and cultural activity (Andrews & Boule, 1999).

Human behavior and cultural practices contribute to the likelihood of acquisition of many, but not all, emerging and re-emerging infectious diseases. Behavior is the process of persons acting or doing something in a certain way—the action, reaction, or response of persons under specified circumstances. Behavior contributes to the formation and ongoing evolution of culture. Culture, reflecting the standard features of everyday life, is "the integrated pattern of human knowledge, belief, and behavior that depends upon the capacity for learning and transmitting knowledge to succeeding generations" (Merriam-Webster OnLine Dictionary).

The purpose of this chapter is to supplement information provided throughout this book and to highlight areas of human behavior and culture that provide considerable influence on emerging and re-emerging disease transmission. This chapter will focus on those topic areas most directly affected by behavioral or cultural practices, including sexual behavior, antibiotic utilization, hygienic practices, travel, nutritional behavior, breast-feeding, immunization behavior, threat of bioterrorism, and other selected behavioral or cultural considerations. Topic areas not addressed in detail are availability of potable water, medical and microbiological technological advances, increasing sensitivity of detection systems, reallocation of funds away from public health and sanitation, deterioration of public health infrastructure, population growth, increased life expectancy, and the shift to an older age composition of the world population.

SEXUAL BEHAVIORS

Sexual behaviors are integral to the perpetuation of sexually transmitted diseases (STDs). The sexual urges that influence sexual behaviors can be quite strong; thus, modifying sexual behavior is difficult not only to discuss but also to effect change and then to sustain changes. Sexual behavior is influenced by multiple interacting behavioral and societal factors, including hormones, emotions, desire to procreate, cultural and family traditions, personal belief systems, religion, financial need or desire, and curiosity. While the practice of abstinence and/or the modification of sexual behavior can substantially reduce the toll of STDs, the morbidity and mortality attributable to sexual behavior are an ongoing concern to health officials worldwide. The STD pandemic shows no signs of slowing. Building an international consensus about appropriate interventions to reduce STD risk and transmission is a daunting task, due in great measure to the diversity and idiosyncrasy of human behavioral, societal, and cultural traditions. Thus, the design, implementation, social acceptance, continuation, and acceptance of activities to reduce transmission of STDs are far from straightforward (Lashley, 2006).

Sexual activity, voluntary and involuntary, is associated with transmission of numerous emerging and reemerging STDs, such as human immunodeficiency virus (HIV), hepatitis B, gonococcal infections, syphilis, and chlamydia (Centers for Disease Control and Prevention [CDC] 1999a, 2001a, 2003b, 2005a). The most common route for HIV transmission remains sexual. In sub-Saharan Africa and other developing countries, HIV transmission occurs primarily through heterosexual contact. The acquired immunodeficiency syndrome (AIDS) pandemic global epicenter remains Africa, especially South Africa, where the 2004 infection rate among pregnant women attending public antenatal clinics was almost one in three. The global numbers for HIV infection remain staggering. At the end of 2005, the Joint United Nations Programme on HIV/AIDS

(UNAIDS, 2006) reported an estimated 38.6 million persons worldwide living with HIV (the majority of these in developing nations). Of these 38.6 million, 4.1 million were new infections, and 2.8 million deaths occurred due to HIV infection. Social instability may encourage sexual activity with multiple partners as migrant workers, refugees, and women resort to prostitution to feed and clothe themselves. Cultural practices may promote sex with multiple partners because in some parts of the world sexual relations with multiple sex partners is considered normal activity. Superstitions also may foster sexual relations with multiple partners; in some areas, intercourse with a virgin is believed to cure an HIV infection (Bartholet, 2000). Other factors that influence the sexual transmission of HIV and other STDs include little or no condom use, low circumcision rates, low literacy rates, religious beliefs, and women's lack of control over the circumstances or safety of sex.

Strategies to address these behavioral and cultural issues are complex, difficult to design, hard to implement, and challenging to sustain. Effective education must be culturally sensitive, presented in native language, readily available to the entire population in the targeted area, and adaptable to different ages. Work to improve social and political problems is dependent on the constructive interactions of entire communities; these constructive interactions can be hard to start and even harder to maintain. Accessibility to health care, medicine, and safe sex barrier supplies must be insured. Infrastructures to provide education and health care need to be developed and sustained. Currently, many parts of the world have inadequate resources for education, are struggling to maintain the local economy, and have inadequate resources to assure access to health care, medicines, and contraceptives.

Despite formidable challenges, UNAIDS (2006) reports positive progress from 126 reporting countries: treatment access expansion (from 240,00 in 2001 to about 1.3 million receiving antiretroviral therapy in low- and middle-income countries); exponential growth in persons using HIV testing and counseling services (more than 70 countries surveyed with growth from about 4 million in 2001 to 16.5 million persons in 2005); a decline in persons having sex before 15 years of age and increased condom use in 8 of 11 sub-Saharan countries; an HIV prevalence decline of 25% or more among 15–24 year olds in capital cities from 6 of 11 African countries with high HIV rates; and increasing coverage of HIV-positive women receiving antiretroviral prophylaxis (up to nearly 60% in some countries). Thus, STD rate reduction via behavioral and cultural practice changes is possible and sustainable (Nelson et al., 1996).

However, in the U.S., although there is an apparent trending towards incidence reduction, from 2001–2004 HIV/AIDS cases have increased among men who have sex with men. Men having sex with men and persons exposed through heterosexual contact accounted for 80% of all HIV/AIDS cases diagnosed in 2004 (CDC 2005a). Whereas the global HIV incidence rate is believed stabilized since the late 1990s, UNAIDS (2006) reports that Bangladesh and Pakistan display signs of HIV outbreaks, and increasing prevalence is noted in China, Indonesia, Papua New Guinea, and Vietnam. There remains pervasive stigma and bias against HIV-positive persons; adequate care and support is wanting for the 15 million AIDS orphan children; and many countries acknowledge policies that interfere with HIV prevention and care measures.

Inroads made with HIV do not necessarily translate to inroads for associated STDs. For example, the trend of HIV transmission reduction among homosexual populations in San Francisco during the late 1980s and early 1990s experienced reversal during the late 1990s, ostensibly associated with a younger homosexual generation that had not experienced firsthand the consequences of HIV infection and thus did not have strong motivation to practice safer sex. A limitation to this finding is that many of the men had longstanding HIV infection before the diagnosis of syphilis (CDC, 2004a). In addition, extreme economic debt and political problems in developing countries impede economic development necessary to stem the STD epidemic. Behavioral approaches to lower STD rates include providing access to, offering education about, and validating proper use of safer sex practices. This approach is dependent upon multiple critical factors, such as adequate sustained financial resources, stable health program infrastructure, and ongoing support from political, religious, and public sources. Learning new patterns of behavior, effectively applying them in culturally appropriate settings, and sustaining them are key to STD transmission management. Integration of knowledge about individual and group dynamics into better STD outcomes will continue to depend on the ability of each community to identify and engage the specific issues germane to its own individual culture or society that contribute to transmission of STDs. Reducing and maintaining reduction of STD transmission is an international public health concern and is slated to remain a high priority for public health program funding and development.

ANTIBIOTIC USE

Chapter 2 provides an excellent summary of the current state of antimicrobial resistance. The current armamentarium of antibiotics continues to become increasingly less effective as a tool to combat infectious diseases; thus, there is an increasing opportunity for the occurrence and transmission of antibiotic resistant new and reemerging diseases (CDC, 2006f). Human behaviors contribute much to antimicrobial resistance.

These include antimicrobial use in agriculture, aquaculture, and animal husbandry; disincentives for pharmaceutical intensive antibacterial research; antimicrobial continued abuse, overuse, and misuse; counterfeit dispensing; treatment guidelines not followed by prescriber or patient; misinformation; economic hardship; employer pressure; inadequate antibiotic supply; lack of access to antibiotics; misdiagnosis; consumption of expired or bogus antibiotics; and pharmaceutical marketing campaigns (Avorn & Solomon, 2000; Cohen & Tartasky, 1997; World Health Organization [WHO], 2000).

Until the early 1990s, the consequences of emerging drug resistance were largely dismissed because new drugs were on the market or in the pharmaceutical pipeline that countered developing resistance. For example, international dissemination of ampicillin-resistant gonococci quickly occurred after initial identification in Thailand and the Philippines. New cephalosporins and beta-lactamase inhibitors were available and provided a "quick fix," and apparently little thought was given to the likelihood that resistance evolution would be ongoing and that the new medication pool might dry up (Brown, Warnnissorn, Biddle, Panikabutra, & Traisupa, 1982). The quick fix approach delayed, but did not prevent, the current situation of increasing resistance and fewer treatment options.

As of 2000, worldwide, about half of all produced antibiotics were used to treat animals, to treat cultivated foodstuffs, and to provide livestock growth promoters (WHO, 2000). One outcome of livestock therapy, prophylaxis, or growth dosing has been the development of bacterial resistance that is transmitted among species. Vancomycin-resistant *Enterococcus* (VRE) *faecium* is the benchmark example of resistant bacteria appearance in livestock with subsequent identification among humans. Widespread use of avoparcin in animals (equivalent to vancomycin in humans) was causally associated with selective pressure that resulted in VRE emergence in livestock.

Research has established a causal link between antibiotic use in animals and agriculture and development of antibiotic-resistant strains of *Salmonella, Campylobacter,* and *Escherichia coli* (U.S. Government Accountability Office [GAO], 1999). *Salmonella* is often found in poultry, eggs, and beef; up to 4 million infections occur each year in the United States. One particular strain, *Salmonella* DT104, is resistant to ampicillin, chloramphenicol, streptomycin, sulfonamides, and tetracycline. Human disease was first reported in the mid-1980s in the United Kingdom, and as of the late 1990s, the United States estimated about 340,000 cases each year. In 1993, England began to use fluoroquinolones to treat poultry; by 1996 the United Kingdom reported that 14% of the *Salmonella* DT104 strains were resistant to fluoroquinolones. The United States approved fluoroquinolones for agricultural and husbandry use in 1995.

Fluoroquinolone-decreased susceptibility is currently rare, but the threat of increasing resistance is real (GAO, 1999).

Campylobacter spp. are often found in poultry, pork, and beef; up to 4 million infections occur each year in the United States (Gupta et al., 2004). In Australia, where fluoroquinolones have never been approved for use in agriculture and husbandry, there are only rare case reports of fluoroquinolone-resistant Campylobacter infection in humans (Unicomb, Ferguson, Riley, & Collignon, 2003). In contrast, shortly after 1995, when the FDA approved fluoroquinolones for use in poultry, the first human case of fluoroquinolone-resistant Campylobacter was identified. Prior to the use of fluoroquinolones in animals, the WHO determined that human resistance had not occurred among persons with no previous exposure to this group of antibiotics. This story is strongly suggestive of direct animal-to-human transmission of Campylobacter fluoroquinolone-resistant strains (GAO, 1999). And concern is growing.

Corrective regulatory measures are under way—albeit much more in developed than in developing nations. The American Veterinary Medical Association advocates integration of four behavioral principles: emphasize hygiene, routine health examinations, and immunization as preferential to rampant antibiotic use; consider therapeutic alternatives for antibiotics; avoid or prudently use antibiotics important in treating human disease (e.g., fluoroquinolones); and avoid inappropriate use of antibiotics (GAO, 1999). The use of antibiotics to promote growth in animal feeds has been banned in some countries. Avoparcin, a widely used animal antibiotic mixed in feed to promote animal growth, was removed from the European market in 1999 (Kopecny, 1999). In the United States, the National Milk Producers Federation and the National Pork Producers Council provide quality assurance programs that instruct on prudent antibiotic use; the National Broiler Council reports thoughtful antibiotic use by poultry producers—one company, Tyson, discontinued antibiotic use to promote animal growth in the mid-1990s (GAO, 1999). Antibiotic residue on produce can promote development of resistance among normal gastrointestinal flora once the coated produce is ingested. In the event that resistant strains do develop, the strains are likely to colonize the gastrointestinal tract. Washing raw fruit and vegetables—a long-standing common sense food preparation practice—is a simple and probably effective technique to remove both antibiotic residues. Despite this ongoing and growing momentum to modify behaviors in agriculture and husbandry, the threat remains (Garau et al., 1999; Prats et al., 2000).

Antibiotic resistance in humans is influenced by economic hardship, misinformation, legal or illegal refugee traffic, as well as other factors. It is not unusual in developing countries for consumers to purchase single medication doses and for consumers to discontinue medication as soon as there is symptom relief (WHO, 2000). In Vietnam, findings from a 1997 study suggested that fully 70% of antimicrobial prescriptions for serious infections were inadequate in quantity and about 25% of antimicrobial prescriptions were considered not necessary. Fully 63% of antimicrobials prescribed in China for confirmed bacterial infections were the wrong choice. Antibiotic overprescription of about 50% was estimated among physicians in the United States and Canada (WHO, 2000).

Drug resistance has been a substantial problem with management of tuberculosis (TB), a reemerging infectious disease (see chapter 20) (CDC, 1992). The persistence of TB and the development of not only multidrug-resistance but also extensive drug resistance is related to drug availability and distribution in developing countries, the choice of regimen based on susceptibility of the organism, whether or not the person has HIV infection, adherence (or lack thereof) to the regimen, and other factors. Issues of reliable drug availability and sustained distribution are ongoing—global health agencies and governing bodies struggle continuously to design, implement, and successfully complete programs. Strategies to promote therapy adherence have included directly observed therapy (DOT), DOT-Plus frameworks for treatment, as well as Stop TB strategies for low- and middle-income countries (CDC, 2006f). These mechanisms are difficult to practice on an international scale and in developing regions of the world and regions impacted by natural disaster, civil unrest, and impoverished public health infrastructures. Nonetheless, experience demonstrates that TB incidence and transmission can be reduced through behavioral and/or practice changes.

TB incidence rates in the United States are now at the lowest rates since national recording began in 1953, although TB rates higher than average continue to be reported in certain racial and ethnic populations (CDC, 1994; CDC, 2005b; CDC, 2005c). A national action plan has been published (CDC, 2005c). The successful TB control program implemented in the United States may be difficult to replicate in all parts of the world (CDC, 2005d). Special consideration has been directed to TB management in correctional and detention facilities, which are noted for relatively high rates of TB and high risk for TB transmission. Behavioral factors that contribute to the relatively high rate include movement of inmates into and out of overcrowded and poorly ventilated facilities, nonreceipt of routine nonemergency medical care before incarceration (e.g., purified protein derivative testing), and incomplete TB contact exposure investigations. The CDC has published recommendations that provide guidelines and a framework to enable effective and sustained prevention and control of TB in these types of facilities (CDC, 2006d).

Excessive antibiotic use is associated with development of antibiotic resistance. In developed countries, a prescription is needed for many antibiotics. Whereas this screening filter should promote judicious antibiotic utilization, the mechanism guarantees neither proper ordering nor proper use. Patients who present to their physician with symptoms tend to expect a prescription, usually for antibiotics, and, if not automatically offered a prescription, tend to request one for antibiotics. This behavior is not rooted in clinical data but rather has long-standing psychosocial and cultural ties (Bell, Kravitz, & Wilkes, 1999; Wilson, Crane, Barrett, & Gonzales, 1999). By readily yielding to this ready fallback, a prescriber achieves benefits such as a rapid office visit, increased office productivity, and a decrease in costs and work time associated with diagnostic testing.

Antibiotics misuse is rampant in hospitals as well as in communities. Stepping into the 21st century, pediatricians continue to report that parents usually expect their child to receive antibiotics, even when not clinically indicated (e.g., to treat upper respiratory viral infections; Stivers, 2002). And misuse is evident in the outpatient setting. A cohort study of outpatient vancomycin use for 297 patients was conducted from 1997 through 2002. Centers for Disease Control and Prevention recommendations were published and distributed, and adherence to these was encouraged (CDC, 1995; Fraser, Stoser, Wang, Allen, & Zembower, 2005). Noncompliance occurred for about 50% of the outpatients, related to prolonged empiric therapy, dosing convenience, and prolonged use after surgery; compliance with recommendations was associated with attempting a microbiologic diagnosis. Current estimates are that each year 1 in 1,000 U.S. patients receives outpatient antibiotic parenteral therapy—this, plus ongoing trends for ever-shorter hospital stays, provides impetus for critical assessment of convenience, cost, and dosing considerations for outpatient parenteral antibiotic therapy (Tice et al., 2004).

A behavior of repeated use of antibiotics, over time, can predispose skin flora and gastrointestinal flora to develop antibiotic resistance. In developing countries, many antibiotics marketed by prescription are available over the counter, increasing the likelihood of antibiotic misuse and the potential for resistance. Misinformation also is a factor. For example, in the Philippines, isoniazid is considered by many to be the equivalent of a vitamin for the pulmonary system, and children often receive this "vitamin." This ongoing subtherapeutic, nonclinically indicated dosing provides selective pressure driving toward antibiotic resistance (WHO, 2000).

There is an ongoing consumer demand for household cleaners and hygiene products that have antibacterial ingredients. Triclosan is a common ingredient in many of these products; some laboratory data suggest a link between exposure to triclosan and other triclosan-related antibacterial ingredients and development of antimicrobial resistance by bacteria (Aiello & Larson, 2003; Levy, 2001). Aiello et al. (2005) conducted a study to examine whether use of antibacterial cleaning products resulted in carriage of antimicrobial-resistant organisms on hands. But the 1-year study did not show a significant increase in antimicrobial resistance. Given the ongoing consumer demand for antibacterial household and hygiene products, further study is indicated on this topic, including study of longer term use of these products and bacterial antibiotic resistance trends among household members.

As with other dimensions of human behavior influencing antibiotic resistance, data demonstrate that the behavior of excessive antibiotic use can be modified. For example, during the late 1980s, Finnish public health officials noted an increase in erythromycin resistance among Group A streptococcal isolates (Seppala et al., 1997). In 1991, to stem the trend, national guidelines were issued that were intended to reduce the use of macrolides in the treatment of respiratory and skin infections. Within a year's time, macrolide use had decreased more than 40%, and significant declines in erythromycin resistance among Group A streptococcal isolates occurred in Finland. A more modest intervention occurred during a 1999 cholera outbreak in Madagascar. The Ministry of Defense erected extensive roadblocks and required all travelers to take oral antibiotics; nonselective antibiotic administration to those without cholera increased selective pressure for antibiotic resistance. The Ministry of Defense subsequently modified the control program such that only travelers reporting diarrhea were given antibiotics (Markon, 2000).

In order to enlist community and health care partnership in reduction of antibiotic resistance, the CDC has launched a multifaceted Campaign to Prevent Antimicrobial Resistance, especially in health care settings. Strategies focus on transmission prevention, prudent antimicrobial selection and use, infection prevention, and tips on infection diagnosis and treatment. Information about this program can be accessed at the CDC's Web site at http://www.cdc.gov/drugresistance/healthcare/default.htm.

HYGIENIC BEHAVIOR: COMMUNITY SETTINGS

Hygienic behaviors (including poor personal hygiene, poor food preparation techniques, and inadequate occupational and environmental hygiene) have been associated with emerging and reemerging disease transmission in the community and home (Scott, 1999). Inadequate hygienic practices have been associated with reemerging foodborne and waterborne transmission of such infections as cholera, E. coli O157:H7 (see chapters 4 and 9), viral gastroenteritis, zoonoses, and hemorrhagic fevers (see chapter 8).

The importance of inadequate hygienic behaviors in the occurrence of reemerging infectious diseases is demonstrated in the African experience with cholera. In Madagascar, only one in three people has access to clean water; only 3% have access to flush toilets; and money is usually not available to purchase charcoal to boil water, a critical step in preventing cholera (Markon, 2000). Poor hygiene, contaminated water, or contaminated soil clinging to vegetables can be vectors for cholera transmission. Effective control measures include public health campaigns that recommend good hygiene, hand washing, boiling water, and sprinkling chlorine in shallow wells. Worldwide, fully one sixth of the world's population—about 1.1 billion persons—lack access to clean water, and even more—about 2.6 billion—do not have access to adequate sanitary facilities (Hughes & Koplan, 2005). Effective strategies include funding to institute and then sustain the control measures and also public health campaigns that promote personal hygiene, hand hygiene, boiling water, clean food preparation areas, and sprinkling chlorine in shallow wells.

Inadequate hygienic practices have also been associated with transmission of Ebola hemorrhagic fever (EHF), an emerging disease first recognized in 1976 (Peters & LeDuc, 1999; see chapter 8). Current theory is that the index patient of an outbreak becomes infected through contact with an infected animal. Other people then become exposed by direct contact with the blood and/or other potentially infectious fluids of the infected person. Thus, the virus readily spreads through families and friends of the infected person because close contact and accidental exposure to infectious fluids is likely to occur while feeding, holding, caring for, or otherwise assisting the infected person and during postmortem body care (Kerstiens & Matthys, 1999). Ebola hemorrhagic fever transmission can occur readily in the community in the absence or use of barrier equipment and hand washing. The exposure among health care workers who do not use personal protective equipment would thus be akin to household exposure with ensuing risk for EHF transmission. For example, in the Kikwit, Democratic Republic of the Congo, EHF outbreak in 1995, before control measures were begun, 67 health care workers became infected with EHF. After interventions were started, only three health care workers developed EHF, and no infections occurred among staff involved with body burial (Kerstiens & Matthys, 1999). Upon initiation of control measures (provision of protective equipment, antiseptics, and barrier-nursing technique training), EHF transmission to health care workers was reduced dramatically during EHF outbreaks (Guimard et al., 1999). Difficulties encountered in maintenance of healthful hygienic practices include limited access to potable water, adequate plumbing facilities, population migration to refugee camps, crowding, and disruption of goods and supplies due to civil unrest, war, or economic hardship. One innovative approach to promoting improved community hygiene is a recently launched Web site (http://www.ifh-homehygiene.org) where the International Scientific Forum on Home Hygiene has provided comprehensive guidelines for the prevention of infection in the domestic environment.

Community hygiene practices can contribute significantly to both increased and decreased transmission risk for emerging respiratory pathogens. The Hong Kong severe acute respiratory syndrome (SARS) experience during 2003, as compared to Hong Kong respiratory virus activity during 1998–2002, serves as a good example (Lo et al., 2005). The etiologic agent for SARS is a coronavirus with transmission including infectious droplet direct contact with mucous membranes and contact with contaminated fomites. During the 2003 SARS outbreak, there were multiple cultural and behavioral changes—various public places were closed, social activities were truncated, schools were suspended, and a majority of the population reported wearing a mask, using soap for hand hygiene, covering the mouth when coughing or sneezing, and washing hands after contact with possibly contaminated fomites (Leisure and Cultural Services Department, 2003). Data from the Government Virus Unit was used in order to ascertain whether these changes impacted overall respiratory virus occurrence. The proportion of positive specimens (PPS) of respiratory viruses from each month of 2003 was compared to the proportion of PPS from 1998 through 2002. A marked decrease in PPS was noted during March to July 2003 compared to the 1998–2002 PPS for influenza virus, parainfluenza virus, respiratory syncytial virus, and adenovirus. This time frame in 2003 corresponded to the interval of most rigorous control measures. Since August 2003, with a decrease in control measures and conclusion of SARS outbreak, there has been an increase in PPS similar to the rate observed during 1998–2002. The observed effects likely were real, as suggested by similar changes not being observed in hepatitis B rates (the transmission route being different than that of SARS and respiratory viruses) and by the effect remaining apparent after controlling for differences in patients' age groups. The take-home message of this observational study is that aggressive population-based behavioral changes can influence and contribute to reduction in transmission of viral respiratory infections (Lau, Yang, Tsui, & Kim, 2005; World Health Assembly, 2003).

Hygienic practices are important to the overall health and health promotion for each individual in the home or community. Personal, family, community, political, religious, and cultural practices influence the type of hygienic practices that are used. Access to usable water, cleaning supplies, and waste disposal systems are also important components of hygienic practices. On a global scale, education is ongoing with increasing attention to culturally and linguistically diverse populations about the chain of infection (host to susceptible host via route of transmission) and the value of hygienic practices to reduce the risk for disease transmission. On an international level, strategies are continuously explored and implemented to assist communities that do not have potable water and access to cleaning supplies.

HYGIENIC BEHAVIOR: HEALTH CARE SETTINGS

Hygienic behavior in the health care setting includes environmental cleaning, hand hygiene, and use of Standard Precautions. A premise is that improvement in hygienic behavior will lead to reduction of CDC estimates that each year nearly 2 million U.S. patients develop infections while in a hospital, with an attributable mortality number of about 90,000 (National Nosocomial Infections Surveillance, 2004; Weinstein, 2001). Environmental surfaces (i.e., floors, walls, furniture, beds, medical equipment) can become contaminated from infected, transiently colonized, or chronically colonized patients, visitors, health care personnel, or pet therapy animals. A contaminated environment can become a source for emerging infectious disease agents, such as vancomycin-resistant enterococci. A study of health clinics in the United Republic of Tanzania provides an interesting example—40% of presumed sterile reusable needles and syringes were contaminated with bacteria; the source of the contamination was not clear, and the variable of a contaminated environment could have been contributory (WHO, 2000). Regularly conducted fomite disinfection, soil removal, and waste removal are necessary to reduce the likelihood of organism transmission from the health care environment (CDC, 2003c). Although sanitizing or disinfecting agents can be used, less expensive nongermicidal cleaning agents are usually sufficient for routine cleaning and are less likely to cause chemical sensitivity reactions. The gold standard is to select the Environmental Protection Agency's registered disinfectants and use them in accordance with the manufacturers' recommendations. The selection of cleaning products should be carefully considered, and decisions should be congruent with public health recommendations (Favero & Bond, 2001; Information Required in a Premarket Notification Submission, 2006; Medical Devices: Adequate Directions for Use, 2006). Health care settings should have written procedures for environmental cleaning that emphasize practices to suppress dust, dirt, and aerosolization (e.g., vacuum cleaners should include exhaust filters). Spill cleanup procedures should specify use of protective barriers to protect staff from exposure to the spill and use of disinfectants that inactivate bloodborne pathogens, for example, a dilute hypochlorite sodium (bleach) solution or a quaternary ammonium compound.

Hand hygiene is the single most important means of preventing the spread of emerging and reemerging infectious diseases and infection in general (Garner & Favero, 1985); the importance of hand hygiene is such that in 2006 the Joint Commission on Accreditation of Healthcare Organizations (JCAHO) established hand hygiene programs as a mandatory standard and elevated the visibility of hand hygiene to the level of a JCAHO National Patient Safety Goal (JCAHO, 2006). The behavior of good hand hygiene reduces carriage of transient flora and thus reduces risk for organism transmission. A causal association between hand hygiene and reduced infection transmission, morbidity, and mortality related to hospital-acquired infections is well established, beginning more than 150 years ago with the eloquent work of Semmelweis (Wiese, 1930) and continuing through ongoing case reports and observational, microbiologic, and epidemiologic study (Bonten, Hayden, Nathan, & Van Voorhis, 1996; Coello et al., 1994; Larson, Early, Cloonan, Sugrue, & Parides, 2000; Wenzel & Edmond, 2001). As of the late 1990s and continuing into the current decade, health care staff hand hygiene practices leave much room and opportunity for improvement (Boyce, 1999). A causal association between hand hygiene failure and the slippery slope descent to ongoing antimicrobial resistance is also well established (Weinstein, 2001). For reasons not fully understood and that remain under active study, hand hygiene adherence varies, influenced by such factors as personal practice, condition of skin, occupation, clinical setting, hand hygiene product availability, time of day, administrative support, and perception of risk to self and others. Health care personnel have reported that nonadherence is attributable to excessive workload and to skin irritation, sensitivity, and dryness caused by hand hygiene (Larson & Killien, 1982; Zimakoff, Kjelsberg, Larsen, & Holstein, 1992). Nonetheless, hand hygiene is an integral component of quality care and patient safety promotion in all health care settings.

In 2002, the CDC (2002) published the landmark "Guideline for Hand Hygiene in Health-Care Settings." This document provides a comprehensive, detailed review of hand hygiene scientific data, including health care personnel practices, lessons learned from behavioral theories, and methods to be considered for use to enhance hand hygiene practices. Hand hygiene research agenda subject matter is summarized. This agenda includes a call for ongoing laboratory-based and epidemiologic research and development, continued research and development on hand hygiene products (e.g., to minimize potential sensitivity and irritation and to promote ease of performing hand hygiene), staff education, and promotion (e.g., to include assessment of key determinants of hand hygiene behavior among different cultures of health care personnel and evaluation of multimodal programs designed to promote hand hygiene). In addition, specific indication recommendations are provided for the following preparations: hand hygiene with an alcohol-based hand rub, nonantimicrobial soap and water, antimicrobial soap and water, hand antisepsis, surgical hand antisepsis, hand hygiene agent selection, skin care, use of gloves, artificial fingernails/extenders and rings in the health care setting, educational and motivational programs, and administrative measures. This document also offers some performance indicators, such as periodic monitoring with data collection and feedback, which may be useful to health care institutions as each develops its own hand hygiene program to be fully compliant with JCAHO standards.

Standard Precautions is an infection control strategy designed to reduce the risk of transmission of bloodborne pathogens as well as pathogens from moist body substances (Occupational Safety and Health Administration, 1991). This concept and practice is firmly entrenched in the United States and is slowly becoming established as an international infection control standard. The behavior patterns specified by Standard Precautions—administrative controls (e.g., annual training, participation in a hepatitis B vaccination program), engineering controls (e.g., access to sharps disposal containers), and thoughtful use of barrier equipment (e.g., gloves, masks, gowns, eyewear)—are designed to reduce risk for organism transmission in the health care setting from patient to staff, staff to patient, and patient to staff to patient. Noncompliance with Standard Precautions can result in disease transmission. A dramatic illustrative case report occurred in October 2004, in Philadelphia (Lewis et al., 2006). An unvaccinated laboratory employee working with vaccinia virus partly outside a biosafety cabinet contracted ocular vaccinia infection. Vaccinia (smallpox) vaccination is recommended for health care and laboratory workers who have occupational exposure to nonattenuated orthopoxviruses (CDC, 1997, 2001f). An investigation was able to pinpoint the infection source to a single experiment; whereas the precise mechanism for organism entry could not be determined, the most likely route was either hand-to-eye inadvertent inoculation or inoculation through aerosolization of the virus. Vaccination—in compliance with Standard Precautions and CDC immunization recommendations—likely would have prevented this infection. In addition, consistent use of safety goggles and performance of all virus manipulation in a biosafety cabinet would further reduce risk for transmission (Isaacs, 2004).

Eventual integration of the precepts and concepts of Standard Precautions to an international health care cultural standard should promote behaviors in all health care settings that lead to reduced transmission of emerging and reemerging infectious diseases. In addition, contact precautions and precautions for organisms disseminated by droplet or aerosol transmission are recommended when appropriate.

INJECTION AND RECREATIONAL DRUG USE

Injection and recreational illicit drug use (primarily cocaine, heroin, and amphetamine) is behavior initiated, maintained, and sustained by each individual person. Cultural, social, and personal bonding to the illicit drug community further entrenches each affected person, very often with associated negative impact on the affected person's partners, children, extended family, livelihood, and economic solvency. The culture and behavior of persons who participate in injection and recreational drug use are extremely complex and the topics of ongoing family angst, community concern, domestic/international activity, research, policy formulation, and legislative activity.

Injection and recreational drug user behavior is well known to contribute to transmission of emerging and reemerging infectious diseases. The ongoing associated practices of sharing unsterile injection equipment and practicing unsafe sex enhance disease transmission risks such as HIV and hepatitis B and C (Cherubin & Sapira, 1993). In the United States, injection drug use is a recognized risk factor for HIV infection, accounting for about 24% of adult AIDS cases reported from 2001 to 2004, without including joint categories such as male to male sexual contact and injection drug use or heterosexual contact with an injection drug user (CDC, 2003b, 2005a). Injection drug use also accounts for about one half of new hepatitis C cases (CDC, 2001d). The strongest predictor among the population with new hepatitis C infection was duration of injection; other associated risk factors were opiate use, heterosexual orientation, and history of incarceration in a prison. Despite ongoing alerts about the dangers for disease transmission via sharing used needles, and despite the implementation of needle-exchange programs in various parts of the world, the sharing behavior persists and disease transmission continues. Since 2003 in Taiwan there has been an ongoing escalation of HIV infection among injecting drug users (Chen et al., 2006). Taiwan's Center for Disease Control reported that HIV injection drug users accounted for 1.75% of reported HIV infections (13/773) in 2002, 8.1% (70/861) in 2003, and most recently 30.3% (462/1,521) in 2004 (Republic of China Centers for Disease Control, 2005). Although the number of drug offenders in the prison system has increased (from 5,988 in 2003 to 9,303 in 2004), and the rate of HIV infection among inmates has increased (from 13.3/100,000 in 2002 to 56.8/100,000 in 2004), prisoners are routinely tested for HIV infection and HIV-positive inmates are segregated from HIV-negative inmates. Thus, prison transmission is unlikely—more likely is the premise that the general Taiwan drug-injecting population is increasing and the HIV-infection rate in this population is exploding (Cohen, 2004).

Immunization is the best preventive measure for hepatitis B infection. Immunization has been recommended since 1982 for injection drug users, yet injection drug user coverage is low and hepatitis B outbreaks persist (Alter et al., 1990). The infection toll is hefty; within 5 years of injection drug use, the hepatitis B infection rate is about 70% (Garfein, Vlahov, Galai, Doherty, & Nelson, 1996). Barriers include absence of health insurance or adequate financial resources, inaccessibility to regular medical care or providers that routinely offer immunization, and ignorance about hepatitis B infection (Stancliff, Salomon, Perlamn, & Russell, 2000). During 2000, in the context of a hepatitis B outbreak mainly among injection drug users, Pierce County in Washington State launched a multidimensional targeted hepatitis B vaccine program (CDC, 2001a). Free vaccine clinics that included travel reimbursement were established at syringe exchange sites, the county health department, and later the soup kitchen, substance abuse treatment program, and county jail. Workers at all sites promoted the free vaccine clinics. About 2,000 persons were immunized during a 7-month period, and during this period the number of new hepatitis B cases decreased from 13 per month to 2 cases per month. The behavioral strategy of incorporation of immunization into preexisting programs, clinics, and public services seems practical and acceptable to the target population, is not new (Trubatch, Fisher, Cagle, & Fenaughty, 2000), and will hopefully become more a part of ongoing sustained collaboration among health departments, correction departments, public service departments, and community organizations.

Inhalation of illicit drugs is another behavior associated with reemergence of TB. "Hotboxing," the behavior of smoking marijuana with others in a vehicle with windows closed and no ventilation so that the smoke is repeatedly inhaled by all persons in the vehicle, has been found contributory to TB transmission during a 2003–2004 outbreak investigation in Washington State (Oeltmann et al., 2006). Similarly, "shotgunning," the behavior of inhaling smoke from illicit drugs and then exhaling the smoke directly into a person's mouth, was linked to TB transmission among a cohort of exotic dancers and their contacts (Perlman et al., 1997). Sharing a "bong," a water pipe, has been linked to TB transmission in Australia (Munckhof, Konstantinos, Wamsley, Mortlock, & Gilpin, 2003).

Illicit drug users are known as a population for whom behavior modification is very difficult to achieve and more difficult to sustain. The simplest and perhaps most controversial is the culture of syringe exchange programs, operating both within and outside legal sanction (e.g., legal, illegal-tolerated, illegal-underground), in various settings (e.g., storefront locations, health clinics, home visits, vans), with some offering other public and social services (CDC, 1998). Interventions to promote achievable risk behavior change among drug-using populations are labor intensive and time intensive. Interventions must entail adequate funding and then sustainability of infrastructure and funding. Specifics include cross-training of substance abuse counselors, provision of substance abuse education among school-aged children, access to trained healthcare personnel, legal efforts to remove illegal drug supplies, availability of instruction on the use of condoms and dentals dams to prevent disease transmission, information about "safer infection techniques," ready nonjudgmental referral and accessibility to substance abuse treatment programs, and ready accessibility to basic health care services.

TRAVEL

The increased ease of travel is associated with an increased risk of transmission of emerging and reemerging diseases (see chapter 25). Refugee traffic—common from locations of military strife (e.g., Iraq, Lebanon), political and civil unrest (e.g., the Philippines), natural disaster (e.g., drought, earthquake, famine, fire, flood, hurricane, tornado, monsoon, tsunami)—and immigrant traffic (legal or illegal, domestic or international) provide obstacles to health care access; medicine and medical supplies; and adequate shelter, nutrition, sanitary services, and potable water. The resultant migration and immigration of large numbers of refugees has resulted in the emergence of infectious diseases in areas where these diseases were previously unknown or rare.

Continued political changes in many parts of the world have eased previous restrictions on travel across borders. Increased ease of travel by land, air, and water has provided a mechanism for rapid dissemination and transmission of infectious agents. Air travel provides service to most global locations within a 24-hour period and thus expands the potential for rapid spread of diseases, examples of which are discussed throughout this book. The Canadian experience with SARS during 2003 is an example (Skowronski et al., 2006). The WHO issued a SARS global alert in March 2003 (WHO, 2003). Unfortunately, prior to this date, travelers with SARS acquired from the Hotel M. cluster in Hong Kong returned to British Columbia and Ontario (Poutanen et al., 2003). Toronto reported three imported cases leading to an additional 243 cases and 43 deaths; Vancouver reported four imported cases and one additional case. Fortunately, the Canadian British Columbia Centre for Disease Control (BC-CDC) already had pandemic threat preparation in place. In mid-February 2003, the BCCDC learned that China was identifying cases of unexplained atypical pneumonia and that Hong Kong was identifying reemergence of influenza A H5N1 and issued its own travel alert. Due to this alert and the hospital's almost immediate implementation of infection control, there was limited transmission. Pandemic preparation in Ontario was not in place, and there was much opportunity for transmission both in the community and the health care setting.

Timely public health alerts, efficient and effective network communication, central sentinel disease management coordination, and local-level baseline preparedness are each essential tools for successful travel-behavior-related emerging and reemerging infectious disease management. Ongoing research, timely epidemiological investigation of unexplained disease clusters and case reports, and travelers' infection transmission management strategy for emerging and reemerging infectious disease transmission likely will remain at the forefront of public health agenda.

NUTRITIONAL BEHAVIOR

"You are what you eat" is an adage that applies to nutritional behavior and is associated with emerging and reemerging disease transmission. The association of nutritional behavior and risk for transmission of *Cyclospora cayetanensis* and *E. coli* O157:H7 are delineated in chapters 6 and 9. A list of emerging and reemerging diseases associated with foodborne transmission is provided in Appendix B. This chapter discusses select topic areas that illustrate the breadth and scope of nutritional behavior in the context of emerging and reemerging diseases.

Creutzfeldt–Jakob disease and variant Creutzfeldt–Jakob disease (vCJD) case reports provide the most prominent examples of nutritional behavior as associated with emerging and reemerging infectious disease transmission. Chapter 21 provides a detailed epidemiologic review of these and other prion diseases (transmissible spongiform encephalopathies). Reports of Creutzfeldt–Jakob disease likely attributable to nutritional behavior are those cases associated with the consumption of the brains of wild goats or squirrels (Kamin & Patten, 1984). Variant Creutzfeldt–Jakob disease, first reported in the United Kingdom in 1996, has been causally linked to ingestion of cattle products contaminated with the bovine spongiform encephalopathy (BSE) agent (Belay & Schonberger, 2005). Due to the newness of vCJD and concern of possible prionemia as vCJD migrates from the gastrointestinal tract to the brain, monitoring for bloodborne transmission began in 1997. The occurrence of bloodborne transmission was confirmed as of 2004—in the United Kingdom 2 of 48 recipients of blood components from donors who subsequently died of vCJD were confirmed to have bloodborne transmission of vCJD (Llewelyn et al., 2004). Behavior to reduce this small risk was rapidly implemented (Alter, 2000). For example, in the United States the FDA instituted a geographic-based donor deferral policy in 1999 (FDA,

1999/2002). As of late 2005 fewer than 200 patients with vCJD have been reported—157 from the United Kingdom, 13 from France, 3 from Ireland, and 1 each from Canada, Italy, Japan, Portugal, Spain, the Netherlands, and the United States. The predominant route of exposure is foodborne, and the predominant exposure is residence in the United Kingdom or after ingestion of imported BSE-contaminated cattle products (Belay et al., 2005; CDC, 2003a). The estimated incubation period for foodborne exposure ranges from 5 years to 21 years.

Foodborne trematodiasis is caused by liver flukes, lung flukes, and intestinal flukes. In some parts of Asia, notably Korea, there has been significant prevalence reduction in foodborne trematodiasis, related to various behavioral and cultural changes such as social and economic development (access to improved sanitation), health education programs, urbanization, food inspections, and use of chemical fertilizers (Fried, Gracyk, & Tamang, 2004; Keiser & Utzinger, 2004). However, in Southeast Asia and the Western Pacific region, foodborne trematodiasis is an emerging infectious disease issue (Keiser & Utzinger, 2005). Aquaculture production is escalating exponentially in these areas, due to global projected demand to maintain food with a high protein value and improved transportation and distribution processes in these regions to bring the aquatic products to local and international markets (Muir, 2005). Behavioral and cultural factors are implicit in transmission of foodborne trematodes—traditional local cuisine in Southeast Asia and the Western Pacific includes partially cooked or raw aquatic products (e.g., raw drunken crabs and raw grass carp in China, raw crab soaked in soy sauce in the Republic of Korea, raw fish in Thailand; Lun et al., 2005; WHO, 1995). In industrialized countries, foreign travel and ingesting imported aquatic foods are frequently associated with infection. In the event that aquaculture escalation is accompanied with tools established as effective for foodborne trematodiasis control (food inspections, education campaigns, disease treatment, access to improved sanitation), then this issue may not remain on the emerging infectious disease menu, but only time, and infectious disease surveillance, will tell.

Breast-feeding for the first 6 months of life is an excellent source of nutrition for neonates and infants. Data consistently indicates that human milk feeding decreases the incidence and/or severity of a wide range of infectious diseases in industrial and developing countries (Dayan, Ortega-Sanchez, LeBaron, Quinlisk, & Iowa Measles Response Team, 2004).

Under certain circumstances, there are situations in which human milk is not recommended (American Academy of Pediatrics, 2005). Medical guidance should be available to help identify clinical conditions or environmental exposures that preclude breast-feeding. In general, infectious conditions for which breast-feeding is not recommended are a mother who is HIV positive, is taking antiretroviral medications, has active untreated tubercular infection, is infected with human T-cell lymphotropic virus 1 or 2, is using/dependent on an illicit drug, is taking chemotherapy agents (e.g., antimetabolites that interfere with cell division and DNA replication), is undergoing radiation therapy (until the milk is free of radiation), and/or has herpes simplex lesions on a breast (Dyan et al., 2004).

The standard of care among industrialized countries is that infants of HIV-infected women should not be breast-fed. Women in industrialized countries are likely to have access to potable water, ample supplies of infant formula, and access to medical resources to help ensure that the formula is properly mixed and administered. This standard seems sensible provided that safe, accessible, and affordable alternative nourishment is available to the infants. However, in parts of the world where malnutrition and infectious diseases are the primary causes of infant mortality, and where a practical, sustainable alternative to breast-feeding is not available, the WHO recommends breast-feeding, regardless of the mother's HIV status (WHO Collaborative Study Team, 2000; WHO, 2001, 2004). In these parts of the world, the drinking water may be laden with disease-causing bacteria, the mother may not have access to or may not be able to afford infant formula, and the mother may not have access to medical resources to insure that the formula is being properly prepared and administered. Data from developing countries consistently indicate that the infant mortality risk associated with alternative feeding is greater than the risk for acquiring infections, such as HIV, from breast-feeding (Mbori-Ngacha et al., 2001; Kourtis, Buteera, Ibegbu, Belec, & Duerr, 2003; WHO Collaborative Study Team, 2000). One study from Africa assessed exclusive breast-feeding by HIV-positive mothers for the first 3 to 6 months of life and HIV-transmission risk (Coutsoudis, Pillay, Spooner, Kuhn, & Coovadia, 1999; Coutsoudis & Rollins, 2003). Infants who exclusively breast-fed did not have increased HIV-infection rate; infants receiving either formula or a combination of breast milk and formula had a higher rate of HIV infection. WHO recommends specific guidance and support for at least the first 2 years of their children's lives for HIV-1-infected women who decide not to breast-feed their children (WHO, 2004).

Before discouraging breast-feeding, mothers must be ensured sustained access to clean water, adequate supplies of formula, and meticulous teaching in formula preparation and administration (Nduati et al., 2000). Each community needs to assess the resources available to HIV-infected mothers, to discuss resource availability with public health officials, and to proceed together with a breast-feeding recommendation that, given data relevant to the individual community, is most likely to promote maternal and infant health and reduce infant morbidity and mortality.

IMMUNIZATION BEHAVIOR

Fewer and fewer diagnosed cases of vaccine-preventable diseases are reported each year, due in large measure to unceasing efforts by the public health international and national communities in partnership with local governments and communities. The outcome of ongoing immunization program success is regions of the world that are free from smallpox, measles, and poliomyelitis and impressive reductions in diphtheria-, tetanus-, and pertussis-attributed morbidity and mortality (CDC, 2006e). The WHO closely monitors vaccine mortality estimates—the number of deaths that might be prevented if vaccine programs were fully practiced. During 2002, WHO estimates that polio claimed fewer than 1,000 lives of children aged younger than 5 years; diphtheria claimed the lives of 4,000 children; yellow fever claimed the lives of 15,000 children; 198,000 children died from tetanus; 294,000 children's lives were lost to pertussis; 386,000 children succumbed to *Hemophilus influenzae* type b; and measles claimed the lives of 540,000 (WHO & United Nations Children's Fund, 2005). For 2003, WHO estimates that vaccination prevented 2 million pediatric deaths (WHO, 2005). Behavioral and cultural factors are contributory to ongoing vaccine-preventable deaths. These include infrastructure development and maintenance to sustain current vaccine levels, as well as strategy development and implementation to vaccinate susceptible populations and susceptible persons beyond infancy. The 2005 WHO Global Immunization Vision and Strategy encourages integration of vaccine programs into preexisting programs. An example of successful meld has been vitamin A supplements administered in conjunction with immunizations (WHO, 2005); during 2004 several countries reported that they provided vitamin A to infants along with routine vaccines.

From 1991 to 1999, Zambia, a southern African country, reported annual measles cases from 1,698 to 23,518 (CDC, 2001c). During 1999–2004 ongoing strategies were implemented to control measles (CDC, 2005e). This campaign remains a work in progress, but indications are very encouraging: 33,628 cases were reported in 2001 compared to 16,793 cases in 2003. In addition, Zambia has achieved a decreasing measles mortality. From 1999 to 2000, the average annual deaths attributed to measles were 217; during 2003, a total of 98 deaths were reported; and during 2004, 3 deaths were reported. Zambia achievement is related to vaccine delivery improvement, surveillance system enhancement, and ongoing vaccine control strategy activity—sustainability of routine measles vaccination (more than 90%) will be an ongoing behavioral and cultural challenge.

Occurrence of worldwide reduction in vaccine-preventable disease morbidity and mortality has a negative flip side. Economically strained households and households lacking sufficient health insurance may cut corners and not obtain recommended vaccinations, relying on herd immunity and the mantra "it will not happen to me" for disease protection. Some people's religious or cultural beliefs do not support immunization activity. Some people lend credence to the theory that the measles-mumps-rubella (MMR) vaccine is a causal factor for autism or the theory that neurodevelopmental disorders (including speech delay, language delay, attention-deficit/hyperactivity disorder, and autism) can be caused by vaccines containing the mercury-based preservative thimerosal. This behavior, in addition to the fact that no vaccine is 100% effective, results in a continuing reservoir of persons susceptible to, at risk for contracting, and potentially able to be sources for continued transmission of vaccine-preventable diseases.

Vaccine safety research surveillance monitoring has repeatedly determined that there is no causal relation between autism, neurodevelopmental disorders, and receipt of the MMR vaccine and thimerosal-containing vaccines. The Institute of Medicine has conducted a comprehensive review of published data and reports on these theories, most recently in 2001 and in 2004. The May 2004 report summarized findings from five new epidemiological studies conducted in Sweden, Denmark, the United States, and the United Kingdom; nine controlled observational studies; three ecological studies; and two studies based on a passive reporting system in Finland (Institute of Medicine, 2004). Nonetheless, parents sometimes or often raise concerns about possible neurological vaccination effects and overall vaccine safety. The behavioral emphasis for pediatricians and family practitioners must be that of open two-way communication in a manner that promotes mutual trust, opinion exchange, and successful communication of vaccine information and the overwhelming health benefit of vaccine program compliance.

Immunization program nonadherence is associated with reemergence of preventable diseases (CDC, 2000). During September 2004–February 2005, an outbreak of pertussis occurred in the United States, in an Amish community in Kent County, Delaware (CDC, 2006c). During May 2005 an imported case of measles occurred in the United States, resulting in the largest U.S. measles outbreak since 1996 (Yip, Papania, & Redd, 2004). During early May an Indiana resident, a measles-susceptible missionary, visited an orphanage in Bucharest, Romania, where a measles outbreak subsequently occurred. The missionary returned to the United States with measles-like symptoms; a rash developed in mid-May and measles was diagnosed retrospectively (CDC, 2005d). Exposure to this index case resulted in a total of 24 cases of measles. One of these cases occurred in a person working in a medical facility. These outbreaks probably reflect the low coverage level for routine childhood vaccination, underscore the importance to heed the Advisory Committee on Immunization Practices' recommendation that all persons who travel internationally and persons who work in medical facilities be vaccinated for measles (Dayan et al., 2005), and highlight the need to promote vaccination through culturally appropriate strategies (CDC, 2006e).

Ongoing information campaigns and continuing education on the personal and public health merits of vaccination foster enduring cooperation with vaccine programs (CDC, 1999b). However, factors other than behavior are involved with failure to immunize—vaccines such as those for hepatitis B and *H. influenzae* are often too costly in developing countries (Okie, 1999). Thus, achieving and sustaining adequate immunization behavior and immunization levels—with positive ongoing momentum worldwide—will continue as a multifaceted international challenge.

BIOTERRORISM

The behavior of bioterrorists is a worrisome global concern (see chapter 27). The underlying unpredictable nature of, and the resultant toll on, the terms of economics, the environment, and quality of life places bioterrorism prominently on the roster of each nation's domestic and international agenda. Bioterrorists intentionally introduce agents with the anticipated highest outcome of morbidity, mortality, societal unease, and economic crippling. Persons engage in this behavior to further ideological, material, or spiritual objectives. The premise of bioterrorism seems to reside in a mantra of greatest damage equating with worldwide attention and eventual worldwide capitulation to ideological, material, or spiritual objectives.

The threat of deployment of biologic weapons on both civilian and military targets has many unknowns—the targets, the agent(s), routes for delivery and distribution, and the ability of public health and health care systems to mount timely and appropriate responses (Breman & Henderson, 1998; English, 1999). The intentional release of *Bacillus anthracis* resulting in 23 cases of both cutaneous and inhalational anthrax by late 2001 spurred countries to accelerate efforts to develop programs to counter bioterrorism. For example, the United States Department of Defense has established a mandatory anthrax vaccination program for military personnel, and organizations (e.g., the CDC and the Association for Professionals in Infection Control and Epidemiology) have published bioterrorism management procedures. Continued preparation for bioterrorism is ongoing and will likely include the development of management procedures for other potential infectious diseases that may be used in bioterrorism.

OTHER BEHAVIORAL AND CULTURAL CONSIDERATIONS

Socioeconomic Change

Socioeconomic changes influence emerging and reemerging disease transmission. In the tropical sector of the world, vector control programs for dengue consistently demonstrate successful prevention via vector control and then subsequent socioeconomic-influenced nonsustainability (Schliessmann et al., 1974; Kouri, Gusman, Bravo, & Triana, 1989; Ooi, Goh, & Gubler, 2006). The Pan American Health Organization conducted an effective elimination campaign in Mexico during the 1950s and 1960s (Pan American Health Organization, 1998). Subsequent social and economic shifts (rural to urban population emigration without adequate housing, water, sewage, and waste management systems; proliferation of nonrecyclable products, which provided plentiful breeding locations for *Aedes aegypti*; diminished public health infrastructure and resources) allowed vector reinfestation and reemergence of dengue (Pan American Health Organization, 1994; Torres-Muñoz, 1995). More recently, after a low incidence for 15 years, dengue (see chapter 7) reemerged in Singapore during the 1990s. Dengue resurgence in the 1990s is multifactorial, with socioeconomic contributors including increased activity outside the home and a cost-driven surveillance shift from vector surveillance toward case identification. Reduction of virus transmission via case identification is cost effective in the short run (coinciding with effective entomologic, surveillance-based vector control) but not so in the long run. In Singapore, loss of entomologic, surveillance-based vector control saves dollars but allows propagation of the host. Moreover, control by case response lacks adequate sensitivity—subacute and mild undifferentiated cases can be easily missed, leading to increased disease transmission (Ooi et al., 2006).

Civil Conflict and Political Instability

Civil conflict and/or political instability, ever present in various parts of the world (e.g., Afghanistan, the Darfur region of Sudan, Iraq, Lebanon, the Philippines, Sierra Leone, Somalia), invites transmission of emerging diseases and reestablishment of formerly controlled infectious diseases (e.g., malaria, typhoid, vaccine-preventable diseases). Resources and organization for public health programs are undermined. Nonadherence to recommended vaccination schedules increases the pool of susceptible persons and the likelihood of vaccine-preventable disease occurrence and transmission. Increased homelessness amplifies the risk for TB transmission. Lack of access to potable water and clean food increases the likelihood of foodborne and waterborne diseases. Interruption of regular market patterns disrupts access to contraceptives and promotes STD transmission.

The recent experience in the Darfur region of Sudan underscores the association of civil conflict and reemerging infectious diseases. Civil conflict during 2003 resulted in internal migration of about 1 million persons and an emigration of about 170,000 persons to Chad. Measles control activities were severely disrupted, and beginning in March 2004 there were reports of measles outbreaks among displaced residents (CDC, 2004b). Despite aggressive vaccination campaigns that included vaccination of about 80,000 children, reports of measles outbreaks continued (Moore et al., 1993; Toole & Waldman, 1993). The WHO and UNICEF conducted a vaccination feasibility study including variables such as the approaching rainy season, displaced persons movements, lack of security, ability to maintain proper vaccine temperature during storage and handling to preserve potency, and vitamin A supplementation for children younger than 5 years. During June 2004, following extensive social mobilization, intensive training sessions, and a negotiation with rebel forces to allow vaccination in the South Darfur conflict areas, a mass measles vaccination campaign was started that resulted in approximately 93% vaccination of accessible population and 77% vaccination of the total target population. Follow-up indicated a reduced morbidity and mortality related to measles. Challenges to surmount include sustainability, re-establishment of routine vaccination and "follow up" campaigns at set intervals.

The International Health Regulations (IHR) 2005 provides tremendous opportunity for global advancement of surveillance and disease response—especially germane to countries dealing with civil unrest and political instability (World Health Assembly, 2005a). Revision of the 1969 IHR was undertaken by the WHO in 1995, with approval of new IHR in 2005 and adoption as an international treaty in 2005 by the World Health Assembly (World Health Assembly, 2005b). The overall surveillance concept and evaluation framework of the IHR are aligned with the CDC surveillance system framework and the public health surveillance definition as "the ongoing systematic collection, analysis, and interpretation of outcome-specific data for use in the planning, implementation, and evaluation of public health practice" (CDC, 2001e, p. 4; Thacker, 2000). Challenges for successful integration of IHR 2005 into global infectious disease activity include financial funding, technological ability, and capability to upgrade (and then sustain) existing surveillance systems, especially in developing countries; administrative and managerial government capability to detect and respond to emerging and reemerging disease challenges; political commitment to report notifiable diseases and to apply trade and travel restrictions; and countries' adjustment of their systems of law and constitutional systems to support IHR 2005 (Baker & Fidler, 2006). The core of IHR 2005 is the establishment of cohesive, efficient global public health surveillance: The potential to institute early control measures for emerging and reemerging infectious diseases is within the realm of reality. Indeed, in May 2006, given the ongoing risk that avian influenza will jump to readily transmissible human infection, the World Health Assembly adopted a resolution for voluntary, immediate compliance by WHO member countries with IHR 2005 (Baker & Fidler, 2006).

Body Art

Body art involves ritual cutting (excludes male circumcision), piercing, tattooing, and branding. Emerging and reemerging disease may occur when nonsterile equipment or poor infection-control technique is used, adequate body art site care is not maintained, and/or the body art office is unlicensed (CDC, 2006b). Body art practitioners are largely unlicensed, unregulated, and not subject to routine health inspections (Braithwaite, Stephens, Sterk, & Braighwait, 1999; Greif & Hewitt, 1998). Body art procedures are associated with transmission of methicillin-resistant *Staphylococcus aureus* (MRSA), tetanus, hepatitis B, hepatitis C, HIV, and other organisms at the time of the procedure and in the course of wound care (CDC, 2006b; Fisman, 1999; Loscalzo, Ryan, Loscalzo, Sarna, & Cadag, 1995; Mamtani, Malhotra, Gupta, & Jain, 1978; MacDonald, Crofts, & Kaldor, 1996; O'Malley, Smith, Braun, & Prevots, 1998; Pugatch, Mileno, & Rich, 1998; Tweeten & Rickman, 1998).

Ritual cutting is not uncommon and can be associated with disease acquisition. An anecdotal report of a 6-week-old infant who developed fatal septicemia with a resistant strain of *Pseudomonas aeruginosa* after ritual cutting illustrates the risk for disease transmission introduced by body art behavior (Mathur & Sahoo, 1984).

Body piercing directly affects subcutaneous body sites and is associated with infectious complications. In the United States only six states have regulatory authority over body-piercing businesses (Akhondi & Rahimi, 2002). Body piercing occurs in private homes, department stores, medical offices, and regulated and nonregulated businesses. Generally, antibiotics are not used, and sterilization procedures vary. Tongue piercing has been associated with *Neisseria* endocarditis (Tronel, Chaudemanche, Pechier, Doutrelant, & Hoen, 2001); nasal piercing has been associated with mitral valve staphylococcal endocarditis (Ramage, Wilson, & Thomson, 1997); nipple piercing has been associated with *Staphylococcus epidermidis* endocarditis (Ochsenfahrt, Friedl, Hannekum, & Schumacher, 2001); and *E. coli* infection is associated with genital piercing—in addition to increased risk for STD due to tissue trauma and possible unwanted pregnancy due to condom rupture (Fiumara & Eisen, 1983). One case report of *Hemophilus aphrophilus* endocarditis illustrates the morbidity induced via body piercing complications (Akhondi & Rahimi, 2002). An adult male with a history of aortic valvuloplasty at 8 years of age presented with 6 days' duration of fever, chills, and rigors. The tongue had been pierced with a bispherical stud 2 months before symptom onset. Blood culture and the stud culture were positive for *H. aphrophilus*. Endocarditis was confirmed via a transesophageal echocardiogram showing a deformed aortic valve with multiple vegetative lesions. The patient received intravenous therapy as an inpatient and then completed a 6-week intravenous antibiotic course at home. Another study of piercing complications in patients with congenital heart disease (Cetta, Graham, & Lichtenberg, 1999) showed about 23% of the study population with earlobe piercing developed piercing-related infections from 1 to 3 weeks after piercing. Fortunately, no endocarditis was reported in this study.

Tattooing complications are well documented. Findings from a 1992–2005 CDC investigation of HIV transmission among male inmates demonstrated that getting a tattoo and engaging in male–male sex were associated with HIV transmission among inmates (CDC, 2006a). Multivariate logistic regression model analysis identified receipt of a tattoo while in prison as one of four covariates significantly associated with HIV seroconversion. However, this report does not constitute documentation of HIV transmission via tattooing. Whereas receipt of a tattoo was associated with seroconversion, further investigation is indicated, for example, tattoo artists' HIV status, sharing of tattoo equipment among HIV-infected and non-HIV-infected inmates, disinfection of tattoo equipment, and commonality in time frame from tattoo receipt to HIV conversion. Another recent CDC investigation of 34 cases of MRSA transmission from body art procedures determined that each case involved unlicensed tattooists; 13 of the 34 reported receiving their tattoos in public places (private residence or park) and use of homemade tattooing equipment (CDC, 2006b). In the United States there is no federal oversight for body art, and laws and regulating authorities vary (Tattooing and Body Piercing of Humans by Nonmedical Personnel for Remuneration, 2005; Tattoo and Body Piercing Services, 1997, 1998; Tattooists and Body Piercers, 2004).

Death Rituals

Death rituals, or "funerary practices," are richly diverse, reflecting the broad international cultural variety enfolding death (Stephen, 1998). Mortuary staff and all persons who wash and drape bodies before burial or cremation are at risk for emerging and reemerging diseases such as hepatitis C, HIV, and EHF (see chapter 8; Gatrad, 1994). Adherence to standard precautions in all funerary practices is essential to maintain a low risk of disease transmission but in many cases is difficult to incorporate because of cultural beliefs and practices.

Human body part consumption traditions (e.g., to attempt to cure illness) are well documented in Chinese and Western cultures (Chen & Chen, 1998; Cooper & Sivin, 1973; MacCulloch, 1925). Although cannibalism is uncommon and unusual, in instances in which it has been practiced, disease transmission has been documented. For example, ritualistic postmortem cannibalism practiced until the late 1950s by the Fore highlanders of New Guinea was directly related to the transmission of kuru, a transmissible, fatal encephalopathy (see chapter 19; Gibbs & Gajdusek, 1978; Gajdusek, 1979). Disease transmission halted when the cultural ritual of postmortem cannibalism was discontinued.

SUMMARY

Consideration of individual, community, and societal behavioral and cultural mores are integral to successful and sustained emerging and reemerging infectious disease management. Emerging and reemerging infectious disease management will depend in large measure on the integration of economic, environmental, medical, political, and social sciences into the structure and function of national and international public health policies and programs. Infant mortality provides an indication of the overall health of populations, and use of this barometer should continue. Prevention through education about high-risk behaviors, cultural reinforcement of preventive behaviors, and health care access for surveillance and immunization remain the best defenses. Acknowledgement of the influence of civil unrest, military strife, human migration, natural disaster, and economic markets into the panorama of emerging and reemerging infectious diseases is critical to facilitate early disease identification and management.

REFERENCES

Aiello, A. E., & Larsen, E. (2003). Antibacterial cleaning and hygiene products as an emerging risk factor for antimicrobial drug resistance in the community. *Lancet Infectious Diseases, 3*, 501–506.

Aiello, A. E., Marshall, B., Levy, S. B., Della-Latta, P., Lin, S. X., & Larson, E. (2005). Antibacterial cleaning products and drug resistance. *Emerging Infectious Diseases, 11*, 1565–1570.

Akhondi, H., & Rahimi, A. R. (2002). *Haemophilus aphrophilus* endocarditis after tongue piercing. *Emerging Infectious Diseases, 8*(8), 850–851.

Retrieved August 04, 2006, from http://www.cdc.gov/nciod/EID/vol8no8/ 01-0458.htm

Alter, M. (2000). How is Creutzfeldt-Jakob disease acquired? *Neuroepidemiology,* *19*(2), 55–61.

Alter, M. D., Hadler, S. C., Margolis, H. S., Alexander, W. J., Hu, P. Y., Judson, F. N., et al. (1990). The changing epidemiology of hepatitis B in the United States. *Journal of the American Medical Association, 263,* 1218–1222.

American Academy of Pediatrics. (2005). Policy statement: Breastfeeding and the use of human milk. *Pediatrics, 115,* 496–506.

Andrews, M. M., & Boule, J. S. (Eds.). (1999). *Transcultural concepts in nursing care* (3rd ed.). Philadelphia: Lippincott Williams & Wilkins.

Avorn, J., & Solomon, D. H. (2000). Cultural and economic factors that (mis)shape antibiotic use. The nonpharmacologic basis of therapeutics. *Annals of Internal Medicine, 133,* 128–135.

Baker, M., & Fidler, D. (2006). Global public health surveillance under new international health regulations. *Emerging Infectious Diseases, 12,* 1058–1065.

Bartholet, J. (2000, January 17). Africa's plague years. *Newsweek,* pp. 32–37.

Belay, E. D., & Schonberger, L. B. (2005). The public health impact of prion diseases. *Annual Review of Public Health, 26,* 191–212.

Belay, E. D., Sejvar, J. J., Shieh, W. J., Wiersma, S. T., Zou, W. Q., Gambetti, P., et al. (2005). Variant Creutzfeldt-Jakob disease death, United States. *Emerging Infectious Diseases, 11,* 1351–1354.

Bell, R. A., Kravitz, R. L., & Wilkes, M. S. (1999). Direct-to-consumer prescription drug advertising and the public. *Journal of General Internal Medicine, 14,* 651–657.

Bonten, M. J. M., Hayden, M. K., Nathan, C., & Van Voorhis, J. (1996). Epidemiology of colonization of patients and environment with vancomycin-resistant enterococci. *Lancet, 348,* 1615–1619.

Boyce, J. M. (1999). Is it time for action: Improving hand hygiene in hospitals. *Annals of Internal Medicine, 130,* 153–155.

Braithwaite, R. L., Stephens, T., Sterk, C., & Braighwait, K. (1999). Risks associated with tattooing and body piercing. *Journal of Public Health Policy, 20,* 459–470.

Breman, J., & Henderson, D. A. (1998). Poxvirus dilemmas—Monkeypox, smallpox, and biologic terrorism. *New England Journal of Medicine, 339,* 557–559.

Brown, S., Warnnissorn, T., Biddle, J., Panikabutra, K., & Traisupa, A. (1982). Antimicrobial resistance of *Neisseria gonorrhoea* in Bangkok: Is single-drug treatment passé. *Lancet, 320,* 1366–1368.

Centers for Disease Control. (1992). National action plan to combat multidrug-resistant tuberculosis. *Morbidity and Mortality Weekly Report, 41*(RR-11), 1–48.

Centers for Disease Control and Prevention. (1994). Guidelines for preventing the transmission of *Mycobacterium tuberculosis* in health-care facilities. *Morbidity and Mortality Weekly Report, 43*(RR-13), 1–132.

Centers for Disease Control and Prevention. (1995). Recommendations for preventing the spread of vancomycin resistance. Recommendations of the

Hospital Infection Control Practices Advisory Committee (HICPAC). *Morbidity and Mortality Weekly Report, 44*(RR-12), 1–13.

Centers for Disease Control and Prevention. (1997). Immunization of health-care workers: Recommendations of the Advisory Committee on Immunization Practices (ACIP) and the Hospital Infection Control Practices Advisory Committee (HICPAC). *Morbidity and Mortality Weekly Report, 46*(RR-18), 1–42.

Centers for Disease Control and Prevention. (1998). Update: Syringe exchange programs—United States, 1997. *Morbidity and Mortality Weekly Report, 47,* 652–655.

Centers for Disease Control and Prevention. (1999a). Resurgent bacterial sexually transmitted disease among men who have sex with men—King County, Washington, 1997–1999. *Morbidity and Mortality Weekly Report, 48,* 773–777.

Centers for Disease Control and Prevention. (1999b). Measles eradication: Experience in the Americas. *Morbidity and Mortality Weekly Report, 48*(SU-01), 57–64.

Centers for Disease Control and Prevention. (2000). *Guidelines for the control of pertussis outbreaks.* Atlanta, GA: U.S. Department of Health and Human Services, CDC. Retrieved August 05, 2006, http://www.cdc.gov/nip/publications/pertussis/guide.htm

Centers for Disease Control and Prevention. (2001a). Outbreak of syphilis among men who have sex with men—Southern California, 2000. *Morbidity and Mortality Weekly Report, 50,* 117–120.

Centers for Disease Control and Prevention. (2001b). Hepatitis B vaccination for injection drug users—Pierce County, Washington, 2000. *Morbidity and Mortality Weekly Report, 50,* 388–390, 399.

Centers for Disease Control and Prevention. (2001c). Measles incidence before and after supplementary vaccination activities—Lusaka, Zambia, 1996–2000. *Morbidity and Mortality Weekly Report, 50,* 513–516.

Centers for Disease Control and Prevention. (2001d). Public health and injection drug use. *Morbidity and Mortality Weekly Report, 50,* 377.

Centers for Disease Control and Prevention. (2001e). Updated guidelines for evaluating public health surveillance systems: Recommendations from the guidelines working group. *Morbidity and Mortality Weekly Report, 50*(RR-13), 1–36.

Centers for Disease Control and Prevention. (2001f). Vaccinia (smallpox) vaccine: Recommendations of the Advisory Committee on Immunization Practices (ACIP), 2001. *Morbidity and Mortality Weekly Report, 50*(RR-10), 1–25.

Centers for Disease Control and Prevention. (2002). Guideline for hand hygiene in health-care settings. Recommendations of the Healthcare Infection Control Practices Advisory Committee and the HICPAC/SHEA/APIC/IDSA Hand Hygiene Task Force. *Morbidity and Mortality Weekly Report, 51*(RR-16), 1–44.

Centers for Disease Control and Prevention. (2003a). Bovine spongiform encephalopathy in a dairy cow—Washington state, 2003. *Morbidity and Mortality Weekly Report, 52,* 1280–1285.

Centers for Disease Control and Prevention. (2003b). HIV diagnoses among injection drug users in states with HIV surveillance—25 sites, 1994–2000. *Morbidity and Mortality Weekly Report, 52*, 634–636.

Centers for Disease Control and Prevention. (2003c). Guidelines for environmental infection control health-care facilities. *Morbidity and Mortality Weekly Report, 52*(RR-10), 1–42.

Centers for Disease Control and Prevention. (2004a). Trends in primary and secondary syphilis and HIV infections in men who have sex with men, San Francisco and Los Angeles, California, 1998–2002. *Morbidity and Mortality Weekly Report, 53*(26), 575–578.

Centers for Disease Control and Prevention. (2004b). Emergency measles control activities—Darfur, Sudan, 2004. *Morbidity and Mortality Weekly Report, 53*, 897–899.

Centers for Disease Control and Prevention. (2005a). *HIV/AIDS surveillance report, 2004* (Vol. 16, pp. 1–45). Atlanta, GA: U.S. Department of Health and Human Services, Centers for Disease Control and Prevention. Retrieved August 1, 2006, from http://www.cdc.gov/hiv/stats/hasrlink.htm.

Centers for Disease Control and Prevention. (2005b). Controlling tuberculosis in the United States. Recommendations from the American Thoracic Society, CDIC, and the Infectious Diseases Society of America. *Morbidity and Mortality Weekly Report, 54*(RR-12), 1–81.

Centers for Disease Control and Prevention. (2005c). Guidelines for preventing the transmission of *Mycobacterium tuberculosis* in health-care settings, 2005. *Morbidity and Mortality Weekly Report, 54*(RR-17), 1–141.

Centers for Disease Control and Prevention. (2005d). Import-associated measles outbreak—Indiana, May–June 2005. *Morbidity and Mortality Weekly Report, 54*(42), 1073–1075.

Centers for Disease Control and Prevention. (2005e). Progress in measles control—Zambia, 1999–2004. *Morbidity and Mortality Weekly Report, 54*, 581–584.

Centers for Disease Control and Prevention. (2006a). HIV transmission among male inmates in a state prison system—Georgia, 1992–2005. 2006. *Morbidity and Mortality Weekly Report, 55*, 421–426.

Centers for Disease Control and Prevention. (2006b). Methicillin-resistant *Staphylococcus aureus* skin infections among tattoo recipients—Ohio, Kentucky, and Vermont, 2004–2005. *Morbidity and Mortality Weekly Report, 55*, 677–679.

Centers for Disease Control and Prevention. (2006c). Pertussis outbreak in an Amish community—Kent County, Delaware, September 2004–February 2006. *Morbidity and Mortality Weekly Report, 55*, 817–821.

Centers for Disease Control and Prevention. (2006d). Prevention and control of tuberculosis in correctional and detention facilities: Recommendations from CDC. *Morbidity and Mortality Weekly Report, 55*(RR-09), 1–44.

Centers for Disease Control and Prevention. (2006e). Vaccine preventable deaths and the global immunization vision and strategy. *Morbidity and Mortality Weekly Report, 55*, 511–515.

Centers for Disease Control and Prevention. (2006f). Emergence of *Mycobacterium tuberculosis* with Extensive Resistance to Second-Line Drugs—Worldwide, 2000–2004. *Morbidity and Mortality Weekly Report, 55*, 301–305.

Cetta, F., Graham, L. C., & Lichtenberg, R. C. (1999). Piercing and tattooing in patients with congenital heart diseases. *Journal of Adolescent Health, 24*, 160.

Chen, T., & Chen, S. Y. (1998, Spring). Medical cannibalism in China: The case of ko-ku. *The Pharos, 23–25*.

Chen, Y. M., Lan, Y. C., Lai, S. F., Yang, J. Y., Tsai, S. F., & Kuo, S. H. (2006). HIV-1 CRF07_BC infections, injecting drug users, Taiwan. *Emerging Infectious Diseases, 12*, 703–705.

Cherubin, C. E., & Sapira, J. D. (1993). The medical complications of drug addiction and the medical assessment of the intravenous drug user: 25 Years later. *Annals of Internal Medicine, 119*, 1017–1128.

Coello, R, Jimenez, J., Garcia, M., Arrovo, P., Minguez, D., Fernandez, C., et al. (1994). Prospective study of infection, colonization and carriage of methicillin-resistant *Staphylococcus aureus* in an outbreak affecting 990 patients. *European Journal of Clinical Microbiology & Infectious Diseases, 13*, 74–81.

Cohen, F. L. & Tartasky, D. (1997). Microbial resistance to drug therapy: A review. *American Journal of Infection Control, 25* (1): 51–64.

Cohen, J. (2004). Asia and Africa: On different trajectories? *Science, 304*, 1932–1938.

Cooper, W. C., & Sivin, N. (1973). Man as a medicine: Pharmacological and ritual aspects of traditional therapy using drugs derived from the human body, in Chinese science. In S. N. Nakayama (Ed.), *Explorations of an ancient tradition* (pp. 203–272). Boston: MIT Press.

Coutsoudis, A., Pillay, K., Spooner, E., Kuhn, L., & Coovadia, H. M. (1999). Influence of infant-feeding patterns on early mother-to-child transmission of HIV-I in Durban, South Africa: A prospective cohort study. South African Vitamin A Study Group. *Lancet, 354, 471–476*.

Coutsoudis, A., & Rollins, N. (2003). Breast-feeding and HIV transmission: The jury is still out. *Journal of Pediatric Gastroenterology and Nutrition, 36*, 434–442.

Dayan, G. Y., Ortega-Sanchez, I. R., LeBaron, C. W., Quinlisk, M. P., & The Iowa Measles Response Team (2005). The cost of containing one case of measles: The economic impact on the public health infrastructure—Iowa, 2004. *Pediatrics, 116*, e1–e4.

English, J. F. (1999). Overview of bioterrorism readiness plan: A template for health care facilities. *American Journal of Infection Control, 27*, 468–469.

Favero, M. S., & Bond, W. W. (2001). Chemical disinfection of medical and surgical materials. In S. S. Block (Ed.), *Disinfection, sterilization and preservation* (5th ed., pp. 881–917). Philadelphia, PA: Lippincott Williams & Wilkins.

Fisman, D. (1999). Infectious complications of body piercing. *Clinical Infectious Diseases, 28*, 1340.

Fiumara, N. J., & Eisen, R. (1983). The titivating penile ring. *Sexually Transmitted Diseases, 10,* 43–44.

Food and Drug Administration. (1999/2002). *Guidance for industry: Revised preventive measures to reduce the possible risk of transmission of Creutzfeldt-Jakob disease (CJD) and variant Creutzfeldt-Jakob disease (vCJD) by blood and blood products* (Rev. ed.). Rockville, MD: Food and Drug Administration, Center for Biologics Evaluation and Research. Retrieved August 3, 2006, from http://www.fda.gov/cber/gdlns/cjdvcjd.htm

Fraser, T. G., Stoser, V., Wang, Q., Allen, A., & Zembower, T. R. (2005). Vancomycin and home health care. *Emerging Infectious Diseases, 11,* 1558–1564.

Fried, B., Gracyk, T. K., & Tamang, L. (2004). Food-borne intestinal trematodiasis in humans. *Parasitology Research, 93,* 159–179.

Gajdusek, D. (1979). Le kuru, in Collogue sur les virus lents, organise le 17 Septembre 1978 a Talloires, France. *Collection Fondation Mérieux*: Talloires, France, pp. 25–57.

Garau, J., Xercavins, M., Rodriquez-Carballeria, M., Gomez-Vera, J. R., Coll, I., Vidal, D., et al. (1999). Emergence and dissemination of quinolone-resistant *Escherichia coli* in the community. *Antimicrobial Agents and Chemotherapy, 43,* 2736–2741.

Garfein, R. S., Vlahov, D., Galai, N., Doherty, M. C., & Nelson, K. E. (1996). Viral infections in short-term injection drug users: The prevalence of the hepatitis C, hepatitis B, human immunodeficiency, and human T-lymphotropic viruses. *American Journal of Public Health, 86,* 655–661.

Garner, J. S., & Favero, M. S. (1985). CDC guidelines for handwashing and hospital environmental control. *Infection Control, 7,* 231–243.

Gatrad, A. (1994). Muslim customs surrounding death, bereavement, postmortem examinations and organ transplants. *British Medical Journal, 309,* 521–523.

Gibbs, C., & Gajdusek, D. C. (1978). Subacute spongiform encephalopathies: The transmissible virus dementias. In P. Katzman, R. D. Terry & K. L Bick (Eds.), *Aging* (Vol. 7, pp. 559–576). New York: Raven Press.

Goh, K. T., Ng, S. K., Chan, Y. C., Lim, S. J., & Chua, E. C. (1987). Epidemiological aspects of an outbreak of dengue fever/dengue hemorrhagic fever in Singapore. *Southeast Asian Journal of Tropical Medicine and Public Health, 18,* 295–302.

Greif, J., & Hewitt, W. (1998). The living canvas. *Advance for Nurse Practitioners, 6*(6), 26–31, 82.

Guimard, Y., Bwaka, M. A., Colebunders, R., Calain, P., Massamba, M., De Roo, A., et al. (1999). Organization of patient care during the Ebola hemorrhagic fever epidemic in Kikwit, Democratic Republic of the Congo, 1995. *Journal of Infectious Diseases, 179* (Suppl 1), S268–273

Gupta, A., Nelson, J. M., Barrett, T. J., Tauze, R. V., Rossiter, S. P., Friedman, C. R., et al. (2004). Antimicrobial resistance among *Campylobacter* strains, United States, 1997–2001. *Emerging Infectious Diseases, 10,* 1102–1109.

Hughes, J. M., & Koplan, J. P. (2005). Saving lives through global safe water. *Emerging Infectious Diseases, 11,* 1636–1637.

Information Required in a Premarket Notification Submission, 21 C.F.R. § 807.87.e (2006).

Institute of Medicine, Board on Health Promotion and Disease Prevention. (2004). *Immunization safety review: Vaccine and autism.* Washington, DC: National Academy Press. Retrieved August 3, 2006, from http://www.iom.edu/CMS/3793/4705/20155.aspx.

Isaacs, S. N. (2004). Working safely with vaccinia virus: Laboratory technique and role of vaccinia vaccination. *Methods in Molecular Biology, 269,* 1–14.

Joint Commission on Accreditation of Healthcare Organizations. (2006). *National safety goals. Facts about 2006 national patient safety goals.* Retrieved August 8, 2006, from http://www.jointcommission.org/PatientSafety/NationalPatientSafetyGoals/06_npsg_facts.htm

Joint United Nations Programme on HIV/AIDS. (2006, May). *2006 report on the global AIDS epidemic.* Geneva, Switzerland: Author.

Kamin, M., & Patten, B. M. (1984). Creutzfeldt-Jakob disease: Possible transmission to humans by consumption of wild animal brains. *American Journal of Medicine, 76,* 142–145.

Keiser, J., & Utzinger, J. (2004). Chemotherapy for major food-borne trematodes: A review. *Expert Opinion on Pharmacotherapy, 5,* 1711–1726.

Keiser, J., & Utzinter, J. (2005). Emerging foodborne trematodiasis. *Emerging Infectious Diseases, 11,* 1507–1514.

Kerstiens, B., & Matthys, F. (1999). Interventions to control virus transmission during an outbreak of Ebola hemorrhagic fever: Experience from Kikwit, Democratic Republic of the Congo, 1995. *Journal of Infectious Diseases, 179*(Suppl. 1), S263–267.

Kopecny, E. (1999, December 21). *Antibiotic in poultry feed discontinued—worldwide.* Retrieved August 6, 2006, from http://www.sare.org/htdocs/hypermail/html-home/41-html/0200.html

Kouri, G. P., Gusman, M. G., Bravo, J. R., & Triana, C. (1989). Dengue hemorrhagic fever/dengue shock syndrome: Lessons from the Cuban epidemic, 1981. *Bulletin of the World Health Organization, 67,* 375–380.

Kourtis, A. P., Buteera, S., Ibegbu, C., Belec, L., & Duerr, A. (2003). Breast milk and HIV-1: Vector of transmission or vehicle of protection? *Lancet Infectious Diseases, 3,* 786–793.

Larson, E., & Killien, M. (1982). Factors influencing handwashing behavior of patient care personnel. *American Journal of Infection Control, 10,* 93–99.

Larson, E. L., Early, E., Cloonan, P., Sugrue, S., & Parides, M. (2000). An organizational climate intervention associated with increased handwashing and decreased nosocomial infections. *Behavioral Medicine, 26,* 14–22.

Lashley, F. R. (2006). Transmission and epimioloy of HIV/AIDS: A global view. *Nursing Clinics of North America, 41,* 339–354.

Lau, J. T., Yang, X., Tsui, H. Y., & Kim, J. H. (2005). Impacts of SARS on health-seeking behaviors in general population in Hong Kong. *Preventive Medicine, 41,* 454–462.

Leisure and Cultural Services Department. (2003, March). *Additional precautionary measures at LCSD facilities and functions* (Press Release 27). Retrieved August 1, 2006, from http://www.info.gov.hk/gia/general/200303/27/0327250.htm

Levy, S. B. (2001). Antibacterial household products: Cause for concern. *Emerging Infectious Diseases, 7,* 512–515.

Lewis, F. M., Chernak, E., Goldman, E., Li, Y., Karem, K., Damon, I. K., et al. (2006). Ocular vaccinia infection in laboratory worker, Philadelphia, 2004. *Emerging Infectious Diseases, 12,* 134–137.

Llewelyn, C. A., Hewitt, P. E., Knight, R. S., Amar, K., Cousens, S., & Mackenzie, J., et al. (2004). Possible transmission of variant Creutzfeldt-Jakob disease by blood transfusion. *Lancet, 363,* 417–421.

Lo, J. Y., Tsang, T. H., Leung, Y. H., Yeung, E. Y., Wu, T., & Lim, W. W. (2005). Respiratory infections during SARS outbreak, Hong Kong, 2003. *Emerging Infectious Diseases, 11,* 1738–1741.

Loscalzo, I., Ryan, J., Loscalzo, J., Sarna, A., & Cadag, S. (1995). Tetanus: A clinical diagnosis. *American Journal of Emerging Medicine, 13,* 488–490.

Lun, Z. R., Gasser, R. B., Lai, D. H., Li, A. X. Z., Zhu, X. Q., Uy, X. B., et al. (2005). Clonorchiasis: A key foodborne zoonosis in China. *Lancet Infectious Diseases, 5,* 31–41.

MacCulloch, J. (1925). Cannibalism. In J. Hastings (Ed.), *Encyclopedia of religion and ethics* (pp. 194–209). New York: Charles Scribner's Sons.

MacDonald, M., Crofts, N., & Kaldor, J. (1996). Transmission of hepatitis C virus: Rates, routes and cofactors. *Epidemiologic Reviews, 18,* 137–147.

Mamtani, R., Malhotra, P., Gupta, P. S., & Jain, B. K. (1978). A comparative study of urban and rural tetanus in adults. *International Journal of Epidemiology, 7,* 185–188.

Markon, C. (2000, March 20). *Cholera, diarrhea and dysentery update.* Retrieved August 1, 2006, from http://www.cnr.berkeley.edu/~slist/ns113/msg00096.html

Mathur, D., & Sahoo, A. (1984). Pseudomonas septicaemia following tribal tattoo marks. *Tropical and Geographical Medicine, 36,* 301–302.

Mbori-Ngacha, D., Nduati, R., John, G., Reilly, M., Richardson, B., Mwatha, A., et al. (2001). Morbidity and mortality in breastfed and formula-fed infants of HIV-1-infected women: A randomized clinical trial. *Journal of the American Medical Association, 286,* 2413–2420.

Medical Devices: Adequate Directions for Use, 21 C.F.R. §§ 801.5, 807.87.e (2006).

Merriam-Webster OnLine Dictionary. Retrieved August 01, 2006, from http://www.m-w.com/

Moore, P. S., Marfin, A. A., Quenemoen, L. E., Gessner, B. D., Ayulo, Y. S., Miller, D. S., et al. (1993). Mortality rates in displaced and resident populations off central Somalia during 1992 famine. *Lancet, 341,* 935–938.

Muir J. (2005). Managing to harvest? Perspectives on the potential of aquaculture. *Philosophical Transactions of the Royal Society of London. Series B, Biological Sciences, 360,* 191–218.

Munckhof, W. J., Konstantinos, A., Wamsley, M., Mortlock, M., & Gilpin, C. (2003). A cluster of tuberculosis associated with use of a marijuana water pipe. *International Journal of Tuberculosis and Lung Disease, 7,* 860–865.

Nduati, R., John, G., Mbori-Ngacha, D., Richardson, B., Overbaugh, J., Mwatha, A., et al. (2000). Effect of breastfeeding and formula feeding on transmission of HIV-1: A randomized clinical trial. *Journal of the American Medical Association, 283,* 1167–1174.

National Nosocomial Infections Surveillance. (2004). National Nosocomial Infections Surveillance (NNIS) System Report, data summary from January 1992 through June 2004, issued October 2004. *American Journal of Infection Control, 32,* 470–485.

Nelson, K. E., Celentano, D. D., Eiumtrakol, S., Hoover, D. R., Beyrer, C., Suprasert, S., et al. (1996). Changes in sexual behavior and a decline in HIV infection among young men in Thailand. *New England Journal of Medicine, 335,* 297–303.

Occupational Safety and Health Administration: Bloodborne Pathogens, 56 Fed. Reg. 64004 (1991) (codified at 29 C.F.R. pt. 1910.1030).

Ochsenfahrt, C., Friedl, R., Hannekum, A., & Schumacher, B. A. (2001). Endocarditis after nipple piercing in a patient with a bicuspid aortic valve. *Annals of Thoracic Surgery, 71,* 1365–1366.

Oeltmann, J. E., Oren, E., Haddad, M. B., Lake, L. K., Harrington, T. A., Ijaz, K., et al. (2006). Tuberculosis outbreak in marijuana users, Seattle, Washington, 2004. *Emerging Infectious Diseases, 12,* 1156–1159.

Okie, S. (1999, August 10). Science races to stem TB's threat. *The Washington Post,* pp. A1, A4.

O'Malley, C., Smith, N., Braun, R., & Prevots, D. R. (1998). Tetanus associated with body piercing. *Clinical Infectious Diseases, 27,* 1343–1344.

Ooi, E.-E., Goh, K.-T., & Gubler, D. J. (2006). Dengue prevention and 35 years of vector control in Singapore. *Emerging Infectious Diseases, 12,* 887–893.

Pan American Health Organization. (1994). Dengue and dengue hemorrhagic fever in the Americas: Guidelines for prevention and control. *Scientific Publication, 548,* 3–22.

Pan American Health Organization. (1998). Measles in the Americas, 1997. *EPI Newsletter, 20*(1), 5–6.

Perlman, D. C., Perkins, M. P., Paone, D., Kochems, L., Salomon, N., Friedmann, P., et al. (1997). "Shotgunning" as an illicit drug smoking practice. *Journal of Substance Abuse Treatment, 14,* 3–9.

Peters, C., & LeDuc, J. W. (1999). An introduction to Ebola: The virus and the disease. *Journal of Infectious Diseases, 179*(Suppl. 1), ix–xvi.

Poutanen, S. M., Low, D. E., Henry, B., Finkelstein, S., Rose, D., Green, K., et al. (2003). Identification of severe acute respiratory syndrome in Canada. *New England Journal of Medicine, 348,* 1995–2005.

Prats, G., Mirelis, B., Llovet, T., Munoz, C., Miro, E., & Navaro, F. (2000). Antibiotic resistance trends in enteropathogenic bacteria isolated in 1985–1987 and 1995–1998 in Barcelona. *Antimicrobial Agents and Chemotherapy, 44,* 1140–1145.

Pugatch, D., Mileno, M., & Rich, J. D. (1998). Possible transmission of human immunodeficiency virus type 1 from body piercing. *Clinical Infectious Diseases, 26,* 767–768.

Ramage, I. J., Wilson, N., & Thomson, R. B. (1997). Fashion victim: Infective endocarditis after nasal piercing. *Archives of Disease in Childhood, 77,* 187.

Republic of China Center for Disease Control, Department of Health. (2005). *Reported cases of HIV/AIDS by year in Taiwan 1984–2004.* Retrieved August 8, 2006, from http://www.cc.gov.tw/en/index/asp

Schliessmann, D. J., & Calherios, L. B. (1974). A review of the status of yellow fever and *Aedes aegypti* eradication program sin the Americas. *Mosquito News, 34,* 1–9.

Scott, E. (1999). Hygienic issues in the home. *American Journal of Infection Control, 27,* S22–25.

Seppala, H., Klaukka, T., Vuopio-Varkila, J., Muotiala, A., Helenius, H., Lager, K., et al., for the Finnish Study Group for Antimicrobial Resistance. (1997). The effect of changes in the consumption of macrolide antibiotics on erythromycin resistance in group A streptococci in Finland. *New England Journal of Medicine, 337,* 441–446.

Skowronski, D. M., Petric, M., Daly, P., Parker, R. A., Bryce, E., Doyle, P. W., et al. (2006). Coordinated response to SARS, Vancouver, Canada. *Emerging Infectious Diseases, 12,* 155–158.

Stancliff, S., Salomon, N., Perlamn, D. C., & Russell, P. C. (2000). Provision of influenza and pneumococcal vaccines to injection drug users at a syringe exchange. *Journal of Substance Abuse Treatment, 18,* 263–265.

Stephen, M. (1998). Consuming the dead: A Kleinian perspective on death rituals cross-culturally. *International Journal of Psychoanalysis, 79,* 1173–1194.

Stivers, D. (2002). Participating in decisions about treatment: Overt parent pressure for antibiotic medication in pediatric encounters. *Social Science and Medicine, 54,* 111–130.

Tattooing and Body Piercing of Humans by Nonmedical Personnel for Remuneration, Ky. Rev. Stat. Ann. § 211.760 (2005).

Tattoo and Body Piercing Services, Ohio Administrative Code § 3701-9 (1998).

Tattoo and Body Piercing Services, Ohio Revised Code §§ 3730.01–3730.11 (1997).

Tattooists and Body Piercers, 26 Vt. Stat. Ann. §§ 79-4101–4109. (2004).

Thacker, S. B. (2000). Historical development. In S. T. Teutsch & R. E. Churchill (Eds.), *Principles and practice of public health surveillance* (pp. 1–16). New York: Oxford University Press.

Tice, A. D., Rehm, S. J., Dalovisio, J. R., Bradley, J. S., Martinelli, L. P., Graham, D. R., et al. (2004). Practice guidelines for outpatient parenteral antimicrobial therapy. *Clinical Infectious Diseases, 38,* 1651–1672.

Toole, M. J., & Waldman, R. J. (1993). Refugees and displaced persons. War, hunger, and public health. *Journal of the American Medical Association, 270,* 600–605.

Torres-Muñoz, A. (1995). La fiebre amarilla en México: Erradiacación del *Aëdes aegypti* [Yellow Fever in Mexico: Eradication of *Aëdes aegypti*]. *Salud Pública de México, 37,* S103–110.

Tronel, H., Chaudemanche, H., Pechier, N., Doutrelant, L., & Hoen, B. (2001). Endocarditis due to *Neisseria* mucosa after tongue piercing. *Clinical Microbiology Infection, 7,* 275–276.

Trubatch, B. N., Fisher, D. G., Cagle, H. H., & Fenaughty, A. M. (2000). Vaccination strategies for targeted and difficult-to-access groups. *American Journal of Public Health, 90,* 447.

Tweeten, S., & Rickman, L. S. (1998). Infectious complications of body piercing. *Clinical Infectious Diseases, 26,* 735–740.

Unicomb, L., Ferguson, J., Riley, T. V., & Collignon, P. (2003). Fluoroquinolone resistance in *Campylobacter* absent from isolates, Australia. *Emerging Infectious Diseases, 9,* 1482–1483.

U.S. Government Accountability Office. (1999). *Food safety. The agricultural use of antibiotics and its implications for human health* (GAO/RCED-99-74). Washington, DC: Author.

Wenzel, R. P., & Edmond, M. B. (2001). The impact of hospital-acquired bloodstream infections. *Emerging Infectious Diseases, 7,* 174–177.

Weinstein, R. A. (2001). Controlling antimicrobial resistance in hospitals: Infection control and use of antibiotics. *Emerging Infectious Diseases, 7,* 188–192.

Wiese, E. R. (1930). Semmelweis. *Annals of Medical History, 2,* 80–88.

Wilson, A. A., Crane, L. A., Barrett, P. H., & Gonzales, R. (1999). Public beliefs and use of antibiotics for acute respiratory illness. *Journal of General Internal Medicine, 14,* 658–662.

World Health Assembly. (2003). *Consensus document on the epidemiology of severe acute respiratory syndrome (SARS)* (Report No. WHO/CDS/CSR/GAR/2003.11). Geneva, Switzerland: Author.

World Health Assembly. (2005a). *Application of the international health regulations* (Resolution No. WHA 59.3). Retrieved May 26, 2006, from http://www.who.int/gb/ebwha/pdf_files/WHA59/WHA59_2-en.pdf

World Health Assembly. (2005b). *Revision of the international health regulations* (Resolution No. WHA58.3). Retrieved January 1, 2006, from http://www.who.int/bg/ebwha/pdf_fies/WHA58-REC1/english/Resolutions.pdf

World Health Organization. (1995). *Control of foodborne trematode infections. Report of a WHO study group.* Geneva, Switzerland: Author.

World Health Organization. (2000). *Overcoming antimicrobial resistance, WHO infectious disease report, 2000.* Geneva, Switzerland: Author.

World Health Organization. (2001, January 15). *New data on the prevention of mother-to-child transmission of HIV and their policy implications.* Geneva, Switzerland: Author. Retrieved January 1, 2006, from www.unaids.org/publications/documents/mtct/MTCT_Consultation_Report. doc

World Health Organization. (2003). Consensus document on the epidemiology of severe acute respiratory syndrome (SARS). Report no. WHO/CDS/CSR/GAR/2003. 11. Geneva: The Organization; 2003.

World Health Organization. (2004). *HIV transmission through breastfeeding: A review of available evidence.* Geneva, Switzerland: Author. Retrieved August 4, 2006, from http://www.who.int/child-adolescent-health/New_Publications/NUTRITION/ISBN_92_4_156271_4.pdf

World Health Organization. (2005). *2004 Global immunization data.* Retrieved August 4, 2006, from http://www.who.int/immunization_monitoring/data/GlobalImmunizationData.pdf

World Health Organization Collaborative Study Team on the role of breast-feeding on the prevention of infant mortality. (2000). Effect of breast-feeding on infant and child mortality due to infectious disease in less developed countries: A pooled analysis. *Lancet, 355,* 451–455.

World Health Organization & United Nations Children's Fund. (2005). *Global immunization vision and strategy, 2006–2015.* Geneva, Switzerland: Author. Retrieved January 1, 2006, from http://www.who.int/vaccines/GIVS/english/GIVS_Final_17Oct05.pdf

Yip, F. Y., Papania, M. J., & Redd, S. B. (2004). Measles outbreak epidemiology in the United States, 1993–2001. *Journal of Infectious Diseases, 189*(Suppl. 1), S54–60.

Zimakoff, J., Kjelsberg, A. B., Larsen, S. O., & Holstein, B. (1992). A multicenter questionnaire investigation of attitudes toward hand hygiene, assessed by the staff in fifteen hospitals in Denmark and Norway. *American Journal of Infection Control, 20,* 58–64.

CHAPTER TWENTY-NINE

Into the Future

C. J. Peters

The public health and the research communities have made strides in responding to emerging infectious diseases, but much more needs to be done. These infections deserve our attention because of trends in our modern world that are placing important evolutionary pressures on microbes. Simultaneously we are providing greater opportunities for the infectious agents to emerge locally as well as moving around the world to set up housekeeping in new places.

The combination of changing ecology and travel and transport of organisms is nowhere seen more clearly than in antibacterial resistance (see chapters 2 and 20). The selective forces of widespread antibiotic use have led to the emergence and movement of populations of resistant bacteria carrying the genetic information to elude our therapeutic efforts. Sometimes, the distance traveled is only from one bed to another in the intensive care unit, but in other cases the movement has been worldwide. Even the pneumococcus is now widely resistant to penicillin, denying us the use of the best antibiotic we have ever developed in treating this common and often life-threatening infectious agent. Simultaneously there is a huge genetic pool of bacteria that are not notable human pathogens but that are subject to selection in human and animal reservoirs and may subsequently transfer their genetic material to other bacteria of more direct importance (see chapter 2).

The role of selection is more subtle but not less important in viral diseases. Some chronic or latent viruses such as herpesviruses or polyomaviruses have coevolved with humans and uncommonly cause serious disease in the normal host. Other viruses are transmitted in nature and infect humans as a sideline. These may be important pathogens when transmitted directly from animals to humans, but they also form a pool of agents that can potentially adapt to interhuman transmission, much as viruses such as measles did centuries ago and human immunodeficiency virus (HIV) has done more recently (Fenner, 1970; Gao et al., 1999). Influenza A could be thought of as an avian virus that periodically generates mutants and reassortants that can adapt to human transmission (Hay, 2001). The flow of viruses between different species and within a single species is critically dependent on selection, ecology, and movement of infected hosts. This drama is being played out today as influenza A strains evolve among wild and domestic fowl; they have the capacity to induce a high mortality in humans (about half die) but have not yet evolved to permit ready interhuman transmissibility (chapter 14).

In the evolutionary game, viruses and bacteria have a marked advantage over us vertebrates. Their generation time is measured in hours and not months or decades. In the case of RNA viruses, their polymerase is very inefficient in faithful replication of progeny, and every new burst of infectious agents contains thousands of mutants. Nevertheless, microorganisms must conform to the iron rules of selection, and they evolve stepwise, although bacteria are much more adept at incorporating plasmids or other groups of genes that change their properties. Interestingly, the role of viral mutants in driving the emergence of disease seems to be relatively small, with the exception of influenza and a few other viruses. Mutations are adaptive and allow the viruses to function in changing situations.

IMPORTANCE OF TRAVEL AND TRANSPORT

Another obvious factor is travel by humans with consequent transport of viruses, vectors, and reservoirs. This became a major factor in the 1500s with the age of exploration. Ships began to traverse the oceans with increasing frequency, and travel and exploration further breached intracontinental barriers. In the last quarter century, we have multiplied the number of ships and further accentuated the process with rapid movement by airplanes.

To illustrate the importance of ecology and the mixing effect of travel and transport, let us consider emergences of hazardous virus diseases over the last 5 years such as hantaviruses, Ebola virus, Hendra virus, Nipah virus, severe adult respiratory syndrome (SARS), smallpox, Rift Valley fever virus, and Marburg virus (see Appendix A, Table A.4). The epidemics these diseases cause are often sufficiently dramatic to motivate a reasonable investigation of the inciting circumstances, and these episodes are one of the categories we should be concerned about in the future. They are usually zoonotic viruses transmitted in nature and often are highly hazardous in the laboratory. These viruses will be used to give a framework for examining emerging infections in general, but the lessons from this group apply broadly to most of the emerging pathogens, particularly the viruses.

HANTAVIRUS PULMONARY SYNDROME: SURPRISES FOR MEDICINE

In 1993 a mysterious epidemic of fatal respiratory disease occurred in the southwestern United States. Investigations were at first stymied but soon discarded a toxin explanation and identified a hantavirus as the cause (Ksiazek et al., 1995; Nichol et al., 1993). In spite of the fact that previously known hantaviruses caused hemorrhagic fever with renal syndrome, the mechanisms underlying the pathogenesis of the mystery disease were consonant with those of other hantavirus infections (Ksiazek et al., 1995; Zaki et al., 1995). In fact, with newer diagnostic approaches and awareness of the clinical syndrome, the American hantaviruses were soon found to be numerous and generally to cause hantavirus pulmonary syndrome, or HPS (Peters, 1998). Several hundred cases have now been diagnosed in North, Central, and South America.

Local outbreaks, including the one that led to the initial registration of HPS were usually precipitated by changes in weather conditions. Longitudinal studies of rodent populations and rodent infection in the southwestern United States have shown a close relationship with rainfall, and this has been driven by the climatic changes following El Niño Southern Oscillation (ENSO) events (Mills, Yates, Ksiazek, Peters, & Childs, 1999; Yates, et al., 2002). There are no practical interventions to protect human populations in rural areas other than rodent proofing of homes (see Appendix C, Table C.6).

A second big surprise from the hantavirus story has been the finding that one of the American hantaviruses, Andes virus, caused a large Argentine epidemic with human-to-human transmission (Wells, Sosa Estani, et al., 1997). Indeed, Andes virus has repeatedly been implicated in interhuman spread in both Argentina and Chile. Such transmission has not been seen with any other hantavirus, including Sin Nombre virus in the United States (Wells, Young, et al., 1997).

NIPAH VIRUS, MONOCULTURES, AND SPECIES JUMPING

Both Hendra and Nipah viruses were discovered during relatively recent epidemics (Chua et al., 2000; Murray et al., 1998). They belong to the scientifically venerable virus family Paramyxoviridae but are sufficiently different from known members that they have been assigned to a new genus in that family. Both viruses apparently have their usual life in megachiropterans, also known as fruit-eating bats or flying foxes. In the case of Hendra virus, a limited number of horses and humans have been infected, and the cause of emergence is unknown. Undoubtedly, the movement of flying foxes into suburban sites (possibly related to habitat destruction) facilitated the equine infections, and the unusual disease in a prominent horse trainer caring for a sick racing horse led to increased interest and could well have been important in the discovery.

In the case of Nipah virus, the proximity of flying foxes to a pig-raising industry that had been modernized, resulting in large numbers of animals in close proximity, seemed to be an important factor. Interestingly, the industrialization of pork production not only set the stage for the emergence of Nipah virus through providing dense populations of a monoculture of pigs, but also assisted in disease recognition by improving veterinary observations and recording of the mortality and health status of the animals. Apparently, economic motivations for porcine public health are more readily perceived than those for international human public health.

Movement of pigs between farms (often clandestine) was felt to be a major factor in spread within Malaysia, and export of pigs to Singapore resulted in disease among abattoir workers there. Virus infection was found in humans (who suffered encephalitis with a high case fatality and sometimes severe residua), horses, dogs, and cats. Genetic analyses of the viruses have not yet shown a signature difference between the virus in its natural reservoir and the virus in its new host; in fact, if differences were found they would most probably be adaptive rather than the origin of the epidemics.

Nipah virus is a very dangerous agent with the capabilities to spread directly from pig to pig and to infect several other species. This ability to cross species is unusual, particularly for a paramyxovirus. Presumably, the availability of a dense monoculture of pigs was the event that led to its ability to adapt from its original flying fox host, and the movement of pigs enhanced its spread within Malaysia and elsewhere. The slaughter of more than a million pigs was needed to control the virus, a feat that would have been much more difficult to accomplish expeditiously in a country such as the United States where more environmental and other regulations are in place. Fortunately, the prompt containment prevented the progress of the disease from peninsular Malaysia to the Asian mainland and thence into China, where pigs are a very important part of the economy and the food supply.

FILOVIRUSES AND INTERHUMAN TRANSMISSION

The filoviruses are undoubtedly viruses with a reservoir in nature, but scientists have been unable to find the source of either of the two major viruses, Ebola virus and Marburg virus (see chapter 8). Recently, Ebola viral RNA has been detected in bats in Africa (Leroy et al., 2005), and epidemiological evidence has suggested multiple Marburg infections of persons entering subterranean mines (Bausch et al., 2006), but the issue of the true reservoir remains unsettled. Both have emerged sporadically from their natural cycles and been brought into contact with multiple humans through the intermediary of nonhuman primates or nosocomial spread (Peters & LeDuc, 1999). One operative mechanism is movement of the primates to Europe or the United States for use in vaccine production and/or biomedical research. Another is the poor hygienic standards in African hospitals. Proper barrier nursing was shown to stop Ebola transmission in Zaire in 1995 (Khan et al., 1999), and this experience has been replicated in epidemics in Gabon and South Africa.

The South African experience is particularly relevant to the United States (Richards et al., 2000). A sick physician from Gabon was admitted to a well-equipped hospital, but the diagnosis was not suspected. He underwent extensive workup and was cared for using routine precautions. One of the nurses who was involved in a cut-down procedure became critically ill, and in an attempt to make a diagnosis, samples were sent for testing for Crimean-Congo hemorrhagic fever, an important pathogen in South Africa. The virus laboratory routinely sought all known viral hemorrhagic fever agents in their examinations and unexpectedly diagnosed the nurse with Ebola. Retrospectively, the index case was identified and confirmed by blood serology and virus isolation from semen. The occurrence of only one secondary case even though no special Ebola-related precautions were taken suggests the pattern we would likely see in the United States if Ebola virus were introduced: very limited spread in hospital staff and intimate contacts (Dowell et al., 1999). Of course, if a known Ebola patient were admitted, any hospital would take special precautions, but an attitude of panic would not be justified (Peters, Jahrling, & Khan, 1996).

Thus, the danger of Ebola virus to humans does not lie in its ability to cause lethal, spreading epidemics that would defy control. In contrast to humans, however, Ebola virus seems to have had a major impact on gorilla populations and may well push this already-endangered species into extinction (Leroy et al., 2004). Filoviruses remain important problems because their reservoir is unknown; thus, we have no way to understand the factors underlying their transition into humans. The epidemics that occur when Ebola or Marburg viruses are introduced into the human population are stalking horses for inadequate hygiene in hospitals, reuse of needles and syringes without sterilization which also contribute to emergent hepatitis and HIV transmission, and inadequate surveillance (Peters, 2005). The potential future danger is that failure to terminate chains of transmission could set the stage for genetic adaptation of the virus to interhuman spread.

RIFT VALLEY FEVER AND VECTORBORNE DISEASES

Rift Valley fever virus is a mosquito-borne pathogen of domestic animals and humans in sub-Saharan Africa (Peters, 1997). It first showed its ability for distant spread in 1977 when it caused a major epidemic in Egypt. After dying out there, it recurred in the 1990s. More recently, it has caused a major epidemic in eastern Africa after the inciting ENSO event in 1997–1998 (Linthicum et al., 1999). The waning of that epidemic was followed by an introduction of the virus into the western coast of the Arabian Peninsula (Shoemaker et al., 2002). The extensive animal and human epidemic claimed more than 120 human lives and established once again the ability of this virus to move to new environments (Shope, Peters, & Davies, 1982).

It is of interest to examine some of the worst offenders among the mosquito-borne viruses for factors that predispose to geographical movement. In the cases of urban yellow fever, dengue, and chikungunya viruses, the vector utilized in its transported mode is *Aedes aegypti,* a mosquito that is capable of living with humans whenever they allow standing water to exist in containers, tires, and other receptacles. In these cycles, humans are the relevant vertebrate host (Peters & Dalrymple, 1990). West Nile virus came to North America and found a home with avian vertebrate hosts, and the ubiquitous *Culex pipiens* mosquito transmits the virus (Despommier, 2001). The American togavirus Venezuelan equine encephalitis seems to be evolving to use equines introduced in post-Columbian times as its vertebrate amplifier and to be transmitted by a variety of relatively common mosquito vectors (Weaver, 1998). Rift Valley fever has also acquired new vertebrate amplifying hosts with the introduction and reintroduction of sheep and cattle to Africa. It also has a very broad range of potential mosquito vectors, specifically including common North American mosquitoes (House, Turell, & Mebus, 1992). This would seem to be a versatile and dangerous virus simply awaiting a stochastic event to cause major problems outside Africa.

SARS: PROTOTYPE OF THE "BAD DREAM"

I believe that most experts would predict that among the known microorganisms the most likely emerging virus would be a new influenza A strain and the most likely emerging bacterial pathogen would be a known agent that has acquired toxin and/or antibiotic resistance genes. However, I have believed for some time that the most likely serious emerging pathogen (particularly among the viruses) will be a "new" virus, possibly from a taxon that had not previously been recognized as a threat (e.g., Marburg virus in 1967, Ebola virus in 1976, American hantaviruses in 1993, Nipah and Hendra viruses in the 1990s). Every emerging virus problem has to have two properties: (a) it has to be able to spread, and for a zoonotic virus that means its zoonotic cycle must be efficient, but the far more threatening situation is for the virus be transmitted directly from person to person; and (b) it has to be virulent. As if in answer to these two criteria, a communicable pneumonic disease appeared in southern China in 2002—SARS (chapter 22). The case-fatality rate was about 10%, principally among older or medically compromised persons. The economic impact was measured in the 10s of billions of U.S. dollars as it spread to several countries. The basic reproductive number (R_0) was ~3, indicating that without intervention it was very likely to spread and establish itself as an endemic disease (Dye & Gay, 2003). In spite of some glitches, the international system succeeded in eliminating the disease through personal protective measures. This episode demonstrated the pervasive need for international surveillance to protect people who may feel safe in their North American homes and the unpredictability of the appearance of new RNA viruses. The best reconstruction of what led to the SARS epidemic is that a coronavirus circulated in nature (perhaps one of a newly discovered group) and infected civets held in crowded food markets in southern China; from the civets it spread to market staff and then to others (Li et al., 2004). Phylogenetic studies on isolates from civets and patients from 2002 to 2004 show a pattern of continuing evolution of the virus as it adapts and spreads within the human population. Our ability to identify this virus rapidly depended on a strong coronavirus research base, solid classical virology and pathology, and international cooperation.

SMALLPOX AND THE RETURN OF OLD FOES

It is ironic that the eradication of a virus could be the cause for even greater anxiety than when it was causing extensive human disease. No one would prefer to have smallpox circulating in human populations, but interruption of its obligatory interhuman transmission chain in 1977 led to a cessation of vaccination that has left humans at risk of extensive epidemics should the virus be reintroduced. The revelations that the virus has been used to produce a biological weapon by the former Soviet Union have led to major concerns in the biomedical community. The belief that the Russian military or other countries may possess smallpox and the rise of concern about bioterrorism have led to the conclusion that defenses against smallpox are needed. A susceptible population, inadequate vaccine stocks, rapid and extensive travel, and loss of medical expertise simply make even the remote possibility of a reintroduction unacceptable. Of the viruses discussed, this is the only one with a proven track record of epidemic interhuman spread, and its roughly 30% mortality rate leaves little doubt as to the human and social impact of a smallpox epidemic.

In the context of smallpox, it is worth remembering other high-hazard viruses could be agents of bioterrorism or biological warfare (see chapter 27). Will they be used, and will they show us new faces of some of the viral hemorrhagic fevers and other lethal viruses (Peters, 2000)?

FORECAST FOR THE FUTURE

The last decade has provided many examples of changes in infectious disease patterns. Some emergences are directly related to the increasing pool of immunosuppressed or otherwise compromised hosts in the human population that provide a substrate for the infecting agent. Other infectious diseases do not represent any change of incidence but rather are a consequence of our improved ability to recognize or test for the condition. At first glance, the latter would not seem to be an emergence, but this situation meets the definition of the Institute of Medicine (IOM) for an emerging infectious disease (Lederberg, Shope, & Oaks, 1992). The inclusion of this category as emerging infections is justified because we must go through the same process of evaluation, public health response, education, and research as for other diseases that represent true increases in incidence. HPS provides an excellent example.

GENETIC CHANGE
    plus
ECOLOGIC CHANGE   *equals*   EVOLUTIONARY
    plus   OPPORTUNITIES FOR
TRAVEL OF HUMANS   MICROBIAL PATHOGENS
    AND
TRANSPORT OF
OTHER SPECIES

Figure 29.1. A schema for emerging infections.

Table 29.1. Some Generally Applicable Factors in Emergence

- New diagnostic methods or recognition of a new syndrome can uncover a common disease not previously appreciated (HPS and all its American relatives).
- "New" agents are still being discovered. Some are doing what they have always done (HPS), but others are changing host range and posing completely new threats (Nipah virus, Andes virus, SARS).
- Most of the viruses are not readily spread from person to person, with the exception of the old pathogen smallpox. Some may be a threat to increase their interhuman capability (filoviruses), and some have been truly surprising (Andes hantavirus, SARS).
- In the case of zoonotic diseases, great fluctuations in incidence can occur depending on climatic conditions; ENSO provides one of the driving forces (HPS, Rift Valley fever).
- Local disturbances in land use or agricultural practices may lead to changes in virus, vector, or reservoir circulation (Rift Valley fever, hantaviruses, Nipah virus).
- Changes in human ecology can favor the emergence of diseases (Ebola and Marburg viruses).
- Local and intercontinental movement of viruses is possible and may cause die-off (filoviruses) or protracted transmission (Rift Valley fever).
- Advances in one country can be major setbacks in another (disposable needles and filoviruses).
- Eradication of a disease brings its own problems, including accumulation of susceptibles, deterioration of vaccine stocks, and changing vaccine standards (smallpox, poliomyelitis).
- Vectors and reservoirs can be subject to distant introduction.
- Study of epidemics yields important information.
- Prediction is an important goal but is not yet accurate.

ENSO = El Niño Southern Oscillation; HPS = hantavirus pulmonary syndrome; SARS = severe adult respiratory syndrome.

The most important challenges for the future are agents that attack the normal host. We have made the case that ecological change provides the selective forces to which viruses and their vectors/reservoirs adapt. Furthermore, the rapidly increasing pace of travel and transport increases the occasions for genetically flexible RNA viruses to exploit opportunities arising through ecological shifts (Figure 29.1; Peters, 2001). Some of the factors that are quite generally related to the increasing pace of infectious disease emergence in humans are exemplified in Table 29.1, mainly considering high-hazard virus disease emergence over the last 5–10 years.

The combined impact of ecological change and travel is multiplied; disturbed environments have long been recognized to be the most receptive to introductions of exotic flora and fauna (Elton, 1958; Vitousek, D'Antonio, Loope, & Westbrooks, 1996). If we look at the total impact of humans on the earth through these processes, we find an alarming

Table 29.2. Human Impact on Earth's Ecology

- Half of land surface is transformed by human action.
- Extinction rates of animal species increased 100–1000 times.

  One fourth of bird species are extinct.
  Many fishing areas are depleted, with many actual and threatened extinctions.

- Biological invasions are common.

  Nonnative plants comprise 20% of continental and 50% of island species.
  West Nile virus is the latest recognized viral invasion to North America.
  Foot and mouth disease invaded the United Kingdom and Europe in 2001.
  SARS spread worldwide in 2002–2003.
  H5 influenza A, which is lethal to humans, emerged from Asia in 2003–2006.

- More than one half of all surface freshwater is used by humans.

  98% of U.S. rivers have at least one major dam.
  Two thirds of all Earth's rivers have at least one dam.
  Shortages of clean water are projected for two thirds of Earth's inhabitants in next quarter century.
  WHO identifies more than 1 billion humans without clean water today.

- Humans have impacted climate and weather.

  Global warming is certain.
  How much is anthropogenic?
  Weekly cycle of rainfall off North American coast demonstrates human impact on weather.

- More nitrogen is fixed by humans than all other sources.

  Humans have had a major impact on sulfur, mercury, lead, and other elements.
  DDT, PCB, and other toxic, slowly degraded compounds made by humans are accumulating in the environment and in living organisms.

SARS = severe adult respiratory syndrome; DDT = dichloro-diphenyl-trichloroethane; PCB = polychlorinated biphenyls.
Sources: Adapted from Holland & Peterson, 1995; Leakey & Lewin, 1995; Vitousek et al., 1997.

degree of change (Table 29.2). From space, satellites show us that more than half of the earth's land surface has been modified by human behavior (Vitousek, Mooney, Lubchenco, & Melillo, 1997).

   We are driving extinction of animals and plants at a rate far greater than ever seen before (Leakey & Lewin, 1995). Water, an essential resource, is being usurped extensively by humans, and it is projected that it will become a limited resource in quantity and quality within a decade or two. These changes are clearly documented, without entering controversial areas such as anthropogenic contributions to global warming or hot-button issues such as old growth forests and the rain forest. The extensive use of our planet's bounty leaves less and less room for any mistakes and fewer avenues of remediation. Increasingly, the old adage about "dilution is the solution to pollution" is no longer valid. In 2001, the United States

Table 29.3. Scientific Tools Helpful in Dealing with Infectious Diseases

---

- Molecular biology, immunology
- Genomics, proteomics
- Bioinformatics
- High-throughput gene chip technology
- Advances in study of veterinary, wildlife, and human diseases
- Remote sensing

---

came face to face with power shortages on the West Coast; increasing hydroelectric power from the northwestern states to alleviate this problem would result in further ecological modifications and additional pressure on endangered species.

The lack of flexible alternatives will become increasingly problematic as world population forces more dependence on modern intensive agriculture. Intensive cultivation of plants and animals will lead to situations in which a single genetically homogenous species will be grown in a limited area, making a perfect target for emerging diseases. This situation has been recognized since the Irish potato famine and amply documented subsequently.

The modification of centuries-old practices of rice growing and irrigation in the island ecosystem of Bali provides an instructive example (Lansing, 1991). In an attempt to increase the production of rice, "green" rice strains and intensive water—fertilizer regimens were introduced. The changes in planting and irrigation practices led to eruptions of pests and the need for intensive pesticide use. Water supplies became inadequate, and the distribution of water was skewed. Crops underwent cycles of infection by fungi and viruses and required repeated introductions of resistant rice strains. This type of problem may be soluble and might lead to increased food production in the long run, but it is sure to introduce vulnerabilities to agricultural diseases. The 2001 outbreak of foot and mouth disease in England and its rapid spread only serve to emphasize the impact of agricultural diseases in today's mobile, intensive food production industry.

If we are going to deal successfully with the increasing amount of change and the accelerating rate of change, we need both local action and technology. Technology (Table 29.3) has given us powerful tools in the struggle, but many of these approaches now are used in a reductionist fashion. For example, molecular biology today often focuses on the individual organism or gene. We need to emphasize, however, the power of integrative approaches in which we use molecular biology to follow the movement of genes and the structure of complex organisms and ecological systems. Genomics so far has been about one genome from a species and not a population of genomes interacting with populations of other species'

Table 29.4. Recognition of Emerging Human Diseases Is Critically Dependent on Local Health Care Services

---

- Competent and alert health care providers
- Pathologists and autopsies
- Routine clinical diagnostic laboratories to identify the usual disease offenders
- Public health institutions to collate information and compare it
- Background surveillance data
- Public health microbiology laboratory backup
- Access to reference capability (clinicians, pathologists, microbiology laboratory, and other expertise) for unusual or complex problems

---

genomes and an environment. Hopefully, in the future high-throughput gene chip technology will lead to an increased capacity to survey for multiple genetic sequences in emerging diseases and to also correlate complex genetic events in hosts and pathogens. As noted in the Bali example, we also have to bear in mind some of the unintended consequences of technology.

The local action needed to recognize emerging infections is fairly well understood (Table 29.4; Peters, 2001; Peters, in press). Indeed, these activities are primarily those of a good health care system and a well-supported public health infrastructure. This is perhaps unfortunate because it might be easier to mobilize the global community for some sort of specialized technological project than to attempt to improve activities that we already know are in various degrees of trouble.

In spite of the positive features in our struggle against infectious diseases, there are some real obstacles. We show no sign of taking important steps to stabilize the world's ecological change or the population growth that is a major driving force for ecological change. The warning call on emerging infections was issued from an IOM committee headed by Joshua Lederberg and Robert Shope (Lederberg et al., 1992). Ten years later, Lederberg and Margret Hamburg headed a committee that revisited the issue (Smolinski, Hamburg, & Lederberg, 2003). The conclusions were not optimistic; the problems seen and foreseen in the first report were largely unameliorated, and indeed the feeling of the committee was that the interactions among the factors leading to emergence were enhancing the danger (Peters, in press).

Bioterrorism and biological warfare are wild cards; will they be used more extensively than merely anthrax spores placed in a few letters? Now that the barrier has been broken and someone with the obvious capability of preparing a dry powder with the very dangerous particle size and aerosol properties of the October 2001 attack is involved, we can most assuredly expect further attempts with anthrax. The former Soviet Union

Table 29.5. Elements for Dealing with Emergence That are Absent From the World Stage

---

- Adequate public health and curative health infrastructure in most countries in the world
- Will to improve public and curative health infrastructure in all countries in the world
- Enough resources and international cooperation for adequate global surveillance
- Research designed to elucidate more of the principles underlying emergence
- Ability to make practical vaccines for human use
- Balanced regulatory atmosphere to facilitate responses to threats

---

prepared literally tons of infectious agents such as tularemia, plague, smallpox virus, and Marburg virus. Massive dissemination of these agents could lead to new patterns of infectious disease distribution (Peters, 2000).

We are faced with critical deficits in a number of areas (Table 29.5), and their reversal is not likely. I think those of us working in the arena of emerging infections are going to be in business for a long time (Peters, in press).

REFERENCES

Bausch, D. G., Nichol, S. T., Muyembe, J. J., Borchert, M., Rollin, P. E., Sleurs, H., et al. (2006). Marburg hemorrhagic fever associated with multiple genetic lineages of virus. *New England Journal of Medicine, 355,* 909–919.

Chua, K. B., Bellini, W. J., Rota, P. A., Harcourt, B. H., Temin, A., Lam, S. K., et al. (2000). Nipah virus: A recently emergent deadly paramyxovirus. *Science, 288,* 1432–1435.

Despommier, D. (2001). *West Nile story.* New York: Apple Trees Productions.

Dowell, S. F., Mukunu, R., Ksiazek, T. G., Khan, A. S., Rollin, P. E., Peters, C. J., et al. (1999). Transmission of Ebola hemorrhagic fever: A study of risk factors in family members, Kikwit, Democratic Republic of the Congo, 1995. *Journal of Infectious Diseases, 179*(Suppl. 1), S87–91.

Dye, C., & Gay, N. (2003). Modeling the SARS epidemic. *Science, 300,* 1884–1885.

Elton, C. S. (1958). *The ecology of invasions by animals and plants.* London: Methuen.

Fenner, F. (1970). The impact of civilization on the biology of man. In S. V. Boyden (Ed.), *The impact of civilization on the biology of man* (pp. 122–147). Canberra: Australian National University Press.

Gao, F., Bailes, E., Robertson, D. L., Chen, Y., Rodenburg, C. M., Michael, S. F., et al. (1999). Origin of HIV-1 in the chimpanzee *Pan troglodytes troglodytes. Nature, 397,* 436–441.

Hay, A. J. (2001). Potential of influenza A viruses to cause pandemics. In W. L. Irving, J. W. McCauley, D. J. Rowlands, & G. L. Smith (Eds.), *New challenges to health: The threat of virus infection, 60th Symposium of the Society for General Microbiology* (pp. 89–104). Cambridge, UK: Cambridge University Press.

Holland, H. D., & Petersen, U. (1995). *Living dangerously: The earth, its resources, and the environment.* Princeton, NJ: Princeton University Press.

House, J. A., Turell, M. J., & Mebus, C. A. (1992). Rift Valley fever: Present status and risk to the Western Hemisphere. *Annals of the New York Academy of Sciences, 653,* 233–242.

Khan, A. S., Tshioko, F. K., Heymann, D. L., Le Guenno, B., Nabeth, P., Kerstiens, B., et al. (1999). The reemergence of Ebola hemorrhagic fever, Democratic Republic of the Congo, 1995. *Journal of Infectious Diseases, 179*(Suppl. 1), S76–86.

Ksiazek, T. G., Peters, C. J., Rollin, P. E., Zaki, S., Nichol, S., Spiropoulou, C., et al. (1995). Identification of a new North American hantavirus that causes acute pulmonary insufficiency. *American Journal of Tropical Medicine and Hygiene, 52,* 117–123.

Lansing, J. S. (1991). *Priests and programmers. Technologies of power in the engineered landscape of Bali.* Princeton, NJ: Princeton University Press.

Leakey, R., & Lewin, R. (1995). *The sixth extinction.* New York: Anchor/Doubleday.

Lederberg, J., Shope, R. E., & Oaks, S. (1992). *Emerging microbial threats.* Washington, DC: U.S. National Academy of Science Press.

Leroy, E. M., Kumulungui, B., Pourrut, X., Rouquet, P., Hassanin, A., Yaba P., et al. (2005). Fruit bats as reservoirs of Ebola virus. *Nature, 438,* 575–576.

Leroy, E. M., Rouquet, P., Formenty, P., Souquiere, S., Kilbourne, A., Froment, J. M., et al. (2004). Multiple Ebola virus transmission events and rapid decline of central African wildlife. *Science, 303,* 387–390.

Li, W., Wong, L., Li, F., Kuhn, F. J., Huang, I., Choe, H., et al. (2004). Animal origins of the severe acute respiratory syndrome coronavirus: Insight from ACE2—S-protein interactions. *Journal of Virology, 303,* 387–390.

Linthicum, K. J., Anyamba, A., Tucker, C. J., Kelley, P. W., Myers, M. F., & Peters, C. J. (1999). Climate and satellite indicators to forecast Rift Valley fever epidemics in Kenya. *Science, 285,* 397–400.

Mills, J. N., Yates, T. L., Ksiazek, T. G., Peters, C. J., & Childs, J. E. (1999). Long-term studies of hantavirus reservoir populations in the southwestern United States. Rationale, potential, and methods. *Emerging Infectious Diseases, 5,* 95–101.

Murray, K., Eaton, B., Hooper, P., Wang, L., Williamson, M., & Young, P. (1998). Flying foxes, horses, and humans: A zoonosis caused by a new member of the *Paramyxoviridae.* In W. M. Scheld, D. Armstrong, & J. M. Hughes (Eds.), *Emerging infections 1* (pp. 43–58). Washington, DC: ASM Press.

Nichol, S. T., Spiropoulou, C. F., Morzunov, S., Rollin, P. E., Ksiazek, T. G., Feldmann, H., et al. (1993). Genetic identification of a hantavirus associated with an outbreak of acute respiratory illness. *Science, 262,* 914–917.

Peters, C. J. (1997). Emergence of Rift Valley fever. In J. F. Saluzzo & B. Dodet (Eds.), *Factors in the emergence of arbovirus diseases* (pp. 253–264). Paris: Elsevier.

Peters, C. J. (1998). Hantavirus pulmonary syndrome in the Americas. In W. M. Scheld, W. A. Craig, & J. M. Hughes (Eds.), *Emerging infections 2* (pp. 17–64). Washington, DC: ASM Press.

Peters, C. J. (2000). Are hemorrhagic fever viruses practical agents for biological terrorism? In W. M. Scheld, W. A. Craig, & J. M. Hughes (Eds.), *Emerging infections 4* (pp. 203–211). Washington, DC: ASM Press.

Peters, C. J. (2001). The viruses in our past, the viruses in our future. In G. L. Smith, W. L. Irving, J. W. McCauley, & D. J. Rowlands (Eds.), *New challenges to health: The threat of virus infection, 60th Symposium of the Society for General Microbiology* (pp. 1–32). Cambridge, UK: Cambridge University Press.

Peters C. J. (2005). Marburg and Ebola—Arming ourselves against the deadly filoviruses. *New England Journal of Medicine, 352,* 2571–2573.

Peters, C. J. (in press). Emerging virus diseases. In D. M. Knipe & P. M. Howley (Eds.), *Field's virology.* Philadelphia: Lippincott, Williams & Wilkins.

Peters, C. J., & Dalrymple, J. M. (1990). Alphaviruses. In B. N. Fields & D. M. Knipe (Eds.), *Virology* (pp. 713–761). New York: Raven Press.

Peters, C. J., Jahrling, P. B., & Khan, A. S. (1996). Management of patients infected with high-hazard viruses: Scientific basis for infection control. *Archives of Virology* (Suppl. 11), 1–28.

Peters, C. J., & LeDuc, J. W. (1999). An introduction to Ebola: The virus and the disease. *Journal of Infectious Diseases, 179*(Suppl. 1), ix–xvi.

Richards, G. A., Murphy, S., Jobson, R., Mer, M., Zinman, C., Taylor, R., et al. (2000). Unexpected Ebola virus in a tertiary setting: Clinical and epidemiologic aspects. *Critical Care Medicine, 28,* 240–244.

Shoemaker, T., Boulianne, C., Vincent, M. J., Pezzanite, L., Al-Qahtani, M. M., Al-Mazrou, Y., et al. (2002). Genetic analysis of viruses associated with emergence of Rift Valley fever in Saudi Arabia and Yemen, 2000–01. *Emerging Infectious Diseases, 12,* 1415–1420.

Shope, R. E., Peters, C. J., & Davies, F. G. (1982). The spread of Rift Valley fever and approaches to its control. *Bulletin of the World Health Organization, 60,* 299–304.

Smolinski, M. S., Hamburg, M. A., & Lederberg, J. (Eds.). (2003). Microbial threats to health: emergence, detection, and response. Report of the Committee on Emerging Microbial Threats to Health in the 21st Century, Institute of Medicine of the National Academies. Washington DC: National Academies Press.

Vitousek, P. M., D'Antonio, C. M., Loope, L. L., & Westbrooks, R. (1996). Biological invasions as global environmental change. *American Scientist, 8,* 468–478.

Vitousek, P. M., Mooney, H. A., Lubchenco, J., & Melillo, J. M. (1997). Human domination of Earth's ecosystems. *Science, 277,* 494–499.

Weaver, S. C. (1998). Recurrent emergence of Venezuelan equine encephalomyelitis. In W. M. Scheld, D. Armstrong, & J. M. Hughes (Eds.), *Emerging Infections 1* (pp. 27–42). Washington, DC: ASM Press.

Wells, R. M., Sosa Estani, S., Yadon, Z. E., Enria, D., Padula, P., Pini, N., et al. (1997). An unusual hantavirus outbreak in southern Argentina. Person-to-person transmission? *Emerging Infectious Diseases, 3,* 171–174.

Wells, R. M., Young, J., Williams, R. J., Armstrong, L. R., Busico, K., Khan, A. S., et al. (1997). Hantavirus transmission in the United States. *Emerging Infectious Diseases, 3,* 361–365.

Yates, T. L., Mills, J. N., Parmenter, C. A., Ksiazek, T. G., Parmenter, R. R., Vande Castle, J. R., et al. (2002). The ecology and evolutionary history of an emergent disease: Hantavirus pulmonary syndrome. *Bioscience, 52,* 989–998.

Zaki, S. R., Greer, P. W., Coffield, L. M., Goldsmith, C. S., Noted, K. B., Foucar, K., et al. (1995). Hantavirus pulmonary syndrome: Pathogenesis of an emerging infectious disease. *American Journal of Pathology, 146,* 552–579.

Appendices

Emerging/Reemerging Infectious Diseases by Organism

Felissa R. Lashley

Table A.1. Examples of Emerging/Reemerging Bacteria*

Bacteria	Major Disease(s)	Comments
Anaplasma phagocytophilum	Human granulocytic anaplasmosis	Identified during 1992–1993 outbreak in Midwest. Formerly known as *Ehrlichia* spp., causing human granulocytic ehrlichiosis. Is a tickborne rickettsiae. Can rarely be transmitted by transfusion. Causes fever, chills, myalgia, headache, and malaise, with rash not usual. Ranges in severity. Can include shock-like syndrome. See chapter 16.
Bartonella clarridgeiae	Cat scratch disease	Identified only recently as a human pathogen. Described in 1995. Found in cats. Can cause cat scratch disease.
Bartonella elizabethae	Endocarditis, bacteremia	Identified as a new species in 1993. Formerly called *Rochalimaea*. Associated with exposure to rats, especially among the homeless or injecting drug users. See chapter 3.
Bartonella grahamii	Endocarditis	Identified recently as a rare human pathogen.

(continued)

Table A.1. *(continued)*

Bacteria	Major Disease(s)	Comments
Bartonella henselae	Bacillary angiomatosis (BA), cat scratch disease, bacteremia, endocarditis, peliosis	Causes cat scratch disease. BA first described in persons with AIDS in 1987. Also causes relapsing fever and endocarditis. The cat is a major reservoir. Children and persons with HIV disease are most susceptible to cat scratch disease. See chapter 3.
Bartonella koehlerae	Endocarditis	Very rare in humans. First case in humans reported in 2004. Cats are a major reservoir.
Bartonella quintana	BA, trench fever, endocarditis, peliosis, bacteremia	BA occurs almost exclusively in immunocompromised persons. BA lesions may be multifocal and highly vascular. Peliosis usually occurs in the immunosuppressed. See chapter 3.
Bartonella vinsonii	Endocarditis	Rare in humans. Has two subspecies. Dogs are an important reservoir.
Bartonella washoensis	Myocarditis	Very rare in humans.
Borrelia burgdorferi	Lyme disease	Recognized in 1978 in Lyme, CT. Transmitted to humans via deer ticks. Can have severe chronic sequelae. Characterized by a skin lesion known as erythema migrans, which appears in about 60% at the site of the tick bite. Other symptoms may include rash, malaise, headache, chills, fever, backache, arthralgia, and myalgia. Later effects may include arthritis and neurological and cardiac manifestations. See chapter 16.
Burkholderia (formerly *Pseudomonas*) *pseudomallei*	Melioidosis	Endemic in Thailand and Guam, and now present in India, the Caribbean, Australia, and Malaysia. Considered a tropical disease. Most persons develop inapparent infection that may be latent, appearing after many years when the person is immunosuppressed. May cause parotid abscess in children and acute septicemia, a neurologic syndrome, or suppuration in the liver or other organ in adults. Persons with cystic fibrosis who travel may be especially susceptible. Considered by some to be reemerging because of geographic spread and antimicrobial resistance, especially to aminoglycosides and most β-lactams.

Table A.1. *(continued)*

Bacteria	Major Disease(s)	Comments
Campylobacter jejuni	Enteritis	A zoonotic infection. Became recognized as a human pathogen in the 1970s. Symptoms include fever, diarrhea (watery or bloody), and abdominal pain. Trigger for Guillain–Barré syndrome.
Chlamydophila (formerly *Chlamydia*) *pneumoniae*	Association with coronary heart disease, pharyngitis, bronchitis, sinusitis, and pneumonia	Considered emerging in context of its association with coronary heart disease. In 1983 was recognized in connection with pneumonia, pharyngitis, and other infections. See chapter 24.
Clostridium histolyticum	Soft tissue inflammation and infection	Outbreak in 2003–2004 among injecting drug users.
Clostridium novyi	Soft tissue inflammation and infection	Outbreak in April 2000 of unexplained illness and deaths in injecting drug users in Great Britain. High mortality rate.
Corynebacterium diphtheriae	Diphtheria	Reemerging in places where public heath systems are in disarray such as the former Soviet Union states. Vaccine preventable. Uncommon forms such as cutaneous diphtheria seen mostly in immigrants to developed countries.
Ehrlichia chaffeensis	Human monocytic ehrlichiosis	Recognized in 1987. Are rickettsiae. Transmitted by ticks and also transfusion, rarely. Illness ranges in severity from mild to severe. Fever, headache, chills, myalgia, malaise with nausea, vomiting, and anorexia. Rash occurs in 20–35%. Multiorgan failure can occur. See chapter 16.
Ehrlichia ewingii	Ehrlichiosis	Identified in patients from Missouri beginning in 1996. Tickborne rickettsiae. Presentation includes fever, headache, and thrombocytopenia. Clinical disease can be identical to that of *E. chaffeensis* or human granulocytic anaplasmosis. See chapter 16.
Ehrlichia sennetsu	Illness similar to mononucleosis	First reported in 1985. Found in Japan and Malaysia.
Enterobacter sakazakii	Meningitis, septicemia, necrotizing enterocolitis	Gram-negative bacillus. Occurs mostly in infants, especially those who are premature or low-birth weight. Few cases in adults. Powdered infant formula has been epidemiologically linked to cases. High fatality rate (40–80%).

(continued)

Table A.1. *(continued)*

Bacteria	Major Disease(s)	Comments
Enterococcus faecalis	Vancomycin-resistant nosocomial surgical infections	Gastrointestinal (GI) tract and skin are reservoirs. Accounts for about 15–18% of vancomycin-resistant enterococci (VRE) infections. See chapter 2.
Enterococcus faecium	Vancomycin-resistant nosocomial surgical infections	Same reservoirs as above. Accounts for 80–85% of VRE infections. See chapter 2.
Escherichia coli O157:H7	Diarrheal illness, hemolytic uremic syndrome	First recognized in outbreak in the early 1980s. Foodborne illness associated with several vehicles including alfalfa sprouts, ground beef, unpasteurized apple juice, and others. Can be waterborne. See chapter 9.
Helicobacter pylori	Peptic ulcer disease, gastritis, mucosa-associated lymphoid tissue gastric lymphoma, gastric adenocarcinoma	Was isolated in 1982 and given its present name in 1989. Has been designated as a class I carcinogen by the WHO. See chapter 24.
Legionella pneumophila	Legionnaires disease (LD), Pontiac fever	LD recognized after infection occurred in attendees at an American Legion convention in Philadelphia in July 1976. May be associated with travel-related infections and spray from such sources as spas and others. Causes pneumonia. See chapters 3 and 15.
Leptospira spp. *L. interrogans,* *L. borgpeter-senii,* *L. weillei, and others*	Leptospirosis	Zoonotic disease of worldwide distribution. Results from exposure to infected animal urine directly or indirectly through contaminated soil or water. Can penetrate skin or mucous membranes. More usual in children and young adult men related to occupational exposure. Is considered reemerging due to outbreaks in Nicaragua (1995) and U.S. travelers to Costa Rica (1996) from contaminated river water during white-water rafting. Two types of illness: one with mild febrile illness without jaundice, and one with jaundice, fever, chills, headache, rash, myalgia, conjunctivitis, and prostration. Icteric form

Table A.1. *(continued)*

Bacteria	Major Disease(s)	Comments
		may have hepatic dysfunction, renal insufficiency, and hemorrhage. Can develop complications (including pulmonary, conjunctival, and GI) and central nervous system (CNS) involvement. See chapter 3.
Listeria monocytogenes	Listeriosis	Gram-positive bacteria only recently considered as causing GI disease, diarrhea, nausea, vomiting, abdominal cramps, and often fever. Most cases of listeriosis occur in immunocompromised persons, the elderly, or pregnant women. Typical illness manifestations are flu-like symptoms, sepsis, or CNS illness. Frequent contaminated foods include deli meats and soft cheeses. See chapter 3.
Mycobacterium avium complex	Pulmonary and disseminated disease in persons with human immun-odeficiency virus (HIV) disease	Ubiquitous soil and water bacteria considered emerging because of the increase in persons with HIV disease. May also affect the GI tract, causing diarrhea, malabsorption, and abdominal pain. Disseminated disease is usually seen in persons with CD4 counts <50 mm^3.
Mycobacterium celatum	Pulmonary and disseminated disease in persons with HIV disease	Usually found in immunosuppressed persons such as those with HIV disease.
Mycobacterium goodii	See comments	Wound infections associated with surgical implants, cellulitis, osteomyelitis, and bursitis.
Mycobacterium genavense	Disseminated disease in patients with HIV disease	Described first in 1990. Accounts for about 13% of disseminated mycobacterial infections in Switzerland. Manifestations include diarrhea, pain, weight loss, fever, anemia, pancytopenia, and hepatosplenomegaly.
Mycobacterium haemophilum	Cutaneous, pulmonary, and disseminated disease; arthritis; osteomyelitis	Usually found in immunosuppressed persons such as those with HIV disease. Described in 1978. Cause of syndrome consisting of a dermatitis and necrotizing painful skin lesions in immunocompetent and

(continued)

Table A.1. *(continued)*

Bacteria	Major Disease(s)	Comments
		immunosuppressed persons who also may have joint infections. Reservoir is unknown. Considered emerging by virtue of increasing infection rates and increase in geographic distribution.
Mycobacterium kansasii	Pulmonary and disseminated disease	Usually found in persons with HIV disease. Considered emerging in that context.
Mycobacterium marinum	Skin lesions	Causes skin nodules or small ulcers on extremities that can take years to heal. May result in some scarring. May disseminate in the immunosuppressed. Transmitted through contaminated water including aquariums. May result following skin abrasions. Emerging by virtue of increasing rates of infection.
Mycobacterium tilburgii	See comments	Found in a few patients with HIV and nonimmunosuppressed persons. Causes GI manifestations. Very rare. Name is proposed.
Mycobacterium tuberculosis	See comments	The extensively drug-resistant XDR-TB strain is resistant to virtually all second-line TB drugs and is emerging in rural South Africa. See chapter 20 for MDR-TB.
Mycobacterium ulcerans	Buruli ulcer	Reservoir is unknown. Primarily in children. Necrotic skin ulcers. Infections may be linked to environmental disturbances such as flooding in Uganda and the use of recycled sewage water to irrigate a golf course in Australia. Scarring during healing. Frequently results in deformities including contracture. Becoming third most prevalent mycobacterial disease.
Mycobacterium wolinskyi	Wound infections	Very rare. Isolated from facial abscess and post-open heart surgery wound infection.
Mycoplasma penetrans	Antiphospholipid syndrome	Has been more frequently described in persons with HIV infection but affects others as well. Characterized by hemocytopenic and vaso-occlusive manifestations, pulmonary and neurologic manifestations including stroke, and myelitis.

Table A.1. *(continued)*

Bacteria	Major Disease(s)	Comments
Rhodococcus equi	Pneumonia most common	First human case reported in 1967 in a person receiving steroids for hepatitis. Most cases occur in persons with AIDS and CD4 counts <200 mm^3. Is considered emerging because of the increase in cases. Extrapulmonary infections can occur, particularly brain and renal abscesses, and osteomyelitis.
Staphylococcus aureus (toxin-producing strains)	Toxic shock syndrome	In 1978, toxic shock syndrome in healthy young women (especially 15–19 years of age) was identified. After a peak in 1980, cases have markedly declined. The illness was associated with the menstrual cycle and rise of superabsorbent tampons and vaginal infection followed by toxin production leading to the syndrome. Nonmenstrually associated cases can occur in both sexes. See chapter 3. Strains are becoming resistant to methicillin and vancomycin (see chapter 2).
Staphylococcus lugdunensis	Abscesses, meningitis, device-related infections, endocarditis	In the past 10 years has been implicated in community-acquired and nosocomial infections.
Stenotrophomonas (formerly *Xanthomonas*) *maltophilia*	Endocarditis, sepsis	This gram-negative bacterium is considered an emerging nosocomial pathogen in immunocompromised people. Its increase is attributed to more immunocompromised hospitalized patients and use of antimicrobial agents. Sources include ice machines and prepackaged salads.
Streptococcus pyogenes	Fasciitis, toxic shock syndrome	Emergence of invasive Group A streptococcal infections in the mid-1980s. See chapter 3.
Streptococcus suis	Septicemia, toxic shock syndrome, arthritis, meningitis, endocarditis	Usually infects pigs with sporadic cases in humans. Large human outbreak occurred in July 2005 in China with about 215 cases identified.

(continued)

Table A.1. *(continued)*

Bacteria	Major Disease(s)	Comments
Vibrio cholerae	Cholera	Cholera is an old disease causing severe diarrheal illness, but the seventh cholera pandemic began in Indonesia in 1961, caused by the *V. cholerae* O1 serogroup, El Tor biotype. The organism is curved and gram negative. In 1992, *V. cholerae* O139 was identified in India. Epidemic cholera appeared in Latin America in 1991 after nearly 100 years of absence. Characterized by "rice water" diarrheal stools. See chapter 4.
Vibrio parahaemolyticus	Gastroenteritis	Rare outbreaks before 1997. In 1998, the first outbreak of serotype O3:K6 occurred in the United States when 416 persons developed gastroenteritis from eating oysters from Galveston Bay in Texas. In 2006, a multistate outbreak resulted from consumption of raw and undercooked seafood from Oregon and Washington.
Vibrio vulnificus	See comments	Emergence reported in 1979. Infections usually result from consumption of shellfish, especially raw oysters from the Gulf of Mexico. An increase is seen in the summer. Infection can result in septicemia with bulbous skin lesions, shock, and rapid death. Persons with iron overload such as hemochromatosis are especially vulnerable. In 2006, cases reported from Rhode Island and Germany as wound infections, especially in those with some immunosuppression.
Yersinia pseudotuberculosis	See comments	Considered as an emerging infection in patients with HIV and causing septicemia in a few cases.

Sources: Boulouis et al., 2005; Bowen & Braden, 2006; Braden, 2006; Brazier et al., 2004; Buller et al., 1999; Centers for Disease Control and Prevention, 2000; Chomel et al., 2006; Dance, 2000; Dobos, Quinn, Ashford, Horsbaugh, & King, 1999; Drudy, Mullane, Quinn, Wall, & Fanning, 2006; French, Benator, & Gordin, 1997; Guerrant, et al., 2006; IARC Working Group on the Evaluation of Carcinogenic Risks To Humans, 1994; Looney, 2005; Paglia et al., 2005; Parola et al., 2005; Pechère et al., 1995; Pepin, 2006; Qureshi, 2005; Seifert, Oltmanns, Becker, Wisplinghoff, & von Eiff, 2005; Singh et al., 2007; Strickland, 2000; Török, 2007; "*Vibrio parahaemolyticus*," 2006; "*Vibrio vulnificus*," 2006; Wagner et al., 2006; Wormser et al., 2006; Yáñez, et al., 1999; Yu et al., 2006;

*See Appendix B, Table B.3, for rickettsioses since they are tickborne.

Table A.2. Selected Emerging/Reemerging Fungal Pathogens*

Organism	Disease	Comments
Aspergillus spp. such as A. *flavus* A. *fumigatus* A. *niger* A. *terreus*	Aspergillosis	Are common ubiquitous, filamentous fungi found in soil and decaying organic matter. Usually affect immunosuppressed persons, especially if neutropenic or on corticosteroid therapy. Affected persons often have hematological disease. Portal of entry is usually respiratory tract. Most common cause of nosocomial fungal pneumonia. Symptoms include pleuritic chest pain, fever, dyspnea, and cough. May disseminate as well as cause severe pulmonary disease.
Candida spp. such as C. *albicans* C. *famata* C. *glabrata* C. *guillier-mondii* C. *kefyr* C. *krusei* C. *lusitaniae* C. *norvegensis* C. *parapsilosis* C. *rugosa* C. *stellatoidea* C. *tropicalis*	Candidiasis	Is a yeast. Formerly considered of minor importance in relation to mucosal surfaces. Increasing in frequency as a nosocomial infection. Most invasive mycosis in developed countries, and one of the leading invasive fungi infections in hospitalized patients. Increased awareness of pathogenicity of non-albicans species. Increase in both superficial and systemic *Candida* infections, especially in those who are immunosuppressed or have medical devices. Can affect oropharynx, eye, esophagus, vagina, and anorectal area and can disseminate.
Cryptococcus gattii	Cryptococcosis	Mostly thought to be restricted to tropical climates. Recently affected previously healthy people on Vancouver Island. Causes pulmonary and neurological disease. Also found in other parts of British Columbia, Washington and Oregon.
Cryptococcus neoformans	Cryptococcal disease	Is an encapsulated yeast found in soil, especially if contaminated with pigeon or chicken droppings, causing disease in both the immunocompetent and immunosuppressed. Overall incidence has increased greatly due to the numbers of human immunodeficiency virus (HIV)-infected persons and transplant recipients. Usually enters through respiratory tract, causing pulmonary disease. May disseminate to extrapulmonary sites. Often causes meningitis and, less commonly, disease in

(continued)

Table A.2. *(continued)*

Organism	Disease	Comments
		nearly any tissue especially joints, oral cavity, skin lesions, pericardium, myocardium, and genitourinary tract. Various varieties and serotypes are known with specific predilections.

Fusarium spp. such as
  F. moniliforme
  F. solani
	Fusariosis	Are common filamentous fungi inhabiting soil. Acquire infection usually by inhalation, direct inoculation, or ingestion of toxin. Are considered representative of emerging hyaline molds. Their toxins are potentially lethal and are monitored in crops. Immunosuppressed persons with neutropenia are most vulnerable. Cause respiratory, skin lesions, paronychia, disseminated infection, and chronic liver infection. Portals of entry may be through catheters, lungs, sinuses, and periunguinal areas. Responsible for outbreak of keratitis in contact lens wearers who used Bausch and Lomb ReNu MoistureLOC solution in 2005–2006.

Penicillium marneffei	Penicillinosis	Most prevalent among HIV-infected persons. In Southeast Asia is considered an acquired immunodeficiency syndrome (AIDS)-indicator disease. Also found in HIV-negative people who traveled in endemic areas such as Thailand, China, Hong Kong, Vietnam, Indonesia, Singapore, and Myanmar (Burma). Signs/symptoms include cough, hepatosplenomegaly, skin lesions (papules, generalized papular rash, nodules), fever, weight loss, anemia, and leukocytosis. May disseminate. First reported human infection in 1959, then no reports until 1984.
Pneumocystis jiroveci (formerly *carinii*)	Pneumocystosis, pneumonia	Classified as a fungus (from a protozoan parasite) relatively recently. Usually seen in immunosuppressed persons and was originally the most frequent opportunistic infection seen in persons with HIV infection. Increased in incidence with HIV epidemic. Most common infection is seen in lungs, causing pneumonia. Other sites are lymph nodes, adrenal glands, liver, eye, ear, thyroid, kidney, spleen, gastrointestinal (GI) sites, skin, mediastinum, and disseminated disease.

Table A.2. *(continued)*

Organism	Disease	Comments
Rhodotorula spp.	See comments	Yeast-like fungi causes invasive disease in immunocompromised patients.
Scedosporium apiospermum *S. prolificans*	See comments	Alkaline mould. First associated with disease in humans in 1984. Usually occurs in immunocompetent person after surgery. Usually localized, often osteoarticular. In the immunosuppressed person is often disseminated.
Sporothrix schenckii	Sporotrichosis	A dimorphic fungus found in soil, sphagnum moss, and hay. Usually localized to skin, subcutaneous tissue and lymphocutaneous disease especially in the immunocompromised. May disseminate. Other forms include pulmonary, meningeal, and osteoarticular.
Trichosporon beigelii	Fungemia and disseminated disease	A yeast infection that usually is invasive in the immunosuppressed, especially those with neutropenia. Also seen in premature infants. Usually enters through the respiratory or GI tract or vascular catheters. May disseminate, causing cutaneous lesions, chorioretinitis, renal failure, cellulitis, meningitis, endocarditis, hepatic disease, and peritonitis. High mortality rate.
Zygomycetes	Zygomycosis	Pathogenic mold. Has become an emerging invasive fungal infection in the last decade. Affects immunosuppressed patients or those receiving broad spectrum antimicrobial drugs. Affects those with hematologic malignancies.

Sources: Chaturvedi, Dyavaiah, Larsen, & Chaturvedi, 2005; Chayakulkeeree, Ghannoum, & Perfect, 2006; Galgiani et al., 2005; Guerrant, Walker, & Weller, 2006; Kauffman, Hajjeh, & Chapman, 2000; Kidd et al., 2007; Kontoyiannis & Lewis, 2006; MacDougall et al., 2007; Mandell, Bennett, & Dolin, 2005; Nucci & Anaissie, 2006; Nucci & Marr, 2005; Reuter et al., 2005; Petrini, 2006; Vanittanakom, Cooper, Fisher, & Sirisanthana, 2006; Zaoutis et al., 2005.

*Most are emerging due to a greater prevalence of persons with altered host immunity.

Table A.3. Selected Emerging/Reemerging Parasites*

Parasite	Disease	Comments
Anncaliia algerae	Keratoconjunctivitis, myositis, skin infection	Formerly known as *Nosema* and *Brachiola*.
Anncaliia connori	See comments	A microsporidia first associated with disease in 1973. Can cause disseminated disease in non-HIV-infected persons. Formerly called *Nosema* and *Brachiola*.
Anncaliia vesicularum	Myositis	Described in 1998 and formerly known as *Brachiola*.
Angiostrongylus and spp.	Angiostrongyliasis	A recent outbreak in China of more than 130 persons from raw/undercooked Amazonia snails resulted in headache and meningitis. Snails become infected by this nematode through eating infected rat feces.
Babesia microti and spp.	Babesiosis	Usually a tickborne disease. Some cases can result from blood transfusion. Manifestations can include fever, chills, malaise, headache, myalgia, abdominal pain, mild hepatosplenomegaly, and depression. Complications can include renal failure, adult respiratory distress syndrome, and myocardial infarction. Can range from asymptomatic to severe disease, especially in the elderly or immunocompromised. See chapter 16.
Cryptosporidium hominis *Cryptosporidium parvum*	Cryptosporidiosis	Causes diarrhea and gastrointestinal (GI) illness. Usually results from contaminated water ingestion, but can be foodborne. Contamination of water supplies or crops can result from leaking septic tanks or runoff from manure in fields after heavy rain. Largest outbreak of about 403,000 was in Milwaukee in 1993. *C. hominis* is designated as Genotype I or the human genotype, and *C. parvum* is designated as Genotype II or the bovine genotype, although it can also cause human infection. See chapter 5.

Table A.3. *(continued)*

Parasite	Disease	Comments
Cyclospora cayetanensis	Cyclosporiasis	A coccidian protozoan first recognized to infect humans in Papua New Guinea. Manifestations include diarrhea, bloating, abdominal pain, fatigue, fever, and weight loss. Outbreaks have been recognized in the United States since the late 1990s. Guatemalan raspberries, mesclun lettuce, and basil have been identified as vehicles in various outbreaks. See chapter 6.
Echinococcus granulosus	Cystic echinococcosis	A tapeworm causing cyst development in liver and lungs. The adult tapeworm lives in dogs, but livestock can be affected, especially sheep. Infection occurs when humans ingest contaminated food or water. Is essentially worldwide, but in the United States most cases are important, and is increasing in the immigrant population.
Echinococcus multilocularis	Alveolar echinococcosis or hydatid disease	A tapeworm infection usually found in foxes. Can be acquired from contaminated hands, fur of infected animals, contaminated food or water, or inhalation of dust containing tapeworm eggs. Occurs in arctic region and northern hemisphere (Canada, U.S.–Canadian border, central Europe, and Siberia). Imported red foxes from these areas to southeastern United States may be infected. Potential for establishing endemic foci there. Maintained in foxes but wolves, coyotes, cats, and dogs are also final hosts. Intermediate hosts include mice, voles, lemmings, and muskrats. Cysts develop in liver and lungs. Can be fatal.
Encephalitozoon cuniculi	Microsporidiosis	Hepatitis, peritonitis, encephalitis, urethritis, cellulitis, keratoconjunctivitis, cystitis, diarrhea, and disseminated disease. Renal insufficiency and cough may follow infection. In the immunocompetent, seizures have been described.

(continued)

Table A.3. *(continued)*

Parasite	Disease	Comments
Encephalitozoon hellem	Usually disseminated infection	Described in humans in 1991. May cause keratoconjunctivitis, sinusitis, prostatitis, pneumonitis, nephritis, urethritis, cystitis, diarrhea, and disseminated infection.
Encephalitozoon intestinalis	Enteritis	Not usually seen in persons not infected with human immunodeficiency virus (HIV). First identified in persons with acquired immunodeficiency syndrome (AIDS) in 1993. Causes chronic diarrhea. Formerly called *Septata intestinalis*. May cause cholangitis in persons with AIDS. See chapter 3.
Enterocytozoon bieneusi	Enteritis, biliary tract disease	First identified in a person with HIV in 1985. Usually limited to GI tract. Can cause diarrhea and cholangitis. Possibility of potential of waterborne transmission. Rarely causes respiratory infection. Can infect immunocompetent persons. See chapter 3.
Gnathostomosis spinigerum and spp.	Gnathostomiasis	This nematode has had a high prevalence in Southeast Asia and is now emerging in South America and Mexico, especially Acapulco. Humans acquire infection from eating raw or undercooked fish containing larvae in their muscles, especially in the form of sashimi or ceviche. In humans, swelling occurs in skin, subcutaneous tissue, and certain organs such as GI tract, liver, eyes, and central nervous system. May see migratory subcutaneous lesions that are caused by larvae migration. Within 24–48 hours of ingestion may see fever, malaise, nausea, vomiting, diarrhea, and pain.
Leishmania spp., especially *L. donovani*	Leishmaniasis	Protozoan infection transmitted by sand flies. Endemic in many areas. Has expanded in range and increased in frequency with deforestation in Latin America. Has increased in fox and pet dog population. Coffee growing

Table A.3. *(continued)*

Parasite	Disease	Comments
		facilitates development of parasites in vectors. Outbreak in southern Sudan due to ecological changes favoring sand flies and waves of nonimmune immigrants. Can cause asymptomatic infection, localized skin lesions, or disseminated infection, which can involve viscera. Seen in travelers returning from Latin America and military returning from Iraq and Afghanistan.
Metorchis conjunctus	Liver disease	A helminth considered to have emerged in 1993. The long-term oncogenic potential is unknown. An outbreak occurred in Montreal from eating contaminated sashimi at a picnic.
Nosema ocularum	Keratoconjunctivitis	A microsporidia. Can cause keratoconjunctivitis in non-HIV-infected persons.
Paragonimus spp.	Paragonimiasis	This lung fluke inhabits freshwater, mainly in parts of Asia, Africa, and South America. Has caused a recent outbreak of disease in California traced to eating imported contaminated raw or undercooked fresh crab.
Plasmodium falciparum *Plasmodium malariae* *Plasmodium ovale* *Plasmodium vivax*	Malaria	Transmitted by mosquitoes (*Anopheles* spp). Is considered emerging because of drug-resistant strains. See chapter 17.
Pleistophora ronneafiei and spp.	Myositis	A microsporidia. Can cause myositis in persons with and without AIDS. Little is known about epidemiology.
Taenia solium	Cysticercosis	Is a pork tapeworm. Neurocysticercosis is becoming the most important parasitic nervous system infection and a cause of epilepsy. Endemic in South America, Africa, and most of Asia. Seen more

(continued)

Table A.3. *(continued)*

Parasite	Disease	Comments
		frequently in Europe, North America, and Australia because of immigration of infected persons and tourism. Increasing numbers of cases have been seen in the United States since the 1970s, and the majority are in persons from Mexico or Central America. In one instance in the early 1990s, a cluster of cases among orthodox Jews in the United States was traced to infected domestic workers from Central America. See chapter 3.
Trachipleistophora hominis	Microsporidiosis	Associated with myositis, keratoconjunctivitis, disseminated disease, and sinusitis, usually in those with AIDS. Identified in 1996.
Trypanosoma cruzi	Chagas disease (American trypanosomiasis)	Acute disease is relatively rare in the United States, with most cases occurring in Texas. However, the number of people with chronic infections is about 100,000 due to immigration, thus posing a potential risk to the blood supply where there is a high concentration of immigrants from endemic areas.
Vittaforma corneae	See comments	A microsporidia first associated with disease in 1973. Can cause disseminated disease in persons with HIV disease. Can cause keratoconjunctivitis in the immunocompetent.

Sources: "*Angiostrongylus* meningitis," 2006; Budke, 2006; Chrieki, 2002; Deplazes, 2006; Didier et al., 2004; Didier & Weiss, 2006; Dumler, 2005; Galgiani et al., 2005; Guerrant, Walker, & Weller, 2006; Kern et al., 2004; Leiby, 2006; MacLean, 1998; Mandell, Bennett, & Dolin, 2005; Mathis, Weber, & Deplazes, 2005; Murray, Berman, Davies, & Saravia, 2005; "*Paragonimus,*" 2006; Rojas-Molina, Pedraza-Sanchez, Torres-Bibiano, Meza-Martinez, & Escobar-Gutierrez, 1999; Strickland, 2000; Wormser et al., 2006.

*Some researchers believe that the microsporidia should be reclassified as fungi (Didier et al., 2004).

Table A.4. Selected Emerging/Reemerging Viruses

Virus	Major Disease Association	Comments
Australian bat lyssavirus	Encephalitis	Virus identified in 1996 in a black flying fox (a bat species) in Australia. Carried by bats. Causes a rabies-like disease. First known human case was in a woman in 1996 who died.
Avian influenza virus	Avian influenza	Is actually a way of referring to the H5N1 strain of the influenza A virus. This outbreak began in Asia and has affected millions of wild birds and poultry. Most of the human cases identified have had close contact with poultry or birds. Human-to-human transmission is not efficient. In most cases, respiratory symptoms are typical and mortality has been high. In a few cases, diarrhea was prominent. There is fear the virus could mutate and become more virulent or more efficient in human-to-human transmission. See chapter 14.
Barmah Forest virus	See comments	Confined to Australia currently. Isolated from mosquitoes in southeastern Australia in 1974. Reported as infecting humans in 1986. Symptoms include arthralgia, myalgia, fever, rash, and lethargy that can last 6 months. Outbreak in 1993–1994.
Cache Valley virus	Cache Valley virus disease	A mosquito-borne bunyavirus. Very rare. Seen in North America. Causes encephalitis. Not commonly screened for.
Chikungunya virus	Chikungunya fever	This alphavirus was first isolated in Tasmania in 1953. Considered as reemerging due to expansion of range into Asia and the Indian Islands. Reunion Island is particularly hard hit. Vectors include *Aedes* spp. mosquitoes. Symptoms include fever, arthralgia, and rash. This outbreak had unreported complications such as vertical transmission, myocarditis, and hepatitis as well as encephalitis.

(continued)

Table A.4. *(continued)*

Virus	Major Disease Association	Comments
Coronavirus HKU1	Respiratory disease	Identified in Hong Kong in 2005. Causes upper and lower respiratory tract disease.
Dengue virus	Dengue and dengue hemorrhagic fever	Has expanded its geographic range beginning in the mid-1970s. Are 4 serotypes. Belongs to the flavivirus family. Transmitted by the *Aedes aegypti* mosquito and others. Worldwide tropical distribution. Causes a spectrum of disease depending on serotype and host characteristics. See chapter 7.
Enterovirus 71	Encephalomyelitis	Isolated as cause of encephalitis in 1969. In 1997 and 1998 caused neurovirulent outbreaks in Asia. Other outbreaks occurred later.
Hantaviruses		
Andes virus	Hantavirus pulmonary syndrome (HPS)	Found in Argentina and Chile. Primary reservoir is *Oligoryzomys longicaudatus* rodent. First seen in 1993.
Bayou virus	HPS	Found in southeastern United States. Reservoir is *Oryzomys palustris* (the rice rat). Renal disease and myositis prominent. Cases have occurred in Louisiana and Texas.
Black Creek Canal virus	HPS	Reservoir is *Sigmodon hispidus* (cotton rat). Found in southeastern United States. First identified in 1993 in Florida. Renal failure can occur. Myositis can be prominent.
Choclo virus	HPS	Reported from Panama. Outbreak in 1999–2000. Reservoir is *Oligoryzomys fulvescens* rodents.
Hantaan virus	Hemorrhagic fever with renal syndrome (HFRS)	A bunyavirus. Most cases in Korea, China, and Japan. Abrupt onset with fever, chills, flushed face and torso, weakness, headache, myalgia, nausea, and vomiting. Hypotension or shock occurs on about Day 5 followed by oliguria. Some patients get hemorrhagic manifestations such as epistaxis and subconjunctival hemorrhage. May

Table A.4. *(continued)*

Virus	Major Disease Association	Comments
		have fluid, electrolyte, and central nervous system (CNS) abnormalities. A diuretic phase then occurs about 2 weeks after onset and convalescence may be associated with polyuria. Mortality is 5–15%.
HV39694 virus	HPS	Found in Argentina. Primary reservoir is unknown.
Juquitiba virus	HPS	Found in Brazil. Primary reservoir is unknown. First recognized in 1993.
Laguna Negra virus	HPS	Found in Paraguay and Bolivia. Primary reservoir is *Calomys laucha*. First seen in 1995.
Lechiguanas virus	HPS	Found in Argentina. First noted in 1988.
Monongahela virus	HPS	Found in eastern United States. Primary reservoir is the rodent *Peromyscus maniculatus*.
New York virus	HPS	Found in eastern United States. Primary reservoir is *Peromyscus leucopus* (white-footed mouse).
Oran virus	HPS	Found in Argentina. Primary reservoir is *O. longicaudatus*. First seen in 1984.
Puumala virus	Nephropathia epidemica/HFRS	Symptoms include fever, abdominal pain, and renal dysfunction. Major reservoir is bank vole. Endemic in northern two thirds of Sweden. May be associated with Guillain–Barré syndrome. Mildest of the old world hantaviruses under HFRS rubric.
Sin Nombre virus	HPS	Recognized in 1993 after a cluster of persons with acute respiratory syndrome occurred in the southwestern United States. Mice are reservoirs. See chapter 11.
Hemorrhagic fever viruses		
Crimean-Congo hemorrhagic fever virus	Crimean-Congo hemorrhagic fever	Tickborne bunyavirus isolated in 1967. Extensive geographic range. Can be spread by person-to-person contact or contact with blood/tissues of infected animals.

(continued)

Table A.4. *(continued)*

Virus	Major Disease Association	Comments
Ebola virus	Ebola hemorrhagic fever	Filovirus identified in 1976 with outbreaks in Zaire. Reservoir unknown. See chapter 8.
Guanarito virus	Venezuelan hemorrhagic fever	Arenavirus recognized in 1989. Main host is cane mouse. Incubation period is 1–2 weeks.
Junín virus	Argentine hemorrhagic fever	Arenavirus isolated in 1958. Main reservoir is corn mouse.
Lassa virus	Lassa hemorrhagic fever	Arenavirus first isolated from a patient in western Africa in 1969. Transmitted to humans via contact with common rodents, infected human secretions, and contaminated needles in hospitals. Fever, weakness, malaise, joint pain, headache, sore throat, and cough. Bleeding occurs in about 20%. Incubation period about 18 days. Ribavirin used in treatment. See chapter 8.
Machupo virus	Bolivian hemorrhagic fever	Large outbreak in 1964. Exposure through bush mice via food, water, or direct contact. Causes fever, myalgia, petechiae, and thrombocytopenia. Most often seen in agricultural workers in spring and summer.
Marburg fever virus	Marburg hemorrhagic fever	A filovirus first isolated in 1967 during an outbreak among laboratory workers, medical personnel, and their families. Other outbreaks have been described in Zimbabwe and Kenya. Large outbreak occurred in Angola in 2005; 252 people were infected and 227 died. See chapter 8.
Sabiá virus	Brazilian hemorrhagic fever	Arenavirus isolated from a human case in 1990. Little known to date.
Hendra virus (formerly called equine morbillivirus)	Encephalitis, respiratory disease	First recognized in Australia in 1995. Reservoir is a type of fruit bat. Humans apparently infected from contact with horses that had been infected by bats. See chapter 3.

Table A.4. *(continued)*

Virus	Major Disease Association	Comments
Hepatitis C virus	Hepatitis C	A flavivirus known to exist since the early 1970s but identified in 1988. Incubation period is 15–150 days. Can cause chronic hepatitis leading to cirrhosis. Many who develop disease are asymptomatic. The disease progresses slowly and insidiously, and many do not know they are infected. See chapter 12.
Hepatitis D virus	See comments	Discovered in 1977 and recognized as causing infection in 1981 in Venezuela. The hepatitis D virus is an RNA virus, and infection with it usually depends on coinfection with hepatitis B. Can cause chronic hepatitis. Transmission is bloodborne and percutaneous with permucosal routes possible. Incubation period is 15–150 days.
Hepatitis E virus	Hepatitis E	A calicivirus detected in a patient with non-A, non-B hepatitis in 1983. May not be new but was not differentiated from hepatitis A and B by previous techniques. Virus characterized in 1990. Believed to be responsible for large epidemics in developing countries, especially in Asia. Fecal–oral route is predominant transmission. Water contaminated by fecal matter is believed to be a primary source of infection.
Hepatitis G virus	Suspected of causing some cases of hepatitis	A bloodborne RNA flavivirus with worldwide distribution but varying prevalence. Its role in causing hepatitis is uncertain, but it is more prevalent in persons with hepatitis than the general population. Discovered in 1995.
Human bocavirus	Acute respiratory illness	A parvovirus recently identified. Believed to cause acute respiratory illness, especially in children, with symptoms of paroxysmal cough, fever, sore throat, flu-like illness, and headache. Illness may require hospitalization.

(continued)

Table A.4. *(continued)*

Virus	Major Disease Association	Comments
Human coronavirus NL-63	Acute respiratory illness	Identified in the Netherlands in 2004. Affects young children and the elderly more frequently.
Human herpesvirus 6	Exanthem subitum (roseola)	Isolated in 1986 from persons with HIV and lymphoproliferative disorders. Believed to cause CNS complications in liver transplant recipients. Was a predictor of invasive fungal infections and was associated with late mortality. Infects most children by 2 years of age.
Human herpesvirus 7	Exanthem subitum (roseola)	Causes roseola and has been implicated in CNS complications, but other disease associations are unknown. Infects most children by 3 years of age.
Human herpesvirus 8	Kaposi sarcoma (KS)	Identified first in 1994. Found in KS lesions of HIV-infected person. Associated also with interstitial pneumonitis, encephalitis, hepatitis, and febrile illness. Can be transmitted through transfusion. See chapter 24.
Human immunodeficiency virus 1 (HIV-1)	HIV disease/acquired immunodeficiency syndrome (AIDS)	A retrovirus first identified in a group of homosexual men in 1981. Results in severe immunodeficiency and alterations leading to various opportunistic infections and neoplasms. See chapter 12.
Human immunodeficiency virus 2 (HIV-2)	HIV disease/AIDS	Identified in 1985. Is largely confined to West Africa. Appears to cause milder disease than HIV-1 and to be somewhat less easily transmitted. See chapter 12.
Human papillomaviruses	Genital warts, anal warts, cervical neoplasia	Was not realized as an etiologic agent of these conditions until 1980s. Closely associated with cervical intraepithelial neoplasia. Also causes anal and genital warts. Many types, but HPV 16 is the most important oncogenic type. A vaccine for certain types has been developed. See chapter 24.

Table A.4. *(continued)*

Virus	Major Disease Association	Comments
Human T-cell lymphotropic virus 1 (HTLV-1)	HTLV-1-associated myelopathy/tropical spastic paraparesis, (HAM/TSP) adult T-cell leukemia/lymphoma (ATL)	Discovered in 1980 after ATL was characterized. A human retrovirus. Has also been linked with uveitis and arthritis. Has worldwide distribution and is endemic in certain locales. See chapter 24.
Human T-cell lymphotropic virus 2	Adult hairy cell leukemia	A human retrovirus. Also associated with a neurologic syndrome similar to HAM/TSP. See chapter 24.
LaCrosse encephalitis virus	California–LaCrosse encephalitis	*Aedes* mosquitoes are reservoir and host. First isolated in 1964. Occurs primarily in children.
Metapneumovirus	Respiratory tract infection	Identified in the Netherlands in 2004. Mainly affects infants, young children, and the elderly. See chapter 18.
Me Tri virus	CNS illness in children	An alphavirus reported from children in Vietnam in 1995.
Monkeypox virus	Monkeypox	An orthopox virus. Detected in 1970 in the Democratic Republic of the Congo. Outbreak in 2003 in the midwestern United States that affected 72 people and resulted from contact with infected prairie dogs that the importer housed with an infected Gambian giant rat. Causes febrile illness with rash, lymphadenopathy, and respiratory symptoms. See chapter 19.
Ngari virus	Hemorrhagic fever	Is a mosquito-borne bunyavirus. True incidence is unknown. Can be neuroinvasive. Identified in 1997–1998 in Africa.
Nipah virus	Encephalitis	A paramyxovirus. Symptoms include fever, headache, dizziness, vomiting, reduced level of consciousness, seizures, focal neurologic signs such as nystagmus, absent or reduced reflexes, tachycardia, abnormal pupils, hypertension, segmental myoclonus, ptosis, thrombocytopenia, and coma. In

(continued)

Table A.4. *(continued)*

Virus	Major Disease Association	Comments
		1998 over 200 residents of a pig farming community in Malaysia were infected. Abbattoir workers in Singapore experienced an outbreak in 1999. In Bangladesh, outbreaks from 2001 to 2004 resulted in case fatality rates of about 75% and documented human-to-human transmission. Incubation period is 1–3 weeks. Bats may be a reservoir. See chapter 3.
Noroviruses	Gastroenteritis	Formerly called Norwalk viruses. First associated with material obtained from a 1968 outbreak of gastroenteritis in Norwalk, OH, in 1972. Causes abrupt-onset diarrhea, nausea, and vomiting with occasional additional symptoms. Is a calicivirus transmitted by fecal-contaminated food and water, aerosolization, and person-to-person contact. Incubation period is 24–48 hours. Usually mild. Has caused outbreaks on cruise ships. Responsible for majority of foodborne gastroenteritis in the United States. See chapter 3.
O'nyong-nyong virus	O'nyong-nyong fever	A mosquito-borne alphavirus in the *Togaviridae* family initially isolated during an epidemic in Uganda in 1959 affecting more than 2 million people. Another major outbreak occurred in 1996–1997, when the virus showed a genetic difference from the earlier outbreak. Signs/symptoms include arthralgia, generalized skin rash, lymphadenopathy, and fever. Usually nonfatal.
Oropouche virus	Oropouche fever	The virus was first isolated in 1955 in Trinidad from a febrile forest worker. The vector is the biting midge and/or mosquitoes. Characterized by fever, headache, ocular pain, myalgia, and arthralgia.

Table A.4. *(continued)*

Virus	Major Disease Association	Comments
Parvovirus B19	Erythema infectiosum (fifth disease)	Primarily infects children. More than 50% of adults have been infected. Identified in 1975. Transmissible only during short period of viremia. Difficult to screen for. Causes self-limited disease associated with mild rash or arthropathy. More chronic or severe manifestation in the immunocompromised and severe aplastic crises in persons with anemia. Fetal infections can cause fetal hydrops and fetal death. Has induced aplastic anemia in some transfusion recipients and symptoms in persons with hemophilia who received contaminated clotting factor.
Rift Valley fever virus	Rift Valley fever	While a few early human cases were recognized, the first large human epidemic was in Egypt in 1977–1978 involving about 200,000 cases and about 600 deaths. In humans signs/symptoms range from flu-like syndrome to hemorrhagic fever, encephalitis, and/or retinitis. East African epidemic took place in 1997–1998 involving Kenya and Somalia. Large outbreak in Kenya in 2006–2007. Is usually a zoonosis affecting sheep and cattle. Transmitted by mosquitoes, aerosol, and contact.
Rocio virus	Encephalitis	A flavivirus detected during an encephalitis outbreak in Brazil in 1975–1976. Transmitted by mosquitoes.
Rotavirus	Diarrheal illness	Rotavirus belongs to the *Reoviridae* family and was identified in 1973 in children with diarrhea in Australia. Worldwide distribution. Infection can be asymptomatic or cause mild to severe diarrheal disease. Incubation usually less than 48 hours with abrupt onset of

(continued)

Table A.4. *(continued)*

Virus	Major Disease Association	Comments
		vomiting and watery diarrhea with or without low-grade fever. Most cases resolve, but in developing countries may be cause of mortality in children under 2 years.
SEN virus	May be associated with non-A–E hepatitis	Transmitted via transfusion but has not yet been proven to be associated with hepatitis.
Severe acute respiratory syndrome (SARS) coronavirus	SARS	Emerged as an atypical pneumonia in the Guangdong province of China in November 2002. Areas most affected were parts of Asia and through travel to Toronto, Canada. Causes influenza-like symptoms such as fever, myalgias, headache, diarrhea, cough, and dyspnea. Pneumonia is common. See chapter 22.
Toscana virus	Febrile disease with or without CNS manifestations	Is a bunyavirus transmitted by the sand fly as a vector. Can be asymptomatic or cause febrile disease with or without CNS manifestations such as meningitis. Found in Italy, Portugal, France, Slovenia, Greece, Cyprus, and Turkey. Symptoms include fever, nausea, vomiting, headache, neck rigidity, and myalgia. Incubation period is a few days to 2 weeks.
TT virus	Unknown at present	Small DNA virus identified in Japan in 1997 and named for the patient, TT. May be transmissible by oral–fecal route and transfusion (not established). Possibly transfusion-hepatitis transmitted.
Venezuelan equine encephalitis virus (VEE)	Encephalitis	VEE virus characterized in 1930s. No outbreaks reported from 1973 to 1992. Large outbreak in 1995 in Venezuela and Colombia affecting humans and horses. Transmitted to humans via mosquitoes. Usually mild infection with headache, chills, fever, myalgia, nausea, and vomiting.

Table A.4. *(continued)*

Virus	Major Disease Association	Comments
West Nile virus	West Nile fever	Mosquito-borne flavivirus. Most infections are mild but can cause encephalitis. Outbreak in New York City in 1999 was first in western hemisphere. Is now endemic in the United States and Canada. See chapter 23.
Whitewater Arroyo virus	Hemorrhagic fever	An arenavirus carried by wood rats and probably transmitted through exposure to rat urine often by aerosol. First found in 1996 in western United States. Associated with human deaths in 1999 and 2000.

Sources: Arnold, Singh, Spector, & Sawyer, 2006; Bastien, Brandt, Dust, Ward, & Li, 2006; Bessaud et al., 2006; Campbell et al. 2006; Centers for Disease Control and Prevention, 2003; Charel et al., 2005; Chew et al., 2000; De Souza Lopes, Coimbra, de Abrev Sacchetta, & Calisher, 1978; Eaton, Broder, Middleton, & Wang, 2006; Gerrard, Li, Barrett, & Nichol, 2004; Guerrant, Walker, & Weller, 2006; Ha, Calisher, Tien, Karabatsos, & Gubler, 1995; Hutson, Atmar, & Estes, 2004; Lewis, 2006; Lindsay, Johansen, Broom, Smith, & Mackenzie, 1995; "Lyssavirus," 1999; Mackenzie, 2005; Mandell, Bennet, & Dolin, 2005; "Marburg Hemorrhagic Fever," 2005; Maunula, Miettinen, & von Bonsdorff, 2005; McJunkin, Khan, & Tsai, 1998; Palacios & Oberste, 2005; Parola et al., 2006; Sanbonmatsu-Gámez et al., 2005; Skowronski et al., 2005; Strickland, 2000; Vincent et al., 2000.

REFERENCES

Angiostrongylus meningitis—China (02). (2006, August 22). *ProMED Digest, 376,* unpaginated.

Arnold, J. C., Singh, K. K., Spector, S. A., & Sawyer, M. H. (2006). Human bocavirus: Prevalence and clinical spectrum at a children's hospital. *Clinical Infectious Diseases, 43,* 283–288.

Bastien, N., Brandt, K., Dust, K., Ward, D., & Li, Y. (2006). Human bocavirus infection, Canada. *Emerging Infectious Diseases, 12,* 848–850.

Bessaud, M., Peyrefitte, C. N., Pastorino, B. A. M., Tock, F., Merle, O., Colpart, J.-J., et al. (2006). Chikungunya virus strains, Reunion Island outbreak. *Emerging Infectious Diseases, 12,* 1604–1606.

Boulouis, H.-J., Chang, C.-C., Henn, J. B., Kasten, R. W., & Chomel, B. B. (2005). Factors associated with the rapid emergence of zoonotic *Bartonella* infections. *Veterinary Research, 36,* 383–410.

Bowen, A. B., & Braden, C. R. (2006). Invasive *Enterobacter sakazakii* disease in infants. *Emerging Infectious Diseases, 12,* 1185–1189.

Braden, C. R. (2006). *Salmonella enterica* serotype Enteritidis and eggs: A national epidemic in the United States. *Clinical Infectious Diseases, 43,* 512–517.

Brazier, J. S., Gal, M., Hall, V., & Morris, T. E. (2004). Outbreak of *Clostridium histolyticum* infections in injecting drug users in England and Scotland. *European Surveillance, 9*(9), 15–16.

Budke, C. M. (2006). Global socioeconomic impact of cystic echinococcosis. *Emerging Infectious Diseases, 12,* 296–303.

Campbell, G. L., Mataczynski, J. D., Reisdorf, E. S., Powell, J. W., Martin, D. A., Lambert, A. J., et al. (2006). Second human case of Cache Valley virus disease. *Emerging Infectious Diseases, 12,* 854–856.

Centers for Disease Control and Prevention. (2000). Update: *Clostridium novyi* and unexplained illness among injecting drug users—Scotland, Ireland and England. *Morbidity and Mortality Weekly Report, 49,* 201–205.

Centers for Disease Control and Prevention. (2003). Multistate outbreak of monkypox—Illinois, Indiana, and Wisconsin, 2003. *Morbidity and Mortality Weekly Report, 52,* 537–540.

Charrel, R. N., Gallian, P., Navarro-Mari, J.-M., Nicoletti, L., Papa, A., Sánchez-Seco, M. P., et al. (2005). Emergence of Toscana virus in Europe. *Emerging Infectious Diseases, 11,* 1657–1663.

Chaturvedi, S., Dyavaiah, M., Larsen, R. A., & Chaturvedi, V. (2005). *Cryptococcus gattii* in AIDS patients, southern California. *Emerging Infectious Diseases, 11,* 1686–1692.

Chayakulkeeree, M., Ghannoum, M. A., & Perfect, J. R. (2006). Zygomycosis: The re-emerging fungal infection. *European Journal of Clinical Microbiology and Infectious Diseases, 25,* 215–229.

Chew, M. H. L., Arguin, P. M., Shay, D. K., Goh, K., Rollin, P. E., Shieh, W., et al. (2000). Risk factors for Nipah virus infection among abattoir workers in Singapore. *Journal of Infectious Diseases, 181,* 1760–1763.

Chomel, B. B., Boulouis, H.-J., Maruyama, S., & Breitschwerdt, E. B. (2006). *Bartonella* spp. in pets and effect on human health. *Emerging Infectious Diseases, 12,* 389–394.

Chrieki, M. (2002). Echinococcosis–an emerging parasite in the immigrant population. *American Family Physician, 66,* 817–820.

Dance, D. A. (2000). Melioidosis as an emerging global problem. *Acta Tropica, 5,* 115–119.

Deplazes, P. (2006). Ecology and epidemiology of *Echinococcus multilocularis* in Europe. *Parassitoloia, 48,* 37–39.

De Souza Lopes, O., Coimbra, T. L., de Abrev Sacchetta, L., & Calisher, C. H. (1978). Emergence of a new arbovirus disease in Brazil, I. Isolation and characterization of the etiologic agent, Rocio virus. *American Journal of Epidemiology, 100,* 444–449.

Didier, E. S., Stovall, M. E., Green, L. C., Brindley, P. J., Sestak, K., & Didier, P. J. (2004). Epidemiology of microsporidiosis: Sources and modes of transmission. *Veterinary Parasitology, 126,* 145–166.

Didier, E. S., & Weiss, L. M. (2006). Microsporidiosis: Current status. *Current Opinion in Infectious Diseases, 19,* 485–492.

Dobos, K. M., Quinn, F. D., Ashford, D. A., Horsbaugh, C. R., & King, H. C. (1999). Emergence of a unique group of necrotizing mycobacterial diseases. *Emerging Infectious Diseases, 5,* 367–378.

Drudy, D., Mullane, N. R., Quinn, T., Wall, P. G., & Fanning, S. (2006). *Enterobacter sakazakii*: An emerging pathogen in powdered infant formula. *Clinical Infectious Diseases, 42,* 996–1002.

Dumler, J. S. (2005). *Anaplasma* and *Ehrlichia* infection. *Annals of the New York Academy of Sciences, 1063,* 361–373.

Eaton, B. T., Broder, C. C., Middleton, D., & Wang, L.-F. (2006). Hendra and Nipah viruses: Different and dangerous. *Nature Reviews Microbiology, 4,* 23–35.

French, A. L., Benator, D. A., & Gordin, F. M. (1997). Nontuberculous mycobacterial infections. *Medical Clinics of North America, 81,* 361–379.

Galgiani, J. N., Ampel, N. M., Blair, J. E., Catanzaro, A., Johnson, R. H., Stevens, D. A., et al. (2005). Coccidioidomycosis. *Clinical Infectious Diseases, 41,* 1217–1223.

Gerrard, S. R., Li, L., Barrett, A. D., & Nichol, S. T. (2004). Ngari virus is a Bunyamwera virus reassortant that can be associated with large outbreaks of hemorrhagic fever in Africa. *Journal of Virology, 78,* 8922–8926.

Guerrant, R. L., Walker, D. H., & Weller, P. F. (Eds.). (2006). *Tropical infectious diseases* (2nd ed.). Philadelphia: Churchill Livingstone Elsevier.

Ha, D. Q., Calisher, C. H., Tien, P. H., Karabatsos, N., & Gubler, D. J. (1995). Isolation of a newly recognized alphavirus from mosquitoes in Vietnam and evidence for human infection and disease. *American Journal of Tropical Medicine and Hygiene, 53,* 100–104.

Hutson, A. M., Atmar, R. L., & Estes, M. K. (2004). Norovirus disease: Changing epidemiology and host susceptibility factors. *Trends in Microbiology, 12,* 279–287.

IARC Working Group on the Evaluation of Carcinogenic Risks to Humans. (1994). *Schistosomes, liver flukes and* Helicobacter pylori: *Views and expert opinions of an IARC Working Group on the Evaluation of Carcinogenic Risks in Humans* (Monograph 61). Lyon, France: International Agency for Research on Cancer.

Kauffman, C. A., Hajjeh, R., & Chapman, S. W. for the Mycoses Study Group. (2000). Practice guidelines for the management of patients with *Sporotrichosis*. *Clinical Infectious Diseases, 30,* 684–687.

Kern, P., Ammon, A., Kron, M., Sinn, G., Sander, S., Petersen, L. R., et al. (2004). Risk factors for alveolar echinococcosis in humans. *Emerging Infectious Diseases, 10,* 2088–2093.

Kidd, S. E., Bach, P. J., Hingston, A. O., Mak, S., Chow, Y., MacDougall, L., et al. (2007). *Cryptococcus gattii* dispersal mechanisms, British Columbia, Canada. *Emerging Infectious Diseases, 13,* 51–57.

Kontoyiannis, D. P., & Lewis, R. E. (2006). Invasive zygomycosis: Update on pathogenesis, clinical manifestations, and management. *Infectious Disease Clinics of North America, 20,* 581–607.

Leiby, D. A. (2006). Babesiosis and blood transfusion: Flying under the radar. *Vox Sanguinis, 90,* 157–165.

Lewis, D. B. (2006). Avian flu to human influenza. *Annual Review of Medicine, 57,* 137–154.

Lindsay, M. D. A., Johansen, C. A., Broom, A. K., Smith, D. W., & Mackenzie, J. S. (1995). Emergence of Barmah Forest virus in Western Australia. *Emerging Infectious Diseases, 1,* 22–26.

Looney, W. J. (2005). Role of *Stenotrophomonas maltophila* in hospital-acquired infection. *British Journal of Biomedical Sciences, 62,* 145–154.

Lyssavirus, bat—Australia. (1999, August 13). *ProMED Digest, 99*(195), unpaginated.

MacDougall, L., Kidd, S. E., Galanis, E., Mak, S., Leslie, M. J., Cieslak, P. R., et al. (2007). Spread of *Cryptococcus gattii* in British Columbia, Canada, and detection in the Pacific Northwest, USA. *Emerging Infectious Diseases, 13,* 42–50.

Mackenzie, J. S. (2005). Emerging zoonotic encephalitis viruses: Lessons from Southeast Asia and Oceania. *Journal of Neurovirology, 11,* 434–440.

Mandell, G. L., Bennett, J. E., & Dolin, R. (Eds.). (2005). *Mandell, Douglas, and Bennett's principles and practice of infectious diseases* (6th ed.). Philadelphia: Churchill Livingstone Elsevier.

Marburg hemorrhagic fever—Angola. (2005). *ProMED Digest,* unpaginated.

Mathis, A., Weber, R., & Deplazes, P. (2005). Zoonotic potential of the microsporidia. *Clinical Microbiology Reviews, 18,* 423–445.

Maunula, L., Miettinen, I. T., & von Bonsdorff, C. H. (2005). Norovirus outbreaks from drinking water. *Emerging Infectious Diseases, 11,* 1716–1721.

McJunkin, J. E., Khan, R. R., & Tsai, T. F. (1998). California–La Crosse encephalitis. *Infectious Disease Clinics of North America, 12,* 83–91.

Murray, H. W., Berman, J. D., Davies, C. R., & Saravia, N. G. (2005). Advances in leishmaniasis. *Lancet, 366,* 1561–1577.

Nucci, M., & Anaissie, E. (2006). Emerging fungi. *Infectious Disease Clinics of North America, 20,* 563–579.

Nucci, M., & Marr, K. A. (2005). Emerging fungal diseases. *Clinical Infectious Diseases, 41,* 521–526.

Paglia, M. G., D'Arezzo, S., Festa, A., Del Borgo, C., Loiacono, L., Antinori, A., et al. (2005). *Yersinia pseudotuberculosis* septicemia and HIV. *Emerging Infectious Diseases, 11,* 1128–1130.

Palacios, G., & Oberste, M. S. (2005). Enteroviruses as agents of emerging infectious diseases. *Journal of Neurovirology, 11,* 424–433.

Paragonimus—US (California). (2006). *ProMED Digest, 372,* unpaginated.

Parola, P., de Lamballerie, X., Jourdan, J., Rovery, C., Vaillant, V., Minodier, P., et al. (2006). Novel Chikungunya virus variant in revelers returning from Indian Ocean islands. *Emerging Infectious Diseases, 12,* 1493–1499.

Parola, P., Paddock, C. D., & Raoult, D. (2005). Tick-borne rickettsioses around the world: Emerging diseases challenging old concepts. *Clinical Microbiology Reviews, 18,* 719–756.

Pechère, M., Opravil, M., Wald, A., Chave, J. P., Bessesen, M., Sievers, A., et al. (1995). Clinical and epidemiologic features of infection with *Mycobacterium genavense*. Swiss HIV Cohort Study. *Archives of Internal Medicine, 155,* 400–404.

Pepin, J. (2006). Improving the treatment of *Clostridium difficile*-associated disease: Where should we start? *Clinical Infectious Diseases, 43,* 553–555.

Petrini, B. (2006). *Mycobacterium marinum*: Ubiquitous agent of waterborne granulomatous infections.

Qureshi, A., Mooney, L., Denton, M., & Kerr, K. G. (2005). *Stenotrophomonas maltophilia* in salad. *Emerging Infectious Diseases, 11,* 1157–1158.

Reuter, C. W., Morgan, M. A., Bange, F. C., Gunzer, F., Eder, M., Hertenstein, B., et al. (2005). *Candida kefyr* as an emerging pathogen causing nosocomial bloodstream infections in neutropenic leukemia patients. *Clinical Infectious Diseases, 41,* 1365–1366.

Rift Valley fever—Kenya (North Eastern Province) (02). (2007). *ProMED Digest, 004,* unpaginated.

Rojas-Molina, N., Pedraza-Sanchez, S., Torres-Bibiano, B., Meza-Martinez, H., & Escobar-Gutierrez, A. (1999). Gnathostomosis, an emerging foodborne zoonotic disease in Acapulco, Mexico. *Emerging Infectious Diseases, 5,* 264–266.

Sanbonmatsu-Gámez, S., Pérez-Ruiz, M., Collao, X., Sánchez-Seco, M. P., Morillas-Márquez, F., de la Rosa-Fraile, M., et al. (2005). Toscana virus in Spain. *Emerging Infectious Diseases, 11,* 1701–1707.

Seifert, H., Oltmanns, D., Becker, K., Wisplinghoff, H., & von Eiff, C. (2005). *Staphyloccus lugdunensis* pacemaker-related infection. *Emerging Infectious Diseases, 11,* 1283–1286.

Singh, J. A., Upshur, R., & Padayatchi, N. (2007). XDR-TB in South Africa: No time for denial or complacency. *PloS Medicine, 4,* e50.

Skowronski, D. M., Astell, C., Brunham, R. C., Low, D. E., Petric, M., Roper, R. L., et al. (2005). Severe acute respiratory syndrome (SARS): A year in review. *Annual Review of Medicine, 56,* 557–581.

Strickland, G. T. (Ed.). (2000). *Hunter's tropical medicine and emerging infectious diseases* (8th ed.). Philadelphia: W. B. Saunders.

Török, M. E. (2007). Neurological infections: Clinical advances and emerging threats. *Lancet Neurology, 6,* 16–18.

Vanittanakom, N., Cooper, C. R., Jr., Fisher, M. C., & Sirisanthana, T. (2006). *Penicillium marneffei* infection and recent advances in the epidemiology and molecular biology aspects. *Clinical Microbiology Reviews, 19,* 95–110.

Vibrio parahaemolyticus, shellfish—USA: Rhode Island. (2006, August 5). *ProMED Digest, 348,* unpaginated.

Vibrio vulnificus—USA (multistate). (2006, August 7). *ProMED Digest, 352,* unpaginated.

Vincent, M. J., Quiroz, E., Gracia, F., Sanchez, A. J., Ksiazek, T. G., Kitsutani, P. T., et al. (2000). Hantavirus pulmonary syndrome in Panama: Identification of novel hantaviruses and their likely reservoirs. *Virology, 277,* 14–19.

Wagner, D., Vos, M., Buiting, A. G., Serr, A., Bergmans, A. M., Kern, W., et al. (2006). "*Mycobacterium tilburgii*" infections. *Emerging Infectious Diseases, 12,* 532–534.

Wormser, G. P., Dattwyler, R. J., Shapiro, E. D., Halperin, J. J., Steere, A. C., Klepner, M. S., et al. (2006). The clinical assessment, treatment, and prevention of Lyme disease, human granulocytic anaplasmosis, and babesiosis: Clinical practice guidelines by the Infectious Diseases Society of America. *Clinical Infectious Diseases, 43,* 1089–1134.

Yañez, A., Cedillo, L., Neyrolles, O., Alonso, E., Prévost, M. C., Rojas, J., et al. (1999). *Mycoplasma penetrans* bacteremia and primary antiphospholipid syndrome. *Emerging Infectious Diseases, 5,* 164–167.

Yu, H., Jing, H., Chen, Z., Zheng, H., Zhu, X., Wang, H., et al. (2006). Human *Streptococcus suis* outbreak, Sichuan, China. *Emerging Infectious Diseases, 12,* 914–920.

Zaoutis, T. E., Argon, J., Chu, J., Berlin, J. A., Walsh, T. J., & Feudtner, C. (2005). The epidemiology and attributable outcomes of candidemia in adults and children hospitalized in the United States: A propensity analysis. *Clinical Infectious Diseases, 41,* 1232–1239.

APPENDIX B

Emerging/Reemerging Infectious Diseases by Modes of Transmission

Felissa R. Lashley

Table B.1. Selected Emerging/Reemerging Foodborne and Waterborne Pathogens

Organism	Comments
Parasitic	
Angiostrongylus spp.	A recent outbreak in China of more than 130 persons from raw/undercooked Amazonia snails is resulting in headache and meningitis. Snails become infected by this nematode through eating infected rat feces.
Cyclospora cayetanensis	Responsible for large multistate and Canadian outbreaks in 1997 and 1998 due to contaminated Guatemalan raspberries, mesclun lettuce, and basil. Later outbreaks tended to involve fresh basil. Causes gastrointestinal illness. See chapter 6.
Cryptosporidium hominis *Cryptosporidium parvum*	A waterborne emerging pathogen implicated in major outbreaks involving both contaminated drinking and recreational water. Causes diarrhea and gastrointestinal illness. See chapter 5.

(continued)

Table B.1. *(continued)*

Organism	Comments
Gnathostomosis spinigerum and spp.	This nematode has had a high prevalence in Southeast Asia and is now emerging in South America and Mexico, especially Acapulco. Humans acquire infection from eating raw or undercooked fish containing larvae in their muscles, especially in the form of sashimi or ceviche. In humans, swelling caused by larvae migration occurs in skin, subcutaneous tissue, and certain organs.
Metorchis conjunctus	A helminth considered to have emerged in 1993. The long-term oncogenic potential is unknown. An outbreak occurred in Montreal from eating contaminated sashimi at a picnic.
Paragonimus spp.	This lung fluke inhabits freshwater mainly in parts of Asia, Africa, and South America. Has caused a recent outbreak of disease in California traced to eating imported contaminated raw or undercooked fresh crab.
Bacterial	
Campylobacter jejuni	A zoonotic infection. Became recognized as a human pathogen in the 1970s. Symptoms include fever, diarrhea (watery or bloody), and abdominal pain. Trigger for Guillain–Barré syndrome. See chapter 24.
Escherichia coli O137:H7	Diarrheal illness and hemolytic uremic syndrome. First recognized in outbreak in the early 1980s. Foodborne illness associated with several vehicles including alfalfa sprouts, lettuce, spinach, ground beef, unpasteurized apple juice, and others. Can be waterborne. See chapter 9.
Legionella pneumophila	Causes Legionnaires disease (LD) and Pontiac fever. LD was recognized after infection occurred in attendees at an American Legion convention in Philadelphia in July 1976. May be associated with travel-related infections and spray from such sources as spas and others. Causes pneumonia. One method of spread is through contaminated water. See chapters 3 and 15.
Listeria monocytogenes	A gram-positive bacteria only recently considered as causing gastrointestinal disease, diarrhea, nausea, vomiting, and abdominal cramps, often with fever. Most cases of listeriosis occur in immunocompromised persons, the elderly, or pregnant women. Is severe in pregnancy and can result in fetal loss. Typical illness manifestations are flu-like symptoms, sepsis, or central nervous system illness. Frequent contaminated foods include deli meats, hot dogs, and soft cheeses. See chapter 3.

Table B.1. *(continued)*

Organism	Comments
Salmonella Enteriditis	A 41-state outbreak occurred in 1995 from ice cream prepared from a premix hauled in tanker trucks previously hauling raw eggs. Raw or undercooked eggs or poultry are frequent vehicles for infection. Causes gastroenteritis. See Chapter 3.
Vibrio cholerae	Cholera is an old disease causing severe diarrheal illness, but the seventh cholera pandemic began in Indonesia in 1961 and was caused by the *V. cholerae* O1 serogroup, El Tor biotype. The organism is curved and gram negative. In 1992, *V. cholerae* O139 was identified in India. Epidemic cholera appeared in Latin America in 1991 after nearly 100 years of absence. Characterized by "rice water" diarrheal stools. See chapter 4.
Vibrio parahaemolyticus	Rare outbreaks before 1997. In 1998, the first outbreak of serotype O3:K6 occurred in the United States when 416 persons developed gastroenteritis from eating oysters from Galveston Bay in Texas. In 2006, widespread outbreak in Oregon, Washington, Canada, and New York from eating undercooked or raw oysters from Washington.
Vibrio vulnificus	Emergence reported in 1979. Infections usually result from consumption of shellfish, especially raw oysters from the Gulf of Mexico. An increase is seen in the summer. Infection can result in septicemia with bulbous skin lesions, shock, and rapid death. Persons with iron overload such as hemochromatosis are especially vulnerable. Recently found in Rhode Island waters.
Yersinia enterocolitica	Increasingly recognized as a source of gastroenteritis sometimes with rectal bleeding and ileal perforation. Symptoms often suggest mesenteric adenitis or appendicitis. Serogroup O:3 is becoming more frequent. Hogs are an important reservoir, and eating pork is a risk factor for infection. Infants have acquired yersiniosis after transfer of the organism from the hands of caretakers who previously prepared chitterlings (pork intestines).
Viral	
Hepatitis A virus	While not an emerging infectious disease, a new vehicle for infection was identified. Frozen strawberries contaminated at the processing company in California and served in U.S. Department of Agriculture-sponsored school lunch

(continued)

Table B.1. *(continued)*

Organism	Comments
	programs in several states in 1997 resulted in cases of hepatitis A in children in two states. Contaminated green onions have also been a source of infection. Infection is by the fecal–oral route.
Noroviruses (formerly Norwalk virus)	Are caliciviruses. Cause gastroenteritis, for example, from eating contaminated raw oysters resulting from oyster gatherers who used toilets without holding tanks on their boats. Also reports of outbreaks from contaminated delicatessen meats, fresh produce items, and frozen raspberries. First visualized in 1972. Have caused many outbreaks on cruise ships.
Other	
Abnormal prions	Agent causes fatal bovine spongiform encephalopathy through contaminated food (mainly beef and beef products), which is manifested as variant Creutzfeldt–Jakob disease in humans. See chapter 21.

Source: "*Angiostrongylus* meningitis," 2006; Blanton et al., 2006; Braden, 2006; Centers for Disease Control and Prevention, 2001; Gottlieb et al., 2006; MacLean, 1998; Mandell, Bennett, & Dolin, 2005; Maunula, Miettinen, & von Bonsdorff, 2005; "*Paragonimus*," 2006; Prier & Solnick, 2000; Rojas-Molina, Pedraza-Sanchez, Torres-Bibiano, Meza-Martinez, & Escobar-Gutierrez, 1999; Strickland, 2000; "*Vibrio parahaemolyticus*," 2006; "*Vibrio vulnificans*," 2006; Wheeler et al., 2005.

Table B.2. Selected Transfusion/Transplantation-Transmissible Emerging/Reemerging Infectious Agents

Agent	Disease	Comments
Viruses		
Hepatitis C virus	Hepatitis C	A flavivirus known to exist since the early 1970s but identified in 1988. Incubation period is 15–150 days. Can cause chronic hepatitis leading to cirrhosis. Many who develop disease are asymptomatic. The disease progresses slowly and insidiously, and many do not know they are infected. See chapter 12.
Hepatitis G virus (GBV-C/HGV)	See comments	May cause some commonly acquired hepatitis. At this time not believed to cause severe liver disease
Human immunodeficiency virus (HIV)	HIV disease/acquired immunodeficiency syndrome	A retrovirus first identified in a group of homosexual men in 1981 for Type 1 and in 1985 in West Africa for Type 2. Results in severe immunodeficiency and alterations leading to various opportunistic infections and neoplasms. See chapter 13.
Human T-cell lymphotropic virus 1 (HTLV-1)	Adult T-cell leukemia/lymphoma and HTLV-1-associated myelopathy/tropical spastic paresis (HAM/TSP)	Identified in 1980. Has also been linked with uveitis and arthritis. Has worldwide distribution and is endemic in certain locales. See chapter 24
HTLV-2	Adult hairy cell leukemia (probable)	Isolated in 1982. A retrovirus that may also play a role in neurologic disease similar to HAM/TSP. Endemic in certain native American and Indian populations in Panama, Brazil, and central Africa. See chapter 24.
Lymphocytic choriomeningitis virus	Central nervous system infection	Is a rodentborne zoonosis. Often occurs in those associated with Syrian hamsters as pets or in the lab. Exposure usually through aerosol, droplet, contact with rodent excreta or blood, and indirect fomite contact. Considered emerging because transmission by organ transplant has been described. Can result in meningitis.

(continued)

Table B.2. *(continued)*

Agent	Disease	Comments
Parvovirus B19	Erythema infectiosum	Identified in 1975. Transmissible only during short period of viremia. Difficult to screen for. Causes self-limited disease associated with mild rash or arthropathy. More chronic or severe manifestation in the immunocompromised and severe aplastic crises in persons with anemia. Fetal infections can cause fetal hydrops and fetal death. Has induced aplastic anemia in some transfusion recipients and symptoms in persons with hemophilia who received contaminated clotting factor.
Rabies	Rabies	Considered emerging because an unusual route of transmission has been found. Has been transmitted via organ transplantation from infected donor to recipients.
TT Virus	Unknown	May be associated with hepatitis.
West Nile virus (WNV)	West Nile fever, neuroinvasive disease	National blood screening for WNV began in 2003. See chapter 23.
Parasites		
Babesia microti and *Babesia* spp.	Babesiosis	About 26 transfusion-transmitted cases reported in the United States as of 1998 from diverse geographical areas including the northeast and the state of Washington. May be tickborne. Symptoms include fever, chills, sweating, malaise, weakness, headache, and myalgia as well as mild hepatosplenomegaly. See chapter 16.
Leishmania donovani	Leishmaniasis	Usually transmitted by sand flies. Endemic in many areas. Has expanded in range and increased in frequency with deforestation in Latin America. Has increased in fox and pet dog population. Coffee growing facilitates development of parasites in vectors. Outbreak in

Table B.2. *(continued)*

Agent	Disease	Comments
		southern Sudan due to ecological changes favoring sand flies and waves of nonimmune immigrants.
Plasmodium vivax Plasmodium falciparum Plasmodium malariae Plasmodium ovale	Malaria	Prevention of transfusion-transmitted malaria depends on donor travel history: 1-year deferral is used for those who traveled to area with endemic malaria and 3 years for those who lived in endemic area or have a history of malaria. About 3 cases of transfusion-transmitted malaria per year in the United States. See chapter 17.
Trypanosoma cruzi	Chagas disease	Overall risk in the United States is relatively low but higher than HIV and HCV, especially in endemic disease areas or where there are high concentrations of immigrants from endemic areas. Acute infection leads to chronic lifelong disease. Cases from both transfusion and organ transplantation have been described.
Bacteria		
Anaplasma phagocytophila	Human granulocytic anaplasmosis	Similar to human granulocytic ehrlichiosis (HGE). Rash is less likely to occur. May exhibit toxic shock-like syndrome, First recognized in 1992–1993. See chapter 16.
Borrelia burgdorferi	Lyme disease	Recognized in 1978 in Lyme, CT. Transmitted to humans via deer ticks. Can have severe chronic sequelae. Characterized by a skin lesion known as erythema migrans that appears in about 60% at the site of the tick bite. Other symptoms may include rash, malaise, headache, chills, fever, backache, arthralgia, and myalgia. Later effects may include arthritis and neurological and cardiac manifestations. See chapter 16.

(continued)

Table B.2. *(continued)*

Agent	Disease	Comments
Ehrlichia chaffeensis	HME	First identified in 1987 in Arkansas. Symptoms include fever, headache, chills, myalgia, arthralgia, malaise, and nausea; vomiting, diarrhea, and weight loss may develop later. A rash may develop in up to 30%. Complications can include renal symptoms, meningoencephalitis and respiratory failure. See chapter 16.
Other		
Abnormal prions	Creutzfeldt–Jakob disease	Iatrogenic disease has resulted from corneal transplant, electroencephalogram electrodes, and dura mater grafts. Agent causes fatal transmissible spongiform encephalopathy. See chapter 21.
Abnormal prions	Variant Creutzfeldt–Jakob disease	Agent causes fatal transmissible spongiform encephalopathy. See chapter 21.

Sources: Alter, Stramer, & Dodd, 2007; Brown, 2000; Busch, Kleinman, & Nemo, 2003; Centers for Disease Control and Prevention, 2006a, 2006b; Dietz et al., 2007; Dodd & Leiby, 2004; Eid, Brown, Patel, & Razonable, 2006; Foster et al., 2006; Guerrant, Walker, & Weller, 2006; Kitchen & Chiodini, 2006; Leiby, 2006; Luban, 2005; Mandell, Bennett, & Dolin, 2005; Montgomery et al., 2006; Parola, Davoust, & Raoult, 2005; Pauli, 2005; Peden, Head, Ritchie, Bell, & Ironside, 2004; Srinivasan et al., 2005.

Table B.3. Selected Emerging/Reemerging Vectorborne Diseases

Disease	Organism	Vector	Clinical Man-ifestation(s)	Comments
Bacterial				
African tick-bite fever	*Rickettsia africae*	*Amblyomma* ticks	Headache, fever, eschar at bite site, regional lymphadenopathy.	Isolated in Zimbabwe in 1990. Also seen in Tanzania, South Africa, and Guadeloupe.
Astrakhan fever	Bacteria closely related to *Rickettsia conorii*	Tick	Eruptive febrile illness occurring in summers.	First observed in 1983; 1989 identification. Reservoir includes dogs. Found near Caspian Sea.
California flea rickettsiosis	*Rickettsia felis*	Flea	Fever, headache, with or without rash. Description is not yet fully known.	Seen in California and Texas.
Flinders Island spotted fever	*Rickettsia honei*	Tick	Rash, fever, enlarged lymph nodes. Eschar may be present.	Agent identified in 1992 in Tasmania. May be related to Queensland tick typhus.
Human ehrlichiosis	*Ehrlichia ewingii*	Ticks (including Lone Star tick)	Fever, chills, headaches, leukopenia, myalgia.	Described in Missouri in 1999. Reservoir includes dogs. See chapter 16.
Human granulocytic anaplasmosis	*Anaplasma phagocytophila*	Ticks	Fever, chills, myalgia, headache, malaise. Rash not usual. Ranges in severity. Case fatality rate can be 10%.	Described in 1992–1993. Formerly known as *Ehrlichia*. See chapter 16.

(continued)

Table B.3. *(continued)*

Disease	Organism	Vector	Clinical Man-ifestation(s)	Comments
Human monocytic ehrlichiosis	*Ehrlichia chaffeensis*	Ticks (Lone Star ticks and American dog ticks)	Fever, headache, chills, myalgia, malaise with nausea, vomiting, anorexia. Rash occurs in 20–30%. Case fatality rate can be 5%. Multiorgan failure can occur.	Described in 1987. Reservoir includes white-tailed deer. See chapter 16.
Israeli spotted fever/Israeli tick typhus	*Rickettsia conorii* variants	Ticks	Mild spotted fever.	Described in 1974. Occurs in Israel and near Caspian sea.
Japanese or Oriental spotted fever	*Rickettsia japonica*	Ticks	Rash, fever, chills. May be black necrotic lesion at bite site.	Recognized in Japan in 1984. Agent isolated in 1986. Reservoir includes mice and other rodents.
Lyme disease	*Borrelia burgdorferi*	Ticks	Rash, fever, chills, malaise, myalgias. May evolve into chronic illness with neurological symptoms and arthritis.	Reservoirs include deer, mice, and birds. See chapter 16.
Marseilles tick- bite fever	*Rickettsia mongoloti-monae*	Ticks	A spotted fever with rash, fever, and headache.	Identified in Mongolia and Marseilles, France. First found in 1996. Reservoirs

Table B.3. *(continued)*

Disease	Organism	Vector	Clinical Manifestation(s)	Comments
				include migratory birds.
Spotted fever rickettsiosis	*Rickettsia parkeri* (and other agents)	Ticks	A spotted fever with rash, fever, headache, myalgia, and multiple eschars.	Recognized as a bacterium in 1939 but not associated with human disease until 2004.
Parasitic				
Babesiosis	*Babesia microti* and other species	Ticks	Manifestations can include fever, chills, malaise, headache, myalgia, abdominal pain, mild hepatosplenomegaly, and depression. Complications can include renal failure, adult respiratory distress syndrome, myocardial infarction. Can range from asymptomatic to severe disease, especially in the elderly or immunocompromised.	See chapter 16.
Leishmaniasis	*Leishmania donovani*	Sand fleas	Malaise, fever, chills.	Causes illness in 500,000 yearly. Possibly emerging in

(continued)

Table B.3. *(continued)*

Disease	Organism	Vector	Clinical Manifestation(s)	Comments
				United States through pet dogs brought back from endemic areas abroad by military families, and now found in fox hounds in United States.
Malaria	*Plasmodium vivax Plasmodium falciparum Plasmodium ovale Plasmodium malariae*	Mosquitoes (*Anopheles* spp)	Chills, fever, anemia. Severity depends on species. See chapter 17.	Drug resistance is becoming problematic. Locally acquired cases have been described in the United States.
Viral				
Cache Valley virus disease	Cache Valley virus	Mosquitoes	Encephalitis	Very rare bunyavirus seen in North America. Not commonly screened for.
California–LaCrosse encephalitis	LaCrosse encephalitis virus	*Aedes* mosquitoes	Encephalitis	First isolated in 1964. Occurs primarily in children.
Chikungunya fever	Chikungunya virus	Mosquitoes *Aedes* spp.	Fever, arthralgia, and rash.	This alphavirus was first isolated in Tasmania in 1953. Considered as reemerging due to expansion of range into Asia and the Indian Islands. Reunion Islands are particularly

Table B.3. *(continued)*

Disease	Organism	Vector	Clinical Man-ifestation(s)	Comments
				hard hit. This outbreak has unreported complications such as vertical transmission, myocarditis, and hepatitis as well as encephalitis.
Crimean-Congo hemor-rhagic fever	Crimean-Congo hemorrhagic fever virus	Ticks	Sudden onset of fever, headache, back and joint pain, red eyes, bleeding man-ifestations such as severe bruising, and nosebleeds.	Bunyavirus. Hard ticks are vectors and reservoir. Isolated in 1967. Treatment is supportive.
Dengue virus	Dengue and dengue hemorrhagic fever	Mosquitoes	See chapter 7.	Has expanded its geographic range beginning in the mid-1970s. Are four serotypes. Belongs to the flavivirus family. Worldwide tropical distribution. Causes a spectrum of disease depending on serotype and host characteristics.
Encephalitis	Rocio virus	Mosquitoes	Encephalitis	A flavivirus detected during an encephalitis outbreak in Brazil in 1975–1976.

(continued)

Table B.3. *(continued)*

Disease	Organism	Vector	Clinical Manifestation(s)	Comments
Encephalitis	Venezuelan equine encephalitis virus (VEE)	Mosquitoes	Usually mild infection with headache, chills, fever, myalgia, nausea, and vomiting.	VEE virus characterized in 1930s. No outbreaks reported from 1973 to 1992. Large outbreak in 1995 in Venezuela and Colombia affecting humans and horses.
Febrile disease with or without central nervous system (CNS) manifestations	Toscana virus	Sand fly	Fever, nausea, vomiting, headache, neck rigidity, and myalgia disease with or without CNS manifestations such as meningitis.	Is a bunyavirus. Can be asymptomatic. Found in Italy, Portugal, France, Slovenia, Greece, Cyprus, and Turkey. Incubation period is a few days to 2 weeks.
O'nyong-nyong fever	O'nyong-nyong virus	Mosquito	Arthralgia, generalized skin rash, lymphadenopathy, fever.	Alphavirus in the *Togaviridae* family initially isolated during an epidemic in Uganda in 1959 affecting more than 2 million people. Another major outbreak occurred in 1996–1997, when the virus showed a genetic difference from the earlier outbreak. Usually nonfatal.

Table B.3. *(continued)*

Disease	Organism	Vector	Clinical Man-ifestation(s)	Comments
Oropouche fever	Oropouche virus	Biting midge, mosquitoes	Fever, headache, ocular pain, myalgia, and arthralgia.	The virus was first isolated in 1955 in Trinidad from a febrile forest worker.
Rift Valley fever	Rift Valley virus	Mosquitoes	Flu-like syndrome to hemorrhagic fever, encephalitis, and/or retinitis.	While a few early human cases were recognized, the first large human epidemic was in Egypt in 1977–1978 involving about 200,000 cases and about 600 deaths. East African epidemic took place in 1997–1998 involving Kenya and Somalia. Is usually a zoonosis affecting sheep and cattle. Transmitted by mosquitoes, aerosol, and contact. An outbreak in Kenya had affected 154 people with 52 deaths as of early January, 2007.

Sources: Bessaud et al., 2006; Buller et al., 1999; Centers for Disease Control and Prevention, 2006b; Dumler, 2005; Enserink, 2000; Goodman, Dennis, & Sonenshine, 2005; Guerrant, Walker, & Weller, 2006; Mandell, Bennett, & Dolin, 2005; Parola et al., 2006; Parola, Paddock, & Raoult, 2005; "Rift Valley fever", 2007; Strickland, 2000; Wormser, 2006.

REFERENCES

Alter, H. J., Stramer, S. L., & Dodd, R. Y. (2007). Emerging infectious diseases that threaten the blood supply. *Seminars in Hematology, 44,* 32–41.

Angiostrongylus meningitis—China (02). (2006). *ProMED Digest, 376,* unpaginated.

Bessaud, M., Peyrefitte, C. N., Pastorino, B. A. M., Tock, F., Merle, O., Colpart, J.-J., et al. (2006). Chikungunya virus strains, Reunion Island outbreak. *Emerging Infectious Diseases, 12,* 1604–1606.

Blanton, L. H., Adams, S. M., Beard, R. S., Wei, G., Bulens, S. N., Widdowson, M.-A., et al. (2006). Molecular and epidemiologic trends of caliciviruses associated with outbreaks of acute gastroenteritis in the United States, 2000–2004. *Journal of Infectious Diseases, 193,* 413–421.

Braden, C. R. (2006). *Salmonella enterica* serotype enteritidis and eggs: A national epidemic in the United States. *Clinical Infectious Diseases, 43,* 512–517.

Brown, P. (2000). The risk of blood-borne Creutzfeldt-Jakob disease. *Developments in Biological Standardization, 102,* 53–59.

Buller, R. S., Arens, M., Hmiel, S. P., Paddock, C. D., Sumner, J. W., & Rikihisa, Y. (1999). *Ehrlichia ewingii,* a newly recognized agent of human ehrlichiosis. *New England Journal of Medicine, 341,* 148–155.

Busch, M. P., Kleinman, S. H., & Nemo, G. J. (2003). Current and emerging infectious risks of blood transfusions. *Journal of the American Medical Association, 289,* 959–962.

Centers for Disease Control and Prevention. (2001). Diagnosis and management of foodborne illnesses: A primer for physicians. *Morbidity & Mortality Weekly Report, 50,* 1–69.

Centers for Disease Control and Prevention. (2006a). Chagas disease after organ transplantation—Los Angeles, California, 2006. *Morbidity & Mortality Weekly Report, 55,* 798–800.

Centers for Disease Control and Prevention. (2006b). Diagnosis and management of tickborne rickettsial diseases: Rocky Mountain spotted fever, ehrlichioses, and anaplasmosis—United States. *Morbidity and Mortality Weekly Report, 55*(RR-4), 1–29.

Dietz, K., Raddatz, G., Wallis, J., Müller, N., Zerr, I., Duerr, H-P, et al. (2007). Blood transfusion and spread of variant Creutzfeldt-Jakob disease. *Emerging Infectious Diseases, 13,* 89–95.

Dodd, R. Y., & Leiby, D. A. (2004). Emerging infectious threats to the blood supply. *Annual Review of Medicine, 55,* 191–207.

Dumler, J. S. (2005). *Anaplasma* and *Ehrlichia* infection. *Annals of the New York Academy of Sciences, 1063,* 361–373.

Eid, A. J., Brown, R. A., Patel, R., & Razonable, R. R. (2006). Parvovirus B19 after transplantation: A review of 98 cases. *Clinical Infectious Diseases, 43,* 40–48.

Enserink, M. (2000). Has leishmaniasis become endemic in the U.S.? *Science, 290,* 1181, 1183.

Foster, E. S., Signs, K. A., Marks, D. R., Kapoor, H., Casey, M., Stobierski, M. G., et al. (2006). Lymphocytic choriomeningitis in Michigan. *Emerging Infectious Diseases, 12,* 851–853.

Goodman, J. L., Dennis, D. T., & Sonenshine, D. E. (Eds.). (2005). *Tick-borne diseases of humans.* Washington, DC: ASM Press.

Gottlieb, S. L., Newbern, E. C., Griffin, P. M., Graves, L. M., Hoekstra, R. M., Baker, N. L., et al. (2006). Multistate outbreak of listeriosis linked to turkey deli meat and subsequent changes in US regulatory policy. *Clinical Infectious Diseases, 42,* 29–36.

Guerrant, R. L., Walker, D. H., & Weller, P. F. (Eds.). (2006). *Tropical infectious diseases* (2nd ed.). Philadelphia: Churchill Livingstone Elsevier.

Kitchen, A. D. & Chiodini, P. L. (2006). Malaria and blood transfusion. *Vox Sanguinis, 90,* 77–84.

Klein, H. G. (2000). Will blood transfusion ever be safe enough? *Journal of the American Medical Association, 284,* 238–240.

Leiby, D. A. (2006). Babesiosis and blood transfusion: Flying under the radar. *Vox Sanguinis, 90,* 157–165.

Luban, N. L. C. (2005). Transfusion safety: Where are we today? *Annals of the New York Academy of Sciences, 1054,* 325–341.

MacLean, J. D. (1998). The North American liver fluke, *Metorchis conjunctus.* In W. M. Scheld, W. A. Craig, & J. M. Hughes (Eds.), *Emerging infections 2* (pp. 243–256). Washington, DC: ASM Press.

Mandell, G. L., Bennett, J. E., & Dolin, R. (Eds.). (2005). *Mandell, Douglas, and Bennett's principles and practice of infectious diseases* (6th ed.). Philadelphia: Churchill Livingstone Elsevier.

Maunula, L., Miettinen, I. T., & von Bonsdorff, C. H. (2005). Norovirus outbreaks from drinking water. *Emerging Infectious Diseases, 11,* 1716–1721.

Montgomery, S. P., Brown, J. A., Kuehnert, M., Smith, T. L., Crall, N., Lanciotti, R. S. et al., (2006). Transfusion-associated transmission of West Nile virus, United States 2003 through 2005. *Transfusion, 46,* 2038–2046.

Paragonimus—US (California). (2006). *ProMED Digest, 372,* unpaginated.

Parola, P., Davoust, B., & Raoult, D. (2005). Tick-and flea-borne rickettsial emerging zoonoses. *Veterinary Research, 36,* 469–492.

Parola, P., de Lamballerie, X., Jourdan, J., Rovery, C., Vaillant, V., Minodier, P., et al. (2006). Novel Chikungunya virus variant in travelers returning from Indian Ocean islands. *Emerging Infectious Diseases, 12,* 1493–1499.

Parola, P., Paddock, C. D., & Raoult, D. (2005). Tick-borne rickettsioses around the world: Emerging diseases challenging old concepts. *Clinical Microbiology Reviews, 18,* 719–756.

Pauli, G. (2005). Tissue safety in view of CJD and variant CJD. *Cell and Tissue Banking, 6,* 191–200.

Peden, A. H., Head, M. W., Ritchie, D. L., Bell, J. E., & Ironside, J. W. (2004). Preclinical CJD after blood transfusion in a PRNP codon 129 heterozygous patient. *Lancet, 364,* 529–531.

Prier, R., & Solnick, J. V. (2000). Foodborne and waterborne infectious diseases. *Postgraduate Medicine, 107,* 245–255.

Rift Valley fever—Kenya (North Eastern Province) (02). (2007). *ProMED Digest, 004,* unpaginated.

Rojas-Molina, N., Pedraza-Sanchez, S., Torres-Bibiano, B., Meza-Martinez, H., & Escobar-Gutierrez, A. (1999). Gnathostomosis, an emerging foodborne zoonotic disease in Acapulco, Mexico. *Emerging Infectious Diseases, 5,* 264–266.

Srinivasan, A., Burton, E. C., Kuehnert, M. J., Rupprecht, C., Sutker, W. L., Ksiazek, T. G., et al. (2005). Transmission of rabies virus from an organ donor to four transplant recipients. *New England Journal of Medicine, 352,* 1103–1111.

Strickland, G. T. (Ed.). (2000). *Hunter's tropical medicine and emerging infectious diseases* (8th ed.). Philadelphia: W. B. Saunders.

Vibrio parahaemolyticus, shellfish—USA: Rhode Island. (2006, August 5). *ProMED Digest, 348,* unpaginated.

Vibrio vulnificus—USA (multistate). (2006, August 7). *ProMED Digest, 352,* unpaginated.

Wheeler, C., Vogt, T. M., Armstrong, G. L., Vaughan, G., Weltman, A., Nainan, O. V., et al. (2005). An outbreak of hepatitis A associated with green onions. *New England Journal of Medicine, 353,* 890–897.

Wormser, G. P. (2006). Early Lyme disease. *New England Journal of Medicne, 354,* 2794–2801.

APPENDIX C

Prevention of Emerging/Reemerging Infectious Diseases

Felissa R. Lashley

Table C.1. Prevention of Foodborne Illness*

- Avoid raw or undercooked meat and poultry. Use a thermometer to measure the internal temperature of meat. Meats should be cooked to an internal temperature of at least 160° F, and poultry to 170° F for turkey breast and 165° F to 180° F for others. Fish should be opaque and firm; shellfish in shells should be cooked until the shells open.
- Cook eggs until the yolks are firm. Avoid raw or undercooked eggs or foods containing raw or lightly cooked eggs, including certain salad dressings, cookie and cake batters, sauces, and beverages such as unpasteurized eggnog. If you use recipes in which eggs remain raw or only partially cooked, use pasteurized eggs.
- Avoid raw or undercooked fish or shellfish, including oysters, clams, mussels, and scallops. Properly cooked fish should be opaque and flake easily with a fork.
- Avoid raw or unpasteurized milk or cheeses.
- Avoid unpasteurized fruit or vegetable juices.
- Make sure there are no cold spots where pathogens can survive when cooking in a microwave oven.
- Bring sauces, soups, and gravies to a boil when reheating. Heat other leftovers thoroughly to at least 165° F.

(continued)

Table C.1. *(continued)*

- Avoid cross-contaminating foods by washing hands, utensils, countertops, and cutting boards with hot, soapy water after they have been in contact with food items and before preparing the next food. If possible, use a different cutting board for raw meat, poultry, and seafood products.
- Rinse poultry before cooking.
- Wash hands with hot, soapy water before preparing and after handling food and after using the bathroom, touching a pet, or changing a diaper.
- Educate food handlers on appropriate hand washing and food preparation procedures as well as personal hygiene.
- Exclude ill employees from food handling and preparation.
- Put cooked meat on a clean platter, rather than back on the one that held the raw meat. Use separate plates for cooked food and raw foods.
- Refrigerate leftovers promptly—do not leave at room temperature. Refrigerate or freeze perishables, prepared foods, and leftovers within 2 hours or sooner.
- Divide large amounts of leftovers into shallow containers for quick cooling in the refrigerator. Do not pack the refrigerator; cool air must circulate to keep food safe.
- Avoid leaving cut produce at room temperature for many hours.
- Do not defrost food at room temperature. Thaw food in the refrigerator, under cold running water, or in the microwave oven.
- Marinate foods in the refrigerator.
- Separate raw meat, poultry, and seafood from other foods in your grocery shopping cart and in your refrigerator.
- Rinse fresh fruits and vegetables in running tap water to remove visible dirt and grime. Do not use soap or detergents. If necessary, use a small vegetable brush to remove surface dirt. Also wash packaged salad mixes even if marked prewashed.
- Be careful not to contaminate foods while slicing them up on the cutting board.
- Avoid preparing food for others if you have a diarrheal illness.
- Avoid eating food prepared from nonlicensed street vendors, particularly in developing countries.
- When eating out, eat in establishments with high ratings from the health department.
- In developing countries, avoid eating cut fresh fruits and vegetables, salads, and nonpeelable fruits and vegetables. Hot foods should be served piping hot.
- Avoid eating food and organ parts from certain high-risk animals including rodents, bushmeat, squirrels, and game animals.

Table C.1. *(continued)*

Special Added Prevention for Immunocompromised Persons

- Educate them and their caregivers about high-risk foods.
- Avoid soft cheeses such as feta, Brie, Camembert, blue-veined, and Mexican-style cheese.
- Avoid getting fluid from hot dog packages on other surfaces or utensils.
- Avoid raw sprouts such as alfalfa, clover, and radish.
- Avoid refrigerated pates or meat spreads and raw or refrigerated lightly smoked fishes such as salmon, trout, whitefish, and mackerel, which may be labeled as lox, kippered, smoked, or jerky.
- Reheat to hot some foods that are bought precooked because they can become contaminated with pathogens after they have been processed and packaged. These foods include hot dogs, luncheon meats (cold cuts), fermented and dry sausage, and other deli-style meat and poultry products.
- Refer to Centers for Disease Control and Prevention, 2002a, for additional preventive measures.

Sources: Centers for Disease Control and Prevention, 2001, 2002a; Gottleib et al., 2006; Guerrant, Walker, & Weller, 2006; Mandell, Bennett, & Dolin, 2005; Strickland, 2000; Talbot, Gagnon, & Greenblatt, 2006.
*Other preventive measures involving the ways in which foods are grown, harvested, stored, prepared, served, packaged, and transported are not covered here.

Table C.2. Measures to Prevent Waterborne Infection

- Store treated water safely.
- Avoid drinking tap water or using ice made from tap water in developing countries.
- Ensure proper treatment of potable water.
- Keep cattle and other such animals away from surface water including rivers or ponds that serve community drinking systems.
- Locate human waste disposal systems such as latrines so that they do not contaminate the water supply by either underground seepage or runoff.
- Wash all fruits and vegetables thoroughly in safe water.
- Wash hands properly and thoroughly:
  - after any contact with animals,
  - after any contact with soil (e.g., gardening),
  - after changing diapers, and
  - before eating or preparing food.
- Avoid drinking water directly from lakes, rivers, ponds, or streams.
- Avoid swallowing water while showering, and use safe water for brushing teeth in developing countries.
- Avoid swimming in water that is likely to be contaminated with human or animal waste and avoid swallowing water during swimming.
- Address cultural practices with the community that include washing in, playing in, and perhaps drinking from the same water where untreated human or animal waste is disposed of or where funeral rites such as washing and preparing the body are carried out.
- Address environmental and policy issues such as proper flood control; proper water treatment and maintenance; replacement of water treatment, storage, and distribution systems; control of animal runoff to surface water and wells; and proper waste elimination from shipping vessels at the appropriate levels.

Additional Measures for Immunocompromised Persons

- Educate yourself specifically about risks and prevention.
- Avoid exposure to young animals such as calves and lambs on farms or at petting zoos.
- Avoid travel in developing countries or use protective measures.
- Avoid sexual practices that may result in exposure to feces.
- Avoid swimming in lakes, rivers, streams, ponds, public swimming pools, or recreational water parks.
- Avoid working with diaper-aged children.
- Avoid contact with feces of all animals, particularly young farm animals such as calves.
- Consume only water that has been purified by boiling for 1 minute or by treatment with certain filters. The CDC AIDS Hotline (1-800-342-2437) has information on filters that remove *Cryptosporidium* from water.

Sources: Centers for Disease Control and Prevention, 2001, 2002a, 2002b, 2004a, 2005a; Guerrant, Weller, & Walker, 2006.

Table C.3. Prevention of Recreational Waterborne Infection

- Provide adequate bathroom facilities including diaper-changing areas at recreational areas.
- Limit the number of swimmers per unit area.
- Educate patrons and operators.
- Improve filtration methods, disinfection methods, and pool design.
- Change recreational water industry practices (e.g., provide specific pools with dedicated filtration systems for children so the water is not mixed with adult pools, limit access of young children to adult pools, and operate filtration systems at higher turnover rates).
- Refrain from swimming when experiencing diarrhea and continue to do so for weeks after the resolution of the diarrhea.
- Swimmers, boaters, rafters, and water-skiers should avoid swallowing recreational water.
- Encourage persons not to enter the water if they have diarrhea because people can spread germs in the water even without having an "accident."
- Wash hands thoroughly after using the toilet or changing diapers, and clean the rectal area thoroughly after a bowel movement.
- Notify lifeguards of fecal matter in the water or persons changing diapers on tables and chairs in pool or beach areas.
- Encourage parents to take children to the toilet for bathroom breaks often.
- Change diapers in a bathroom, not near the pool or shore.
- Wash children thoroughly (especially their bottoms) with soap and water before swimming because everyone has invisible amounts of fecal matter on his or her bottom that ends up in the water.
- Include in education programs that swim diapers or pants to keep fecal matter from leaking into the water are not leakproof.

Note: Technical information on filtration and disinfection may be obtained from the Environmental Protection Agency. Immunocompromised persons may need special precautions.
Sources: Centers for Disease Control and Prevention [CDC], 2002a, 2004b, 2005a. Information about preventing recreational waterborne illness is available from the CDC's Web site at http://www.cdc.gov/healthyswimming.

Table C.4. Measures to Prevent Tickborne Infectious Diseases

- Avoid tick-infested areas when possible.
- Walk in the middle of trails and avoid side vegetation.
- Wear appropriate barrier clothing.
- Remove any attached ticks carefully, promptly, and properly.
- Wear long pants.
- Tuck pant legs into socks.
- Tuck shirt into pants.
- Wear hat.
- Use appropriate tick repellants correctly.
- Treat clothing with permethrin repellant.
- Apply DEET insect repellant to outdoor clothing and exposed skin using appropriate precautions.
- Do body checks for ticks at least once per day and more often if necessary.
- Wear light-colored clothing so ticks are visible in contrast.
- Pull back long hair.
- Clear brush and leaf litter from around houses, and keep grassy areas mowed.
- Limit food available to rodents from house areas such as keeping bird feeders distant from houses.
- Keep wildlife such as deer away from houses and gardens.
- Remove ticks from household pets promptly.

Sources: Buckingham, 2005; Centers for Disease Control and Prevention, 2006; Guerrant, Walker, & Weller, 2006.

Table C.5. Preventing Mosquito Bites

- Use good screens on windows and doors.
- Limit time outside during peak mosquito activity such as dawn and dusk.
- Sleep in an air-conditioned, well-screened area whenever possible.
- Keep unscreened windows closed.
- Use a mosquito net saturated with permethrin (e.g., Elimite, Nix) if screens or pyrethrin insecticides are not available (nets are available at camping supply retailers).
- Use permethrin spray on clothes to repel mosquitoes (e.g., tick repellents, Duranon, Permanonel).
- Use an aerosol "knock-down" spray in the rooms, including shower areas.
- Always wear dark-colored, long-sleeved clothing and long pants, especially at night.
- Spray an insecticide or repellent on clothing because mosquitoes may bite through thin clothing.
- Apply an insect repellent that contains either N, N-diethyl-*m*-toluamide (DEET) or dimethyl phthalate to exposed areas such as wrists and ankles.
- Be watchful for mosquitoes, especially in the evening.
- Avoid using perfume or any other kind of scented cosmetics.
- Use household insecticides for flying insects in a hotel room.
- Travel during low transmission seasons when possible.
- Seek accommodation in facilities at higher elevations, if possible.
- Use burning coils or candles formulated with mosquito repellents for outdoor lounging.
- Try to stay in air-conditioned or well-screened quarters.
- Change water in birdbaths regularly.
- Cover stored water in receptacles tightly.
- Eliminate potential mosquito breeding sites such as old tires, tree holes, flower pots, wading pools, and any open containers that collect water.
- Dispose of refuse promptly and appropriately.
- Campaign aggressively for education about the above items.

Note: Vitamin B and ultrasound devices do not prevent mosquito bites. Environmental methods of mosquito control are not covered here.

Sources: Centers for Disease Control and Prevention, 2005b, 2005c; Guerrant, Walker & Weller, 2006.

Table C.6. Prevention of Rodentborne Infection

Around the Home
    Wash dishes and clean floors and counters.
    Discard leftover pet food and empty water bowls at night inside and
        outside the home.
    Store food and garbage in containers with tight lids inside and outside the
        home.
    Clear brush and grass from foundations.
    Seal holes and cracks or use metal flashing around base of buildings.
    Conduct ongoing trapping if plague is a problem.
    Spread flea powder in area, and be careful to follow directions to protect
        humans and domestic animals.
    Elevate hay, wood piles, and garbage cans and locate them 100 feet from
        the house.
    Remove junk or things that provide shelter to rodents.
    Store animal feed in containers with lids.

When Cleaning Rodent-Infested Areas
    Air out the area before entering.
    Wear rubber gloves.
    Do not stir up or breathe in dust.
    Soak contaminated areas with disinfectant (e.g., Lysol, bleach solution).
    Dispose of dead animals properly; do not handle dead animals with bare
        hands; and bury, burn, or use double plastic bags for disposal in trash.
    Disinfect and dispose of used gloves.

When Camping or Hiking
    Air out abandoned or unused cabins.
    Inspect cabins for rodent infestation; if present, do not use if possible.
    Check potential outdoor sleeping areas for rodent droppings and burrows.
    Do not disturb rodent burrows or dens.
    Do not sleep near woodpiles or garbage areas.
    Avoid sleeping on bare ground; use mats or elevated cots.
    Store all food in rodent-proof containers and promptly discard, bury, or
        burn garbage.
    Do not handle wild rodents even if friendly like chipmunks, ground
        squirrels, and others.

Sources: Centers for Disease Control and Prevention, 2002b; Guerrant, Walker, & Weller, 2006.

REFERENCES

Buckingham, S. C. (2005). Tick-borne infections in children. *Pediatric Drugs, 7,* 163–176.

Centers for Disease Control and Prevention. (2001). Diagnosis and management of foodborne illnesses: A primer for physicians. *Morbidity and Mortality Weekly Report, 50,* 1–69.

Centers for Disease Control and Prevention. (2002a). Guidelines for preventing opportunistic infections among HIV-infected persons—2002 recommendations of the U.S. Public Health Service and the Infectious Disease Society of America. *Morbidity and Mortality Weekly Report, 51*(RR-8), 1–52.

Centers for Disease Control and Prevention. (2002b). Hantavirus pulmonary syndrome—United States: Updated recommendations for risk reduction. *Morbidity and Mortality Weekly Report, 51*(RR-9), 1–15.

Centers for Disease Control and Prevention. (2004a). Surveillance for waterborne-disease outbreaks associated with drinking water—United States, 2001–2002. *Morbidity and Mortality Weekly Report, 53*(SS-8), 23–44.

Centers for Disease Control and Prevention. (2004b). Surveillance for waterborne-disease outbreaks associated with recreational water—United States, 2001–2002. *Morbidity and Mortality Weekly Report, 53*(SS-8), 1–22.

Centers for Disease Control and Prevention. (2005a, August 19). *Fact sheet. Preventing cryptosporidiosis: A guide for people with compromised immune systems.* Atlanta, GA: Author.

Centers for Disease Control and Prevention. (2005b, October 5). *Information for the public: Prescription drugs for malaria.* Retrieved August 9, 2006, from http://www.cdc.gov/travel/malariadrugs.htm

Centers for Disease Control and Prevention. (2005c, August 22). *West Nile virus. Fight the bite. Avoid mosquito bites to avoid infection.* Retrieved July 26, 2006, from http://www.cdc.gov/ncidod/dvbid/westnile/prevention_info.htm

Centers for Disease Control and Prevention. (2006). *National Center for Infectious Diseases infectious disease information.* Available from http://www.cdc.gov/ncidod/index.htm

Gottlieb, S. L., Newbern, E. C., Griffin, P. M., Graves, L. M., Hoekstra, R. M., Baker, N. L., et al. (2006). Multistate outbreak of listeriosis linked to turkey deli meat and subsequent changes in US regulatory policy. *Clinical Infectious Diseases, 42,* 29–36.

Guerrant, R. L., Walker, D. H., & Weller, P. F. (Eds.). (2006). *Tropical infectious diseases* (2nd ed.). Philadelphia: Churchill Livingstone Elsevier.

Mandell, G. L., Bennett, J. E., & Dolin R. (Eds.). (2005). *Mandell, Douglas and Bennett's principles and practice of infectious discuses* (6th ed.). Philadelphia: Churchill Livingstone Elsevier.

Strickland, G. T. (Ed.). (2000). *Hunter's tropical medicine and emerging infectious diseases* (8th ed.). Philadelphia: W. B. Saunders.

Talbot, E. A., Gagnon, E. R., & Greenblatt, J. (2006). Common ground for the control of multidrug-resistant *Salmonella* in ground beef. *Clinical Infectious Disease, 42,* 1455–1462.

APPENDIX D

Selected Resources

Jerry D. Durham and Felissa R. Lashley

The resources listed include Web sites, organizations, government agencies, universities, and publications. Information on the majority of these topics can also be obtained through the Centers for Disease Control and Prevention (CDC) Web site at http://www.cdc.gov; the World Health Organization (WHO) Web site at http://www.who.int/home_page; and the National Institute of Allergy and Infectious Diseases (NIAID), a division of the National Institutes of Health, Web site at http://www.niaid.nih.gov. Thus, these particular resources are not repeated under each listed topic. State health departments are an additional source of information.

SELECTED WEB SITES FOR SPECIFIC DISEASES/TOPICS

Acquired Immunodeficiency Syndrome (AIDS): See human immunodeficiency virus.
Anaplasmosis: See Lyme disease.
Antimicrobial Resistance

- CDC Antibiotic/Antimicrobial Resistance
  http://www.cdc.gov/drugresistance/
- CDC Antimicrobial Resistance Action Plan
  http://www.cdc.gov/drugresistance/actionplan/index.htm
- Committee to Reduce Infection Deaths
  http://www.hospital-infection.org

- FDA, Center for Veterinary Medicine, National Antimicrobial Monitoring System
  http://www.fda.gov/cvm/narms_pg.html
- U.S. Food and Drug Administration (FDA)
  http://www.fda.gov/cvm/antimicrobial.html

Avian Influenza

- CDC
  http://www.cdc.gov/flu/avian/
- NIAID
  http://www3.niaid.nih.gov/news/focuson/flu/
- U.S. Government Pandemic Flu Home Page
  http://www.pandemicflu.gov/
- WHO
  http://www.who.int/csr/disease/avian_influenza/en/

Babesia: See also Lyme disease.

- American Medical Association
  http://www.ama-assn.org/ama/pub/category/6667.html
- Babesia project
  http://www.vetmed.ucdavis.edu/vbdp/babesia.htm

Bioterrorism

- CDC
  http://www.bt.cdc.gov/bioterrorism/overview.asp
- Department of Homeland Security
  http://www.dhs.gov/xprepresp/committees/editorial_0566.shtm
- National Library of Medicine
  http://www.nlm.nih.gov/medlineplus/biodefenseandbioterrorism.html

Bovine Spongiform Encephalopathy: See Creutzfeldt–Jakob disease and prion diseases.
Cholera

- CDC
  http://www.cdc.gov/ncidod/dbmd/diseaseinfo/cholera_g.htm
- WHO Report on Global Surveillance of Epidemic-Prone Infectious Diseases
  http://www.who.int/csr/resources/publications/cholera/CSR_ISR_2000_1/en/index.html

Clostridium difficile

- CDC, Healthcare-Associated Infections
  http://www.cdc.gov/ncidid/dhqp/id_Cdiff.html
- Clostridium difficile Support Group
  http://cdiffsupport.com

Creutzfeldt–Jakob Disease: See also prion diseases.

- CJD Support Network
  http://www.patient.co.uk
- UK Creutzfeldt-Jakob Disease Surveillance Unit
  http://www.cjd.ed.ac.uk/
- WHO Variant Creutzfeldt-Jakob Disease
  http://www.who.int/mediacentre/factsheets/fs180/en/

Cryptosporidiosis

- Parasitology link
  http://www.k-state.edu/parasitology/

Cyclospora cayatenensis: See also parasites.

- *Cyclospora*
  http://www.k-state.edu/parasitology/cyclospora/cyclospora.html

Dengue Fever

- CDC Handbook
  http://www.cdc.gov/ncidod/dvbid/dengue/
- Directors of Health Promotion and Education
  http://www.astdhpphe.org.infect/dengue.html
- National Institute of Allergy and Infectious Disease
  http://www.niaid.nih.gov/factsheets/dengue/htm
- National Library of Medicine
  http://www.nlm.nih.gov/medlineplus/dengue.html
- WHO
  http://www.who.int/topics/dengue/en/

Ebola Virus

- CDC
  http://www.bt.cdc.gov/agent/vhf
  http://www.cdc.gov/ncidod/dvrd/spb/mnpages/dispages/ebola.htm

- WHO, Communicable Disease Surveillance and Response (CSR)
  http://www.who.int/csr/diseases/ebola/en/

Escherichia coli

- CDC
  http://www.cdc.gov/ncidod/dbmd/diseaseinfo/escherichiacoli_g.ht
- Environmental Protection Agency
  http://www.epa.gov.safewater/ecoli.html
- Food Safety News on the Net
  http://www.mednews.net/bacteria/
- U.S. FDA, Center for Food Safety and Applied Nutrition
  http://vm.cfsan.fda.gov/~mow/chapl5.html

Foodborne Diseases

- CDC site provides an abundance of information on food safety
  http://www.cdc.gov/foodsafety
- Food Safety Research Information Office
  http://www.nal.usda.gov/fsrio/
- Gateway to Government Food Safety Information
  http://www.foodsafety.gov

Hantavirus

- American Lung Association
  http://www.lungusa.org/site/pp.asp?c=dvLUK9O0E&b=35428
- Canada's National Occupational Health and Safety Resource
  http://www.ccohs.ca/oshanswers/diseases/hantavir.html
- CDC, National Center for Infectious Diseases (NCID)
  http://www.cdc.gov/ncidod/discases/hanta/hps/index.htm
- Tropical Diseases Web Ring
  http://www.hantavirus.net/

Hepatitis C

- Hepatitis Foundation International
  http://www.hepfi.org/
- National Digestive Diseases Information Clearinghouse
  http://www.niddk.nih.gov/ddiseases/pubs/chronichepc/index.htm
- National Hepatitis C Coalition
  http://nationalhepatitis-c.org/

Human Immunodeficiency Virus (HIV)

- AIDS Education Global Information System
  http://www.aegis.com/
- AIDSinfo
  http://www.aidsinfo.nih.gov
- AIDS Research Information Center
  http://www.critpath.org/aric/
- AIDS Treatment Information Service
  http://www.hivatis.org
- CDC
  http://www.cdc.gov/hiv/
- CDC, National Prevention Information Network
  http://www.cdcnpin.org/
- HIV InSite Gateway to HIV and AIDS Knowledge
  http://hivinsite.ucsf.edu
- International Association of AIDS Physicians
  http://www.iapac.org
- National Library of Medicine, Specialized Information Services
  http://sis.nlm.nih.gov/HIV/HIVMain.html
- NIAID, Division of Acquired Immunodeficiency Syndrome, NIH
  http://www.niaid.nih.gov/daids/default.htm

Immunocompromised Persons

- Immune Deficiency Foundation
  http://www.primaryimmune.org/
- NIAID, National Institutes of Health
  http://www.niaid.nih.gov/Publications

Lassa Virus

- CDC Lassa Fever Online Slide Set
  http://www.cdc.gov/ncidod/dvrd/spb/mnpages/dispages/
  lassaf.htm

Legionellosis

- The *Legionella* Experts
  http://www.legionella.org
- Legionellosis Resource Site
  http://www.cdc.gov/legionella/

- *Legionella* Risk Management
  http://www.legionellarm.com/faq/faq.htm
- Occupational Safety and Health Administration
  http://www.q-net.net.au/~legion/Legionnaire%60s_Disease_
  Links.htm

Lyme Disease

- American Lyme Disease Foundation, Inc.
  http://www.aldf.com/lyme/stml
- CDC, Division of Vector-Borne Infectious Diseases
  http://www.cdc.gov/ncidod/dvbid/lymeinfo.htm
- International Lyme and Associated Diseases Society
  http://www.ilads.org/
- Lyme Disease Resource Center
  http://www.lymedisease.org/
- Links on Lyme Disease
  http://www.geocities.com/HotSprings/Oasis/6455/lyme-
  links.html

Malaria

- CDC
  http://www.cdc.gov/malaria
- Deployment Health Clinical Center
  http://www.pdhealth.mil/malaria.asp
- Division of Parasitic Disease, CDC
  http://www.dpd.cdc.gov/dpdx/html/malaria.htm
- Malaria Foundation International
  http://www.malaria.org/
- Malaria Genome Project
  http://www.sanger.ac.uk/Projects/P_falciparum/
- Malaria Links
  http://www.geocities.com/aaadeel/malaria.html
- Medline Plus
  http://www.nlm.nih.gov/medlineplus/malaria.html
- Multilateral Initiative on Malaria
  http://www.mim.su.se/english/index.asp
- WHO
  http://www.who.int/topics/malaria/en/
  http://www.who.int/malaria

Marburg Virus

- CDC
  http://www.cdc.ncidod/dvrd/spb/mnpages/dispages/marburg/htm
  http://www.bt.cdc.gov/agent/vhf

Monkeypox

- CDC
  http://www.cdc.gov/ncidod/monkeypox/clinicians.htm
- MedlinePlus
  http://www.nlm.nih.gov/medlineplus/monkeypoxvirusinfections.
  html
- U.S. FDA
  http://www.fda.gov/cber/infosheets/monkeypox.htm

Plague

- CDC
  http://www.cdc.gov/ncidod/dvbid/plague/
  http://www.bt.cdc.gov/agent/plague
- MedlinePlus
  http://www.nlm.nih.gov/medlineplus/plague.html
- NIAID
  http://www.niaid.nih.gov/factsheets/plague.htm
- WHO, Communicable Disease and Surveillance Response
  http://www.who.int/csr/diseases/plague/

Prion Diseases

- British Medical Journal's BSE-CJD Homepage
  http://www.bmj.com/cgi/collection/mad_cow
- CJD Foundation
  http://www.cjdfoundation.org/
- Department of Environment, Food and Rural Affairs, United
  Kingdom
  http://www.defra.gov.uk/animalh/bse/index.html
- FDA, Center for Veterinary Medicine
- National Institute of Neurological Disorders and Stroke
  http://www.ninds.nih.gov/
- National Organization for Rare Disorders
  http://www.rarediseases.org/

- The Official Mad Cow Disease Home Page
  http://www.mad-cow.org
- Prionics AG, University of Zurich
  http://www.prionics.ch/review_e.html
- The UK Creutzfeldt-Jacob Disease Surveillance Unit, Western General Hospital, Edinburgh
  http://www.cjd.ed.ac.uk/
- U.S. Department of Agriculture (USDA)
  http://www.aphis.usda.gov/newsroom/hot_issues/bse.shtml
- U.S. FDA
  http://www.fda.gov/cvm/bsefact.html

Severe Acute Respiratory Syndrome

- CDC
  http://www.cdc.gov/ncidod/sars/
- NIAID
  http://www.niaid.nih.gov/publications/sars.htm
- WHO
  http://www.who.int/csr/sars/en/

Streptococcus pneumoniae

- National Foundation for Infectious Diseases (NFID)
  http://www.nfid.org/factsheets/pneumofacts.html

Travel/Recreation-Associated Diseases

- CDC, NCID: Travelers' Health
  http://www.cdc.gov/travel/index.htm
- International Society of Travel Medicine
  http://www.istm.org/
- The International Travel Medicine Clinic
  http://www.hsc.unt.edu/
- Medical College of Wisconsin: Travel Medicine
  http://healthlink.mcw.edu/content/topic/Travel_Medicine
- Travel Health Online
  http://www.tripprep.com/
- U.S. Department of State
  http:// www.travel.state.gov/travel/cis_pa_tw/tw/tw_1764.html
- WHO, International Travel and Health
  http://www.who.int/ith/en/

Tuberculosis (TB)

- CDC
  http://www.cdc.gov/nchstp/tb/
- National Tuberculosis Curriculum Consortium
  http://ntcc.ucsd.edu/
- Stop TB Partnership
  http://www.stoptb.org/
- WHO Drug-and Multidrug-Resistant Tuberculosis
  http://www.who.int/tb/dots/dotsplus/en/
- WHO Global Tuberculosis Programme
  http://www.who.int/tb/en/

Vancomycin-Resistant *Enterococci*

- CDC, Division of Healthcare Quality Promotion
  http://www.cdc.gov/ncidod/dhqp/ar_vre.html

West Nile Virus

- American Mosquito Control Association
  http//www.mosquito.org
- CDC
  http://www.cdc.gov/niosh/topics/westnile/
  http://www.cdc.gov/ncidod/dvbid/westnile/education.htm
- Cornell University
  http://www.environmentalrisk.cornell.edu/WNV/
- Department of Defense Global Emerging Infections System
  http://www.geis.fhp.osd.mil/GEIS/SurveillanceActivities/WNV/
  WNVmenu.asp
- National Atlas
  http://www.nationalatlas. gov/virusmap.html
- National Pesticide Telecommunications Network
  http://www.ace.orst.edu/info/nptn/wnv/
- New York State Department of Health
  http://www.health.state.ny.us/nysdoh/westnile/index.html
- USDA
  http://www.aphis.usda.gov/vs/nahss/equine/wnv/
- U.S. FDA
  http://www.fda.gov/oc/opacom/hottopics/westnile.html
- U.S. Geological Survey
  http://www.usgs.gov/west_nile_virus.html

SELECTED GENERAL RESOURCES INCLUDING GROUPS AND ORGANIZATIONS FOCUSING ON EMERGING INFECTIOUS DISEASES

American Medical Association: Infectious Diseases. This resource was developed by the American Medical Association to provide physicians and interested consumers with scientifically accurate information on current and relevant issues in infectious disease (ID).
http://www.ama-assn.org/ama/pub/category/1797.html

American Society for Microbiology. This is the oldest and largest single life science membership organization in the world. Its mission is to promote the microbiological sciences and their applications for the common good. They publish various professional journals and books.
http://www.asm.org

Association of State and Territorial Directors of Health Promotion and Public Health. This organization's Web site provides information on various specific emerging IDs (EIDs).
http://www.astdhpphe.org/

Center for Complex Infectious Diseases (CCID). The primary mission of the CCID is to determine the nature, origin, disease associations, modes of transmission, methods of diagnosis, and responses to therapy of complex IDs and to disseminate such information. The CCID is currently specializing in the detection and characterization of viruses that have undergone a "stealth" adaptation to avoid elimination by the immune system.
http://www.ccid.org/

CDC. The CDC is an agency of the Department of Health and Human Services that promotes health and quality of life by preventing and controlling disease, injury, and disability. The CDC has various divisions including the NCID, which specifically deals with EIDs.
http://www.cdc.gov/

Under the NCID, the Division of Vector-Borne Infectious Diseases serves as a national and international reference center for vectorborne viral and bacterial diseases.
http://www.cdc.gov/ncidod/dvbid/

The Division of Viral and Rickettsial Diseases includes the Special Pathogens Branch.
http://www.cdc.gov/ncidod/dvrd/spb

The Division of Bacterial and Mycotic Diseases has information on those pathogens.
http://www.cdc.gov/ncidod/dbmd

The Division of Parasitic Diseases has information on parasitic diseases.
http://www.cdc.gov/ncidod/dpd

The National Center for HIV, STD, and TB Prevention is responsible for public health surveillance, prevention research, and programs to prevent and control HIV infection and AIDS, other sexually transmitted diseases, and TB.
http://www.cdc.gov/nchstp

Council of State and Territorial Epidemiologists (CSTE). The surveillance and epidemiology of IDs, chronic diseases and conditions, and environmental health concerns are priority areas for the CSTE. Over 150 members serve as special topic consultants for a broad range of public health concerns such as HIV/AIDS and vaccine-preventable diseases.
http://vzww.cste.org

EuroSurveillance. This is a European Union project dedicated to the surveillance, prevention, and control of infectious and communicable disease. EuroSurveillance produces a monthly and weekly bulletin.
http://www.eurosurveillance.org

Federation of American Scientists. This organization's ProMED project is focused on surveillance of emerging human, animal, and plant IDs around the world. ProMED, the Program for Monitoring Emerging Diseases, is the premier discussion group for specialists in EIDs.
http://www.fas.org/promed/

Hardin MetaDirectory of Internet Health Sources. This resource's Web site offers extensive links to ID and microbiology sites as well as access to electronic journals and Medline. Access is free, with no registration required.
http://www.lib.uiowa.edu/hardin/md/micro.html

Infection Control Nurses Association (ICNA). The ICNA works in collaboration with medical, nursing, professions allied to medicine, and commercial companies in the fight to control infection using a multinational approach to ID control.
http://www.icna.co.uk/

Infectious Diseases Society of America. This organization strives to promote and recognize excellence in patient care, education, research, public health, and the prevention of IDs. Information on the Society, its meetings, and other related information can be found on its Web site.
http://www.idsociety.org

International Society for Infectious Diseases. This society brings together all individuals interested in ID. It aims to increase the knowledge base of IDs through research and to enhance the professional development of the individual in this discipline; to extend and transfer technical expertise in microbiology and IDs; and to develop, through partnerships, strategies for control and cost-effective management of IDs.

http://www.isid.org/

Ket-On-Line. This Web site is an educational service designed to encourage peer-to-peer exchange of information in the specialty of IDs and antimicrobial therapy. It includes a moderated group discussion, topical news summaries, resource links, and self-guided clinical cases.

http://www.ket-on-line.com

National Center for Infectious Disease. The NCID at the CDC conducts surveillance, epidemic investigations, epidemiologic and laboratory research, training, and public education programs to develop, evaluate, and promote prevention and control strategies for IDs.

http://www.cdc.gov/ncidod

National Foundation for Infectious Diseases. The NFID supports basic and clinical research on IDs, sponsors public and professional education programs, and aids in the prevention of IDs.

http://www.nfid.org

NIAID, National Institutes of Health. This organization provides the major support for scientists conducting research aimed at developing better ways to diagnose, treat, and prevent infectious, immunologic, and allergic diseases.

http://www.niaid.nih.gov

Open Directory Project. This resource is a comprehensive directory of ID sites available online. No registration is required.

http://dmoz.org/Health/Conditions_and_Diseases/Infectious_ Diseases/

Pan American Health Organization. This is an international public health agency working to improve health and living standards of the countries of Central and Latin America.

http://www.paho.org/

Partnership for Food Safety Education. This is a public–private partnership created to reduce the incidence of foodborne illness by educating Americans about safe food-handling practices.

http://www.fightbac.org

Pediatric Infectious Disease Society. This organization works toward the advancement of knowledge of pediatric IDs and its application to the care of children, including diagnosis, treatment, and prevention of IDs.

http://www.pids.org/

U.S. Army Medical Research Institute for Infectious Diseases (USAM-RIID). As the Department of Defense's lead laboratory for the medical aspects of biological warfare defense, USAMRIID conducts research to develop vaccines, drugs, and diagnostics for laboratory and field use. In addition to developing medical countermeasures, USAMRIID formulates strategies, information, procedures, and training programs for medical defense against biological threats.
  http://www.usamriid.army.mil

WHO. The WHO promotes technical cooperation for health among nations, carries out programs to control and eradicate disease, and strives to improve the quality of human life.
  http://www.who.int

WHO's CSR. This program's mission is to strengthen national and international capacity in the surveillance and control of IDs that represent new, emerging, and reemerging public health problems and to mobilize a team of experts to outbreak locations. Access to the global ID situation from the Disease Outbreak News is provided.
  http://www.who.int/emc/

PUBLICATIONS: JOURNALS

Some of the journals listed here are specific to IDs, and others frequently have related materials. Other journals such as *Annals of Internal Medicine* are more general sources. Only a few of these are mentioned below. Some in this list are in print and some are online. The online references are given to aid the reader in locating the journal.

American Journal of Epidemiology: http://www.aje.oupjournals.org
American Journal of Infection Control: http://www.apic.org/ajic/
American Society for Microbiology Journals Online: http://www.journals.asm.org
Annals of Epidemiology: http://www.elsevier.com
Antimicrobial Agents and Chemotherapy: http://aac.asm.org/
Canadian Journal of Infectious Diseases: http://www.pulsus.con/INFDIS/home.html
Clinical Infectious Diseases: http://www.journal-s.uchicago.edu/CID/home.html
Current Clinical Topics in Infectious Diseases: http://www.medirect.com
Current Opinion in Infectious Diseases: http://www.co-infectiousdiseases.com

Diagnostic Microbiology and Infectious Disease: http://www.elsevier.
com/locate/diagmicrobio

Emerging Infectious Diseases: http://www.cdc.gov/ncidod/eid/index.html

European Journal of Clinical Microbiology and Infectious Disease: http://
link.springer.de/link/service/journals/10096/

Infection: http://link.springer.de/link/service/Joumals/15010/index.htm

Infection and Immunity: http://iai.asm.org/

Infectious Disease Alert: http://www.ahcpub.com/Ahc_root_html/
products/newsletters/ida.html

Infectious Disease Clinics of North America: http://www.harcourthealth.
com

Infectious Diseases in Children: http://www.slackinc.com/child/idc/
idchome.htm

Infectious Diseases in Clinical Practice: http://www.infectdis.com

Infecto.com: http://www.infecto.com

International Journal of Antimicrobial Agents: http://ees.elsevier.com/ijaa

Journal of Antimicrobial Chemotherapy: http://www.jac.oupjournals.
org/

Journal of Applied Microbiology: http://www.blackwell-science.com

Journal of Bacteriology: http://jb.asm.org/

Journal of Clinical Microbiology: http://jcm.asm.org/misc/about.shtml

Journal of General Virology: http://vir.sgmjournals.org/

Journal of Hospital Infection: http://www.harcourt-international.com/
journals/jhin

Journal of Infection: http://www.harcourt-International.com/journals/
jinf/

Journal of Infection and Chemotherapy: http://www.harcourt-internatio-
nal.com/journals/jinf/default.cfm?

Journal of Infectious Diseases: http://www.journals.uchicago.edu/JID/

Journal of Medical Microbiology: http://jmm.sgmjournals.org

Journal of Medical Virology: http://www.interscience.wiley.com/jpages/
0146-6615/

Journal of Travel Medicine: http://www.blackwellpublishing.com/
journal.asp?ref=1195-1982&site=1

Journal of Virology: http://jvi.asm.org/misc/About.shtml

Journal Watch: Infectious Diseases: http://www.jwatch.org/id/

Medical Microbiology and Immunology: http://www.link.springer.de/
link/service/journals/00430/index.htm

Microbes and Infection: http://www.pasteur.fr/infosci/publisci/mic-aims.
html

Morbidity and Mortality Weekly Report: http://www.cdc.gov/mmwr

Pediatric Infectious Disease Journal: http://www.pidj.com

Reviews in Tropical Medicine and International Health: http://www.
blackwell-science.com/

PUBLICATIONS: BULLETINS, NEWSLETTERS, REPORTS, AND FACT SHEETS

Current Infectious Disease Reports. These present the views of experts on current advances in infectious diseases and provide selections of the most important papers from the great wealth of original publications, annotated by experts. Manuscripts printed in this journal are available only to paid subscribers.
http://www.current-reports.com/cr_aims.cfm

Disease Outbreak News. Maintained by WHO, this online bulletin offers pertinent information about worldwide communicable disease outbreaks.
http://www.who.int/disease-out-break-news/

Double Helix. This is the official newsletter of NFID.
http://www.nfid.org/

Emerging and Other Communicable Diseases Surveillance and Control (EMC). This program provides fact sheets and references on worldwide emerging and reemerging infectious diseases.
http://www.who.int/emc/index.html

Ket-On-Line Newsletter: This series provides highlights from key international scientific meetings relevant to infectious disease researchers and clinicians.
http://www.ket-on-line.com

NFID. This organization provides fact sheets about infectious diseases, appropriate for reproduction and distribution to patients.
http://www.nfid.org/library/

ProMED Digest. The International Society for Infectious Diseases' Program for Monitoring Emerging Diseases (ProMED) produces an online, daily updated synopsis of current discussions on EIDs.
http://www.promedmail.org

Science Central. Health Sciences: Infectious Disease and Epidemiology: This Web site provides science news alerts, research news, and infectious disease resources available in full text with a searchable index.
http://www.sciquest.com/

Weekly Epidemiological Record (*WER*). This publication serves as an essential instrument for the rapid and accurate dissemination of epidemiological information on cases and outbreaks of diseases under the International Health Regulations; other communicable diseases of public health importance, including the newly emerging or reemerging infections; noncommunicable diseases; and other health problems.

     http://www.who.int/wer/

Glossary

aerobic organisms—organisms that live and thrive in an oxygenated environment

aerosol—fine mist containing minute particles

anaerobic organisms—organisms that need little or no oxygen

arbovirus—virus borne by arthropod vectors

arenavirus—virus family whose members are usually transmitted to humans via rodents; members include the Lassa, Junin, Machupo, and Guanarito viruses, each causing a type of hemorrhagic fever

arthropod—vector belonging to the phylum Arthropoda that transmits an organism from one host to another

autochthonous—locally acquired

biosafety level—specific combinations of work practices, safety equipment, and facilities to minimize exposure of workers to infectious agents; these range from Level 1, which are agents not usually causing human disease, to Level 4, which are for agents posing a high risk of life-threatening disease, such as the Ebola virus

biotype—organisms sharing a specific genotype

bunyavirus—virus family among whose members are the hantaviruses and the Rift Valley fever virus

clade—group or subtype of organisms of related isolates that are classified by genetic similarities

coronavirus—virus family with enveloped ribonucleic acid strains of which usually cause the common cold but a strain was recently identified as the causative agent in the 2003 SARS outbreak

endemic disease—disease that is consistently present in a population or geographic location

endotoxin—toxin of internal origin that is separated from a microorganism on disintegration

epidemic disease—disease that occurs suddenly in numbers in excess of what is usually expected

epizootic—epidemic in an animal population

exotoxin—toxin produced during microbial growth and released without disintegration

filovirus—virus family infecting primates and humans that has only two members, Ebola and Marburg viruses

flavivirus—virus family whose members include the dengue virus, West Nile virus, and the hepatitis C virus

fomite—inanimate object on which pathogens live

host—organism on or within which microorganisms live

immunocompetent—person with a functional immune system

immunocompromised—person whose immune system does not function properly

incidence—measure of frequency with which a new case of a specific condition or disease occurs in a specified time period

incubation period—time from exposure to appearance of disease

index case—earliest recognized case of a disease

isolate—particular strain of a microorganism taken from an individual

microbe—microscopic living organisms such as bacteria, protozoa, and fungi

nosocomial infection—infection that develops and is recognized in patients and employees in a health care institution

outbreak—occurrence of an unusually large number of cases of disease in a short period of time

pandemic—epidemic disease of widespread prevalence usually in more than one continent

pathogen—microorganism causing disease

pathogenicity—ability of an infectious agent to produce disease in a susceptible host

prevalence—number or proportion of persons in a given time period with a specific condition or disease protozoa

protozoa—type of parasite

recurrence—return of a disease or condition thought to be in remission

reservoir for infection—organism such as a human, animal, plant, or inanimate material (often called fomite) in which a microbial agent normally lives and multiplies

retrovirus—virus that has ribonucleic acid as its genetic material and uses reverse transcriptase to copy its genome into host deoxyribonucleic acid; human immunodeficiency virus belongs to this group

serogroup—group of closely related microbes distinguished by a characteristic set of antigens

serotype—particular strain of a microorganism

source of infection—organism or inanimate object or substance from which a microbial agent passes to a host

sporozoa—nonmotile protozoan parasites

vector—living organism, usually an arthropod, that can transfer a microbe from one host to another

virulence—degree of pathogenicity

zoonosis—animal disease transmitted from animals to humans; their ongoing reservoir is in nonhuman animals, and arthropods are usually involved in their transmission

Index

Essentials of Clinical Genetics in Nursing Practice

Felissa R. Lashley, PhD, RN, ACRN, FAAN, FACMG

Refresh your genetic knowledge and enhance your patient care...

We now know that genetic factors can cause disease or affect an individual's susceptibility or resistance to disorders and even to treatment. To provide the best nursing care, it is therefore essential that practitioners and students have a basic knowledge of the science of genetics and how it affects the major areas of nursing expertise.

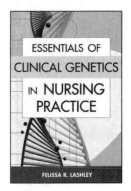

To address this need, Dr. Felissa Lashley has created this "essentials" guide specifically for nurses. From genetic factors and trends affecting health care today, to the more complex discussions of human variation, every genetic topic critical to the practice of nursing and nursing education is covered, including:

- Prevention of Genetic Disease
- Genetic Testing and Treatment
- Genetic Counseling
- Maternal-Child Nursing
- Psychiatric/Mental Health Nursing
- Community/Public Health Nursing
- Trends, Policies, and Social and Ethical Issues

Each chapter examines how genetic information influences treatment and management and is intended to further the development of a nurse's "genetic eye" in the daily care of patients.

2006 · 352pp · softcover · 978-0-8261-0222-5

Health Literacy in Primary Care

A Clinician's Guide

Gloria G. Mayer, RN, EdD, FAAN
Michael Villaire, MSLM

At the intersection of health care delivery and practice there lies a large area of patient care with no manual: how to provide the best care to patients who have a critically low level of comprehension and literacy. Because all patients play a central role in the outcome of their own health care, competent health care becomes almost impossible for caregivers when the boundary of low literary skills is present.

Gloria G. Mayer
Michael Villaire

Health Literacy in Primary Care

A Clinician's Guide

In a concise and well-written format you will learn:
- Common myths about low literacy
- How to recognize patients with low literacy
- Strategies to help patients with low literacy and reduce medical errors
- Cultural issues in health literacy
- Ways to create a patient-friendly office environment
- Guidelines to target and overcome common problems practitioners encounter

This clear, well written book is packed with examples and tips and will serve as a much needed guide for primary care providers, nurse practitioners, hospital administrators, and others who are looking for ways to improve their communication with patients and provide the most beneficial health care to their low-literacy patients.

Table of Contents

- Understanding Health Literacy
- Creating a Patient-Friendly Environment
- Assessing Patients' Literacy Levels
- Understanding and Avoiding Medical Errors
- Factoring Culture into the Care Process
- Improving Patient-Provider Communication

- Designing Easy-to-Read Patient Education Materials
- Principles of Writing for Low Literacy
- Using Alternative Forms of Patient Communication
- Interpreters and Their Role in the Health Care Setting

April 2007 · 312 pp · Softcover · 978-0-8261-0229-4

11 West 42nd Street, New York, NY 10036-8002 • Fax: 212-941-7842
Order Toll-Free: 877-687-7476 • Order Online: www.springerpub.com

Disaster Nursing and Emergency Preparedness for Chemical, Biological, and Radiological Terrorism and Other Hazards

Second Edition

Tener Goodwin Veenema, PhD, MPH, MS, Editor

Disaster planning and emergency preparedness have never been more critical to the nurses who serve as our front-line response. Today's pandemic threats of global terrorism, disease, and natural disasters make this comprehensive handbook of best practices a necessity—meeting the need for a nursing workforce that is adequately prepared to respond to any disaster or public health emergency.

SECOND EDITION

DISASTER NURSING
and **EMERGENCY**
PREPAREDNESS
for Chemical, Biological,
and Radiological Terrorism
and Other Hazards

TENER GOODWIN VEENEMA
EDITOR

In addition to a thorough update based on the most recent recommendations, this second edition contains six new chapters:
- Emergency Health Services (EMS and other first responders)
- Burn Assessment and Management
- Explosive & Traumatic Terrorism
- Caring for High-Risk, High-Vulnerability Patients
- Emerging Infectious Disease (avian and other flu pandemics)
- Chemical Decontamination

All content reflects the guidelines provided in the Federal Disaster Response Plan and the National Incident Management System (NIMS) and therapeutic recommendations from the national Centers for Disease Control and Prevention.

Disaster Nursing will prepare any nurse or EMS team to provide health care under a variety of disaster conditions.

June 2007 · 664pp · Hardcover · 978-0-8261-2144-8

11 West 42nd Street, New York, NY 10036-8002 • Fax: 212-941-7842
Order Toll-Free: 877-687-7476 • Order Online: www.springerpub.com